NURSE'S 5-MINUTE CLINICAL CONSULT

Diagnostic Tests

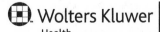 Wolters Kluwer | Lippincott Williams & Wilkins
Health

Philadelphia · Baltimore · New York · London
Buenos Aires · Hong Kong · Sydney · Tokyo

Library of Congress
Cataloging-in-Publication Data

Nurse's 5-minute clinical consult. Diagnostic tests.
    p. ; cm.
    Includes bibliographical references and index.
    1. Nursing diagnosis—Handbooks, manuals, etc. I. Lippincott Williams & Wilkins.   II. Title: Nurse's five-minute clinical consult. III. Title: Diagnostic tests.
    [DNLM: 1. Diagnostic Tests, Routine—nursing—Handbooks.
    WB 39 N9745 2007]
    RT48.6.N84 2007
    616.07'5—dc22
ISBN13 978-1-58255-514-0
ISBN10 1-58255-514-1 (alk. paper)   2006031950

Contents

Contributors and consultants

Elizabeth (Libby) A. Archer, RN, EdD
Associate Professor
Baptist College of Health Sciences
Memphis

Debra F. Chastang, APRN, CNS, MSN, CS-C
Clinical Nurse Specialist—Orthopaedics and Pain Management
Providence Hospital
Mobile, Ala.

Lillian Craig, RN, MSN, FNP-C
Nursing Instructor
Oklahoma Panhandle State University
Goodwill

Peggy S. Denning, RN, MSN
Assistant Director of Nursing
Tri-State School of Practical Nursing
Erie, Pa.

April N. Hart, RN, MSN, FNP,BC
Assistant Professor
Bethel College
Mishawaka, Ind.

Rebecca E. Heyne, RN, MSN
Clinical Instructor, Nursing
Walsh University
North Canton, Ohio

Julia Anne Isen, FNP, MS, CNS
Assistant Clinical Professor
University of California at San Francisco School of Nursing

Jaclynn A. Johnson, RNC, MSN
Lead Instructor Freshman Nursing
Otero Junior College
La Junta, Colo.

Christine Kennedy, RN, MSN
Nursing Instructor
Eli Whitney Technical School
Hamden, Conn.

Carol T. Lemay, RN
Consultant
Brattleboro, Vt.

Kendra S. Seiler, RN, MSN
Nursing Instructor
Rio Hondo Community College
Whittier, Calif.

Georgia Simmons, RN, BSN
Practical Nursing Instructor
Ivy Tech State College
Madison, Ind.

Allison J. Terry, RN, MSN, PhD
Director of Center for Nursing Workforce Research
Alabama Board of Nursing
Montgomery

Janet E. Williams, RN, BSN
Assistant Master Technical Instructor
University of Texas at Brownsville and Texas Southmost College
Brownsville

Diagnostic Tests

ABO blood typing

DESCRIPTION
- Classifies blood according to the presence of major antigens A and B on red blood cell (RBC) surfaces
- Classifies blood according to serum antibodies anti-A and anti-B

PURPOSE
- To establish a patient's blood group according to the ABO system
- To check the compatibility of donor and recipient blood before a transfusion

PREPARATION
- No dietary restrictions are required.
- Check the patient's history for recent administration of blood, dextran, or I.V. contrast media.

Teaching points
- Tell the patient that the test requires a blood sample and he may experience slight discomfort from the tourniquet and needle puncture.
- Tell him that this test determines his blood group and may also be used to determine the donor's blood type.
- Explain who will perform the test and where it'll be done.
- Tell the patient that he need not restrict food or fluids.
- Tell him that the procedure usually takes less than 5 minutes.

KEY STEPS
- Confirm the patient's identity using two patient identifiers according to facility policy.
- Perform a venipuncture and collect the sample in a 10-ml tube without additives, following standard precautions.
- Label the sample with the patient's name, the hospital or blood bank number, the date, and the phlebotomist's initials.
- Immediately send the sample to the laboratory with a properly completed laboratory request indicating the amount and type of blood component needed.

POSTPROCEDURE CARE
- Apply direct pressure to the venipuncture site until the bleeding stops.

PRECAUTIONS
- Follow standard precautions with collection of sample.
- Handle the sample gently to prevent hemolysis, and send it to the laboratory immediately after collection.

WARNING *If more than 72 hours have elapsed since an earlier transfusion, previously crossmatched donor blood must be recrossmatched with a new recipient serum sample to detect newly acquired incompatibilities before transfusion.*

COMPLICATIONS
- Hematoma at the venipuncture site

NORMAL RESULTS
- In forward typing, if agglutination occurs when the patient's RBCs are mixed with anti-A serum, the A antigen is present, and the blood is type A.
- In forward typing, if agglutination occurs when the patient's RBCs are mixed with anti-B serum, the B antigen is present, and blood is type B.
- In forward typing, if agglutination occurs in both mixes, A and B antigens are present, and the blood is type AB.
- In forward typing, if agglutination doesn't occur in either mix, no antigens are present, and the blood is type O.
- In reverse typing, if agglutination occurs when B cells are mixed with the patient's serum, anti-B is present, and the blood is type A.
- In reverse typing, if agglutination occurs when A cells are mixed with the patient's serum, anti-A is present, and the blood is type B.
- In reverse typing, if agglutination occurs when A and B cells are mixed with the patient's serum, anti-A and anti-B are present, and the blood is typed O.
- In reverse typing, if agglutination doesn't occur when A and B cells are mixed with the patient's serum, neither anti-A nor anti-B is present, and the blood is type AB.

ABNORMAL RESULTS
None known

Acetaminophen level test

DESCRIPTION

- Determines the amount of serum acetaminophen, an analgesic used for fever and pain relief
- Rapidly absorbed from the GI tract, reaching peak concentration in 30 to 60 minutes
- Signs of intoxication appearing 24 to 48 hours after ingestion
- High levels possibly toxic and causing liver toxicity

PURPOSE

- To monitor for acetaminophen overdose

PREPARATION

- No dietary restrictions are required.

Teaching points

- Explain to the patient that this test shows the amount of acetaminophen in the blood.
- Tell the patient that he need not restrict food or fluids.
- Tell the patient that the test requires a blood sample and he may experience slight discomfort from the tourniquet and the needle puncture.
- Explain who will perform the test and where it'll be done.
- Tell the patient that the test should take less than 5 minutes.

KEY STEPS

- Confirm the patient's identity using two patient identifiers according to facility policy.
- Explain to the patient that he may experience slight discomfort from the tourniquet and the needle puncture.
- Perform a venipuncture and collect the sample in a 5-ml tube.

POSTPROCEDURE CARE

- Observe venipuncture site for bleeding or hematoma formation.

PRECAUTIONS

- Maintain standard precautions while collecting the sample.
- Transport the sample to the laboratory immediately after collection.

COMPLICATIONS

- Hematoma at the venipuncture site

NORMAL RESULTS

- Results at the therapeutic dose are 10 to 20 mcg/ml (SI, 66.2 to 132.4 µmol/L).

ABNORMAL RESULTS

- Results greater than 200 mcg/ml (SI, > 1,324 µmol/L) 4 hours after ingestion or greater than 50 mcg/ml (SI, > 331 µmol/L) 12 hours after ingestion signify toxicity and potential for liver damage.

Acetylcholine receptor antibody test

DESCRIPTION

- Most useful immunologic test for confirming acquired (autoimmune) myasthenia gravis
- Two test methods: A binding assay and a blocking assay
- Determines the relative concentration of acetylcholine receptor (AChR) antibodies in serum
- Helps monitor the effectiveness of immunosuppressive therapy for myasthenia gravis

PURPOSE

- To confirm the diagnosis of myasthenia gravis
- To monitor the effectiveness of immunosuppressive therapy for myasthenia gravis

PREPARATION

- Check the patient's history for immunosuppressive drugs that may affect the test results, and note such use on the laboratory request.

Teaching points

- Explain to the patient that this test helps confirm the diagnosis of myasthenia gravis. If appropriate, also explain that it assesses the effectiveness of treatment.
- Inform the patient that he need not restrict food or fluids.
- Tell the patient that the test requires a blood sample and he may experience slight discomfort from the tourniquet and the needle puncture.
- Tell the patient who will perform the test and where it'll be done.
- Explain to the patient how long to keep the bandage on the site and what signs and symptoms of infection to report.

KEY STEPS

- Confirm the patient's identity using two patient identifiers according to facility policy.
- Perform a venipuncture, and collect the sample in a 7-ml tube without additives.
- Keep the sample at room temperature and send it to the laboratory immediately.

POSTPROCEDURE CARE

- Apply direct pressure to the venipuncture site until the bleeding stops.
- Keep a clean, dry bandage over the site for at least 24 hours.
- Check the venipuncture site for infection that might arise because of the patient's compromised immune system, and promptly report changes.

PRECAUTIONS

- Maintain standard precautions when performing the procedure and handling samples.

COMPLICATIONS

- Hematoma at the venipuncture site

NORMAL RESULTS

- The lack of AChR-binding antibodies and AChR-blocking antibodies indicates a normal test result.

ABNORMAL RESULTS

- The presence of positive AChR antibodies in symptomatic adults confirms the diagnosis of myasthenia gravis.
- Patients with ocular symptoms have lower antibody titers than those with generalized symptoms.

INTERFERING FACTORS *Amyotrophic lateral sclerosis (false-positive result)*

Acid mucopolysaccharides test

OVERVIEW

DESCRIPTION

◆ Quantitative test that measures the urine level of acid mucopolysaccharides, a group of polysaccharides (carbohydrates)
◆ Helps detect mucopolysaccharidosis, a rare disorder that may affect the skeleton; joints; liver; spleen; eye; ear; skin; teeth; and the cardiovascular, respiratory, and central nervous systems

PURPOSE

◆ To diagnose mucopolysaccharidosis in infants with a family history of the disease

PREPARATION

◆ No dietary restrictions are required.
◆ If the child is receiving therapy with heparin and must continue it, note this on the laboratory request.

Teaching points

◆ Explain to the infant's parents that the acid mucopolysaccharide test helps to determine the efficiency of carbohydrate metabolism.
◆ Inform them that they need not restrict the child's food or fluid intake.
◆ Tell the parents that the test requires urine collection for 24 hours, and instruct them on how to collect the specimen properly at home.

DIAGNOSTIC PROCEDURE

KEY STEPS

◆ Confirm the patient's identity using two patient identifiers according to facility policy.
◆ Collect the urine over a 24-hour period, discarding the first specimen and retaining the last.
◆ Add 20 ml of toluene (as a preservative) to the collection container at the start of the collection.
◆ Indicate the patient's age on the laboratory request.
◆ Send the specimen to the laboratory immediately after the 24-hour collection period.
◆ Refrigerate the specimen or place it on ice during the collection period.

POSTPROCEDURE CARE

◆ Remove all of the urine collector adhesive from the infant's perineum.
◆ Wash the area gently with soap and water; watch for irritation.

PRECAUTIONS

◆ Use standard precautions when performing the procedure and handling specimens.
◆ Collect the urine for 24 hours, and refrigerate the specimen or keep it on ice.

COMPLICATIONS

None known

INTERPRETATION

NORMAL RESULTS

◆ Value is expressed as milligrams of glucuronic acid divided by the amount of creatinine in the same specimen (which reflects glomerular filtration rate); this compensates for irregularities in the 24-hour urine collection.
◆ Normal acid mucopolysaccharide values for adults are < 13.3 mg glucuronic acid/mg creatinine/ 24 hours.
◆ Child values vary with age.

ABNORMAL RESULTS

◆ Elevated acid mucopolysaccharide levels reliably indicate mucopolysaccharidosis.
◆ Supplementary quantitative analysis and detailed blood studies can identify the defective enzyme.

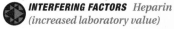 **INTERFERING FACTORS** *Heparin (increased laboratory value)*

Acid perfusion (Bernstein) test

DESCRIPTION

- Helps to distinguish the pain caused by esophagitis (burning epigastric or retrosternal pain that radiates to the back or arms) from pain caused by angina pectoris or other cardiac disorders
- Requires perfusion of saline and acidic solutions into the esophagus through a nasogastric (NG) tube

PURPOSE

- To distinguish chest pain caused by esophagitis from chest pain caused by cardiac disorders

PREPARATION

- The patient should have no antacids for 24 hours before the test, no food for 12 hours before the test, and no fluids or smoking for 8 hours before the test.
- Just before the test, check the patient's pulse rate and blood pressure. Ask him whether he's experiencing heartburn and, if so, to describe it.
- Make sure that the patient or a responsible family member has signed an informed consent form.
- Tell the patient that, when the liquid is being poured through the tube into the esophagus, he should immediately report any pain or burning.

Teaching points

- Tell the patient that the acid perfusion test helps distinguish heartburn from the pain caused by angina pectoris and other cardiac disorders.
- Explain that the test involves passing a tube through his nose into his esophagus and that he may experience some discomfort, a desire to cough, or a gagging sensation during tube passage.
- Explain who will perform the test and where it'll be done.
- Tell the patient that the test takes 1½ to 2 hours.

KEY STEPS

- Confirm the patient's identity using two patient identifiers according to facility policy.
- Mark an NG tube at 12″ (30.5 cm) from the tip.
- After the patient is seated, insert the NG tube into his stomach. Attach a 20-ml syringe to the tube, and aspirate the stomach contents. Withdraw the tube into the esophagus up to the 12″ mark.
- Hang labeled containers of normal saline solution and a prescribed acidic solution (such as a mild hydrochloric acid) on an I.V. pole behind the patient, and then connect the NG tube to the I.V. tubing.
- Open the line from the normal saline solution, and infuse at a rate of 60 to 120 drops/minute. Continue perfusion for 5 to 10 minutes.
- Ask the patient whether he's experiencing discomfort, and record his response.
- Without the patient's knowledge, close the line from the normal saline solution and open the line from the acidic solution. Infuse the acidic solution into the esophagus at the same rate used for the normal saline solution. Continue perfusion for 30 minutes.
- Ask the patient again whether he's experiencing discomfort, and record his response.
- Assess the patient's pulse rate and rhythm to detect any arrhythmia that may develop.
- If the patient experiences discomfort, close the line from the acidic solution immediately and open the line from the normal saline solution. Continue to perfuse this solution until the discomfort subsides.
- If ordered, repeat perfusion of the acidic solution to verify the patient's response. If this isn't required or if the patient experiences no discomfort after perfusion of the acidic solution for 30 minutes, stop the solution and withdraw the NG tube.

POSTPROCEDURE CARE

- If the patient complains of pain or burning, give him an antacid. If he complains of a sore throat, provide soothing lozenges or obtain an order for an ice collar.
- Instruct the patient that he may resume his usual diet and medications, as ordered.

PRECAUTIONS

- Maintain standard precautions when performing the procedure and handling specimens.
- The acid perfusion test is contraindicated in the patient with esophageal varices, heart failure, acute myocardial infarction, or other cardiac disorders.
- Clamp the tube before removing it, to prevent fluid aspiration into the lungs.

COMPLICATIONS

- Tube entering trachea instead of esophagus during intubation (withdraw the tube immediately if the patient develops cyanosis or paroxysmal coughing)

NORMAL RESULTS

- Absence of pain or burning during perfusion of either solution indicates a healthy esophageal mucosa.

ABNORMAL RESULTS

- In the patient with esophagitis, the acidic solution causes pain or burning, while the normal saline solution produces no adverse effects.
- Occasionally, both solutions cause pain in the patient with esophagitis. It's also possible for the patient with asymptomatic esophagitis not to experience pain with either solution.

Acid phosphatase level test

OVERVIEW

DESCRIPTION
- Measures total acid phosphatase and the prostatic fraction in serum
- Prostatic isoenzyme more specific for prostate cancer than erythrocytic isoenzyme
- Increased level more likely if cancer is widespread

PURPOSE
- To detect prostate cancer
- To monitor the patient's response to therapy for prostate cancer (successful treatment decreases acid phosphatase levels)

PREPARATION
- No dietary restrictions are required.
- Notify the laboratory and practitioner of drugs the patient is taking that may affect test results. The drugs may need to be restricted.

Teaching points
- Tell the patient that this test evaluates prostate function.
- Explain that it requires a blood sample and he may experience slight discomfort from the tourniquet and the needle puncture.
- Explain who will perform the test and where it'll be done.
- Tell the patient that he need not restrict food or fluids.
- Tell him that the test should take less than 5 minutes.

DIAGNOSTIC PROCEDURE

KEY STEPS
- Confirm the patient's identity using two patient identifiers according to facility policy.
- Perform a venipuncture, and collect the sample in a 4-ml tube without additives.
- Don't draw the sample within 48 hours of prostate manipulation (rectal examination).
- Send the sample to the laboratory immediately. Acid phosphatase levels decrease by 50% within 1 hour if the sample remains at room temperature without a preservative or if it isn't packed on ice.

POSTPROCEDURE CARE
- Apply direct pressure to the venipuncture site until the bleeding stops.
- Instruct the patient that he may resume medications stopped before the test.

PRECAUTIONS
- Maintain standard precautions when performing the procedure and handling samples.
- Handle the sample gently to prevent hemolysis.
- Don't leave the sample at room temperature for greater than 1 hour.

COMPLICATIONS
- Hematoma at the venipuncture site

INTERPRETATION

NORMAL RESULTS
- Serum values for total acid phosphatase depend on the assay method and range from 0 to 3.7 units/L (SI, 0 to 3.7 units/L).

ABNORMAL RESULTS
- High prostatic acid phosphatase levels generally indicate the presence of a tumor that has spread beyond the prostatic capsule. If the tumor has metastasized to bone, high acid phosphatase levels are accompanied by high alkaline phosphatase (ALP) levels, reflecting increased osteoblastic activity.
- Acid phosphatase levels rise moderately in prostatic infarction, Paget's disease (some cases), Gaucher's disease and, occasionally, other conditions such as multiple myeloma.
- High ALP levels can produce false results because acid phosphatase and ALP are similar, differing mainly in their optimum pH ranges.

INTERFERING FACTORS *Prostate massage, catheterization, or rectal examination within 48 hours of the test; benign prostatic hypertrophy*

Acid-fast stain

DESCRIPTION
- Helps identify organisms of the genus *Mycobacterium* (including pathogens of tuberculosis and leprosy) because they retain carbolfuchsin stain after treatment with acid-alcohol solution
- Particularly useful for identifying mycobacteria in sputum specimens, which may contain many different organisms

PURPOSE
- To examine a specimen for the presence of microorganisms, specifically mycobacteria (which include the bacteria that cause tuberculosis)

PREPARATION
- Preparation for the test depends on the type of specimen to be collected.

Teaching points
- Tell the patient the purpose of the test, the type of test he'll receive, and how it's performed.
- Explain that blood, urine, stool, sputum, bone marrow, or tissue specimens may be collected, depending on the location of the suspected infection. In some cases, a tissue biopsy or an aspiration with a needle may be necessary.
- Explain that the amount of discomfort depends on the type of sampling procedure.
- Inform the patient who will perform the test and where it'll be done.
- Tell the patient that it may take several weeks to receive the results of the test.

KEY STEPS
- Confirm the patient's identity using two patient identifiers according to facility policy.
- Collect the specimen, or assist with its collection. The type of specimen collected will be determined by the location of the suspected infection.
- Send the specimen to the microbiology laboratory.

POSTPROCEDURE CARE
- Check the site of specimen collection for signs of infection.
- After the test, instruct the patient or parent to report adverse effects.

PRECAUTIONS
- Maintain standard precautions, as well as airborne precautions if indicated.
- Clearly indicate the source of the specimen.

COMPLICATIONS
None known

NORMAL RESULTS
- Absence of acid-fast bacteria on the stained specimen is normal.

ABNORMAL RESULTS
- Presence of acid-fast bacteria (including *Nocardia* species and bacteria that cause tuberculosis and nontuberculous infections) is abnormal.

Acoustic admittance test

DESCRIPTION

- Evaluates middle ear function by measuring the flow of sound energy into the ear (admittance)
- Commonly measured by tympanometry and acoustic reflex testing
- Tympanometry: measures middle ear admittance to changes in air pressure in the ear canal
- Acoustic reflex testing: measures the change in admittance produced by the reflex contraction of the stapedius muscle in response to an intense sound
- Reflex decay, part of the acoustic reflex test: is a function of cranial nerve (CN) VIII adaptation or fatigue in response to a sustained reflex-eliciting stimulus

PURPOSE

- *Tympanometry:* To assess the continuity and admittance of the middle ear and evaluate the status of the tympanic membrane
- *Acoustic reflex testing:* To distinguish between cochlear and retrocochlear lesions; to differentiate CN VIII or peripheral brain stem lesions from intra-axial brain stem lesions and locate CN VII lesions relative to stapedius muscle innervation; and to confirm conductive hearing loss and help confirm nonorganic loss

PREPARATION

- Make sure that the ear is free from significant cerumen accumulation.
- Ask the patient to remain still during testing.

Teaching points

- Describe the procedure to the patient and explain that acoustic admittance tests evaluate the condition of the middle ear.
- Tell the patient that he'll feel pressure in the ear but that it won't be painful.
- Explain who will perform the test and where it'll be done.
- Tell the patient that the test should take just a few seconds.

DIAGNOSTIC PROCEDURE

KEY STEPS

- Confirm the patient's identity using two patient identifiers according to facility policy.

Tympanometry

- An otoscopic examination is performed to verify whether impacted cerumen or other obstructions are in the ear canal.
- The size and shape of the canal are checked to select the appropriate-sized probe tip, which is then attached to the probe.
- The probe tip is inserted into the ear canal, while the auricle is pulled upward and back to create a proper seal.
- A graphic display of the results (tympanogram) is obtained. If there's pressure in the middle ear, a clear peak will be present, and the pressure will print out with the test results.
- If there's no change in admittance, the tympanogram appears flat. The possibility that the probe tip rested against the canal wall must be ruled out. A small ear canal (volume of ≤ 0.3 ml) is more likely to cause a flat tympanogram.

Acoustic reflex testing

- The admittance probe is positioned in the ear (same as for tympanometry), but the probe is fixed to the patient's head to reduce the chance of other factors affecting the test results.
- For threshold testing, stimuli of progressively louder levels are introduced until the reflex contraction (if present) occurs.
- Acoustic reflex decay testing presents a tone that's 10 decibels (dB) above the reflex threshold at one or more frequencies (1,000 hertz and below) for 10 seconds. The time the auditory system sustains the contraction at a level of one half-strength or greater is measured.
- Reflexes and reflex decay can be measured ipsilaterally (the probe is in the same ear that receives the tone) or contralaterally (the probe is in the ear opposite to the one that receives the tone).

POSTPROCEDURE CARE
None indicated

PRECAUTIONS

- Obtain medical clearance before performing admittance tests in the patient who has head trauma, a possible labyrinthine fistula, or a history of recent middle ear surgery.

COMPLICATIONS
None known

NORMAL RESULTS

- *Tympanometry:* A type A tympanogram is normal.
- *Acoustic reflex testing:* Normal reflexes are present at an intensity of 65 to 100 dB.

ABNORMAL RESULTS

Tympanometry

- Evidence that doesn't reflect a type A tympanogram is abnormal.

Acoustic reflex testing

- Ears that have conductive involvement commonly have absent reflexes. If the conductive loss is unilateral, presentation of the reflex tone to the involved ear, with measurement contralaterally, may reveal a reflex at an elevated hearing level.
- If the cochlea is the site of a lesion, reflexes may be present, elevated, or absent at normal hearing levels. The more severe the hearing loss, the more likely the finding of an absent reflex.
- Acoustic reflexes are present in most patients with mild to moderately severe hearing losses.
- Absent acoustic reflexes may indicate a retrocochlear lesion, if conductive involvement or severe cochlear loss isn't present.
- Acoustic reflex decay may indicate retrocochlear involvement.
- Reflexes below the admitted threshold indicate a nonorganic problem.

Activated clotting time

DESCRIPTION
- Measures whole-blood clotting time
- Commonly performed during procedures that require extracorporeal circulation, such as cardiopulmonary bypass, ultrafiltration, hemodialysis, and extracorporeal membrane oxygenation (ECMO), and during invasive procedures, such as cardiac catheterization and percutaneous transluminal coronary angioplasty

PURPOSE
- To monitor the effect of heparin on blood coagulation
- To monitor the effect of protamine sulfate in heparin neutralization
- To detect severe deficiencies in clotting factors (except factor VII)

PREPARATION
- If the sample is drawn from a line with a continuous infusion, stop the infusion before drawing the sample.

Teaching points
- Tell the patient that the activated clotting time test monitors the effect of heparin on the blood's ability to coagulate.
- Explain that the test requires two blood samples, usually drawn from an existing vascular access site; no venipuncture is necessary. The first blood sample will be discarded so that any heparin in the tubing won't interfere with the results.
- Explain who will perform the test and where it'll be done (usually at bedside).

KEY STEPS
- Confirm the patient's identity using two patient identifiers according to facility policy.
- Withdraw 5 to 10 ml of blood from the line and discard it.
- Withdraw a clean sample of blood into the special tube containing celite that's provided with the activated clotting time unit.
- Start the activated clotting time unit, and wait for the signal before inserting the tube.
- Flush the vascular access site according to your facility's policy.

POSTPROCEDURE CARE
- Instruct the patient to report discomfort at the site.
- If a venipuncture was performed, monitor the site for signs of bleeding.

PRECAUTIONS
- Maintain standard precautions when performing the procedure and handling samples.
- To avoid contamination when obtaining blood from a venous access device used for heparin infusion, draw and discard at least 5 ml of blood before collecting the test sample.
- Place the sample on ice immediately, if sending it to the laboratory.
- Handle the sample gently to prevent hemolysis.

COMPLICATIONS
- Contamination with heparin, if drawn from a vascular access site used for infusing heparin

NORMAL RESULTS
- In a nonanticoagulated patient, normal activated clotting time is 107 seconds, plus or minus 13 seconds (SI, 107 ± 13 seconds).
- During cardiopulmonary bypass, heparin is titrated to maintain an activated clotting time of 400 to 600 seconds (SI, 400 to 600 seconds).
- During ECMO, heparin is titrated to maintain an activated clotting time of 220 to 260 seconds (SI, 220 to 260 seconds).

ABNORMAL RESULTS
- An elevated result in a nonanticoagulated patient may indicate clotting factor deficiency; further testing is needed.

Adenovirus antibody test

DESCRIPTION
- Determines the presence of an adenovirus, an infection spread through droplet, and also contact, vectors; one of the most frequent causes of viral disease in the respiratory tract

PURPOSE
- To determine if the patient has a current or recent adenovirus infection

PREPARATION
- No dietary restrictions are required.

Teaching points
- Explain to the patient that this test determines if he currently has or has recently had an adenovirus infection.
- Tell the patient that the test requires a blood sample and he may experience slight discomfort from the tourniquet and needle puncture.
- Explain who will perform the test and where it'll be done.
- Tell the patient that he need not restrict food or fluids.
- Explain that the test should take less than 5 minutes.

KEY STEPS
- Confirm the patient's identity using two patient identifiers according to facility policy.
- Perform a venipuncture, and collect the sample in a 5-ml tube without additives.

POSTPROCEDURE CARE
- Apply direct pressure to the venipuncture site until the bleeding stops.

PRECAUTIONS
- Maintain standard precautions when performing the procedure and handling samples.
- Handle the sample gently to prevent hemolysis.
- Send the sample to the laboratory immediately after collection.
- The sample is stable for up to 48 hours, if refrigerated.

COMPLICATIONS
- Hematoma at the venipuncture site

NORMAL RESULTS
- A titer of < 1:8 is normal.

ABNORMAL RESULTS
- A titer of $\geq$ 1:64 indicates a recent or current adenovirus infection.
- A titer of 1:8 to 1:32 may indicate recent infection, and further testing is recommended.
- If the patient is immunocompromised, a culture test may be required to determine if viral infection is present.

Alanine aminotransferase level test

OVERVIEW

DESCRIPTION

- Serum alanine aminotransferase (ALT): one of two enzymes that catalyze a reversible amino group transfer reaction in the Krebs cycle
- An enzyme necessary for tissue energy production
- An enzyme found primarily in the liver, with lesser amounts in the kidneys, heart, and skeletal muscles (a sensitive indicator of acute hepatocellular disease)

PURPOSE

- To detect acute hepatic disease, especially hepatitis and cirrhosis without jaundice, and to evaluate its treatment
- To distinguish between myocardial and hepatic tissue damage (used with aspartate aminotransferase)
- To assess the hepatotoxicity of some drugs

PREPARATION

- No dietary restrictions are required.
- Notify the laboratory and practitioner of drugs the patient is taking that may affect test results. These drugs may need to be restricted.

Teaching points

- Explain to the patient that this test assesses liver function.
- Tell the patient that the test requires a blood sample and he may experience slight discomfort from the tourniquet and needle puncture.
- Explain who will perform the test and where it'll be done.
- Tell the patient that the test should take less than 5 minutes.
- Explain to the patient that he need not restrict food or fluids.

DIAGNOSTIC PROCEDURE

KEY STEPS

- Confirm the patient's identity using two patient identifiers according to facility policy.
- Perform a venipuncture, and collect the sample in a 4-ml tube without additives.

POSTPROCEDURE CARE

- Apply direct pressure to the venipuncture site until the bleeding stops.
- Tell the patient that he may resume medications stopped before the test.

PRECAUTIONS

- Maintain standard precautions when performing the procedure and handling samples.
- Handle the sample gently to prevent hemolysis.
- Monitor a patient with liver dysfunction for prolonged bleeding at the venipuncture site.
- ALT activity is stable in serum for up to 3 days at room temperature.

COMPLICATIONS

- Hematoma at the venipuncture site

INTERPRETATION

NORMAL RESULTS

- Levels of 8 to 50 International Units (SI, 0.14 to 0.85 µkat/L) are normal.

ABNORMAL RESULTS

- Very high ALT levels (up to 50 times normal) suggest viral or severe drug-induced hepatitis or other hepatic disease with extensive necrosis.
- Moderate to high levels may indicate infectious mononucleosis, chronic hepatitis, intrahepatic cholestasis or cholecystitis, early or improving acute viral hepatitis, or severe hepatic congestion from heart failure.
- Slight to moderate elevations of ALT may appear in any condition that produces acute hepatocellular injury, such as active cirrhosis and drug-induced or alcoholic hepatitis.
- Marginal elevations occasionally occur in acute myocardial infarction, reflecting secondary hepatic congestion or the release of small amounts of ALT from myocardial tissue.

Albumin level test

OVERVIEW

DESCRIPTION
- Measures the amount of albumin in serum
- Albumin: Most abundant protein, composing almost 54% of plasma proteins; helps maintain hydrostatic pressure in the capillary system (see *Fluid movement through capillary walls*)

PURPOSE
- To help determine whether a patient has liver disease or kidney disease
- To determine whether enough protein is being absorbed by the body

PREPARATION
- No dietary restrictions are required.
- Because anabolic steroids, androgens, growth hormones, and insulin can increase albumin levels, the patient may need to stop these drugs before the test.

Teaching points
- Explain the purpose of the test and how it's done.
- Tell the patient that the test requires a blood sample and he may experience slight discomfort from the tourniquet and needle puncture.
- Explain who will perform the test and where it'll be done.
- Explain that anabolic steroids, androgens, growth hormones, and insulin can increase albumin levels. The patient may need to stop these drugs before the test.
- Tell the patient that the test should take less than 5 minutes.
- Tell the patient that he need not restrict food or fluids.

DIAGNOSTIC PROCEDURE

KEY STEPS
- Confirm the patient's identity using two patient identifiers according to facility policy.
- Perform a venipuncture, and collect 5 to 10 ml in a red-top tube.
- Follow standard precautions when collecting the sample.

POSTPROCEDURE CARE
- Apply direct pressure to the venipuncture site until the bleeding stops.
- Encourage the patient to eat a high-protein diet, if not contraindicated.

PRECAUTIONS
- Maintain standard precautions when performing the procedure and handling samples.

COMPLICATIONS
- Hematoma at the venipuncture site

INTERPRETATION

NORMAL RESULTS
- Levels of 3.4 to 5.4 g/dl (SI, 34 to 54 g/L) are normal for adults.
- Levels of 4.0 to 5.8 g/dl (SI, 40 to 58 g/L) are normal for children.
- Levels of 4.4 to 5.4 g/dl (SI, 44 to 54 g/L) are normal for infants.
- Levels of 2.9 to 5.4 g/dl (SI, 29 to 54 g/L) are normal for neonates.

ABNORMAL RESULTS
- A decreased level (hypoalbuminemia) may indicate cirrhosis, acute liver failure, severe burns, severe malnutrition, or ulcerative colitis.
- An elevated level (hyperalbuminemia) may indicate dehydration, severe vomiting, or severe diarrhea.

Fluid movement through capillary walls

The movement of fluids through capillaries—a process called capillary filtration—results from blood pushing against the walls of the capillary. That pressure, called hydrostatic or fluid-pushing pressure, forces fluids and solutes through the capillary wall.

When the hydrostatic pressure inside a capillary is greater than the pressure in the surrounding interstitial space, fluids and solutes inside the capillaries are forced out into the interstitial space, as shown here. When the pressure inside the capillary is less than the pressure outside, fluids and solutes move back into it.

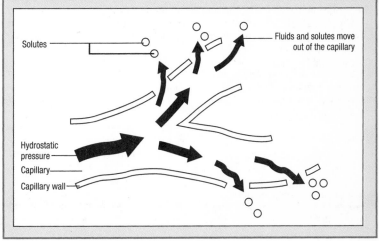

Aldosterone (serum, urine) test

DESCRIPTION

- Measures serum aldosterone levels by quantitative analysis and radioimmunoassay
- Measures urine levels of aldosterone, the principal mineralocorticoid secreted by the adrenal cortex
- Aldosterone: Regulates ion transport across cell membranes in the renal tubules to promote reabsorption of sodium and chloride in exchange for potassium and hydrogen ions; helps to maintain blood pressure and volume and to regulate fluid and electrolyte balance

PURPOSE

- To aid in the diagnosis of primary and secondary aldosteronism, adrenal hyperplasia, hypoaldosteronism, and salt-losing syndrome

PREPARATION

- This test requires a low-carbohydrate, normal-sodium diet (135 mEq or 3 g/day) for at least 2 weeks, preferably for 30 days, before the test.
- Withhold drugs that alter fluid, sodium, and potassium balance — especially diuretics, antihypertensives, steroids, hormonal contraceptives, and estrogens — for at least 2 weeks, preferably for 30 days, before the test.
- Withhold renin inhibitors for 1 week before the test. If the patient must continue them, note this on the laboratory request.
- The patient should avoid licorice for at least 2 weeks before the test because it produces an aldosterone-like effect.
- Strenuous physical exercise and stressful situations should be avoided during the collection period.

Teaching points

- Explain that this test helps determine if the patient's symptoms are from improper hormonal secretion.
- Instruct the patient to maintain a low-carbohydrate, normal-sodium diet for 2 to 4 weeks before the test.

He should also avoid licorice for at least 2 weeks before the test.
- Tell the patient to avoid strenuous physical exercise and stress during the collection period.
- Inform the patient having the serum test that he may experience slight discomfort from the tourniquet and the needle puncture.
- Inform the patient having the urine test that the test requires the collection of urine over 24 hours, and teach him the proper collection technique.
- Explain who will perform the test and where it'll be done.

KEY STEPS

- Confirm the patient's identity using two patient identifiers according to facility policy.

Serum

- Perform a venipuncture while the patient is still supine after a night's rest.
- Collect the sample in a 7-ml clot activator tube, and send it to the laboratory immediately.
- Draw another sample 4 hours later, while the patient is standing and after he has been up and about, to evaluate the effect of postural change.
- Record on the laboratory request whether the patient was supine or standing during the venipuncture.
- If the patient is a premenopausal female, specify the phase of her menstrual cycle because aldosterone levels fluctuate.

Urine

- Collect the patient's urine over a 24-hour period, discarding the first specimen and retaining the last. Use a bottle containing a preservative, such as boric acid, to keep the specimen at a pH of 4.0 to 4.5.
- Refrigerate or place the specimen on ice during the collection period.
- Send the specimen to the laboratory as soon as the collection is complete.

POSTPROCEDURE CARE

- Apply direct pressure to the venipuncture site until the bleeding stops.
- After the test, instruct the patient to resume his usual diet and medications, as ordered.

PRECAUTIONS

- Maintain standard precautions while collecting the sample.
- Handle the sample gently to prevent hemolysis.

COMPLICATIONS

- Hematoma at the venipuncture site

NORMAL RESULTS

Serum

- Laboratory results vary with time of day and posture.
- In people standing upright, normal results are 7 to 30 ng/dl (SI, 190 to 832 pmol/L).
- In people in the supine position, normal results are 3 to 16 ng/dl (SI, 80 to 440 pmol/L).

Urine

- Results of 3 to 19 mcg/24 hours (SI, 8 to 51 nmol/day) are considered normal.

ABNORMAL RESULTS

- Excessive aldosterone secretion may indicate a primary or secondary disease.
- Low serum aldosterone levels may indicate primary hypoaldosteronism, salt-losing syndrome, eclampsia, or Addison's disease.
- Low urine aldosterone levels may result from Addison's disease, salt-losing syndrome, or toxemia of pregnancy. These levels normally rise during pregnancy but rapidly decline after delivery.

Alkaline phosphatase level test

OVERVIEW

DESCRIPTION

- Measures serum levels of alkaline phosphatase (ALP), an enzyme that influences bone calcification as well as lipid and metabolite transport
- Reflects the combined activity of several ALP isoenzymes found in the liver, bones, kidneys, intestinal lining, and placenta
- Particularly sensitive to mild biliary obstruction; a primary indicator of space-occupying hepatic lesions
- Most useful for diagnosing metabolic bone disease

PURPOSE

- To detect and identify skeletal diseases characterized primarily by marked osteoblastic activity
- To detect focal hepatic lesions causing biliary obstruction, such as tumors or an abscesses
- To assess the patient's response to vitamin D in the treatment of rickets
- To supplement information from other liver function studies and GI enzyme tests

PREPARATION

- This test requires an 8-hour fast because fat intake stimulates intestinal ALP secretion.

Teaching points

- Explain to the patient that this test assesses liver and bone function.
- Tell the patient that the test requires a blood sample and that he may experience slight discomfort from the tourniquet and needle puncture.
- Explain who will perform the test and where it'll be done.
- Instruct the patient to fast for at least 8 hours before the test.
- Tell the patient that the test should take less than 5 minutes.

DIAGNOSTIC PROCEDURE

KEY STEPS

- Confirm the patient's identity using two patient identifiers according to facility policy.
- Perform a venipuncture, and collect the sample in a 4-ml clot activator tube.
- Send the sample to the laboratory immediately; ALP activity increases at room temperature because of a rise in pH.

POSTPROCEDURE CARE

- Apply direct pressure to the venipuncture site until the bleeding stops.
- Tell the patient he may resume his usual diet after the test.

PRECAUTIONS

- Maintain standard precautions while collecting and transporting the sample.
- Handle the sample gently to prevent hemolysis.

COMPLICATIONS

- Hematoma at the venipuncture site

INTERPRETATION

NORMAL RESULTS

- Levels of 45 to 115 International Units/ml (SI, 45 to 115 units/L) are normal.

ABNORMAL RESULTS

- Although significant ALP elevations are possible with diseases that affect many organs, they usually indicate skeletal disease or extrahepatic or intrahepatic biliary obstruction causing cholestasis.
- Many acute hepatic diseases cause ALP elevations before they affect serum bilirubin levels.
- Moderate increases in ALP levels may reflect acute biliary obstruction from hepatocellular inflammation in active cirrhosis, mononucleosis, or viral hepatitis.
- Moderate increases are also seen in osteomalacia and deficiency-induced rickets.
- Sharp elevations in ALP levels may indicate complete biliary obstruction by malignant or infectious infiltrations or fibrosis, most common in Paget's disease and, occasionally, in biliary obstruction, extensive bone metastasis, and hyperparathyroidism.
- Metastatic bone tumors resulting from pancreatic cancer raise ALP levels without a concomitant rise in serum alanine aminotransferase levels.
- Isoenzyme fractionation and additional enzyme tests (gamma-glutamyl transferase, lactate dehydrogenase, 5'-nucleotidase, and leucine aminopeptidase) are sometimes performed when the cause of ALP elevations is in doubt.
- Rarely, low levels of serum ALP are linked to hypophosphatasia and protein or magnesium deficiency.

Alpha$_1$-antitrypsin level test

DESCRIPTION

◆ Alpha$_1$-antitrypsin (AAT): A major component of alpha$_1$-globulin; inhibits the release of protease into the body by dying cells
◆ Congenital absence or deficiency of AAT linked to high susceptibility to emphysema in adults and cirrhosis of the liver in children

PURPOSE

◆ To screen the patient at high risk for emphysema
◆ To use as a nonspecific method of detecting inflammation, severe infection, and necrosis
◆ To test for congenital AAT deficiency

PREPARATION

◆ This test requires drug and tobacco restriction and an 8-hour fast.

Teaching points

◆ Explain the purpose of the test and how it's done.
◆ Tell the patient that the test requires a blood sample and he may experience slight discomfort from the tourniquet and needle puncture.
◆ Explain who will perform the test and where it'll be done.
◆ Tell the patient to fast for at least 8 hours before the test.
◆ Tell the patient to avoid hormonal contraceptives and steroids for 24 hours before the test.
◆ Also tell the patient to avoid smoking before the test because tobacco will affect test results.

KEY STEPS

◆ Confirm the patient's identity using two patient identifiers according to facility policy.
◆ Perform a venipuncture, and collect the sample in a 4-ml tube without additives.

POSTPROCEDURE CARE

◆ Apply direct pressure to the venipuncture site until the bleeding stops.
◆ Instruct the patient that he may resume his usual diet and medications discontinued before the test as ordered.

PRECAUTIONS

◆ Maintain standard precautions while collecting the sample.
◆ Handle the sample gently to prevent hemolysis.
◆ Send the sample to the laboratory immediately after collection.

COMPLICATIONS

◆ Hematoma at the venipuncture site

NORMAL RESULTS

◆ AAT levels vary by age, but the normal range is 110 to 200 mg/dl (SI, 1.1 to 2 g/L).

ABNORMAL RESULTS

◆ Decreased AAT levels may occur in early-onset emphysema and cirrhosis, nephrotic syndrome, malnutrition, congenital alpha$_1$-globulin deficiency, and transiently, in the neonate.
◆ Increased AAT levels may occur in chronic inflammatory disorders, necrosis, pregnancy, acute pulmonary infections, respiratory distress syndrome in infants, hepatitis, systemic lupus erythematosus, and rheumatoid arthritis.

INTERFERING FACTORS *Corticosteroids, hormonal contraceptives, smoking before the test (possible false-high result)*

Alpha-fetoprotein level test

OVERVIEW

DESCRIPTION
- Measures the serum and amniotic fluid levels of this protein, which rise during fetal development, cross the placenta, and appear in maternal serum

PURPOSE
- To monitor the effectiveness of therapy in malignant conditions, such as hepatomas and germ cell tumors, and certain nonmalignant conditions such as ataxia-telangiectasia
- To screen for those patients needing amniocentesis or high-resolution ultrasonography during pregnancy

PREPARATION
- No dietary restrictions are required.
- A venipuncture will be performed and a blood sample taken.

Teaching points
- Explain that this test helps in monitoring fetal development, screens for a need for further testing, helps detect possible congenital defects in the fetus, and monitors the mother's response to therapy by measuring a specific blood protein, as appropriate.
- Inform the patient that she need not restrict food, fluids, or medications.
- Tell the patient that the test requires a blood sample and she may experience slight discomfort from the tourniquet and needle puncture.
- Explain who will perform the test and where it'll be done.
- Tell the patient that the test should take less than 5 minutes.

DIAGNOSTIC PROCEDURE

KEY STEPS
- Confirm the patient's identity using two patient identifiers according to facility policy.
- Perform a venipuncture, and collect the sample in a 7-ml clot activator tube.
- Record the patient's age, race, weight, and week of gestation on the laboratory request.

POSTPROCEDURE CARE
- Apply direct pressure to the venipuncture site until the bleeding stops.

PRECAUTIONS
- Maintain standard precautions while collecting and transporting the sample.
- Handle the sample gently to prevent hemolysis.

COMPLICATIONS
- Hematoma at the venipuncture site

INTERPRETATION

NORMAL RESULTS
- When tested by immunoassay, alpha-fetoprotein (AFP) values are less than 15 ng/ml (SI, < 15 mg/L) in men and nonpregnant women. Values in maternal serum are less than 2½ multiples of median for fetal gestational age.

ABNORMAL RESULTS
- Elevated maternal serum AFP levels may suggest neural tube defects or other tube anomalies. Maternal AFP levels rise sharply in the maternal blood of about 90% of women carrying a fetus with anencephaly and in 50% of those carrying a fetus with spina bifida.
- Definitive diagnosis requires ultrasonography and amniocentesis.
- High AFP levels may indicate intrauterine death. Sometimes, high levels indicate other anomalies, such as duodenal atresia, omphalocele, tetralogy of Fallot, and Turner's syndrome.
- Elevated serum AFP levels occur in 70% of nonpregnant patients with hepatocellular carcinoma.
- Elevated serum AFP levels are also related to germ cell tumor of gonadal, retroperitoneal, or mediastinal origin.
- Serum AFP levels rise in ataxia-telangiectasia and sometimes in cancer of the pancreas, stomach, or biliary system and in nonseminiferous testicular tumors.
- Transient modest elevations may occur in nonneoplastic hepatocellular disease, such as alcoholic cirrhosis and acute or chronic hepatitis.
- Elevation of AFP levels after remission suggests tumor recurrence.
- In hepatocellular carcinoma, a gradual decrease in serum AFP levels indicates a favorable response to therapy. In germ cell tumors, serum AFP levels and serum human chorionic gonadotropin levels should be measured concurrently.

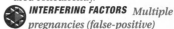 **INTERFERING FACTORS** *Multiple pregnancies (false-positive)*

Alpha$_1$-globulin and alpha$_2$-globulin level test

DESCRIPTION
◆ Roughly measures the various protein fractions in the serum portion of a blood sample

PURPOSE
◆ To aid in ruling out inflammatory disease
◆ To help detect the presence of inflammation

PREPARATION
◆ A venipuncture will be performed and a blood sample taken.

Teaching points
◆ Explain to the patient that the test helps detect inflammatory diseases.
◆ Tell the patient that the test requires a blood sample and that he may experience slight discomfort from the tourniquet and needle puncture.
◆ Explain who will perform the test and where it'll be done.

KEY STEPS
◆ Confirm the patient's identity using two patient identifiers according to facility policy.
◆ Perform the venipuncture according to protocol.

POSTPROCEDURE CARE
◆ Apply direct pressure to the venipuncture site until the bleeding stops.

PRECAUTIONS
◆ Maintain standard precautions while collecting and transporting the sample.

COMPLICATIONS
◆ Hematoma at the venipuncture site

NORMAL RESULTS
◆ Levels of 0.1 to 0.3 g/dl for alpha$_1$-globulin are considered normal.
◆ Levels of 0.6 to 1.0 g/dl for alpha$_2$-globulin are considered normal.

ABNORMAL RESULTS
◆ Increased alpha$_1$-globulin proteins may indicate chronic inflammatory disease (for example, rheumatoid arthritis, systemic lupus erythematosus), acute inflammatory disease, or malignancy.
◆ Decreased alpha$_1$-globulin proteins may indicate an alpha$_1$-antitrypsin deficiency.
◆ Increased alpha$_2$-globulin proteins may indicate acute or chronic inflammation.
◆ Decreased alpha$_2$-globulin proteins may indicate hemolysis.

Aluminum level test

DESCRIPTION

- Measures the level of aluminum in the body, to which it's exposed in a variety of sources
- Aluminum: Excreted in the urine in patients with normal renal function; accumulates in high levels in the tissue in patients with renal failure; and may play a role in Alzheimer's disease

PURPOSE

- To determine the serum aluminum level

PREPARATION

- This test requires a venipuncture.
- The patient should avoid antacids containing aluminum for 24 hours before the test.

Teaching points

- Explain that this test will measure the amount of aluminum in the blood.
- Inform the patient that this test requires a venipuncture and that he may experience slight discomfort from the tourniquet and needle puncture.
- Instruct the patient to avoid taking antacids that contain aluminum for 24 hours before the test.
- Explain who will perform the test and where it'll be done.

KEY STEPS

- Confirm the patient's identity using two patient identifiers according to facility policy.
- Perform the venipuncture using a 7-ml metal-free tube with no additives.

POSTPROCEDURE CARE

- Apply direct pressure to the venipuncture site until the bleeding stops.

PRECAUTIONS

- Maintain standard precautions while collecting and transporting the sample.
- Transport the sample to the laboratory immediately after collection.

COMPLICATIONS

- Hematoma at the venipuncture site

NORMAL RESULTS

- Normal range is 3 to 10 mcg/L (SI, 0.11 to 0.37 µmol/L).

ABNORMAL RESULTS

- Hemodialysis patients should have a level of less than 40 mcg/L.
- Increased aluminum may contribute to dialysis dementia and dialysis osteodystrophy.
- Chronic toxicity may result in several metabolic imbalances.

Alveolar-to-arterial oxygen gradient test

DESCRIPTION

◆ Using calculations based on the patient's laboratory values, helps identify the cause of hypoxemia and intrapulmonary shunting by approximating the partial pressure of oxygenation of the alveoli and arteries

◆ May help differentiate the causes of ventilated alveoli but not perfusion, unventilated alveoli with perfusion, and collapse of the alveoli and capillaries

PURPOSE

◆ To evaluate the efficiency of gas exchange
◆ To assess the integrity of the ventilatory control system
◆ To monitor respiratory therapy

PREPARATION

◆ The test requires a blood sample.
◆ No dietary restrictions are required.

Teaching points

◆ Explain to the patient that the test evaluates how well the lungs are delivering oxygen to the blood and eliminating carbon dioxide.
◆ Tell the patient that the test requires a blood sample.
◆ Inform the patient that he need not restrict food or fluids.
◆ Instruct the patient to breathe normally during the test, and warn him that he may experience cramping or throbbing pain at the puncture site.
◆ Explain who will perform the test and where it'll be done.
◆ Tell the patient that the test should take less than 20 minutes.

KEY STEPS

◆ Confirm the patient's identity using two patient identifiers according to facility policy.
◆ Perform Allen's test to determine arterial perfusion.
◆ Perform an arterial puncture, or draw blood from an arterial line using a heparinized blood gas syringe.
◆ Eliminate all air from the sample, and place it on ice immediately.
◆ Before sending the sample to the laboratory, note on the laboratory request whether the patient was breathing room air or receiving oxygen therapy when the sample was collected.
◆ If the patient was receiving oxygen therapy, note the flow rate and method of delivery. If he was on a ventilator, note the fraction of inspired oxygen, tidal volume, mode, respiratory rate, and positive end-expiratory pressure.
◆ Note the patient's temperature.

POSTPROCEDURE CARE

◆ Apply pressure to the puncture for 3 to 5 minutes or until bleeding has stopped.
◆ Place a gauze pad over the site and tape it in place, but don't tape the entire circumference.
◆ Monitor vital signs and observe for signs of circulatory impairment, such as swelling, discoloration, pain, numbness, and tingling in the bandaged arm or leg.

PRECAUTIONS

◆ Maintain standard precautions while collecting and handling the sample.

COMPLICATIONS

◆ Bleeding from the puncture site

NORMAL RESULTS

◆ Alveolar-to-arterial oxygen gradient (A-aDo$_2$) at rest in room air is less than 10 mm Hg; at maximum exercise, it's 20 to 30 mm Hg.

ABNORMAL RESULTS

◆ Increased values may result from mucus plugs, bronchospasm, or airway collapse (asthma, bronchitis, emphysema).
◆ Hypoxemia results in increased A-aDo$_2$ and may result from arterial septal defects, pneumothorax, atelectasis, emboli, or edema.

Amino acid screening

DESCRIPTION
- Qualitative screen for inborn errors of metabolism of amino acids, the chief components of all proteins and polypeptides
- Amino acids: Ten of at least 20 amino acids in the body not formed in the body and needing to be acquired through diet
- Amino acid accumulation or deficiency resulting from congenital enzyme deficiencies that interfere with normal metabolism of these amino acids

PURPOSE
- To screen for inborn errors of amino acid metabolism

PREPARATION
- The infant must fast for 4 hours before the test.
- A heelstick is required.

Teaching points
- Explain to the parents that plasma amino acid screening determines how well their infant metabolizes amino acids.
- Instruct the parents that the infant must fast for 4 hours before the test.
- Tell the parents that a small amount of blood is drawn from the infant's heel, but that collecting the sample takes only a few minutes.
- Explain who will perform the heelstick and where it'll be done.

KEY STEPS
- Confirm the patient's identity using two patient identifiers according to facility policy.
- Perform a heelstick, and collect 0.1 ml of blood in a heparinized capillary tube.

POSTPROCEDURE CARE
- Apply direct pressure to the venipuncture site until the bleeding stops.
- Tell the parents to resume the feeding of their infant's usual diet.

PRECAUTIONS
- Maintain standard precautions while collecting and transporting the sample.
- Handle the sample gently to prevent hemolysis.

COMPLICATIONS
- Hematoma at the heelstick site

NORMAL RESULTS
- Chromatography shows a normal plasma amino acid pattern.

ABNORMAL RESULTS
- Excessive accumulation of amino acids typically produces overflow aminoaciduria.
- Congenital abnormalities of the amino acid transport system in the kidneys produce a second group of disorders called renal aminoaciduria.
- Comparisons of blood and urine chromatography can help distinguish between the two types of aminoaciduria.
- The plasma amino acid pattern is normal in renal aminoaciduria and abnormal in overflow aminoaciduria.

Ammonia level test

DESCRIPTION

- Measures plasma levels of ammonia, a nonprotein nitrogen compound that helps maintain acid-base balance
- Ammonia: Bypasses the liver and accumulates in the blood in diseases such as cirrhosis of the liver
- Possibly helpful in indicating the severity of hepatocellular damage

PURPOSE

- To help monitor the progression of severe hepatic disease and the effectiveness of therapy
- To recognize impending or established hepatic coma

PREPARATION

- The test requires a venipuncture and a blood sample.
- No dietary restrictions are required.
- Notify the laboratory and practitioner of drugs the patient is taking that may affect the test results; it may be necessary to restrict such drugs.

Teaching

- Explain to the patient (or to a family member, if the patient is comatose) that the plasma ammonia test is used to evaluate liver function.
- Explain that the test requires a blood sample and that the patient may experience slight discomfort from the tourniquet and needle puncture.
- Explain who will perform the test and where it'll be done.
- Explain that no dietary restrictions are needed.

KEY STEPS

- Confirm the patient's identity using two patient identifiers according to facility policy.
- Notify the laboratory before performing the venipuncture, so that preliminary preparations can begin.
- Perform a venipuncture, and collect the sample in a 10-ml heparinized tube.
- Pack the specimen in ice, and send it to the laboratory immediately.

POSTPROCEDURE CARE

- Apply direct pressure to the venipuncture site until the bleeding stops.

PRECAUTIONS

- Maintain standard precautions while collecting and transporting the sample.
- Place the sample on ice immediately after collection.
- Handle the sample gently to prevent hemolysis.

COMPLICATIONS

- Hematoma at the venipuncture site
- Signs of impending or established hepatic coma, if plasma ammonia levels are high

NORMAL RESULTS

- In adults, levels of 15 to 45 mcg/dl (SI, 11 to 32 μmol/L) are considered normal.

ABNORMAL RESULTS

- Elevated plasma ammonia levels are common in severe hepatic disease, such as cirrhosis and acute hepatic necrosis, and can lead to hepatic coma.
- Elevated levels may also occur in Reye's syndrome, severe heart failure, GI hemorrhage, and erythroblastosis fetalis.

Amniotic fluid analysis

DESCRIPTION
- Indicated if the patient is age 35 or older; has a family history of genetic, chromosomal, or neural tube defects; or has had a miscarriage
- Repeated if results are abnormal or tissue cultures fail to grow

PURPOSE
- To detect fetal abnormalities, particularly chromosomal and neural tube defects
- To detect hemolytic disease of the neonate
- To diagnose metabolic disorders, amino acid disorders, and mucopolysaccharidosis
- To determine fetal age and maturity
- To assess fetal health by detecting the presence of meconium or blood or measuring amniotic levels of estriol and fetal thyroid hormone
- To identify fetal gender when one or both parents are carriers of a sex-linked disorder

PREPARATION
- No dietary restrictions are required.
- Ask the patient to void just before the test to minimize the risk of puncturing the bladder.
- Ask the patient to call the practitioner if she notices any fluid loss, bleeding, pain, decreased fetal movement, or an increase in temperature after the test.

Teaching points
- Explain procedure and answer patient's questions.
- Inform the patient that she need not restrict food or fluids.
- Explain to the patient that she'll feel a stinging sensation when the local anesthetic is injected.
- Explain who will perform the test and where it'll be done.
- Tell the patient that the test usually takes less than 1 hour.

KEY STEPS
- Confirm the patient's identity using two patient identifiers according to facility policy.
- After fetal and placental position are determined, a pool of amniotic fluid is located, usually through palpation and ultrasonic visualization.
- The skin is prepared with antiseptic and alcohol, and 1 ml of lidocaine 1% is injected with a 25G needle, first intradermally and then subcutaneously.
- A 20G spinal needle with a stylet is inserted into the amniotic cavity, and the stylet is withdrawn.
- A 10-ml syringe is attached to the needle; then the fluid is aspirated and placed in an amber or a foil-covered test tube.
- The needle is withdrawn and an adhesive bandage placed over the needle insertion site.
- The fetal heart rate and maternal vital signs are monitored every 15 minutes for at least 30 minutes.

POSTPROCEDURE CARE
- Instruct the patient to immediately report abdominal pain or cramping, chills, fever, vaginal bleeding or leakage of serous vaginal fluid, or fetal hyperactivity or unusual fetal lethargy.

PRECAUTIONS
- Place the specimen in a light-resistant container, to prevent breakdown of bilirubin.

COMPLICATIONS
- Spontaneous abortion, fetal or placental trauma, bleeding, premature labor, infection, and Rh sensitization resulting from fetal bleeding into maternal circulation

NORMAL RESULTS
- Normal amniotic fluid is clear but may contain white flecks of vernix caseosa when the fetus is near term.

ABNORMAL RESULTS
- "Port-wine" fluid may be a sign of abruptio placentae, and blood of fetal origin may indicate damage to the fetal, placental, or umbilical cord vessels by the amniocentesis needle.
- Large amounts of bilirubin may indicate hemolytic disease of the neonate.
- Meconium in the amniotic fluid produces a peak at 410 mμ on the spectrophotometric analysis. If meconium is present during labor, the neonate's nose and throat require thorough cleaning to prevent meconium aspiration.
- High amniotic fluid levels indicate neural tube defects; the alpha-fetoprotein (AFP) level may remain normal if a defect is small and closed.
- Elevated AFP levels may result from a multiple pregnancy; from an omphalocele, congenital nephrosis, esophageal or duodenal atresia, cystic fibrosis, exomphalos, Turner's syndrome, and fetal bladder neck obstruction with hydronephrosis; and from an impending fetal death.
- Severe erythroblastosis fetalis, familial hyperuricemia, and Lesch-Nyhan syndrome tend to increase the uric acid level; severe erythroblastosis fetalis decreases the estriol level.
- The lecithin-sphingomyelin (L/S) ratio confirms fetal pulmonary maturity (L/S ratio > 2) or suggests a risk of respiratory distress (L/S ratio < 2).
- A glucose level greater than 45 mg/dl indicates poor maternal and fetal blood glucose control.
- Elevated acetylcholinesterase levels may occur with neural tube defects, exomphalos, and other serious malformations.

Amsler's grid

DESCRIPTION

- Easiest test for detecting central field deficits caused by macular degeneration
- Composed of a central black dot and horizontal and vertical lines that form 5-mm squares (grid helps find central scotomas — blind or partially blind spots in the macular area of the retina)
- Detects microscopic areas of macular or perimacular edema that cause visual distortions
- Only a screening test that must be supplemented by other tests, such as ophthalmoscopy, visual field testing, and fluorescein angiography, to determine the cause of abnormal vision

PURPOSE

- To detect central scotomas
- To evaluate the stability or progression of macular disease

PREPARATION

- If the patient normally wears corrective lenses, he should keep them on during the test.

Teaching points

- Explain to the patient that this test evaluates his central field of vision.
- If he normally wears corrective lenses, instruct him to keep them on during the test.
- Explain who will perform the test and where it'll be done.
- Tell the patient that the test should take less than 10 minutes.

DIAGNOSTIC PROCEDURE

KEY STEPS

- Confirm the patient's identity using two patient identifiers according to facility policy.
- Occlude one of the patient's eyes and hold Amsler's grid at his customary reading distance, about 11″ to 12″ (28 to 30.5 cm) in front of the unoccluded eye.

- Tell the patient to stare at the central dot on the grid, and then ask these questions: Can you see the black dot in the center? When you look directly at the dot, can you see all four sides of the grid? All of the little squares? Do all the lines appear ruler-straight? Is there any blurring, distortion, or movement?
- If the patient answers yes to any of these questions, ask him to elaborate.
- Give him a pencil and paper, and encourage him to outline and describe the specific areas that appear distorted.
- After recording the patient's observations, occlude the other eye and repeat the procedure.
- Remind the patient to keep his unoccluded eye fixed on the central black dot on the grid.
- Perform this test before dilating the patient's pupils and before performing a funduscopic examination or the refraction test.

POSTPROCEDURE CARE

- Support the patient throughout testing.

PRECAUTIONS

- Make sure the patient is wearing corrective lenses, if applicable.

COMPLICATIONS

None known

INTERPRETATION

NORMAL RESULTS

- Patient should be able to see the central black dot and, while staring at the dot, all four sides of the grid and all the small squares. All the lines should appear ruler-straight. He shouldn't see blurring, distortion, or missing squares. (See *Amsler's grid: Normal and abnormal views.*)

ABNORMAL RESULTS

- The inability to see the black dot in the center of the grid suggests a central scotoma.
- If any of the lines don't appear ruler-straight to the patient, metamorphopsia (distorted perception of objects) may be indicated.
- Blurring, distortion, or movement may signal an imminent scotoma.
- Further evaluation by ophthalmoscopy, visual field testing, and fluorescein angiography is needed for abnormal findings.

Amsler's grid: Normal and abnormal views

The illustration on the left shows a normal view of Amsler's grid. The illustration on the right shows a grid as it might look to a patient with a central scotoma caused by a macular hole. The center dot is entirely absent, as are the lines around it. The lines of the periphery of the scotoma appear bowed asymmetrically.

NORMAL VIEW

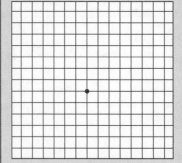

ABNORMAL VIEW

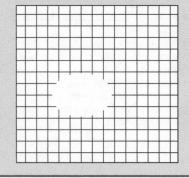

Amylase (serum) level test

DESCRIPTION
◆ Most important laboratory test in patients suspected of having acute pancreatic disease

PURPOSE
◆ To diagnose acute pancreatitis
◆ To distinguish between acute pancreatitis and other causes of abdominal pain that require immediate surgery
◆ To evaluate possible pancreatic injury caused by abdominal trauma or surgery

PREPARATION
◆ This test requires a blood sample.
◆ Abstinence from alcohol is necessary for 24 hours before the test.
◆ Notify the laboratory and practitioner of drugs the patient is taking that may affect test results; it may be necessary to restrict such drugs

Teaching points
◆ Explain to the patient that this test assesses pancreatic function.
◆ Tell the patient that this test requires a blood sample and that he may experience slight discomfort from the tourniquet and the needle puncture.
◆ Inform the patient that he need not fast before the test but must abstain from alcohol for 24 hours before the test.
◆ Explain who will perform the test and where it'll be done.

KEY STEPS
◆ Confirm the patient's identity using two patient identifiers according to facility policy.
◆ Perform a venipuncture, and collect the sample in a 4-ml clot activator tube.
◆ If the patient has severe abdominal pain, draw the sample before diagnostic or therapeutic intervention. For accurate results, it's important to obtain an early sample.

POSTPROCEDURE CARE
◆ Apply direct pressure to the venipuncture site until the bleeding stops.

PRECAUTIONS
◆ Maintain standard precautions while collecting the sample.
◆ Handle the sample gently to prevent hemolysis.

COMPLICATIONS
◆ Hematoma at the venipuncture site

NORMAL RESULTS
◆ Levels of 26 to 102 units/L (SI, 0.4 to 1.74 μkat/L) for adults age 18 and older are considered normal.

ABNORMAL RESULTS
◆ After the onset of acute pancreatitis, amylase levels begin to rise within 2 hours, peak within 12 to 48 hours, and return to normal within 3 to 4 days.
◆ Determination of urine amylase levels should follow normal serum results, to rule out pancreatitis.
◆ Moderate serum amylase elevations may accompany common bile duct, pancreatic duct, or ampulla of Vater obstruction; pancreatic injury from a perforated peptic ulcer; pancreatic cancer; and acute salivary gland disease.
◆ Impaired kidney function may increase serum amylase levels.
◆ Levels may be slightly elevated in a patient who's asymptomatic or responding unusually to therapy.
◆ Decreased serum amylase levels can occur in patients with chronic pancreatitis, pancreatic cancer, cirrhosis, hepatitis, and toxemia of pregnancy.

Amylase (urine) level test

DESCRIPTION

- Method for determining urine amylase levels; the dye-coupled starch method.

PURPOSE

- To diagnose acute pancreatitis when serum amylase levels are normal or borderline
- To aid in the diagnosis of chronic pancreatitis and salivary gland disorders

PREPARATION

- No dietary restrictions are required.
- Notify the laboratory and practitioner of drugs the patient is taking that may affect test results; it may be necessary to restrict such drugs.

Teaching points

- Explain to the patient that this test evaluates the function of the pancreas and the salivary glands.
- Inform the patient that he need not restrict food or fluids.
- Tell the patient that the test requires urine collection for 2, 6, 8, or 24 hours, and teach him how to collect a timed specimen.
- Instruct the patient to empty his bladder, and then begin timing the collection.
- Tell the patient to keep the urine refrigerated during the collection period.

KEY STEPS

- Confirm the patient's identity using two patient identifiers according to facility policy.
- Collect the patient's urine during 2-, 6-, 8-, or 24-hours.
- A 2-hour test is usually performed because collecting urine for a 2-hour period produces fewer errors than a more diagnostic 24-hour collection.
- Cover and refrigerate the specimen during the collection period.
- If the patient is catheterized, keep the collection bag on ice.
- Send the specimen on ice to the laboratory as soon as the test is complete.

POSTPROCEDURE CARE

- Instruct the patient not to contaminate the specimen with toilet tissue or stool.

PRECAUTIONS

- Keep specimen refrigerated or on ice.

COMPLICATIONS

None known

NORMAL RESULTS

- Urine amylase is reported in various units of measure, so values differ among laboratories. The Mayo Clinic reports normal urinary excretion of 1 to 17 units/hour (SI, 0.017 to 0.29 µkat/hour).

ABNORMAL RESULTS

- Urine amylase levels increase in acute pancreatitis; obstruction of the pancreatic duct, intestines, or salivary duct; cancer of the head of the pancreas; mumps; acute injury of the spleen; renal disease, with impaired absorption; perforated peptic or duodenal ulcer; and gallbladder disease.
- Urine amylase levels decrease in chronic pancreatitis, cachexia, alcoholism, liver cancer, cirrhosis, hepatitis, and hepatic abscess.

Amyloid beta-protein precursor test

OVERVIEW

DESCRIPTION
- Assesses the extracellular deposition of amyloid beta-peptide, a major neuropathologic sign of Alzheimer's disease
- Amyloid beta-peptide: from the large beta-amyloid precursor protein (APP)
- APP: major protein subunit of the vascular and plaque amyloid filaments in those with Alzheimer's disease

PURPOSE
- To help in the diagnosis of Alzheimer's disease
- To monitor the progression of Alzheimer's disease and the effectiveness of its treatment

PREPARATION
- The test requires a sample of cerebrospinal fluid (CSF), which is obtained by lumbar puncture.
- No dietary restrictions are required.
- Make sure that the patient or a responsible family member has signed an informed consent form.

Teaching points
- Explain to the patient that this test may help determine if he has Alzheimer's disease.
- Tell the patient that the test requires a sample of CSF, which is obtained by lumbar puncture.
- Tell the patient that no dietary restrictions are required with this test.
- Advise the patient that although a headache is the most common adverse effect of this test, his cooperation during the test can help minimize this effect.
- Explain who will perform the test and where it'll be done.
- Tell the patient that the test should take less than 30 minutes.

DIAGNOSTIC PROCEDURE

KEY STEPS
- Confirm the patient's identity using two patient identifiers according to facility policy.
- Position the patient on his side at the edge of the bed, with his knees drawn up to his abdomen and his chin tucked against his chest (the fetal position), or position the patient sitting while leaning over a bedside table.
- If the patient is in a supine position, provide pillows to support the spine on a horizontal plane.
- The skin site is prepared and draped.
- A local anesthetic is injected.
- The spinal needle is inserted in the midline between the spinous processes of the vertebrae (usually between the third and fourth lumbar vertebrae or between the fourth and fifth).
- The stylet is removed from the needle; CSF drips out of the needle if properly positioned.
- Specimens are collected and placed in the appropriate containers.
- The needle is removed and a small sterile dressing applied.
- Record the collection time on the test request form. Send the form and labeled specimen to the laboratory immediately after collection.

WARNING *Watch the patient for complications of lumbar puncture, such as reaction to the anesthetic, meningitis, bleeding into the spinal canal, cerebellar tonsillar herniation, and medullary compression.*

POSTPROCEDURE CARE
- Keep the patient lying flat for 4 to 6 hours.
- Inform him that he can turn from side to side.
- Encourage the patient to drink fluids, and assist him as needed.
- Give analgesics.
- Monitor the patient's vital signs, neurologic status, and intake and output.
- Monitor the puncture site for redness, swelling, and drainage.

PRECAUTIONS
- Maintain sterile technique during the procedure.
- During the procedure, observe closely for adverse reactions, such as elevated pulse rate, pallor, or clammy skin. Report any significant changes immediately.
- Send specimen to the laboratory immediately after collection.

COMPLICATIONS
- Adverse reaction to the anesthetic
- Infection
- Meningitis
- Bleeding into the spinal canal
- Leakage of CSF
- Cerebellar herniation
- Medullary compression

INTERPRETATION

NORMAL RESULTS
- Levels greater than 450 units/L are considered normal.

ABNORMAL RESULTS
- Decreased levels indicate Alzheimer's disease.

Androstenedione level test

DESCRIPTION

◆ Helps identify disorders related to altered hormone levels, such as female virilization syndromes and polycystic ovary (Stein-Leventhal) syndrome
◆ Possible secretion by tumors of the ovaries or adrenal glands of excessive amounts of androstenedione, which then converts to testosterone, resulting in virilizing symptoms, such as hirsutism and sterility

PURPOSE

◆ To help determine the cause of gonadal dysfunction, menstrual or menopausal irregularities, virilizing symptoms, and premature sexual development

PREPARATION

◆ The test requires a blood sample.
◆ No dietary restrictions are required.
◆ Withhold steroid and pituitary-based hormones. If the patient must continue them, note this on the laboratory request.
◆ The test should occur 1 week before or after the patient's menstrual period, and it may be necessary to repeat the test.

Teaching points

◆ Explain to the patient that this test will help determine the cause of her symptoms.
◆ Tell the patient that the test requires a blood sample and that she may experience slight discomfort from the tourniquet and needle puncture.
◆ Tell the patient that she need not restrict food or fluids.
◆ Explain that the test should occur 1 week before or after her menstrual period and that it may be necessary to repeat the test.
◆ Explain who will perform the venipuncture and where it'll be done.

KEY STEPS

◆ Confirm the patient's identity using two patient identifiers according to facility policy.
◆ Perform a venipuncture, and collect a serum sample in a 7-ml clot activator tube or collect a plasma sample in a green-top tube. If a plasma sample is taken, refrigerate it or place it on ice.
◆ Label the sample appropriately, and send it to the laboratory immediately.
◆ Record the patient's age, sex, and (if appropriate) phase of her menstrual cycle on the laboratory request.

POSTPROCEDURE CARE

◆ Apply direct pressure to the venipuncture site until the bleeding stops.
◆ Instruct the patient that she may resume medications stopped before the test.

PRECAUTIONS

◆ Maintain standard precautions while collecting the sample.
◆ Handle the sample gently to prevent hemolysis.

COMPLICATIONS

◆ Hematoma at the venipuncture site

NORMAL RESULTS

◆ Levels of 85 to 275 ng/dl (SI, 3.0 to 9.6 nmol/L) for women are considered normal.
◆ Levels of 75 to 205 ng/dl (SI, 2.6 to 7.2 nmol/L) for men are considered normal.

ABNORMAL RESULTS

◆ Elevated androstenedione levels are linked to polycystic ovary (Stein-Leventhal) syndrome; Cushing's syndrome; ovarian, testicular, and adrenocortical tumors; ectopic corticotropin-producing tumors; late-onset congenital adrenal hyperplasia; and ovarian stromal hyperplasia.
◆ Elevated levels result in increased estrone levels, causing premature sexual development in children; menstrual irregularities in premenopausal women; bleeding, endometriosis, and polycystic ovaries in postmenopausal women; and feminizing signs, such as gynecomastia, in men.
◆ Decreased levels occur in patients with hypogonadism.

Angioedema panel

DESCRIPTION

- Includes test for C1 esterase inhibitor protein, C1q complement protein, and C4D fragment
- C1 esterase inhibitor protein: A serum component that inhibits the complement proteases C1R and C1S, along with other proteases in the blood clotting system
- C1q complement: Plays a role in the inflammation process
- C4D fragment: Helps determine if classic complement action is present

PURPOSE

- To determine if angioedema is hereditary or acquired
- To exclude rheumatoid arthritis and systemic lupus erythematosus from diagnoses

PREPARATION

- The test requires a blood sample.
- The patient shouldn't eat or drink for 8 hours before the test.

Teaching points

- Explain to the patient that this test helps to determine the cause of the angioedema.
- Tell the patient that the test requires a blood sample and that he may experience slight discomfort from the tourniquet and the needle puncture.
- Instruct the patient not to eat or drink for 8 hours before the test.
- Explain who will perform the venipuncture and where it'll be done.

KEY STEPS

- Confirm the patient's identity using two patient identifiers according to facility policy.
- Perform a venipuncture, and collect a serum sample in a tube without additives.
- Place the sample on ice immediately.
- Label the sample appropriately, and send it to the laboratory immediately.

POSTPROCEDURE CARE

- Apply direct pressure to the venipuncture site until the bleeding stops.

PRECAUTIONS

- Maintain standard precautions while collecting the sample.
- Handle the sample gently to prevent hemolysis.
- Place the sample on ice immediately after collection and while being transported.

COMPLICATIONS

- Hematoma at the venipuncture site

NORMAL RESULTS

- C1 esterase inhibitor protein is functional
- Levels of C1q complement ranging from 7 to 15 mg/dl are considered normal.
- Levels of C4D fragment ranging from 16 to 47 mg/dl are considered normal.
- C4D levels in the normal range exclude rheumatoid arthritis and systemic lupus erythematosus from the causes of angioedema.

ABNORMAL RESULTS

- An abnormal C1 esterase inhibitor protein level is indicative of hereditary angioedema.
- A decreased C1q level may indicate acquired angioedema.

Angiotensin-converting enzyme level test

DESCRIPTION

◆ Measures serum levels of angiotensin-converting enzyme (ACE), which is found in lung capillaries and, in lesser concentrations, in blood vessels and kidney tissue
◆ Monitors response to treatment in sarcoidosis and helps confirm a diagnosis of Gaucher's disease or leprosy

PURPOSE

◆ To aid in the diagnosis of sarcoidosis, especially pulmonary sarcoidosis
◆ To monitor the patient's response to therapy for sarcoidosis
◆ To help confirm Gaucher's disease or leprosy

PREPARATION

◆ The patient must fast for 12 hours before the test.
◆ The test requires a blood sample.
◆ Note the patient's age on the laboratory request. The test may have to be postponed if the patient is younger than age 20 because of the variable ACE levels in this age-group.

Teaching points

◆ Explain the purpose of the test and how it's done.
◆ Inform the patient that he must fast for 12 hours before the test.
◆ Explain that the test requires a blood sample and he may experience slight discomfort from the tourniquet and needle puncture.
◆ Tell the patient that the test should take less than 5 minutes.

KEY STEPS

◆ Confirm the patient's identity using two patient identifiers according to facility policy.
◆ Perform a venipuncture, and collect the sample in a 7-ml clot activator tube.
◆ Avoid using a tube with ethylenediaminetetraacetic acid because this can decrease ACE levels, altering test results.
◆ Send the sample to the laboratory immediately or freeze it until the time of testing.

POSTPROCEDURE CARE

◆ Apply direct pressure to the venipuncture site until the bleeding stops.

PRECAUTIONS

◆ Maintain standard precautions while collecting the sample.
◆ Handle the sample gently to prevent hemolysis.
◆ Immediately place sample on ice or freeze it.

COMPLICATIONS

◆ Hematoma at the venipuncture site

NORMAL RESULTS

◆ In the colorimetric assay, normal results for serum ACE in patients age 20 and older range from 8 to 52 units/L (SI, 0.14 to 0.88 µkat/L).

ABNORMAL RESULTS

◆ Elevated serum ACE levels may indicate sarcoidosis, Gaucher's disease, or leprosy, but results must be correlated with the patient's clinical condition.
◆ In some cases, elevated ACE levels may result from hyperthyroidism, diabetic retinopathy, or hepatic disease.
◆ Serum ACE levels decline as the patient responds to steroid or prednisone therapy for sarcoidosis.

Anion gap test

DESCRIPTION

- Measures the gap between measured cation and anion levels, which are usually equal (making serum electrically neutral), and provides information about the level of anions (including sulfate; phosphate; organic acids, such as ketone bodies and lactic acid; and proteins) that aren't routinely measured in laboratory tests.
- Helps to identify the type of metabolic acidosis and its possible causes.
- Determining the specific cause of metabolic acidosis usually requiring further tests

PURPOSE

- To distinguish among types of metabolic acidosis
- To monitor renal function and total parenteral nutrition

PREPARATION

- The test requires a blood sample.
- No dietary restrictions are required.
- Notify the laboratory and practitioner of drugs the patient is taking that may affect test results; it may be necessary to restrict such drugs.

Teaching points

- Explain to the patient that the anion gap test determines the cause of acidosis.
- Tell the patient that a blood sample is needed and that he may experience slight discomfort from the tourniquet and needle puncture.
- Tell the patient that he need not restrict food or fluids.
- Explain who will perform the venipuncture and where it'll be done.
- Explain that the test should take less than 5 minutes.

KEY STEPS

- Confirm the patient's identity using two patient identifiers according to facility policy.
- Perform a venipuncture, and collect the sample in a 3- or 4-ml clot activator tube.

POSTPROCEDURE CARE

- Apply direct pressure to the venipuncture site until the bleeding stops.
- Instruct the patient to resume medications stopped before the test.

PRECAUTIONS

- Maintain standard precautions while performing the test.
- Handle the sample gently to prevent hemolysis.

COMPLICATIONS

- Hematoma at the venipuncture site

Anion gap and metabolic acidosis

Metabolic acidosis with a normal anion gap (8 to 14 mEq/L) occurs when bicarbonate is lost, as in:

- hypokalemic acidosis caused by renal tubular acidosis, diarrhea, or ureteral diversions
- hyperkalemic acidosis caused by acidifying agents (for example, ammonium chloride, hydrochloric acid), hydronephrosis, or sickle cell nephropathy.

Metabolic acidosis with an increased anion gap (> 14 mEq/L) occurs when organic acids, sulfates, or phosphates accumulate, as in:

- renal failure
- ketoacidosis caused by starvation, diabetes mellitus, or alcohol abuse
- lactic acidosis
- ingestion of toxins, such as salicylates, methanol, ethylene glycol (antifreeze), and paraldehyde.

NORMAL RESULTS

- Anion gap levels of 8 to 14 mEq/L (SI, 8 to 14 mmol/L) are considered normal.

ABNORMAL RESULTS

- An increased anion gap level indicates an increase in one or more of the unmeasured anions: sulfate; phosphates; organic acids, such as ketone bodies and lactic acid; and proteins. This may occur with acidoses that are characterized by excessive organic or inorganic acids, such as lactic acidosis or ketoacidosis.
- Acidosis from an accumulation of metabolic acids (for example, in lactic acidosis) increases the anion gap (> 14 mEq/L), because the unmeasured anion level increases. Metabolic acidosis resulting from this accumulation is called high anion gap acidosis.
- A decreased anion gap level is rare but may occur with hypermagnesemia and paraproteinemic states, such as multiple myeloma and Waldenström's macroglobulinemia. (See *Anion gap and metabolic acidosis*.)

Antegrade pyelography

DESCRIPTION

- Examines the upper collecting system when ureteral obstruction rules out retrograde ureteropyelography or when cystoscopy is contraindicated
- Depends on percutaneous needle puncture for injection of contrast medium into the renal pelvis or calyces
- Allows measurement of renal pressure
- Facilitates cultures, cytologic studies, and evaluation of the renal functional reserve before surgery through urine collection

PURPOSE

- To evaluate upper collecting system obstruction by stricture, calculus, clot, or tumor
- To evaluate hydronephrosis revealed during excretory urography or ultrasonography and to enable placement of a percutaneous nephrostomy tube
- To evaluate the function of the upper collecting system after ureteral surgery or urinary diversion
- To assess renal functional reserve before surgery

PREPARATION

- The patient may need to fast for 6 to 8 hours before the test.
- A needle will be inserted into the patient's kidney after he receives a sedative and local anesthetic.
- Check the patient's history for hypersensitivity reactions to contrast media, iodine, or shellfish. Mark sensitivities clearly on the chart. Also check his history and recent coagulation study results for indications of bleeding disorders.
- Give the patient a sedative just before the procedure, if needed, and check that pretest blood work has been performed, if ordered.

Teaching points

- Explain the purpose of the test to the patient.
- Explain that the test involves insertion of a needle into the kidney after the patient receives a sedative and local anesthetic. Explain that urine may be collected from the kidney for testing and that, if necessary, a tube will be left in the kidney for drainage.
- Tell the patient that he may feel mild discomfort during injection of the local anesthetic and contrast medium and that he may also feel transient burning and flushing from the contrast medium.
- Tell the patient that he may need to fast for 6 to 8 hours before the test.
- Explain who will perform the test and where it'll be done.
- Explain to the patient that the test may take 1 to 2 hours.

KEY STEPS

- Confirm the patient's identity using two patient identifiers according to facility policy.
- The patient is placed in a prone position on the X-ray table. The skin over the kidney is cleaned with antiseptic solution, and a local anesthetic is injected.
- Previous urographic films or ultrasound recordings are studied for anatomic landmarks. (If the kidney in question isn't in the normal position, the angle of needle entry may be adjusted during percutaneous puncture.)
- Under guidance of fluoroscopy or ultrasonography, the percutaneous needle is inserted below the 12th rib at the level of the transverse process of the 2nd lumbar vertebra. Aspiration of urine confirms that the needle has reached the dilated collecting system — $2\frac{3}{4}''$ to $3\frac{1}{8}''$ (7 to 8 cm) below the skin surface in adults.
- Flexible tubing is connected to the needle to prevent displacement during the procedure. If intrarenal pressure is to be measured, the manometer is connected to the tubing as soon as it's in place. Urine specimens are taken, if needed.
- An amount of urine equal to the amount of contrast medium to be injected is withdrawn to prevent overdistention of the collecting system.
- The contrast medium is injected under fluoroscopic guidance. Ureteral peristalsis is observed to evaluate obstruction.
- A percutaneous nephrostomy tube is inserted if drainage is needed because of increased renal pressure, dilation, or intrarenal reflux.

POSTPROCEDURE CARE

- Check the patient's vital signs every 15 minutes for the first hour, every 30 minutes for the second hour, and then every 2 hours for the next 24 hours.

- During each vital signs check, inspect the dressings for bleeding, hematoma, or urine leakage at the puncture site.
- Report urine leakage or the patient's failure to void within 8 hours.
- Monitor the patient's fluid intake and urine output for 24 hours.
- Observe each specimen for hematuria. Report hematuria if it persists after the third voiding.
- If a nephrostomy tube is inserted, make sure it's patent and draining well. Irrigate tube, to maintain patency.
- Give prescribed antibiotics for several days after the procedure, along with prescribed analgesics.
- If hydronephrosis is present, monitor intake and output, edema, hypertension, flank pain, acid-base status, and glucose level.

PRECAUTIONS

Inform the practitioner of:
- the patient's history of bleeding disorders
- the potential for pregnancy
- any history of hypersensitivity reactions to contrast media, iodine, or shellfish.

COMPLICATIONS

- Bleeding at the puncture site
- Hematoma
- Sepsis or extravasation of contrast medium

WARNING *Watch for and report signs that adjacent organs have been punctured, such as pain in the abdomen or flank, or pneumothorax.*
- Hypersensitivity to the contrast medium

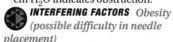

INTERPRETATION

NORMAL RESULTS

- The upper collecting system fills uniformly and appears normal in size and course.
- Normal structures are clearly outlined.

ABNORMAL RESULTS

- Enlargement of the upper collecting system and parts of the ureteropelvic junction indicate obstruction.
- In hydronephrosis, the ureteropelvic junction shows marked distention.
- Intrarenal pressure greater than 20 cm H_2O indicates obstruction.

INTERFERING FACTORS *Obesity (possible difficulty in needle placement)*

Antibody screening

DESCRIPTION
- Also called the *indirect Coombs' test*
- Detects unexpected circulating antibodies
- Detects 95% to 99% of the circulating antibodies

PURPOSE
- To detect unexpected circulating antibodies to red blood cell (RBC) antigens in the recipient's or donor's serum before transfusion
- To determine the presence of anti-D antibody in maternal blood
- To evaluate the need for $Rh_o(D)$ immune globulin
- To aid in the diagnosis of acquired hemolytic anemia

PREPARATION
- The test requires a blood sample.
- No dietary restrictions are required.
- Check the patient's history for recent administration of blood, dextran, or I.V. contrast media.

Teaching points
- Explain to the prospective blood recipient that the antibody screening test helps evaluate the possibility of a transfusion reaction or determines whether fetal antibodies are in the patient's blood and whether treatment is necessary.
- If the test is for a patient who's anemic, explain to him that it helps identify the type of anemia.
- Tell the patient that the test requires a blood sample and that he may experience slight discomfort from the tourniquet and the needle puncture.
- Inform the patient that he need not restrict food or fluids.
- Explain who will perform the test and where it'll be done.
- Tell the patient that the test should take less than 5 minutes.

KEY STEPS
- Confirm the patient's identity using two patient identifiers according to facility policy.
- Perform a venipuncture, and collect the sample in two 10-ml tubes. If the antibody screen is positive, antibody identification is performed on the blood.
- Label the sample with the patient's name, the hospital or blood bank number, the date, and the phlebotomist's initials. Be sure to include on the laboratory request the patient's diagnosis and pregnancy status, history of transfusions, and current drug therapy.
- Send the sample to the laboratory immediately.

POSTPROCEDURE CARE
- Apply direct pressure to the venipuncture site until the bleeding stops.

PRECAUTIONS
- Maintain standard precautions while collecting the sample.
- Handle the sample gently to prevent hemolysis.

COMPLICATIONS
- Hematoma at the venipuncture site

NORMAL RESULTS
- Agglutination doesn't occur, indicating that the patient's serum contains no circulating antibodies other than anti-A or anti-B.

ABNORMAL RESULTS
- A positive result indicates the presence of unexpected circulating antibodies to RBC antigens, which demonstrates donor and recipient incompatibility.
- A positive result in a pregnant patient with Rh-negative blood may indicate the presence of antibodies to the Rh factor from an earlier transfusion with incompatible blood or from a previous pregnancy with an Rh-positive fetus.
- A positive result indicates that the fetus may develop hemolytic disease of the newborn. As a result, repeated testing throughout the pregnancy is necessary to evaluate the development of circulating antibody levels.

Anticardiolipin antibody test

DESCRIPTION

- Identifies the presence of anticardiolipin antibodies, which include immunoglobulin (Ig) G and IgM
- Positive test results occurring in about 40% of patients who have been diagnosed with systemic lupus erythematous
- Patients with these antibodies at higher risk for developing antiphospholipid antibody syndrome, which includes recurring thrombosis (venous and arterial), psychiatric disorders, and thrombocytopenia

PURPOSE

- To detect the presence of anticardiolipin antibodies

PREPARATION

- No dietary restrictions are required.
- A blood sample is required.

Teaching points

- Explain to the patient that the test determines if he has anticardiolipin antibodies.
- Inform the patient that he need not restrict food or fluids.
- Tell the patient that the test requires a blood sample and that he may experience slight discomfort from the tourniquet and needle puncture.
- Explain who will perform the test and where it'll be done.
- Tell the patient that the test should take less than 5 minutes.

KEY STEPS

- Confirm the patient's identity using two patient identifiers according to facility policy.
- Perform a venipuncture, and collect 2 to 6 ml of blood in a tube with a clot activator.

POSTPROCEDURE CARE

- Apply direct pressure to the venipuncture site until the bleeding stops.

PRECAUTIONS

- Maintain standard precautions while collecting the sample.
- Handle the sample gently to prevent hemolysis.

COMPLICATIONS

- Hematoma at the venipuncture site

NORMAL RESULTS

- Negative anticardiolipin antibody results (< 23 GPL for IgG, < 11 MPL for IgM) are considered normal.

ABNORMAL RESULTS

- A positive result indicates the presence of anticardiolipin antibodies.
- A positive result indicates the patient is at higher risk for thrombosis; thrombocytopenia; and spontaneous fetal loss, if pregnant.
- A positive result may be seen in lupus, syphilis, and acute infections and is a normal finding in elderly patients.

Anticentromere antibody test

DESCRIPTION

◆ Centromeres existing as the primary constrictions of a chromosome, dividing the chromosome into arms
◆ Test detecting the presence of anticentromere antibodies, which are one form of antinuclear antibodies
◆ Positive test results occurring in a large number of patients with CREST syndrome, a disease characterized by calcinosis cutis, Raynaud's phenomenon, esophageal dysfunction, sclerodactyly, and telangiectasia
◆ A very small percentage of patients with scleroderma testing positive for anticentromere antibodies (distinguishing CREST from scleroderma based on symptoms alone is difficult)

PURPOSE

◆ To determine the presence of anticentromere antibodies
◆ To help make a differential diagnosis of CREST and scleroderma

PREPARATION

◆ The test requires a blood sample.
◆ No dietary restrictions are required.

Teaching points

◆ Explain to the patient that this test helps diagnose the cause of his illness.
◆ Inform the patient that he need not restrict food or fluid intake.
◆ Tell the patient that the test requires a blood sample and that he may experience slight discomfort from the tourniquet and needle puncture.
◆ Explain who will perform the test and where it'll be done.
◆ Tell the patient that the test should take less than 5 minutes.

KEY STEPS

◆ Confirm the patient's identity using two patient identifiers according to facility policy.
◆ Perform a venipuncture, and collect the sample in a 5-ml tube with gel separator and clot activator.

POSTPROCEDURE CARE

◆ Apply direct pressure to the venipuncture site until the bleeding stops.

PRECAUTIONS

◆ Maintain standard precautions while collecting the sample.
◆ Handle the sample gently to prevent hemolysis.

COMPLICATIONS

◆ Hematoma at the venipuncture site

NORMAL RESULTS

◆ Test results indicating a lack of anticentromere antibodies are normal.

ABNORMAL RESULTS

◆ A positive titer indicates the presence of anticentromere antibodies.
◆ The presence of anticentromere antibodies allows the differential diagnosis of CREST syndrome.

Antideoxyribonucleic acid antibody test

DESCRIPTION

◆ Serum anti–double-stranded deoxyribonucleic acid (dsDNA) levels directly relating to the extent of damage caused by renal or vascular disease
◆ Measures and differentiates levels of these antibodies in a serum sample, using radioimmunoassay, agglutination, complement fixation, or immunoelectrophoresis
◆ Counts oversized complexes too large to pass through a membrane filter, formed by antibodies combining with native DNA

PURPOSE

◆ To confirm a diagnosis of systemic lupus erythematosus (SLE)
◆ To monitor the response of the patient with SLE to therapy and determine the prognosis

PREPARATION

◆ No dietary restrictions are required.
◆ The test requires a blood sample.
◆ Ask the patient if she has had a recent radioactive test; if so, note this on the laboratory request.

Teaching points

◆ Explain to the patient that this test helps diagnose and determine the appropriate therapy for SLE.
◆ Inform the patient that she need not restrict food or fluids.
◆ Tell the patient that the test requires a blood sample and that she may experience slight discomfort from the tourniquet and needle puncture.
◆ Explain who will perform the test and where it'll be done.
◆ Tell the patient that the test should take less than 5 minutes.

KEY STEPS

◆ Confirm the patient's identity using two patient identifiers according to facility policy.
◆ Perform a venipuncture, and collect the sample in a 7-ml tube without additives. Some laboratories may specify a tube with ethylenediaminetetraacetic acid or sodium fluoride and potassium oxalate added.

POSTPROCEDURE CARE

◆ Apply direct pressure to the venipuncture site until the bleeding stops.

PRECAUTIONS

◆ Maintain standard precautions while collecting the sample.
◆ Handle the sample gently to prevent hemolysis.

COMPLICATIONS

◆ Hematoma at the venipuncture site

NORMAL RESULTS

◆ Anti-dsDNA antibody levels less than 25 International Units/ml (SI, < 25 kIU/L) are considered negative for SLE.

ABNORMAL RESULTS

◆ Elevated anti-dsDNA antibody levels may indicate SLE.
◆ Values of 25 to 30 International Units/ml (SI, 25 to 30 kIU/L) are considered borderline positive.
◆ Values of 31 to 200 International Units/ml (SI, 31 to 200 kIU/L) are considered positive, and those greater than 200 International Units/ml (SI, > 200 kIU/L) are considered strongly positive.
◆ Depressed anti-dsDNA levels may follow immunosuppressive therapy, demonstrating effective treatment of SLE.

Antidiuretic hormone (serum) test

OVERVIEW

DESCRIPTION

- Rare quantitative analysis of serum antidiuretic hormone (ADH) levels that may identify diabetes insipidus and other causes of severe homeostatic imbalance
- May be part of dehydration testing or hypertonic saline infusion testing to determine the body's response to hyperosmolality

PURPOSE

- To aid in the differential diagnosis of pituitary diabetes insipidus, nephrogenic diabetes insipidus (congenital or familial), and syndrome of inappropriate antidiuretic hormone (SIADH)

PREPARATION

- The patient needs to fast and limit physical activity for 10 to 12 hours before the test.
- Withhold drugs that may cause SIADH before the test. If the patient must continue them, note this on the laboratory request.
- Make sure that the patient is relaxed and recumbent for 30 minutes before the test.

Teaching points

- Explain to the patient that this test, which measures hormonal secretion levels, may aid in identifying the cause of his symptoms.
- Tell the patient that the test requires a blood sample and that he may experience slight discomfort from the tourniquet and needle puncture.
- Instruct the patient to fast and limit physical activity for 10 to 12 hours before the test.
- Explain who will perform the test and where it'll be done.
- Tell the patient that the test should take less than 1 hour.

DIAGNOSTIC PROCEDURE

KEY STEPS

- Confirm the patient's identity using two patient identifiers according to facility policy.
- Perform a venipuncture, and collect the sample in a plastic collection tube (without additives) or a chilled ethylenediaminetetraacetic acid tube.
- Immediately send the sample to the laboratory, where serum must be separated from the clot within 10 minutes.
- Perform a serum osmolality test at the same time to help interpret the ADH test results.
- Make sure to use a syringe and collection tube made of plastic because the fragile ADH degrades on contact with glass.

POSTPROCEDURE CARE

- Apply direct pressure to the venipuncture site until the bleeding stops.
- Instruct the patient that he may resume his usual diet, activities, and medications that were stopped before the test.

PRECAUTIONS

- Maintain standard precautions while collecting the sample.
- Use only a plastic syringe and collection tube.
- Send the sample to the laboratory within 10 minutes of collection.

COMPLICATIONS

- Hematoma at the venipuncture site

INTERPRETATION

NORMAL RESULTS

- Serum ADH values ranging from 1 to 5 pg/ml (SI, 1 to 5 mg/L) are considered normal.
- Levels may also be evaluated in light of serum osmolality: if serum osmolality is less than 285 mOsm/kg, ADH is normally less than 2 pg/ml (SI, < 2 mg/L); if serum osmolality is greater than 290 mOsm/kg, ADH may range from 2 to 12 pg/ml (SI, 2 to 12 mg/L).

ABNORMAL RESULTS

- Absent or below-normal ADH levels indicate pituitary diabetes insipidus, resulting from a neurohypophyseal or hypothalamic tumor, viral infection, metastatic disease, sarcoidosis, tuberculosis, Hand-Schüller-Christian disease, syphilis, neurosurgical procedures, or head trauma.
- Normal ADH levels in the presence of signs of diabetes insipidus (such as polydipsia, polyuria, and hypotonic urine) may indicate the nephrogenic form of the disease, marked by renal tubular resistance to ADH; however, levels may rise if the pituitary gland tries to compensate.
- Elevated ADH levels may also indicate SIADH, possibly as a result of bronchogenic carcinoma, acute porphyria, hypothyroidism, Addison's disease, cirrhosis of the liver, infectious hepatitis, severe hemorrhage, or circulatory shock.

Antiglobulin test (direct)

DESCRIPTION

- Also called the *direct Coombs' test*
- Detects the presence of immuno-globulins (antibodies) on the surface of red blood cells (RBCs)
- Immunoglobins coat RBCs when they become sensitized to an antigen (such as Rh factor)

PURPOSE

- To diagnose hemolytic disease of the newborn
- To investigate hemolytic transfusion reactions
- To aid in the differential diagnosis of hemolytic anemias, which may be congenital or may result from an autoimmune reaction or use of certain drugs

PREPARATION

- No dietary restrictions are required.
- The test requires a blood sample.
- Withhold medications that may interfere with test results, including quinidine, methyldopa, cephalosporins, sulfonamides, chlorpromazine, diphenylhydantoin, ethosuximide, hydralazine, levodopa, mefenamic acid, melphalan, penicillin, procainamide, rifampin, streptomycin, tetracyclines, and isoniazid.

Teaching points

- Explain that the test helps determine whether the condition results from an abnormality of the body's immune system, the use of certain drugs, or an unknown cause.
- Explain to the parent of a neonate that the test helps diagnose hemolytic disease in the newborn.
- Explain to the patient that the test requires a blood sample and he may experience a slight discomfort from the tourniquet and needle puncture.
- Inform the patient that he need not restrict food or fluids.
- Explain who will perform the test and where it'll be done.
- Give the patient a list of the medications he must stop taking before the test.

KEY STEPS

- Confirm the patient's identity using two patient identifiers according to facility policy.
- Perform a venipuncture, and collect the sample in two 5-ml EDTA tubes

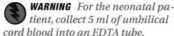 **WARNING** *For the neonatal patient, collect 5 ml of umbilical cord blood into an EDTA tube.*

POSTPROCEDURE CARE

- Apply direct pressure to the venipuncture site until the bleeding stops.
- Instruct the patient to resume medications stopped before the test as ordered.

PRECAUTIONS

- Maintain standard precautions while collecting the sample.
- Handle the sample gently to prevent hemolysis.
- Send the sample to the laboratory immediately.

COMPLICATIONS

- Hematoma at the venipuncture site

NORMAL RESULTS

- A negative test result, in which neither antibodies nor complements appear on the RBCs, is considered normal.

ABNORMAL RESULTS

- A neonatal positive test result indicates that maternal antibodies have crossed the placenta and coated the fetal RBCs, causing hemolytic disease of the neonate.
- In other patients, a positive test result may indicate hemolytic anemia and may help differentiate between autoimmune and secondary hemolytic anemia.
- A positive test result may also indicate sepsis.
- A weakly positive test result may indicate a transfusion reaction, in which the patient's antibodies reacted with transfused RBCs that contained the corresponding antigen.

Anti-insulin antibody test

DESCRIPTION
◆ Detects insulin antibodies in the blood of a diabetic patient who takes insulin

PURPOSE
◆ To determine insulin allergy
◆ To confirm insulin resistance
◆ To determine if hypoglycemia results from insulin overuse

PREPARATION
◆ The test requires a blood sample.
◆ No dietary restrictions are required.
◆ Ask the patient if he has had a radioactive test recently; if so, note this on the laboratory request.

Teaching points
◆ Explain to the patient that this test determines the most appropriate treatment for his diabetes and determines whether he has insulin resistance or an allergy to insulin.
◆ Tell the patient that the test requires a blood sample and that he may experience slight discomfort from the tourniquet and needle puncture.
◆ Inform the patient that he need not restrict food or fluids.
◆ Explain who will perform the test and where it'll be done.

KEY STEPS
◆ Confirm the patient's identity using two patient identifiers according to facility policy.
◆ Perform a venipuncture, and collect the sample in a 7-ml tube without additives.

POSTPROCEDURE CARE
◆ Apply direct pressure to the venipuncture site until the bleeding stops.

PRECAUTIONS
◆ Handle the sample gently to prevent hemolysis.

COMPLICATIONS
◆ Hematoma at the venipuncture site

NORMAL RESULTS
◆ Less than 3% binding of the patient's serum with labeled beef, human, and pork insulin is considered normal.

ABNORMAL RESULTS
◆ Elevated anti-insulin antibody levels may occur in insulin allergy or resistance and in factitious hypoglycemia.

Antimitochondrial antibody test

DESCRIPTION

◆ Detects antimitochondrial antibodies in serum by indirect immunofluorescence
◆ Usually performed with the anti-smooth muscle antibodies test

PURPOSE

◆ To aid in the diagnosis of primary biliary cirrhosis
◆ To distinguish between extrahepatic jaundice and biliary cirrhosis

PREPARATION

◆ The test requires a blood sample.
◆ No dietary restrictions are required.
◆ Check the patient's drug history for oxyphenisatin use, and report it to the laboratory, because it may produce antimitochondrial antibodies.

Teaching points

◆ Explain to the patient that this test evaluates liver function.
◆ Inform the patient that he need not restrict food or fluids.
◆ Tell the patient that the test requires a blood sample and that he may experience slight discomfort from the tourniquet and needle puncture.
◆ Explain who will perform the test and where it'll be done.
◆ Tell the patient that the test should take less than 5 minutes.

KEY STEPS

◆ Confirm the patient's identity using two patient identifiers according to facility policy.
◆ Perform a venipuncture, and collect the sample in a 7-ml tube with no additives.

POSTPROCEDURE CARE

◆ Because the patient with hepatic disease may bleed excessively, apply pressure to the venipuncture site until bleeding stops.

PRECAUTIONS

◆ Maintain standard precautions while collecting the sample.
◆ Handle the sample gently to prevent hemolysis.

COMPLICATIONS

◆ Hematoma at the venipuncture site

NORMAL RESULTS

◆ Serum is normally negative for antimitochondrial antibodies.
◆ Positive test results are titered.

ABNORMAL RESULTS

◆ Although antimitochondrial antibodies appear in 79% to 94% of patients with primary biliary cirrhosis, this test alone doesn't confirm the diagnosis. Further tests, such as serum alkaline phosphatase, serum bilirubin, aspartate aminotransferase, alanine aminotransferase, and possibly liver biopsy or cholangiography, may also be necessary.
◆ The antimitochondrial antibodies may also appear in some patients with chronic active hepatitis, drug-induced jaundice, and cryptogenic cirrhosis.
◆ Antimitochondrial antibodies seldom appear in patients with extrahepatic biliary obstruction, and a positive test result helps to rule out this condition.

Antimyocardial antibody test

DESCRIPTION

- Antimyocardial antibodies present in autoimmune causes of myocardial injury, such as rheumatic heart disease, cardiomyopathy, postthoracotomy syndrome, and postmyocardial infarction syndrome
- Antimyocardial antibodies associated with pericarditis, which can damage the heart tissue
- Antimyocardial antibodies found in up to 40% of patients after cardiac surgery and in some patients following myocardial infarction

PURPOSE

- To detect antimyocardial antibodies in the blood

PREPARATION

- The test requires a blood sample.
- No dietary restrictions are required.

Teaching points

- Explain to the patient that this test determines if there are antimyocardial antibodies in the blood.
- Tell the patient that the test requires a blood sample and that he may experience slight discomfort from the tourniquet and needle puncture.
- Inform the patient that he need not restrict food or fluids.
- Explain who will perform the test and where it'll be done.
- Tell the patient that the test should take less than 5 minutes.

KEY STEPS

- Confirm the patient's identity using two patient identifiers according to facility policy.
- Perform a venipuncture, and collect the sample in a 4-ml tube with no additives.

POSTPROCEDURE CARE

- Apply direct pressure to the venipuncture site until the bleeding stops.

PRECAUTIONS

- Maintain standard precautions while collecting the sample.
- Handle the sample gently to prevent hemolysis.

COMPLICATIONS

- Hematoma at the venipuncture site

NORMAL RESULTS

- Negative test results, in which no antimyocardial antibodies are seen, are considered normal.
- Positive test results are titered.

ABNORMAL RESULTS

- Positive test results indicate the presence of antimyocardial antibodies, confirming that the cause of the patient's myocardial injury or disease is most likely due to an autoimmune reaction.

Antinuclear antibody test

DESCRIPTION

- Measures relative level of antinuclear antibodies (ANAs) in a serum sample through indirect immunofluorescence
- If serum contains ANAs: antigen-antibody complexes formed with the substrate
- If ANAs are found during ultraviolet microscope examination: complexes fluoresce
- Involves titer being taken at the greatest dilution that shows the reaction

PURPOSE

- To screen for systemic lupus erythematosus (SLE) (failure to detect ANAs essentially rules out active SLE)
- To monitor the effectiveness of immunosuppressive therapy for SLE

PREPARATION

- The test requires a blood sample.
- No dietary restrictions are required.
- Check the patient's history for drugs that may affect test results, such as isoniazid and procainamide. Note these findings on the laboratory request.

Teaching points

- Explain that this test evaluates the immune system and that further testing is usually required for diagnosis.
- Tell the patient that the test requires a blood sample and that he may experience slight discomfort from the tourniquet and needle puncture.
- Inform the patient that he need not restrict food or fluids.
- Explain who will perform the test and where it'll be done.
- Tell the patient that the test should take less than 5 minutes.
- Inform the patient that the test may have to be repeated to monitor his response to therapy.

KEY STEPS

- Confirm the patient's identity using two patient identifiers according to facility policy.
- Perform a venipuncture, and collect the sample in a 7-ml tube without additives.

POSTPROCEDURE CARE

- Apply direct pressure to the venipuncture site until bleeding stops.
- Because a patient with an autoimmune disease has a compromised immune system, observe the venipuncture site for signs of infection.
- Keep a clean, dry bandage over the venipuncture site for at least 24 hours.

PRECAUTIONS

- Maintain standard precautions while collecting the sample.
- Handle the sample gently to prevent hemolysis.

COMPLICATIONS

- Hematoma at the venipuncture site

NORMAL RESULTS

- No ANAs are found.

ABNORMAL RESULTS

- Staining pattern and titer are noted.
- Low titers may occur in patients with viral diseases, chronic hepatic disease, collagen vascular disease, and autoimmune diseases and in some healthy adults; incidence increases with age.
- The higher the titer, the more specific the test is for SLE.
- Pattern of nuclear fluorescence helps identify type of immune disease present. (See *Incidence of antinuclear antibodies in various disorders.*)
- A peripheral staining pattern almost exclusively indicates SLE.
- A homogeneous, or diffuse, staining pattern is also associated with SLE as well as with related connective tissue disorders; a nucleolar staining pattern, with scleroderma; and a speckled, irregular staining pattern, with infectious mononucleosis and mixed connective tissue disorders.
- In addition, as serum dilution increases, the fluorescent pattern may change, because different antibodies are reactive at different titers.

Incidence of antinuclear antibodies in various disorders

This chart indicates the percentage of patients with certain disorders whose serum contains antinuclear antibodies (ANAs). About 40% of elderly people and 5% of the general population also have positive ANA findings.

DISORDER	POSITIVE ANA
Systemic lupus erythematosus (SLE)	95% to 100%
Lupoid hepatitis	95% to 100%
Felty's syndrome	95% to 100%
Progressive systemic sclerosis (scleroderma)	75% to 80%
Drug-associated SLE-like syndrome (hydralazine, procainamide, isoniazid)	About 50%
Sjögren's syndrome	40% to 75%
Rheumatoid arthritis	25% to 60%
Healthy family member of SLE patient	About 25%
Chronic discoid lupus erythematosus	15% to 50%
Juvenile arthritis	15% to 30%
Polyarteritis nodosa	15% to 25%
Miscellaneous diseases	10% to 50%
Dermatomyositis, polymyositis	10% to 30%
Rheumatic fever	About 5%

Antismooth muscle antibody test

DESCRIPTION

- Measures the relative level of antismooth muscle antibodies in serum, using indirect immunofluorescence; usually performed with the antimitochondrial antibodies test
- Exposes the serum sample to a thin section of smooth muscle and incubates it; then a fluorescent-labeled antiglobulin is added
- Antiglobulin binding only to antibodies that have complexed with smooth muscle and appear fluorescent when viewed through the microscope under ultraviolet light (see *Serum antibodies in various disorders*)

PURPOSE

- To aid in the diagnosis of active chronic hepatitis and primary biliary cirrhosis

PREPARATION

- The test requires a blood sample.
- No dietary restrictions are required.

Teaching points

- Explain to the patient that this test helps evaluate liver function.
- Inform the patient that he need not restrict food or fluids.
- Tell the patient that the test requires a blood sample and that he may experience slight discomfort from the tourniquet and needle puncture.
- Expain who will perform the test and where it'll be done.
- Tell the patient that the test should take less than 5 minutes.
- Hematoma at the venipuncture site

DIAGNOSTIC PROCEDURE

KEY STEPS

- Confirm the patient's identity using two patient identifiers according to facility policy.
- Perform a venipuncture, and collect the sample in a 7-ml tube without additives.

POSTPROCEDURE CARE

- Because the patient with hepatic disease may bleed excessively, apply direct pressure to the venipuncture site until the bleeding stops.

PRECAUTIONS

- Maintain standard precautions while collecting the sample.
- Handle the sample gently to prevent hemolysis.

COMPLICATIONS

- Hematoma at the venipuncture site

INTERPRETATION

NORMAL RESULTS

- A normal titer of antismooth muscle antibodies is negative.

ABNORMAL RESULTS

- Positive test results are titered.
- The test for antismooth muscle antibodies isn't specific; these antibodies appear in many patients with chronic active hepatitis and in fewer patients with primary biliary cirrhosis.
- Antismooth muscle antibodies may also be present in patients with infectious mononucleosis, acute viral hepatitis, a malignant tumor of the liver, and intrinsic asthma.

Serum antibodies in various disorders

This table shows the percentage of patients with certain disorders who have antimitochondrial or anti–smooth muscle antibodies in their serum. Patients with these antibodies in the serum need further testing to confirm the diagnosis. Up to 1% of healthy people also have antimitochondrial antibodies.

DISORDER	ANTIMITOCHONDRIAL ANTIBODIES	ANTI–SMOOTH MUSCLE ANTIBODIES
Primary biliary cirrhosis	75% to 95%	0% to 50%*
Chronic active hepatitis	0% to 30%	50% to 80%
Extrahepatic biliary obstruction	0% to 5%	0%
Cryptogenic cirrhosis	0% to 25%	0% to 1%
Viral (infectious) hepatitis	0%	1% to 2%†
Drug-induced jaundice	50% to 80%	
Intrinsic asthma		20%
Rheumatoid arthritis and other collagen diseases	1% to 2%	
Systemic lupus erythematosus	3% to 5%††	0%

* In chronic disease, values fall at upper end of range.
† Much higher incidence occurs with hepatic damage.
†† Much higher incidence occurs with renal involvement.

Antispermatozoal antibody test

DESCRIPTION

◆ Antispermatozoal antibodies possibly resulting in decreased fertility
◆ Men with blocked efferent ducts possibly having the antibodies present in the blood as a result of the sperm being reabsorbed through the duct and the sperm antigens reacting with the immune system
◆ Antispermatozoal antibodies also found in women (the clinical significance of this isn't known)
◆ Antispermatozoal antibodies found in the sperm of men and in the cervical mucosa of infertile women

PURPOSE

◆ To detect the presence of antispermatozoal antibodies in men and women to help determine the cause of infertility

PREPARATION

◆ The sperm specimen may be collected by masturbation, coitus interruptus, or the use of a condom.
◆ The test requires a blood sample.

Teaching points

◆ Provide the patient with written instructions, and inform him that the most desirable specimen requires masturbation, ideally in a practitioner's office or laboratory.
◆ Tell the patient to follow the written instructions about the period of sexual continence before the test because this may increase his sperm count.
◆ If the patient prefers to collect the specimen at home, emphasize the importance of delivering the specimen to the laboratory within 1 hour after collection. Warn him not to expose the specimen to extreme temperatures or to direct sunlight.
◆ During cold weather, suggest that the patient keep the specimen container in a coat pocket on the way to the laboratory to protect the specimen from exposure to cold.

◆ For collection by coitus interruptus, instruct the patient to withdraw immediately before ejaculation and to deposit the ejaculate in a suitable specimen container.
◆ For collection by condom, tell the patient to first wash the condom with soap and water, rinse it thoroughly, and allow it to dry completely. (Powders or lubricants applied to the condom may be spermicidal.) Special sheaths that don't contain spermicide are also available for semen collection. Instruct the patient to tie the condom after collection, place it in a glass jar, and promptly deliver it to the laboratory.
◆ Inform the patient that he may feel slight discomfort from the tourniquet and needle puncture.
◆ If obtaining a vaginal sample from a woman, instruct the couple to abstain from intercourse for 2 days and then to have sexual intercourse 2 to 8 hours before the examination. Explain to the patient that she'll be placed in the lithotomy position and that a speculum will be inserted into the vagina to collect the specimen. Tell her that she may feel some pressure but no pain.
◆ Tell the patient that the results should be available within 2 days.

KEY STEPS

◆ Confirm the patient's identity using two patient identifiers according to facility policy.
◆ Ask the patient to collect semen in a clean plastic specimen container.
◆ Before postcoital examination, the examiner wipes excess mucus from the external cervix and collects the specimen by direct aspiration of the cervical canal, using a 1-ml tuberculin syringe without a cannula or needle.
◆ Never lubricate the vaginal speculum. Instead, moisten the speculum with water or physiologic saline solution.

◆ Prepare direct smears on glass microscopic slides after labeling the frosted end. Immediately place smeared slides in Coplin jars containing 95% ethanol.
◆ Perform a venipuncture and collect 5 ml of blood from both the man and the woman.

POSTPROCEDURE CARE

◆ Apply pressure to the venipuncture site.
◆ Answer questions for the couple and provide emotional support.

PRECAUTIONS

◆ If the patient prefers to collect the specimen during coitus interruptus, tell him he must prevent the loss of any of the sperm during ejaculation.
◆ All sperm specimens should be delivered to the laboratory within 1 hour of collection.

COMPLICATIONS

◆ Hematoma at the venipuncture site

NORMAL RESULTS

◆ Test results showing the lack of antispermatozoal antibodies are considered normal.
◆ Positive test results are titered.
◆ A low titer isn't an uncommon finding in men with normal fertility.
◆ A positive antibody test result in a woman isn't an indication of infertility.

ABNORMAL RESULTS

◆ The presence of antispermatozoal antibodies in a man is highly indicative of infertility.
◆ The presence of IgG antispermatozoal antibodies suggests a problem with sperm-ovum fusion.
◆ The presence of IgA antispermatozoal antibodies suggests a problem with motility and penetration of the cervix.

Anti-SS antibody test

DESCRIPTION
- Types of antinuclear antibodies (anti-SS-A, anti-SS-B, and anti-SS-C) used to diagnose Sjögren's syndrome
- Anti-SS-A antibodies occurring in 70% of patients with Sjögren's syndrome without the occurrence of another autoimmune disorder (primary Sjögren's syndrome)
- Anti-SS-B antibodies occurring in 50% of patients with primary Sjögren's syndrome (not regularly found with any other disorders)
- The presence of anti-SS-A and anti-SS-B antibodies indicating Sjögren's syndrome
- Anti-SS-C antibodies occurring in 75% of patient's with Sjögren's syndrome and rheumatoid arthritis (used to differentiate between primary and secondary Sjögren's syndrome)

PURPOSE
- To diagnose Sjögren's syndrome
- To differentiate between primary and secondary Sjögren's syndrome

PREPARATION
- The test requires a blood sample.
- No dietary restrictions are required.

Teaching points
- Explain to the patient that this test helps to diagnose Sjögren's disease and to determine if it occurs alone or with another autoimmune disorder.
- Inform the patient that he need not restrict food or fluids.
- Tell the patient that the test requires a blood sample and that he may experience slight discomfort from the tourniquet and needle puncture.
- Explain who will perform the test and where it'll be done.
- Tell the patient that the test should take less than 5 minutes.

KEY STEPS
- Confirm the patient's identity using two patient identifiers according to facility policy.
- Perform a venipuncture, and collect the sample in a 7-ml tube without additives.

POSTPROCEDURE CARE
- Apply direct pressure to the venipuncture site until the bleeding stops.

PRECAUTIONS
- Maintain standard precautions while collecting the sample.
- Handle the sample gently to prevent hemolysis.

COMPLICATIONS
- Hematoma at the venipuncture site

NORMAL RESULTS
- Negative test results for anti-SS antibodies are considered normal.

ABNORMAL RESULTS
- Test results showing the presence of anti-SS antibodies are considered abnormal.
- The presence of anti-SS-A antibodies may indicate lupus or Sjögren's syndrome.
- The presence of anti-SS-B antibodies indicates primary Sjögren's syndrome.
- The presence of anti-SS-C antibodies indicates Sjögren's syndrome along with other autoimmune disorders.
- The anti-SS antibody titer decreases with therapy for Sjögren's syndrome.

Antistreptolysin-O level test

DESCRIPTION
- Measures the relative levels of the antibody to streptolysin-O (ASO)
- Involves the dilution of serum sample with a commercial preparation of ASO and incubation
- End point is read in Todd units (the reciprocal of the highest dilution [titer] that inhibits hemolysis)

PURPOSE
- To confirm recent or ongoing streptococcal infection
- To help diagnose rheumatic fever and poststreptococcal glomerulonephritis in the presence of symptoms
- To distinguish between rheumatic fever and rheumatoid arthritis when joint pains are present

PREPARATION
- The test requires a blood sample.
- No dietary restrictions are required.
- Check the patient's history for use of drugs that may suppress the streptococcal antibody responses. If the patient must continue these drugs, note this on the laboratory request.

Teaching points
- Explain to the patient that this test detects an immunologic response to certain bacteria (streptococci).
- Inform the patient that he need not restrict food or fluids.
- Tell the patient that the test requires a blood sample and that he may experience slight discomfort from the tourniquet and needle puncture.
- If the test will be repeated at regular intervals to identify active and inactive states of rheumatic fever or to confirm acute glomerulonephritis, tell the patient that measuring the changes in antibody levels helps determine the effectiveness of therapy.
- Explain who will perform the test and where it'll be done.
- Tell the patient that the test should take less than 5 minutes.

KEY STEPS
- Confirm the patient's identity using two patient identifiers according to facility policy.
- Perform a venipuncture, and collect the sample in a 7-ml tube without additives.

POSTPROCEDURE CARE
- Apply direct pressure to the venipuncture site until the bleeding stops.

PRECAUTIONS
- Maintain standard precautions while collecting the sample.
- Handle the sample gently to prevent hemolysis.

COMPLICATIONS
- Hematoma at the venipuncture site

NORMAL RESULTS
- Even healthy people have some detectable ASO titers from previous minor streptococcal infections.
- The normal ASO titers for school-age children is 170 Todd units/ml; for preschoolers and adults, the normal titer is 85 Todd units/ml.

ABNORMAL RESULTS
- High ASO titers usually occur only after prolonged or recurrent infections.
- Generally, a titer higher than 166 Todd units/ml is considered a definite elevation.
- A low titer is good evidence of the absence of active rheumatic fever.
- A higher titer doesn't necessarily mean that rheumatic fever or glomerulonephritis is present; however, it does indicate the presence of a streptococcal infection.
- Serial titers, determined at 10- to 14-day intervals, provide more reliable information than a single titer. An increase in titer 2 to 5 weeks after the acute infection, which peaks 4 to 6 weeks after the initial increase, confirms poststreptococcal disease.

Antithrombin III level test

DESCRIPTION

- Measures levels of antithrombin III, an alpha$_2$-globulin produced in the liver that inhibits serum protease involved in coagulation
- Coagulation system homeostasis resulting from a balance of antithrombin III and thrombin
- Deficiency of antithrombin III leading to an increase in coagulation
- Hereditary antithrombin III deficiency characterized by venous thromboembolic events, usually beginning while the patient is in his 20s
- Acquired antithrombin III deficiency possibly a result of cirrhosis, liver failure, carcinoma, nephrotic syndrome, disseminated intravascular coagulation (DIC), and acute thrombosis
- Antithrombin III needed for heparin to exert its anticoagulant effects (a patient with a low antithrombin III level may require increased doses of heparin to achieve a therapeutic effect)

PURPOSE

- To determine the levels of antithrombin III present

PREPARATION

- The test requires a blood sample.
- No dietary restrictions are required.

Teaching points

- Tell the patient that the test evaluates how his blood clots.
- Inform the patient that he need not restrict food or fluids.
- Tell the patient that the test requires a blood sample and that he may experience slight discomfort from the tourniquet and needle puncture.
- Explain who will perform the test and where it'll be done.
- Tell the patient that the test should take less than 5 minutes.

KEY STEPS

- Confirm the patient's identity using two patient identifiers according to facility policy.
- Perform a venipuncture, and collect the sample in a 7-ml tube with sodium citrate.

POSTPROCEDURE CARE

- Apply direct pressure to the venipuncture site until the bleeding stops.

PRECAUTIONS

- Maintain standard precautions while collecting the sample.
- Handle the sample gently to prevent hemolysis.
- Send the sample to the laboratory immediately.

COMPLICATIONS

- Hematoma at the venipuncture site

NORMAL RESULTS

- Plasma values should be greater than 50% of control values (*Note:* values vary according to laboratory methods used).
- Serum levels should be 15% to 34% lower than plasma values.
- Immunologic values should be 17 to 30 mg/dl (SI, 170 to 300 mg/L).
- Functional levels should be 80% to 120%.

ABNORMAL RESULTS

- Decreased levels of antithrombin III are associated with hypercoagulation states, DIC, hepatic disorders, nephrotic syndrome, protein-wasting disorders, and hereditary deficiencies of antithrombin III.
- If the patient has a low level of antithrombin III, warfarin therapy may be started prophylactically.
- Increased levels of antithrombin III are associated with acute hepatitis, renal transplant, inflammation, obstructive jaundice, and vitamin K deficiency.

INTERFERING FACTORS *Hormonal contraceptives (decreased antithrombin III levels); pregnancy in the last trimester (unreliable results)*

Antithyroid antibody test

DESCRIPTION
- Tanned red cell hemagglutination test detecting antithyroid antibodies, specifically antithyroglobulin and antimicrosomal antibodies
- Indirect immunofluorescence also detecting antimicrosomal antibodies

PURPOSE
- To detect circulating antithyroid antibodies when clinical evidence indicates Hashimoto's thyroiditis, Graves' disease, or other thyroid diseases

PREPARATION
- The test requires a blood sample.
- No dietary restrictions are required.

Teaching points
- Tell the patient that the test evaluates thyroid function.
- Inform the patient that he need not restrict food or fluids.
- Tell the patient that the test requires a blood sample.
- Explain to the patient that he may experience slight discomfort from the tourniquet and needle puncture.
- Explain who will perform the test and where it'll be done.
- Tell the patient that the test should take less than 5 minutes.

KEY STEPS
- Confirm the patient's identity using two patient identifiers according to facility policy.
- Perform a venipuncture, and collect the sample in a 7-ml tube without additives.

POSTPROCEDURE CARE
- Apply direct pressure to the venipuncture site until the bleeding stops.

PRECAUTIONS
- Maintain standard precautions while collecting the sample.
- Handle the sample gently to prevent hemolysis.
- Send the sample to the laboratory immediately.

COMPLICATIONS
- Hematoma at the venipuncture site

NORMAL RESULTS
- The normal titer is less than 1:100 for antithyroglobulin and antimicrosomal antibodies.

ABNORMAL RESULTS
- The presence of antithyroglobulin or antimicrosomal antibodies in serum may indicate subclinical autoimmune thyroid disease, Graves' disease, or idiopathic myxedema.
- Titers of 1:400 or greater for both antibodies strongly suggest Hashimoto's thyroiditis.
- Antithyroglobulin antibodies may also occur in some patients with other autoimmune disorders, such as systemic lupus erythematosus, rheumatoid arthritis, and autoimmune hemolytic anemia.

Apolipoprotein A1 level test

DESCRIPTION
◆ Measures the levels of apolipoprotein A1 (apoA1), one of the surface particles of lipoproteins
◆ ApoA1 existing as the main component of high-density lipoprotein (HDL) (the less apoA1 in the blood, the more that's bound to HDL)
◆ ApoA1 deficiency associated with premature cardiovascular disease

PURPOSE
◆ To measure the amount of apoA1 in the blood
◆ To provide a potentially better index of arthrogenic risk than the HDL assay

PREPARATION
◆ The test requires a blood sample.
◆ The patient needs to restrict food for 12 hours before the test, but water is allowed.
◆ The patient must not smoke before the test.

Teaching points
◆ Tell the patient that the test helps to determine his risk for cardiovascular disease.
◆ Inform the patient that he'll need to restrict food for 12 hours before the test but that water is allowed.
◆ Tell the patient that he may not smoke before the test.
◆ Tell the patient that the test requires a blood sample and that he may experience slight discomfort from the tourniquet and needle puncture.
◆ Explain who will perform the test and where it'll be done.
◆ Tell the patient that the test should take less than 5 minutes.

KEY STEPS
◆ Confirm the patient's identity using two patient identifiers according to facility policy.
◆ Perform a venipuncture, and collect the sample in a 7-ml tube without additives.

POSTPROCEDURE CARE
◆ Apply direct pressure to the venipuncture site until the bleeding stops.

PRECAUTIONS
◆ Maintain standard precautions while collecting the sample.
◆ Handle the sample gently to prevent hemolysis.
◆ Send the sample to the laboratory immediately.

COMPLICATIONS
◆ Hematoma at the venipuncture site

NORMAL RESULTS
◆ ApoA1 levels of 94 to 172 mg/dl (SI, 0.94 to 1.72 g/L) for women are considered normal .
◆ ApoA1 levels of 90 to 155 mg/dl (SI, 0.90 to 1.55 g/L) for men are considered normal.
◆ Women have slightly higher levels of HDL, so they have higher levels of apoA1.

ABNORMAL RESULTS
◆ Increased levels of apoA1 are seen in familial hyperalphalipoproteinemia.
◆ Decreased levels of apoA1 indicate an increased risk of coronary artery disease, ischemic coronary disease, myocardial infarction, and hypertriglyceridemia.
◆ Decreased levels of apoA1 are also seen in apoC-II deficiency, apoA-I Melano disease, apoA-I-C-III deficiency, poorly controlled diabetes, nephrotic syndrome, and renal failure.
◆ Decreased levels of apoA1 are also associated with diets that are high in polyunsaturated fats.

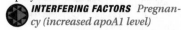 **INTERFERING FACTORS** *Pregnancy (increased apoA1 level)*

Apolipoprotein B level test

DESCRIPTION

- Measure the levels of apolipoprotein B (apoB) one of the surface particles of lipoproteins
- ApoB existing as the main component of low-density lipoprotein (LDL) and very-low-density lipoprotein (VLDL)
- ApoB helping to regulate cholesterol and metabolism and playing a role in the catabolism of LDL

PURPOSE

- To measure the amount of apoB in the blood

PREPARATION

- The test requires a blood sample.
- The patient must restrict food for 12 hours before the test, but water is allowed.
- The patient must not smoke before the test.

Teaching points

- Tell the patient that the test will help determine his risk for cardiovascular disease.
- Inform the patient that he'll need to restrict food for 12 hours before the test but that water is allowed.
- Tell the patient that he may not smoke before the test.
- Tell the patient that the test requires a blood sample and that he may experience slight discomfort from the tourniquet and needle puncture.
- Explain who will perform the test and where it'll be done.
- Tell the patient that the test should take less than 5 minutes.

KEY STEPS

- Confirm the patient's identity using two patient identifiers according to facility policy.
- Perform a venipuncture, and collect the sample in a 7-ml tube without additives.

POSTPROCEDURE CARE

- Apply direct pressure to the venipuncture site until the bleeding stops.

PRECAUTIONS

- Maintain standard precautions while collecting the sample.
- Handle the sample gently to prevent hemolysis.
- Send the sample to the laboratory immediately.

COMPLICATIONS

- Hematoma at the venipuncture site

NORMAL RESULTS

- Levels of apoB of 45 to 110 mg/dl (SI, 0.45 to 1.10 mg/L) in women are considered normal.
- Levels of apoB of 55 to 100 mg/dl (SI, 0.55 to 1.00 mg/L) in men are considered normal.

ABNORMAL RESULTS

- Increased levels of apoB are seen in diabetes, hypothyroidism, biliary obstruction, and coronary artery disease (CAD).
- Increased levels of apoB indicate an increased risk of CAD.
- Decreased levels of apoB are associated with hyperthyroidism, malnutrition, inflammatory joint disease, and chronic anemia.
- Decreased levels of apoB are also see in type I hyperlipidemia and apolipoprotein C-II deficiency.
- A diet that's high in saturated fat and cholesterol may increase apoB levels.

INTERFERING FACTORS Pregnancy (increased apoB level)

Apt test

DESCRIPTION

- Performed on fetal stool to determine if the blood is from the neonate or is maternal blood
- Neonates possibly passing blood in the stool around the third day of life
- Blood most commonly resulting from delivery or from a fissure on the mother's nipple, causing the neonate to swallow blood
- Possible development of internal bleeding, such as rectal bleeding or GI hemorrhage, in the neonate
- Most commonly performed on stool but can also be performed on amniotic fluid or vomitus

PURPOSE

- To determine if blood in the stool of a neonate is fetal or maternal blood

PREPARATION

- Monitor the vital signs of the neonate.

Teaching points

- Explain the purpose of the test to the parents.
- Explain what a positive test result will mean for the infant and the parents.

DIAGNOSTIC PROCEDURE

KEY STEPS

- Confirm the patient's identity using two patient identifiers according to facility policy.
- Collect a small amount of stool or vomitus from the infant. The specimen must have gross blood present.

POSTPROCEDURE CARE

- Continue to monitor the infant for signs of internal bleeding.
- If infant blood is found in the specimen, make sure that the neonate has adequate venous access.
- If maternal blood is found in the specimen, evaluate the mother for cracked nipples and offer support and comfort measures.

PRECAUTIONS

- The specimen must have gross blood present; black, tarry stools aren't tested.
- Transport the specimen to the laboratory immediately.

COMPLICATIONS

- None known

INTERPRETATION

NORMAL RESULTS

- Normal test results show no fetal blood, but maternal blood may be present.

ABNORMAL RESULTS

- The presence of fetal blood indicates active GI bleeding in the neonate.
- The patient and parents should be prepared for further diagnostic procedures to determine the exact cause of the bleeding.

Arginine level test

DESCRIPTION

- Also known as *human growth hormone (hGH) stimulation test*
- Measures hGH levels after I.V. administration of arginine, an amino acid that normally stimulates hGH secretion
- Identifies pituitary dysfunction in infants and children with growth retardation and confirms hGH deficiency
- May be given with an insulin tolerance test or after administration of other hGH stimulants, such as glucagon, vasopressin, and levodopa

PURPOSE

- To aid in the diagnosis of pituitary tumors
- To confirm hGH deficiency in infants and children with low baseline levels

PREPARATION

- The patient must fast and limit physical activity for 10 to 12 hours before the test.
- Withhold all steroid drugs, including pituitary-based hormones. If the patient must continue to take these drugs, record this on the laboratory request.
- Insert an indwelling venous catheter if not already present.

Teaching points

- Explain to the patient, or his parents, that this test identifies hGH deficiency.
- Explain that the patient must fast and limit physical activity for 10 to 12 hours before the test.
- Explain that this test requires I.V. infusion of a drug and collection of several blood samples and *that it lasts at least 2 hours.*
- Explain who will perform the test and where it'll be done.
- Tell the patient to lie down and relax for at least 90 minutes before the test.

KEY STEPS

- Confirm the patient's identity using two patient identifiers according to facility policy.
- Between 6 a.m. and 8 a.m., perform a venipuncture, and collect 6 ml of blood (basal sample) in a clot activator tube.
- Use an indwelling venous catheter to avoid repeated venipunctures. Start I.V. infusion of arginine (0.5 g/kg of body weight) in normal saline solution, and continue for 30 minutes.
- Stop the I.V. infusion, and then draw a total of three 6-ml samples at 30-minute intervals. Collect each sample in a clot activator tube, and label it appropriately.
- Collect each sample at the scheduled time, and specify the collection time on the laboratory request.
- Send each sample to the laboratory immediately because hGH has a half-life of only 20 to 25 minutes.

POSTPROCEDURE CARE

- Apply direct pressure to the venipuncture site until the bleeding stops.
- Tell the patient that he may resume his usual diet, activities, and medications stopped before the test, as ordered.

PRECAUTIONS

- Maintain standard precautions while collecting the sample.
- Handle the sample gently to prevent hemolysis.
- Send the sample to the laboratory immediately.

COMPLICATIONS

- Hematoma at the I.V. or venipuncture site

NORMAL RESULTS

- Arginine should raise hGH levels to more than 10 ng/ml (SI, > 10 mcg/L) in men, to more than 15 ng/ml (SI, > 15 mcg/L) in women, and to more than 48 ng/ml (SI, > 48 mcg/L) in children. Such an increase may appear in the first sample collected 30 minutes after arginine infusion is stopped or in the samples collected 60 and 90 minutes afterward.

ABNORMAL RESULTS

- Levels that rise during fasting or during sleep help to rule out hGH deficiency.
- Failure of hGH levels to increase after arginine infusion indicates decreased anterior pituitary hGH reserve. In children, this deficiency causes dwarfism; in adults, it can indicate panhypopituitarism. When hGH levels fail to reach 10 ng/ml, retesting is required at the same time of day as the original test.

Arterial blood gas analysis

OVERVIEW

DESCRIPTION
- Measures the partial pressure of arterial oxygen (Pao_2), the partial pressure of arterial carbon dioxide ($Paco_2$), and the pH of an arterial sample
- Measures oxygen content (O_2CT), arterial oxygen saturation (Sao_2), and bicarbonate (HCO_3^-) values
- Pao_2: Amount of oxygen the lungs deliver to the blood
- $Paco_2$: How efficiently the lungs eliminate carbon dioxide
- pH: Acid-base level of the blood, or the hydrogen ion (H^+) level
- Acidity indicates H^+ excess; alkalinity, H^+ deficit

PURPOSE
- To evaluate the efficiency of pulmonary gas exchange
- To assess the integrity of the ventilatory control system
- To determine the acid-base level of the blood
- To monitor respiratory therapy

PREPARATION
- The test requires a blood sample.
- No dietary restrictions are required.

Teaching points
- Explain that arterial blood gas analysis evaluates how well the lungs are delivering oxygen to the blood and eliminating carbon dioxide.
- Tell the patient that the test requires a blood sample.
- Instruct the patient to breathe normally during the test, and warn him that he may experience a brief cramping or throbbing pain at the puncture site.
- Inform the patient that he need not restrict food or fluids.
- Explain who will perform the arterial puncture, when it will occur, and the puncture site location (radial, brachial, or femoral artery).
- Tell the patient that the procedure takes less than 10 minutes.

DIAGNOSTIC PROCEDURE

KEY STEPS
- Confirm the patient's identity using two patient identifiers according to facility policy.
- Wait at least 20 minutes before drawing arterial blood when starting, changing, or discontinuing oxygen therapy; after initiating or changing settings of mechanical ventilation; or after extubation.
- Use a heparinized blood gas syringe to draw the sample.
- If using the radial artery, perform the Allen test to determine arterial perfusion.
- Perform an arterial puncture, or draw blood from an arterial line.
- Eliminate air from the sample, place it on ice immediately, and prepare to transport it for analysis.
- Before sending the sample to the laboratory, note on the laboratory request whether the patient was breathing room air or receiving oxygen therapy when the sample was collected.
- Note the flow rate of oxygen therapy and method of delivery. If the patient was on a ventilator, note the fraction of inspired oxygen, tidal volume mode, respiratory rate, and positive end-expiratory pressure.
- Note the patient's temperature.

POSTPROCEDURE CARE
- After applying pressure to the puncture site for 3 to 5 minutes or until bleeding has stopped, tape a gauze pad firmly over it.
- If the puncture site is on the arm, don't tape the entire circumference; this may restrict circulation.
- If the patient is receiving anticoagulants or has coagulopathy, apply pressure to the puncture site longer than 5 minutes, if necessary.
- Monitor vital signs, and observe for signs of circulatory impairment, such as swelling, discoloration, pain, numbness, and tingling in the bandaged arm or leg.

PRECAUTIONS
- Place the sample on ice immediately.
- Exposing the sample to air affects the Pao_2 and $Paco_2$, interfering with accurate results.
- Maintain standard precautions while collecting or handling the sample.

COMPLICATIONS
- Bleeding from the puncture site

INTERPRETATION

NORMAL RESULTS
- Pao_2 levels of 80 to 100 mm Hg (SI, 10.6 to 13.3 kPa) are considered normal.
- $Paco_2$ levels of 35 to 45 mm Hg (SI, 4.7 to 5.3 kPa) are considered normal.
- pH levels of 7.35 to 7.45 (SI, 7.35 to 7.45) are considered normal.
- O_2CT levels of 15% to 23% (SI, 0.15 to 0.23) are considered normal.
- Sao_2 levels of 94% to 100% (SI, 0.94 to 1) are considered normal.
- HCO_3^- levels of 22 to 25 mEq/L (SI, 22 to 25 mmol/L) are considered normal.

ABNORMAL RESULTS
- Decreased Pao_2, O_2CT, and Sao_2 levels and increased $Paco_2$ levels may result from conditions that impair respiratory function, such as respiratory muscle weakness or paralysis, respiratory center inhibition (from head injury, brain tumor, or drug abuse), and airway obstruction (possibly from mucus plugs or a tumor).
- Decreased levels may result from bronchiole obstruction caused by asthma or emphysema; from an abnormal ventilation-perfusion ratio caused by partially blocked alveoli or pulmonary capillaries; or from alveoli that are damaged or filled with fluid because of disease, hemorrhage, or near drowning. (See *Acid-base disorders*.)

Acid-base disorders

DISORDERS AND ARTERIAL BLOOD GAS FINDINGS	POSSIBLE CAUSES	SIGNS AND SYMPTOMS
Respiratory acidosis (excess CO_2 retention)		
pH < 7.35 (SI, < 7.35) HCO_3^- > 26 mEq/L (SI, > 26 mmol/L) (if compensating) $Paco_2$ > 45 mm Hg (SI, > 5.3 kPa)	◆ Central nervous system depression from drugs, injury, or disease ◆ Asphyxia ◆ Hypoventilation due to pulmonary, cardiac, musculoskeletal, or neuromuscular disease ◆ Obesity ◆ Postoperative pain ◆ Abdominal distention	Diaphoresis, headache, tachycardia, confusion, restlessness, apprehension
Respiratory alkalosis (excess CO_2 excretion)		
pH > 7.45 (SI, > 7.45) HCO_3^- < 22 mEq/L (SI, < 22 mmol/L) (if compensating) $Paco_2$ < 35 mm Hg (SI, < 4.7 kPa)	◆ Hyperventilation due to anxiety, pain, or improper ventilator settings ◆ Respiratory stimulation caused by drugs, disease, hypoxia, fever, or high room temperature ◆ Gram-negative bacteremia ◆ Compensation for metabolic acidosis (chronic renal failure)	Rapid, deep breathing; paresthesia; light-headedness; twitching; anxiety; fear
Metabolic acidosis (HCO_3^- loss, acid retention)		
pH < 7.35 (SI, < 7.35) HCO_3^- < 22 mEq/L (SI, < 22 mmol/L) $Paco_2$ < 35 mm Hg (SI, < 4.7 kPa) (if compensating)	◆ HCO_3^- depletion due to renal disease, diarrhea, or small-bowel fistulas ◆ Excessive production of organic acids due to hepatic disease; endocrine disorders, including diabetes mellitus, hypoxia, shock; and drug intoxication ◆ Inadequate excretion of acids due to renal disease	Rapid, deep breathing; fruity breath; fatigue; headache; lethargy; drowsiness; nausea; vomiting; coma (if severe)
Metabolic alkalosis (HCO_3^- retention, acid loss)		
pH > 7.45 (SI, > 7.45) HCO_3^- > 26 mEq/L (SI,> 26 mmol/L) $Paco_2$ > 45 mm Hg (SI, > 5.3 kPa)	◆ Loss of hydrochloric acid from prolonged vomiting or gastric suctioning ◆ Loss of potassium due to increased renal excretion (as in diuretic therapy) or steroid overdose ◆ Excessive alkali ingestion ◆ Compensation for chronic respiratory acidosis	Slow, shallow breathing; hypertonic muscles; restlessness; twitching; confusion; irritability; apathy; tetany; seizures; coma (if severe)

◆ When inspired air contains insufficient oxygen, Pao_2, O_2CT, and Sao_2 levels decrease, but $Paco_2$ levels may be normal. Such findings are common in pneumothorax, impaired diffusion between alveoli and blood (for example, caused by interstitial fibrosis), or an arteriovenous shunt that permits blood to bypass the lungs.

◆ Low O_2CT (with normal Pao_2, Sao_2, and possibly $Paco_2$) values may result from severe anemia, decreased blood volume, or reduced hemoglobin oxygen-carrying capacity.

INTERFERING FACTORS *Exposing the sample to air (increase or decrease in Pao_2 and $Paco_2$); venous blood in the sample (possible decrease in Pao_2 and increase in $Paco_2$)*

Arterial-to-alveolar oxygen ratio

DESCRIPTION

◆ Helps identify the cause of hypoxemia and intrapulmonary shunting by providing an approximation of the partial pressure of oxygenation of the alveoli and arteries
◆ May help differentiate the cause of hypoxemia and intrapulmonary shunting: ventilated alveoli but no perfusion, unventilated alveoli with perfusion, or collapse of the alveoli and capillaries

PURPOSE

◆ To evaluate the efficiency of gas exchange
◆ To assess the integrity of the ventilatory control system
◆ To monitor respiratory therapy

PREPARATION

◆ The test requires a blood sample.
◆ No dietary restrictions are required.

Teaching points

◆ Explain to the patient that the arterial-to-alveolar ratio test evaluates how well the lungs deliver oxygen to the blood and eliminate carbon dioxide.
◆ Tell the patient that the test requires a blood sample.
◆ Inform the patient that he need not restrict food or fluids.
◆ Instruct the patient to breathe normally during the test, and warn him that he may experience cramping or throbbing pain at the puncture site.
◆ Explain who will perform the arterial puncture and where it'll be done.
◆ Tell the patient that the test should take less than 20 minutes.

KEY STEPS

◆ Confirm the patient's identity using two patient identifiers according to facility policy.
◆ If using the radial artery, perform the Allen test to determine arterial perfusion.
◆ Perform an arterial puncture, or draw blood from an arterial line using a heparinized blood gas syringe.
◆ Eliminate all air from the sample, and place it on ice immediately.
◆ Before sending the sample to the laboratory, note on the laboratory request whether the patient was breathing room air or receiving oxygen therapy when the sample was collected.
◆ If the patient was receiving oxygen therapy, note the flow rate and method of delivery. If he was on a ventilator, note the fraction of inspired oxygen, tidal volume, mode, respiratory rate, and positive end-expiratory pressure.
◆ Note the patient's temperature.

POSTPROCEDURE CARE

◆ Apply pressure to the puncture site for 3 to 5 minutes or until bleeding stops.
◆ Place a gauze pad over the site and tape it in place, but don't tape the entire circumference.
◆ Monitor vital signs, and observe for signs of circulatory impairment, such as swelling, discoloration, pain, numbness, and tingling in the bandaged arm or leg.

PRECAUTIONS

◆ Maintain standard precautions while collecting the sample.
◆ Place the sample on ice immediately.

COMPLICATIONS

◆ Bleeding from the puncture site

NORMAL RESULTS

◆ A normal arterial-to-alveolar oxygen ratio is 75%.

ABNORMAL RESULTS

◆ Increased values may result from mucus plugs, bronchospasm, or airway collapse (asthma, bronchitis, emphysema).
◆ Hypoxemia results in an increased alveolar-to-arterial oxygen gradient and may result from arterial septal defects, pneumothorax, atelectasis, emboli, or edema.

Arthrocentesis

DESCRIPTION
- Synovial fluid aspiration
- Involves obtaining a fluid specimen by inserting a needle into a joint space, most commonly the knee, under sterile conditions
- Indicated in undiagnosed articular disease and symptomatic joint effusion

PURPOSE
- To analyze synovial fluid
- To aid in the differential diagnosis of arthritis, especially septic or crystal-induced arthritis
- To identify the cause or nature of joint effusion
- To relieve pain and distention from joint effusion
- To administer drugs, such as corticosteroids, locally

PREPARATION
- Make sure the patient has signed a consent form.
- Note and report allergies.
- If glucose testing of synovial fluid is ordered, advise fasting for 6 to 12 hours before the test; otherwise, there's no need to restrict food or fluids before the test.
- Give the patient a sedative.

Teaching points
- Explain the purpose of the test and how it's done.
- If glucose testing of synovial fluid is ordered, advise fasting for 6 to 12 hours before the test; otherwise, there's no need to restrict food or fluids before the test.
- Inform the patient that failure to adhere to dietary restrictions can affect glucose levels.
- Warn the patient that transient pain may occur when the needle penetrates the joint capsule.
- Explain who will perform the test and where it'll be done.
- Tell the patient that the test should take less than 15 minutes.

DIAGNOSTIC PROCEDURE

KEY STEPS
- Confirm the patient's identity using two patient identifiers according to facility policy.
- The test shouldn't be performed near skin or wound infections.
- Strict sterile technique used during aspiration prevents contamination of joint space or synovial fluid specimen.
- The patient is positioned properly and told to maintain this position during the procedure.
- The skin over the puncture site is cleaned and prepared.
- A local anesthetic is given; an aspirating needle is inserted quickly through the skin, subcutaneous tissue, and synovial membrane into the joint space.
- As much fluid as possible, preferably at least 15 ml, is aspirated into the syringe.
- The joint (except the area around the puncture site) is bandaged to compress the free fluid into this portion of the sac, ensuring maximal collection of fluid.
- If a corticosteroid is injected, the syringe is detached, leaving the needle in the joint. The syringe containing the steroid is attached to the needle, and the steroid is injected.
- The needle is withdrawn, and pressure is applied to the puncture site until bleeding stops.
- The puncture site is cleaned, and sterile dressing is applied.
- A venipuncture is performed to obtain a blood glucose analysis specimen, if synovial fluid glucose is being measured.
- The properly labeled specimens should be sent to the laboratory immediately. If a white blood cell count is ordered, the specimen should be clearly labeled "Synovial fluid" and "Caution: Don't use acid diluents" because these can alter the count.

POSTPROCEDURE CARE
- Apply cold to the affected joint for 24 to 36 hours after aspiration, to decrease pain and swelling.
- Use pillows to support the joint.
- If a large quantity of fluid was aspirated, apply an elastic bandage to prevent fluid from accumulating again.
- Have the patient resume normal activities and diet immediately after the procedure, if his condition permits.
- Warn the patient to avoid excessive use of the joint for a few days after the test, even if pain and swelling have subsided.
- Excessive use can cause transient pain, swelling, and stiffness.
- Watch for and immediately report increased pain and fever, which could indicate joint infection.

PRECAUTIONS
- Use strict sterile technique throughout the test.
- Send the specimen to the laboratory immediately.

COMPLICATIONS
- Joint infection
- Hemorrhage
- Hemarthrosis

INTERPRETATION

NORMAL RESULTS
- Colorless to pale yellow synovial fluid specimens are normal.
- Synovial fluid specimens should be clear.
- Synovial fluid volumes of 0.3 to 3.5 ml (in knee) are normal.
- pH levels of 7.2 to 7.4 are normal.
- Specimens should demonstrate a good mucin clot.

ABNORMAL RESULTS
- Abnormal specimen results may indicate inflammatory disease (systemic lupus erythematosus, rheumatic fever, pseudogout, gout, and rheumatoid arthritis), noninflammatory disease (traumatic arthritis and osteoarthritis), or septic disease (tuberculous and septic arthritis).

Arthrography

DESCRIPTION

- Radiographic examination of a joint after injection of a radiopaque dye, air, or both (double-contrast arthrography)
- Contraindicated in pregnancy and in patients with active arthritis, joint infection, and previous hypersensitivity to iodinated contrast media

PURPOSE

- To outline joint contour and soft-tissue structures
- To evaluate persistent unexplained joint discomfort or pain
- To identify acute or chronic abnormalities of the joint capsule or supporting ligaments of the knee, shoulder, ankle, hip, or wrist
- To detect internal joint derangements
- To locate synovial cysts
- To evaluate damage from recurrent dislocations

PREPARATION

- Make sure the patient has signed an appropriate consent form.
- Note and report allergies.
- No dietary restrictions are required.
- Check patient history for sensitivity to iodine or contrast media. If sensitivity exists, clearly mark the patient's chart.

Teaching points

- Explain the purpose of the test and how it's done.
- Inform the patient that he need not restrict food or fluids.
- Explain who will perform the test and where it'll be done.
- Warn the patient that a tingling sensation, burning, or pressure in the joint may occur with the contrast injection.
- Explain that some swelling, discomfort, or crepitant noises may occur in the joint after the study and that these usually disappear after 1 to 2 days. Tell the pateint to contact his practitioner if symptoms persist.

- Tell the patient that the test will take about 45 minutes.

DIAGNOSTIC PROCEDURE

KEY STEPS

- Confirm the patient's identity using two patient identifiers according to facility policy.
- The skin around the puncture site is cleaned with an antiseptic solution, and a local anesthetic is injected.
- A needle is then inserted into the joint space.
- Fluid may then be aspirated and sent to the laboratory for analysis.
- When fluoroscopic examination shows correct needle placement, a contrast medium is injected into the joint space.
- The needle is removed, and the puncture site is covered with a sterile dressing.
- The joint is put through its range of motion to distribute the contrast medium within the joint space.
- A series of X-rays is taken rapidly, before the joint tissue can absorb the contrast medium.

POSTPROCEDURE CARE

- Tell the patient to rest the joint for 6 to 12 hours.
- Wrap the knee in an elastic bandage for several days, if knee arthrography was performed.
- Apply ice to the joint for swelling.
- Give the patient an analgesic.
- Ask the patient to report signs and symptoms of infection.

PRECAUTIONS

- Arthrography is contraindicated during pregnancy and in the patient with active arthritis, joint infection, or previous sensitivity to radiopaque material.

COMPLICATIONS

- Hypersensitivity reactions to contrast medium
- Persistent joint swelling, pain, or crepitus
- Infection

NORMAL RESULTS

- A knee arthrogram showing a characteristic wedge-shaped shadow pointed toward the interior of the joint indicates a normal medial meniscus.
- A shoulder arthrogram showing the bicipital tendon sheath, redundant inferior joint capsule, and intact subscapular bursa is considered normal.

ABNORMAL RESULTS

- Structural abnormalities of the knee commonly suggest tears and lacerations of the meniscus.
- Extrameniscal lesions may suggest osteochondral fractures, cartilaginous abnormalities, synovial abnormalities, cruciate ligament tears, and joint capsule and collateral ligament disruptions.
- Shoulder abnormalities may suggest adhesive capsulitis, bicipital tenosynovitis or rupture, and rotator cuff tears.

Arthroscopy

DESCRIPTION
- Visual examination of the interior of a joint using a fiber-optic endoscope
- Most commonly used to examine the knee joint
- Permits concurrent surgery or biopsy using triangulation, in which instruments are passed through separate cannulae
- Usually an outpatient procedure

PURPOSE
- To evaluate suspected or confirmed joint disease
- To provide a safe, convenient alternative to open surgery (arthrotomy) and separate biopsy
- To detect, diagnose, treat, and monitor therapy for meniscal, patellar, condylar, extrasynovial, and synovial diseases

PREPARATION
- Make sure the patient has signed a consent form.
- Note and report allergies.
- The patient must fast after midnight before the procedure.
- Check the patient's history for hypersensitivity to the anesthetic.

Teaching points
- Explain the purpose of the test and how it's done.
- Tell the patient to fast after midnight before the procedure.
- Explain who will perform the test and where it'll be done.
- Warn the patient that he may feel discomfort from the injection of the anesthetic and tourniquet pressure.
- Explain that the patient may feel a thumping sensation as the cannula is inserted into the joint.
- Advise the patient to avoid tub baths until after the postoperative visit, although showers are allowed 48 hours after the test.
- Tell the patient that the test takes about 1 hour.

KEY STEPS
- Confirm the patient's identity using two patient identifiers according to your facility policy.
- Shave and prepare an area 5" (12.7 cm) above and below the joint.
- Give the patient a sedative.
- A local or regional anesthetic is given; general anesthesia is for more extensive surgery.
- As much blood as possible is usually drained from the leg by wrapping it in an elastic bandage and elevating it.
- A mixture of lidocaine, epinephrine, and sterile normal saline solution may be injected to distend the knee, reduce bleeding, and provide a better view.
- A cannula is passed through a small incision and positioned in the joint cavity.
- The arthroscope is inserted through the cannula and the knee structures are visually examined.
- Photographs are taken for further study, if indicated.
- A synovial biopsy or appropriate surgery is performed, if indicated.
- The arthroscope is removed, and the joint is irrigated.
- An adhesive strip and compression bandage are applied to the site.

POSTPROCEDURE CARE
- Administer analgesics.
- Elevate the leg and apply ice for the first 24 hours.
- Report fever, bleeding, drainage, or increased swelling or pain in the joint.
- Limit weight bearing by using a walker, cane, or crutches for 48 hours.
- Apply an immobilizer, if ordered.
- Have the patient resume his usual diet.
- Monitor the extremity for neurovascular impairment.

PRECAUTIONS
- Arthroscopy is contraindicated in patients with local skin or wound infections and in patients with fibrous ankylosis with flexion less than 50 degrees.

COMPLICATIONS
- Infection
- Hematoma
- Thrombophlebitis
- Joint injury

NORMAL RESULTS
- Normal study results show a diarthrodial joint surrounded by muscles, ligaments, cartilage, and tendons that's lined with synovial membrane.

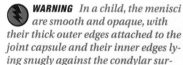 **WARNING** *In a child, the menisci are smooth and opaque, with their thick outer edges attached to the joint capsule and their inner edges lying snugly against the condylar surfaces, unattached.*

- Articular cartilage appears smooth and white.
- Ligaments and tendons appear cablelike and silvery.
- The synovium is smooth and marked by a fine vascular network.
- Degenerative changes begin during adolescence.

ABNORMAL RESULTS
- Meniscal abnormalities may suggest a torn meniscus.
- Patellar abnormalities may suggest chondromalacia, dislocation, subluxation, fracture, or parapatellar synovitis.
- Condylar abnormalities may suggest degenerative articular cartilage, osteochondritis dissecans, or loose bodies.
- Extrasynovial abnormalities may suggesit torn anterior cruciate or tibial collateral ligament, Baker's cyst, or ganglion cyst.
- Synovial abnormalities may suggest synovitis, rheumatoid arthritis, or degenerative arthritis.
- Foreign bodies may suggest gout, pseudogout, or osteochondromatosis.

Aspartate aminotransferase level test

OVERVIEW

DESCRIPTION

- Aspartate aminotransferase (AST) found in the cytoplasm and mitochondria of many cells, primarily in the liver, heart, skeletal muscles, kidneys, pancreas, and red blood cells (also released into serum in response to cellular damage)
- Elevated AST levels highly correlated with myocardial infarction (MI) but sometimes superfluous for diagnosing MI, because it isn't specifically for the heart (doesn't differentiate between acute MI and the effects of hepatic congestion caused by heart failure)

PURPOSE

- To aid in the detection and differential diagnosis of acute hepatic disease
- To monitor patient progress and prognosis in cardiac and hepatic diseases
- To aid in the diagnosis of MI in correlation with creatine kinase and lactate dehydrogenase levels

PREPARATION

- No dietary restrictions are required.
- This test requires blood samples.
- Notify the laboratory and practitioner of drugs the patient is taking that may affect test results; it may be necessary to restrict these drugs.

Teaching points

- Explain to the patient that this test assesses heart and liver function.
- Inform the patient that the test usually requires three venipunctures (one on admission and one each day for the next 2 days). Explain to the patient that he may experience slight discomfort from the tourniquet and needle puncture.
- Tell the patient that he need not restrict food or fluids.
- Explain who will perform the test and where it'll be done.

DIAGNOSTIC PROCEDURE

KEY STEPS

- Confirm the patient's identity using two patient identifiers according to facility policy.
- Perform a venipuncture, and collect the sample in a 4-ml clot activator tube.

POSTPROCEDURE CARE

- Apply direct pressure to the venipuncture site until the bleeding stops.
- Instruct the patient that he may resume medications stopped before the test.

PRECAUTIONS

- Maintain standard precautions while collecting the sample.
- Handle the sample gently to prevent hemolysis.
- To avoid missing peak AST levels, draw serum samples at the same time each day.
- Send the sample to the laboratory immediately.

COMPLICATIONS

- Hematoma at the venipuncture site

INTERPRETATION

NORMAL RESULTS

- AST levels of 12 to 31 units/L (SI, 0.14 to 0.78 µkat/L) are considered normal.

ABNORMAL RESULTS

- AST levels fluctuate in response to the extent of cellular necrosis, being transiently and minimally increased early in the disease process and extremely increased during the most acute phase. Depending on when the initial sample is drawn, AST levels may increase, indicating increasing disease severity and tissue damage, or may decrease, indicating disease resolution and tissue repair.
- Maximum elevations (more than 20 times normal) may indicate acute viral hepatitis, severe skeletal muscle trauma, extensive surgery, drug-induced hepatic injury, or severe passive liver congestion.
- High levels (10 to 20 times normal) may indicate severe MI, severe infectious mononucleosis, or alcoholic cirrhosis.
- High levels also occur during the prodromal or resolving stages of conditions that cause maximum elevations.
- Moderate to high levels (5 to 10 times normal) may indicate dermatomyositis, Duchenne's muscular dystrophy, or chronic hepatitis.
- Moderate to high levels also occur during the prodromal or resolving stages of diseases that cause high elevations.
- Low to moderate levels (2 to 5 times normal) occur at some time during the preceding conditions or may indicate hemolytic anemia, metastatic hepatic tumors, acute pancreatitis, pulmonary emboli, delirium tremens, or fatty liver. AST levels rise slightly after the first few days of biliary duct obstruction.

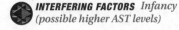 **INTERFERING FACTORS** *Infancy (possible higher AST levels)*

Atrial natriuretic factor test

DESCRIPTION

◆ Radioimmunoassay that measures the plasma level of atrial natriuretic peptide, or atriopeptin
◆ Possibly providing a marker for early asymptomatic left ventricular dysfunction and increased cardiac volume

PURPOSE

◆ To confirm heart failure
◆ To identify asymptomatic cardiac volume overload

PREPARATION

◆ The patient must fast for 12 hours before this test.
◆ This test requires a blood sample.
◆ Check the patient's history for drugs that can influence test results.
◆ Withhold beta-adrenergic blockers, calcium antagonists, diuretics, vasodilators, and cardiac glycosides for 24 hours before collection of the blood sample.

Teaching points

◆ Explain the purpose of the test to the patient, as appropriate.
◆ Inform the patient that he must fast for 12 hours before the test.
◆ Tell the patient the test requires a blood sample and that he may experience slight discomfort from the tourniquet and needle puncture.
◆ Explain who will perform the test and where it'll be done.
◆ Tell the patient that the test should take less than 5 minutes.
◆ Tell the patient that test results will be available within 4 days.

KEY STEPS

◆ Confirm the patient's identity using two patient identifiers according to facility policy.
◆ Perform a venipuncture, and collect the sample in a prechilled potassium EDTA tube.
◆ After chilled centrifugation, promptly freeze the EDTA plasma and send it to the laboratory.

POSTPROCEDURE CARE

◆ Apply direct pressure to the venipuncture site until the bleeding stops.
◆ Instruct the patient that he may resume his usual diet and medications stopped before the test.

PRECAUTIONS

◆ Maintain standard precautions while collecting the sample.
◆ Handle the sample gently to prevent hemolysis.

COMPLICATIONS

◆ Hematoma at the venipuncture site

NORMAL RESULTS

◆ Atrial natriuretic factor levels should be 20 to 77 pg/ml (SI, 20 to 77 ng/L).

ABNORMAL RESULTS

◆ Increased levels may indicate heart failure or elevated cardiac filling pressure.

Auditory brain stem evoked-response test

DESCRIPTION

- Test measuring auditory brain stem evoked response (ABR), also called *brain stem auditory evoked response*
- Most common form of auditory evoked potentials testing
- Analyzes traces to determine if a response is present; analyzes characteristics

PURPOSE

- To screen neonatal hearing, with the goal of providing amplification by age 6 months
- To estimate or confirm the extent of hearing loss in infants and toddlers
- To estimate the threshold in other difficult-to-test patients, such as those with developmental disabilities and those suspected of having nonorganic hearing loss
- To evaluate cranial nerve (CN) VIII and lower brain stem auditory synchronization, which is abnormal when lesions exist in this area or when auditory neuropathy is present (auditory dyssynchronization)

PREPARATION

- Clean ear canals are required for this test and are particularly important when referring for electrocochleography.

⚡ **WARNING** *Depending on a child's age, sedation may be necessary, in which case a health care facility must perform this test. In other facilities, a child may have to undergo sleep deprivation to make sure he sleeps during testing.*

Teaching points

- Advise the patient to dress comfortably and to avoid wearing foundation makeup. Inform the patient that, although the test is painless, electrodes will be applied to the skin.
- Explain the purpose of the test and how it's done.
- Explain who will perform the test and where it'll be done.
- Tell the patient that the test may take 1 to 1½ hours to complete.

KEY STEPS

- Confirm the patient's identity using two patient identifiers according to facility policy.
- Electrodes are connected to a physiologic amplifier and signal-averaging computer.
- Threshold estimation is conducted by an audiologist. The intensity of the signal is varied until the response threshold is obtained. The response threshold is slightly above the hearing threshold, but estimation is possible if the patient has normal hearing.
- In testing for CN VIII and auditory brain stem response, click signals must be made that are clearly audible and occur at different rates. Rapid clicks may reveal a pathology more readily. A click stimulus is presented at a supra-threshold level. The time at which wave V occurs in each ear, the time difference between the evoked waves I and V in each ear, and the time difference between both of these measures is used to indicate the probability of retrocochlear pathology.
- Assessment of central auditory processing ability involves assessing brain stem potentials and one or more of the potentials generated by the neural structures superior to the brain stem.

POSTPROCEDURE CARE

- If the patient was sedated, monitor him until he completely recovers.

PRECAUTIONS

- The patient must cooperate for test results to be accurate.

COMPLICATIONS

- Skin abrasion from electrode placement, causing irritation and minor allergic reactions

NORMAL RESULTS

- ABR wave latencies occur at predictable times for the patient who has normal hearing or who has cochlear loss but hears signals that are above the hearing threshold. The latency between waves I and V is about 4.0 ms. The interaural latency difference of wave V and the I-V interaural latency differences are small, generally less than 0.3 or 0.4 ms.
- The threshold of the ABR is about 10 to 20 decibels (dB) normal hearing level (nHL) for click or high-frequency stimuli, and 20 or 30 dB nHL for lower-frequency stimuli.

ABNORMAL RESULTS

- Cochlear loss increases the threshold of the ABR response.
- The time between waves I and V is unaffected or shortens with cochlear loss; establishing wave I may be more difficult.
- Prolonged I-V interpeak latency is an indicator of CN VIII or lower brain stem pathology.
- Asymmetry of the I-V interpeak interval between ears is also a strong sign of a retrocochlear disorder.

Avian flu virus RNA test

DESCRIPTION

- Determines exposure to avian influenza, an infection that causes viruses in birds
- Wild birds as carriers of the disease but able to transmit the disease to domesticated birds
- Possible transmission of the H5N1 virus from a sick bird to humans (more than one-half of the more-than-100 diagnosed cases of H5N1 have resulted in death)
- Genetic studies showing that H5N1 is able to rapidly mutate, causing concern regarding a potential pandemic outbreak of the flu

PURPOSE

- To detect the presence of H5N1 ribonucleic acid (RNA)

PREPARATION

- No dietary restrictions are required.

Teaching points

- Determine if the patient has been exposed to infected poultry recently.
- Explain that this test helps to determine exposure to the avian flu.
- Tell the patient that the test is performed with a nasal swab.
- Tell the patient that he need not restrict food or fluids.
- Tell the patient that if the test result is positive, this will be reported to the Centers for Disease Control and Prevention (CDC) and the World Health Organization (WHO), and further testing may be done.
- Explain who will perform the test and where it'll be done.
- Tell the patient that the test should take less than 5 minutes.

KEY STEPS

- Confirm the patient's identity using two patient identifiers according to facility policy.
- Obtain a nasal culture from both nostrils.
- Place the swab into a container containing 3 ml of sterile saline solution.
- Place the specimen on ice.

POSTPROCEDURE CARE

- Answer the patient's questions.

PRECAUTIONS

- Maintain standard precautions while collecting the specimen.
- Immediately place the specimen on ice and transport it to the laboratory.

COMPLICATIONS

None known

NORMAL RESULTS

- The presence of H5N1 RNA isn't detected.

ABNORMAL RESULTS

- The presence of H5N1 RNA indicates that the patient has been exposed to the avian flu virus. Immediately contact the CDC and the WHO, and be prepared to ship samples to a designated WHO laboratory.
- A positive test result requires further testing.

Barium enema

DESCRIPTION

- Radiographic examination of the large intestine after rectal instillation of barium sulfate (single-contrast technique) or barium sulfate and air (double-contrast technique)
- Single-contrast technique providing a profile view of the large intestine
- Double-contrast technique providing profile and frontal views

PURPOSE

- To aid in the diagnosis of colorectal cancer and inflammatory disease
- To detect polyps, diverticula, and structural changes in the large intestine

PREPARATION

- Common bowel preparation includes restricted intake of dairy products and maintenance of a liquid diet for 24 hours before the test. The patient is encouraged to drink five 8-oz glasses of water or clear liquids 12 to 24 hours before the test.
- A GoLYTELY preparation isn't recommended because it leaves the bowel too wet for the barium to coat the walls of the bowel.

Teaching points

- Explain that the test permits examination of the large intestine through X-rays taken after a barium enema.
- Tell the patient to restrict intake of dairy products and maintain a liquid diet for 24 hours before the test. Tell him to drink five 8-oz glasses of water or clear liquids 12 to 24 hours before the test.
- Advise the patient to give himself enemas until the return is clear.
- Tell the patient not to eat breakfast before the procedure; if the test is scheduled for late afternoon, he may have clear liquids.
- Tell the patient that he may experience cramping pains or the urge to defecate as the barium or air is introduced into the intestine. Instruct him to breathe deeply and slowly through his mouth to ease the discomfort.
- The patient must contract his anal sphincter tightly against the rectal tube.
- Stress the importance of retaining the barium.
- Explain who will perform the test and where it'll be done.
- Tell the patient that the test takes between 30 and 45 minutes.
- Explain that stools will be light-colored for 24 to 72 hours after the test.

DIAGNOSTIC PROCEDURE

KEY STEPS

- Confirm the patient's identity using two patient identifiers according to facility policy.
- After the patient is in a supine position on a tilting X-ray table, spot films of the abdomen are taken.
- The patient is assisted to the Sims position; a well-lubricated rectal tube is inserted through the anus. For anal sphincter atony or severe mental or physical debilitation, a rectal tube with a retaining balloon is inserted.
- The barium is given slowly. The filling process is monitored fluoroscopically. To aid filling, the table is tilted or the patient is assisted to supine, prone, and lateral decubitus positions. (See *A look at barium enema*.)
- As barium flow is observed, significant spot films are taken.
- The rectal tube is withdrawn, and the patient is escorted to a toilet or given a bedpan to expel as much barium as possible.
- After evacuation, additional overhead film is taken to record mucosal pattern and evaluate the efficiency of colonic emptying.
- A double-contrast barium enema may directly follow the examination or may occur separately. If the enema is performed immediately, a thin film of barium remains in the intestine, coating the mucosa, and air is carefully injected to distend the bowel lumen.
- If a double-contrast technique is performed separately, a colloidal barium suspension is instilled, and the intestine is filled to either the splenic flexure or the middle of the transverse colon. The suspension is then aspirated, and air is forcefully injected into the intestine. If the intestine is filled to the lower descending colon, air should be injected forcefully without the suspension first being aspirated.

- The patient is assisted to erect, prone, supine, and lateral decubitus positions in sequence. Filling is monitored fluoroscopically, and spot films are taken of significant findings.
- After films are taken, the patient is escorted to a toilet or provided with a bedpan.

POSTPROCEDURE CARE

- Make sure that the patient isn't to have further studies before allowing him to have food or fluids. Encourage him to take extra fluids because the bowel preparation and test itself can cause dehydration.
- Encourage the patient to rest because the bowel preparation and test are exhausting.
- Barium retention can cause an intestinal obstruction or fecal impaction. If this happens, give a mild cathartic or enema. The patient's stools will be light-colored for 24 to 72 hours. Record and describe stools.

PRECAUTIONS

- Flexible sigmoidoscopy provides the best view of the rectosigmoid region, where most colon cancers occur.
- Barium enemas should precede barium swallow and the upper GI and small-bowel series because retained barium in the GI tract may interfere with subsequent radiographic studies.
- Contraindications include fulminant ulcerative colitis associated with systemic toxicity and megacolon, suspected bowel perforation, and pregnancy.

COMPLICATIONS

- Perforation of the colon, water intoxication, barium granulomas, intraperitoneal and extraperitoneal extravasation of barium, and barium embolism

INTERPRETATION

NORMAL RESULTS

- *Single-contrast enema:* Barium uniformly fills the intestine, and colonic haustral markings are clearly apparent. The intestinal walls collapse as the patient expels the barium, and the mucosa has a regular, feathery appearance on the postevacuation film.
- *Double-contrast enema:* The intestines uniformly distend with air and have a thin layer of barium, providing excellent detail of the mucosal pattern.

ABNORMAL RESULTS

- An adenocarcinoma or sarcoma occurring higher in the intestine may be identified.
- Abnormal results may indicate a carcinoma, as either a localized filling defect with a sharp transition between normal and necrotic mucosa or circumferential with an "apple core" appearance (characteristics that help distinguish a carcinoma from the more diffuse lesions of inflammatory disease).
- Inflammatory disease, such as diverticulitis, ulcerative colitis, and granulomatous colitis, may be identified.
- Saccular adenomatous polyps, broad-based villous polyps, structural changes in the intestine (such as intussusception, sigmoid volvulus, sigmoid torsion, gastroenteritis, irritable colon, and vascular injury) may be identified.

A look at barium enema

Anteroposterior X-ray of the large intestine after a barium enema. Air has been introduced into the intestine through the enema tube after evacuation of most of the barium.

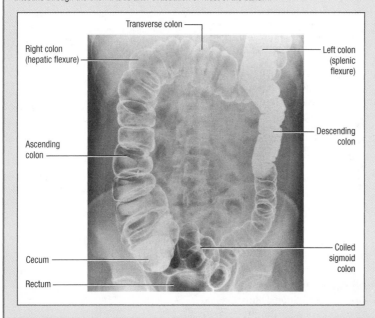

Transverse colon

Right colon (hepatic flexure)

Left colon (splenic flexure)

Ascending colon

Descending colon

Cecum

Coiled sigmoid colon

Rectum

Barium swallow test

DESCRIPTION

◆ Examination of the pharynx and esophagus after ingesting thick and thin mixtures of barium sulfate
◆ Usually part of the upper GI series; indicated in patients with histories of dysphagia and regurgitation

PURPOSE

◆ To diagnose hiatal hernia, diverticula, and varices
◆ To detect strictures, ulcers, tumors, polyps, and motility disorders

PREPARATION

◆ The patient must fast after midnight the night before the test.
◆ The patient's diet is restricted for 2 to 3 days before the test.
◆ The patient will first receive a thick mixture, then a thin one; he must drink 12 to 14 oz (360 to 420 ml) during the examination.
◆ Reassure the patient about safety precautions regarding the tilting X-ray table.
◆ Instruct the patient to put on a gown without snap closures and to remove jewelry, dentures, hair clips, or other radiopaque objects.

Teaching points

◆ Explain that this test evaluates the function of the pharynx and esophagus.
◆ Instruct the patient to fast after midnight the night before the test.
◆ Explain that the patient may be given a restricted diet for 2 to 3 days before the test.
◆ Describe the milk shake consistency and chalky taste of the barium preparation and that it may be unpleasant to swallow.
◆ Inform the patient that he'll be placed in various positions on a tilting X-ray table and that X-rays will be taken.
◆ Explain who will perform the test and where it'll be done.
◆ Tell the patient that the test takes about 30 minutes.

◆ Explain that stools will be chalky and light-colored for 24 to 72 hours after the test.

KEY STEPS

◆ Confirm the patient's identity using two patient identifiers according to facility policy.
◆ The patient is placed in an upright position behind the fluoroscopic screen, and his heart, lungs, and abdomen are examined.
◆ The patient is instructed to take one swallow of the thick barium mixture; pharyngeal action is recorded using cineradiography.
◆ The patient is instructed to take several swallows of the thin barium mixture. Passage of the barium is examined fluoroscopically.
◆ To accentuate small strictures or demonstrate dysphagia, the patient may be asked to swallow a "barium marshmallow" (soft white bread soaked in barium) or a barium pill.
◆ The patient is then secured to the X-ray table and rotated to Trendelenburg's position to evaluate esophageal peristalsis or demonstrate hiatal hernia and gastric reflux.
◆ The patient is instructed to take several swallows of barium while the esophagus is examined fluoroscopically.
◆ After the table is rotated to a horizontal position, the patient takes several swallows of barium so that the esophagogastric junction and peristalsis may be evaluated.
◆ Passage of the barium is fluoroscopically observed, and spot films are taken with the patient in the supine and prone positions.
◆ During fluoroscopic examination of the esophagus, the stomach and duodenum are also carefully studied because neoplasms in these areas may invade the esophagus and cause obstruction.

POSTPROCEDURE CARE

◆ Ensure that additional films and fluoroscopic evaluation haven't been ordered before allowing the patient to resume his usual diet.
◆ Instruct the patient to drink plenty of fluids, unless contraindicated, to help eliminate the barium.
◆ Give a cathartic, if prescribed. Tell the patient to notify the practitioner if he fails to expel the barium in 2 or 3 days.

PRECAUTIONS

◆ A poor swallowing reflex can lead to aspiration of the barium.

COMPLICATIONS

◆ Possible hardening of barium retained in the intestine, causing obstruction or fecal impaction
◆ Abdominal distention and absent bowel sounds, which may indicate constipation and suggest barium impaction

NORMAL RESULTS

◆ The swallowed barium bolus pours over the base of the tongue into the pharynx.
◆ A peristaltic wave propels the bolus through the entire length of the esophagus in about 2 seconds.
◆ When the wave reaches the base of the esophagus, the cardiac sphincter opens, allowing the bolus to enter the stomach. After passage of the bolus, the cardiac sphincter closes.
◆ The bolus evenly fills and distends the lumen of the pharynx and esophagus, and the mucosa appears smooth and regular.

ABNORMAL RESULTS

◆ Hiatal hernia, diverticula, and varices may be diagnosed; pulmonary aspiration may occur in patients with dysphagia.
◆ Strictures, tumors, polyps, ulcers, and motility disorders may be detected (definitive diagnosis requires further testing).

Basal gastric secretion test

DESCRIPTION

- Measures basal secretion during fasting by aspiration of stomach contents through a nasogastric (NG) tube
- Indicated in the patient with obscure epigastric pain, anorexia, and weight loss

PURPOSE

- To determine gastric output while the patient is fasting

PREPARATION

- The test requires insertion of a tube through the patient's nose and into his stomach.
- The patient must restrict food for 12 hours, and fluids and smoking for 8 hours, before the test.
- Notify the laboratory and practitioner of drugs the patient is taking that may affect test results; it may be necessary to restrict these drugs. If the patient must continue these drugs, note this on the laboratory request.
- Check the patient's pulse rate and blood pressure just before the test.
- Encourage the patient to relax.

Teaching points

- Explain that the test measures the stomach's secretion of acid.
- Instruct the patient to restrict food for 12 hours, and fluids and smoking for 8 hours, before the test.
- Inform the patient that the test requires insertion of a tube through his nose and into his stomach, that he may initially experience discomfort, and that he may cough or gag.
- To prevent contamination of the specimens with saliva, instruct the patient to expectorate excess saliva.
- Explain who will perform the test and where it'll be done.
- Tell the patient that the test takes about 1½ hours.

DIAGNOSTIC PROCEDURE

KEY STEPS

- Confirm the patient's identity using two patient identifiers according to facility policy.
- Insert the NG tube after seating the patient comfortably.
- Attach a 20-ml syringe to the tube, and aspirate the stomach contents.
- Ensure complete emptying of the stomach by asking the patient to assume three positions in sequence — supine and right and left lateral decubitus — while aspirating the stomach contents.
- Label the specimen container "residual contents."
- Connect the NG tube to the suction machine. Aspirate the gastric contents by continuous low suction for 1 hour. It's also possible to perform aspiration manually with a syringe.
- Collect a specimen every 15 minutes, but discard the first two; this eliminates the specimens that could be affected by the stress of intubation.
- Record the color and odor of each specimen, and note the presence of food, mucus, bile, or blood.
- Label these specimens "basal contents," and number them 1 through 4.
- Measure secretion volume and acid concentration.
- Monitor the patient's vital signs during the intubation, and observe for arrhythmias.

POSTPROCEDURE CARE

- If the NG tube will remain in place, clamp it or attach it to low intermittent suction.
- Provide soothing lozenges for a sore throat.
- Instruct the patient that he may resume his usual diet and medications, unless the gastric acid stimulation test will also be performed.

PRECAUTIONS

- Instruct the patient to expectorate excess saliva to prevent contamination of gastric specimens with saliva.

- Send the specimen to the laboratory as soon as the collection is completed.

COMPLICATIONS

- Nausea, vomiting, and abdominal distention or pain after removal of the NG tube
- NG tube entering the trachea instead of the esophagus during insertion; remove NG tube immediately, if the patient develops cyanosis or paroxysmal coughing

NORMAL RESULTS

- Basal gastric secretion levels of 1 to 5 mEq/hour, for men, are considered normal.
- Basal gastric secretion levels of 0.2 to 3.3 mEq/hour, for women, are considered normal.

ABNORMAL RESULTS

- Abnormal findings are nonspecific and must be considered with the results of the gastric acid stimulation test.
- Elevated secretion levels may suggest a duodenal or jejunal ulcer (after partial gastrectomy); markedly elevated secretion suggests Zollinger-Ellison syndrome.
- Depressed secretion levels may indicate gastric carcinoma or a benign gastric ulcer.
- The absence of secretion may indicate pernicious anemia.

INTERFERING FACTORS *Cholinergics, reserpine, alcohol, adrenergic-receptor blockers, and adrenocorticosteroids (possible increase); antacids, anticholinergics, histamine-2 receptor blockers, and proton pump inhibitors (possible decrease)*

Basophil count

DESCRIPTION
- Measures peripheral serum basophils, which increase in number during infection and accumulate at the site of infection or inflammation

PURPOSE
- To determine the number of basophils in a peripheral blood smear
- To aid in determining specific conditions related to basophil counts such as myeloproliferative disease

PREPARATION
- This test requires a blood sample.
- No dietary restrictions are required.

Teaching points
- Explain the purpose of the test and how it's done.
- Explain to the patient that the test requires a blood sample and that he may experience slight discomfort from the tourniquet and needle puncture.
- Explain who will perform the test and where it'll be done.
- Tell the patient he need not restrict food or fluids.
- Tell the patient that the test should take less than 5 minutes.

KEY STEPS
- Confirm the patient's identity using two patient identifiers according to facility policy.
- Perform a venipuncture to collect the sample.

POSTPROCEDURE CARE
- Apply direct pressure to the venipuncture site until bleeding stops.

PRECAUTIONS
- Maintain standard precautions while collecting the sample.

COMPLICATIONS
- Hematoma at the venipuncture site

NORMAL RESULTS
- A normal peripheral blood smear infrequently contains basophils.

ABNORMAL RESULTS
- Basophilic leukocytosis is linked to myeloproliferative disease (myelofibrosis, agnogenic myeloid metaplasia, and polycythemia vera).
- A rapid decrease in basophils is linked to an anaphylactic reaction.

Bence Jones protein (urine) level test

DESCRIPTION

◆ Detects the presence of Bence Jones proteins, which are abnormal low-molecular-weight, light-chain immunoglobulins derived from the clone of a single plasma cell
◆ Appear in the urine of 50% to 80% of patients with multiple myeloma and that of most patients with Waldenström's macroglobulinemia
◆ Thermal coagulation and Bradshaw's tests used for screening for Bence Jones proteins, but urine immunoelectrophoresis preferred for quantitative studies (serum immunoelectrophoresis less sensitive than other tests)
◆ Urine and serum studies usually used together when multiple myeloma is suspected

PURPOSE

◆ To confirm the presence of multiple myeloma in the patient with symptoms such as bone pain (especially in the back and the thorax) and persistent anemia and fatigue

PREPARATION

◆ The test requires an early-morning urine specimen.

Teaching points

◆ Explain that this test detects an abnormal protein level in the urine.
◆ Explain to the patient that the test requires an early-morning urine specimen; teach him how to collect a midstream clean-catch specimen.

KEY STEPS

◆ Confirm the patient's identity using two patient identifiers according to facility policy.
◆ Instruct the patient to collect an early-morning urine specimen of at least 50 ml.
◆ Instruct the patient not to contaminate the urine specimen with toilet tissue or feces.
◆ Send the specimen to the laboratory immediately after collection, or refrigerate it if transport is delayed.
◆ Ensure that a refrigerated specimen is analyzed within 24 hours, or arrange for it to be discarded.

POSTPROCEDURE CARE

◆ Answer the patient's questions.

PRECAUTIONS

◆ Maintain standard precautions while handling the specimen.
◆ Send the specimen to the laboratory immediately.

COMPLICATIONS

◆ None known

NORMAL RESULTS

◆ The absence of Bence Jones proteins in a urine specimen is considered normal.

ABNORMAL RESULTS

◆ The presence of Bence Jones proteins in a urine specimen suggests multiple myeloma or Waldenström's macroglobulinemia.
◆ A low level of Bence Jones proteins in the urine of asymptomatic patients may result from benign monoclonal gammopathy.

Beta-hydroxybutyrate assay

DESCRIPTION

- Measures serum levels of beta-hydroxybutyric acid (beta-hydroxybutyrate), one of the three ketone bodies
- Acetoacetate and acetone making up the other two ketone bodies
- Accumulation of all three ketone bodies resulting in ketosis; excessive formation of ketone bodies in the blood resulting in ketonemia

PURPOSE

- To diagnose carbohydrate deprivation, which may result from starvation, digestive disturbances, dietary imbalances, or frequent vomiting
- To aid in the diagnosis of diabetes mellitus resulting from decreased carbohydrate intake
- To aid in the diagnosis of glycogen storage diseases, specifically von Gierke's disease
- To diagnose or monitor the treatment of metabolic disorders, such as diabetic ketoacidosis or lactic acidosis

PREPARATION

- This test requires a blood sample.
- No dietary restrictions are required.

Teaching points

- Explain that this test evaluates ketones in the blood.
- Tell the patient that the test requires a blood sample and that he may experience slight discomfort from the tourniquet and the needle puncture.
- Inform the patient that he need not restrict food or fluids.
- Explain who will perform the test and where it'll be done.
- Tell the patient that the test should take less than 5 minutes.

KEY STEPS

- Confirm the patient's identity using two patient identifiers according to facility policy.
- Perform a venipuncture, and collect the sample in a 5-ml clot activator tube.
- Allow the sample to clot.
- If an acetone level is requested, have this analysis performed first.
- Keep in mind that serum beta-hydroxybutyrate remains stable for at least 1 week at 25.6° to 46.4° F (–3.6° to 8° C). Plasma is also an acceptable sample for beta-hydroxybutyrate analysis.

POSTPROCEDURE CARE

- Apply direct pressure to the venipuncture site until bleeding stops.

PRECAUTIONS

- Maintain standard precautions while collecting the sample.
- Send the sample to the laboratory immediately.

COMPLICATIONS

- Hematoma at the venipuncture site

NORMAL RESULTS

- Levels of beta-hydroxybutyrate of less than 0.4 mmol/L (SI, < 0.4 mmol/L) are considered normal.

ABNORMAL RESULTS

- Increased levels may suggest worsening ketosis. If the reference values are greater than 2 mmol/L (SI, > 2 mmol/L), report this to the patient's practitioner immediately.

Bilirubin level test

DESCRIPTION
◆ Measures serum levels of bilirubin, the predominant pigment in bile
◆ Especially significant in neonates because elevated unconjugated bilirubin can accumulate in the brain, causing irreparable damage

PURPOSE
◆ To evaluate liver function
◆ To aid in the differential diagnosis of jaundice and monitor its progress
◆ To aid in the diagnosis of biliary obstruction and hemolytic anemia
◆ To determine whether a neonate requires an exchange transfusion or phototherapy because of dangerously high unconjugated bilirubin levels

PREPARATION
◆ This test requires a blood sample. If the patient is an infant, the sample will be drawn from his heel.
◆ The adult patient should fast for at least 4 hours before the test; fasting isn't required for the neonate.

Teaching points
◆ Explain that this test evaluates liver function and the condition of red blood cells.
◆ Tell the patient that the test requires a blood sample and that he may experience slight discomfort from the tourniquet and the needle puncture

⚡ **WARNING** *If the patient is an infant, tell the parents that a small amount of blood will be drawn from his heel.*

◆ Inform the adult patient that he need not restrict fluids, but he should fast for at least 4 hours before the test. Fasting isn't necessary for the neonate.
◆ Explain who will perform the test and where it'll be done.
◆ Tell the patient that the test should take less than 5 minutes.

KEY STEPS
◆ Confirm the patient's identity using two patient identifiers according to facility policy.
◆ If the patient is an adult, perform a venipuncture, and collect the sample in a 3- or 4-ml clot activator tube.
◆ If the patient is an infant, perform a heelstick, and fill the microcapillary tube to the designated level with blood.

POSTPROCEDURE CARE
◆ Apply direct pressure to the venipuncture site until bleeding stops.

PRECAUTIONS
◆ Maintain standard precautions while collecting the sample.
◆ Handle the sample gently to prevent hemolysis.
◆ Protect the sample from light.
◆ Send the sample to the laboratory immediately.

COMPLICATIONS
◆ Hematoma at the venipuncture or heelstick site

NORMAL RESULTS
◆ Indirect serum bilirubin levels of 1.1 mg/dl (SI, 19 µmol/L) and direct serum bilirubin levels of less than 0.5 mg/dl (SI < 6.8 µmol/L), in adults, are considered normal.
◆ Total serum bilirubin levels of 2 to 12 mg/dl (SI, 34 to 205 µmol/L), in neonates, are considered normal.

ABNORMAL RESULTS
◆ Elevated indirect serum bilirubin levels usually indicate hepatic damage.
◆ High levels of indirect serum bilirubin are also likely in severe hemolytic anemia.
◆ If hemolysis continues, direct and indirect bilirubin levels may rise.
◆ Other causes of elevated indirect serum bilirubin levels include congenital enzyme deficiencies such as Gilbert syndrome.
◆ Elevated direct serum bilirubin levels usually indicate biliary obstruction.
◆ If obstruction continues, direct and indirect bilirubin levels may rise.
◆ In severe chronic hepatic damage, direct serum bilirubin concentrations may return to normal or near-normal levels, but indirect bilirubin levels remain elevated.
◆ In neonates, total serum bilirubin levels of 15 mg/dl (SI, 257 µmol/L) or more indicate the need for an exchange transfusion.

Bioterrorism infectious agents test

DESCRIPTION

◆ Identifies organisms associated with bioterrorism, which most commonly include botulism, anthrax, hemorrhagic fever, Hantaan virus, Ebola virus, yellow fever, plague, smallpox, and tularemia
◆ Collection of specimen varying based on agent and site of entry (see *Understanding bioterrorism infectious agents*)
◆ Collection methods including cultures from blood, sputum, urine, emesis or gastric aspirate, stools, lymph node aspirate, and scraping of lesions

PURPOSE

◆ To isolate and identify the causative organism

PREPARATION

◆ No dietary restrictions are required.
◆ If botulism is suspected, electromyography may be done to identify the cause of acute flaccid paralysis.

Teaching points

◆ Explain that this test is used to help identify the organism causing the patient's signs and symptoms.
◆ Inform the patient that he need not restrict food or fluids.
◆ Explain who will perform the test and where it'll be done.
◆ Explain to the patient how many samples will need to be collected.
◆ Tell the patient that suspected cases of infection must be reported to local, state, and federal health departments.

DIAGNOSTIC PROCEDURE

KEY STEPS

◆ Confirm the patient's identity using two patient identifiers according to facility policy.
◆ Obtain the specimens as ordered based on the specific infectious agent suspected.
◆ Place blood samples on ice; refrigerate all specimens for botulinum toxin testing.
◆ Send the specimen to the laboratory for a mouse assay to evaluate for botulinum toxin.
◆ Collect vesicular fluid from a previously unopened lesion on at least one culture swab when testing for cutaneous anthrax and smallpox.
◆ Obtain three blood cultures, along with specimens of gastric aspirate, stools, or food, if GI anthrax is suspected.

Understanding bioterrorism infectious agents

The table below lists several possible bioterrorism infectious agents along with the modes of transmission and entry and what specimens may be collected for testing.

INFECTIOUS AGENT	MODE OF TRANSMISSION	MODE OF ENTRY	SPECIMEN FOR TESTING
Clostridium botulinum (spore-forming obligate anaerobe causing botulism)	◆ Soil ◆ Undercooked food not kept warm	◆ Mucosal surface (GI tract, lung) ◆ Wound	◆ Blood, stool, gastric aspirate, emesis ◆ Suspected contaminated food substance
Bacillus anthracis (spore-forming, gram-positive bacillus causing anthrax)	◆ Undercooked meat from infected animals ◆ Inhalation of animal products such as the animal's wool ◆ Intentional release of spores	◆ Skin ◆ Inhalation ◆ GI tract	◆ Blood, sputum, or stool ◆ Fluid from lesion
Viruses causing hemorrhagic fever and yellow fever (including Hantaan virus, Ebola virus)	◆ Bite of infected animal, rodent, or insect	◆ Skin	◆ Blood, sputum, tissue, or urine
Yersinia pestis (causing plague)	◆ Infected flea bite	◆ Skin	◆ Blood, sputum, or lymph node aspirate
Variola virus (causing smallpox)	◆ Airborne via coughing ◆ Direct contact ◆ Contaminated clothing or bedding	◆ Lungs	◆ Fluid from lesion
Francisella tularensis (intracellular parasite causing tularemia)	◆ Infected animals, such as mice, squirrels, or rabbits ◆ Contaminated water, soil, or vegetation	◆ Skin, mucous membranes ◆ Lungs ◆ GI tract	◆ Respiratory secretions and blood ◆ Lymph node biopsy ◆ Lesion scrapings

- When obtaining specimens for tularemia, have the patient provide a forced deep cough for a sputum specimen; obtain a lesional specimen from the leading edge of the lesion.
- Send food that's being tested for botulism in its original container.

POSTPROCEDURE CARE
- If a blood sample is obtained, apply pressure at the venipuncture site until bleeding stops.
- Notify appropriate local, state, and federal health agencies of suspected infection.
- Provide emotional support to the patient.

PRECAUTIONS
- Maintain standard precautions during collection of sample.
- Institute airborne precautions and use negative pressure rooms for patients with suspected infection of hemorrhagic fever, Hantaan virus, Ebola virus, and yellow fever.
- Make sure that specimens being examined for smallpox are performed in a Biosafety laboratory (level 4); specimens for other infections are performed in a Biosafety laboratory (level 2).

COMPLICATIONS
- Not adhering to strict infection precautions
- Hematoma at venipuncture site, if blood is drawn
- Transmission of disease

INTERPRETATION

NORMAL RESULTS
- Normal culture results are negative for the suspected organism.
- The response to repetitive nerve stimulation reveals no increase, if electromyography is done for suspected botulism.

ABNORMAL RESULTS
- Evidence of growth of the causative agent indicates infection.

Bladder tumor markers

OVERVIEW

DESCRIPTION
◆ Substances produced and secreted by bladder tumor cells that help determine tumor activity
◆ Include two urine tumor markers specific for bladder cancer — bladder tumor antigen (BTA) and nuclear matrix protein 22 (NMP22)
◆ BTA produced by bladder cancer cells
◆ NMP22 excreted in the urine when the nucleus of the bladder cancer cells becomes disrupted
◆ NMP22 found in patients who are at high risk for recurrence of bladder cancer and in those who are at risk for developing bladder cancer

PURPOSE
◆ To monitor for and detect bladder cancer recurrence
◆ To identify individuals at risk for bladder cancer

PREPARATION
◆ The test may be helpful in monitoring the patient's disorder.
◆ No dietary restrictions are required.

Teaching points
◆ Explain that this test may be helpful in monitoring the patient's disorder.
◆ Inform the patient that the procedure involves collecting a urine specimen.
◆ Tell the patient that he need not restrict food or fluids.
◆ Explain how to collect the urine specimen and when it'll be done.
◆ Explain that the test should take less than 10 minutes.

DIAGNOSTIC PROCEDURE

KEY STEPS
◆ Confirm the patient's identity using two patient identifiers according to facility policy.
◆ Obtain a random voided urine specimen before noon.

POSTPROCEDURE CARE
◆ Answer the patient's questions.

PRECAUTIONS
◆ Send the specimen to the laboratory immediately.
◆ Refrigerate the specimen if there will be a delay in transport.

COMPLICATIONS
◆ None known

INTERPRETATION

NORMAL RESULTS
◆ Levels of BTA of less than 14 units/ml and of NMP22 of less than 10 units/ml are considered normal.
◆ Normal levels indicate a low risk of bladder cancer or the absence of bladder cancer.

ABNORMAL RESULTS
◆ Elevated BTA and NMP22 levels indicate bladder cancer.
◆ Elevated NMP22 levels alone may be associated with a high risk of bladder cancer.

Bleeding time test

DESCRIPTION

- Measures the duration of bleeding after a measured skin incision
- Three methods of measuring bleeding: template, Ivy, and Duke
- Template method the most common and the most accurate because the incision size is standardized
- Depends on the elasticity of the blood vessel wall and on the number and functional capacity of platelets
- Most commonly for the patient with a personal or family history of bleeding disorders but also useful for preoperative screening
- Usually not recommended for a patient with a platelet count of less than $75 \times 10^3/\mu l$ (SI, $75 \times 10^9/L$).

PURPOSE

- To assess overall hemostatic function (platelet response to injury and functional capacity of vasoconstriction)
- To detect platelet function disorders

PREPARATION

- No dietary restrictions are required.
- Notify the laboratory and practitioner of drugs the patient is taking that may affect test results; it may be necessary to restrict these drugs.

Teaching points

- Explain to the patient that the bleeding time test measures the time it takes to form a clot and stop bleeding.
- Inform the patient that he need not restrict food or fluids.
- Inform the patient that he may feel some discomfort from the incisions, the antiseptic, and the tightness of the blood pressure cuff.
- Inform the patient that, depending on the method used, incisions or punctures may leave tiny scars that should be barely visible when healed.
- Explain who will perform the test and where it'll be done.
- Tell the patient that the test should take less than 30 minutes.

KEY STEPS

- Confirm the patient's identity using two patient identifiers according to facility policy.
- *Template method:* Wrap the blood pressure cuff around the upper arm, and inflate the cuff to 40 mm Hg. Select an area on the patient's forearm with no superficial veins; clean it with antiseptic. Allow the skin to dry completely before making the incision. Apply the appropriate template lengthwise onto the forearm. Use a lancet to make two incisions (1 mm deep and 9 mm long). Start the stopwatch. Without touching the cuts, gently blot the drops of blood with filter paper every 30 seconds until the bleeding stops in both cuts. Average the bleeding times of the two cuts, and record the result.
- *Ivy method:* After applying the blood pressure cuff and preparing the test site, make three small puncture wounds with a disposable lancet. Start the stopwatch immediately. Taking care not to touch the wounds, blot each site with filter paper every 30 seconds until the bleeding stops. Average the bleeding times of the three wounds, and record the result.
- *Duke method:* Drape the patient's shoulder with a towel. Clean the earlobe, and let it air-dry. Make a puncture wound 2 to 4 mm deep on the earlobe with a disposable lancet. Start the stopwatch. Being careful not to touch the ear, blot the site with filter paper every 30 seconds until the bleeding stops. Record the bleeding time.
- Be sure to maintain the cuff pressure at 40 mm Hg throughout the template and Ivy method tests.
- If bleeding hasn't slowed after 15 minutes, stop the test and apply direct pressure to the site.

POSTPROCEDURE CARE

- In a patient with a bleeding tendency (hemophilia), maintain a pressure bandage over the incision for 24 to 48 hours to prevent further bleeding.

Check the test area frequently; keep the edges of the cuts aligned, to minimize scarring.

- In other patients, a piece of gauze held in place by an adhesive bandage is sufficient.
- Instruct the patient that he may resume medications stopped before the test.

PRECAUTIONS

- Maintain standard precautions throughout the test.

 WARNING *If the bleeding doesn't stop in 15 minutes, stop the test.*

COMPLICATIONS

- Bleeding that doesn't slow after 15 minutes

NORMAL RESULTS

- Normal bleeding times are 3 to 6 minutes (SI, 3 to 6 minutes) in the template method; 3 to 6 minutes (SI, 3 to 6 minutes) in the Ivy method; and 1 to 3 minutes (SI, 1 to 3 minutes) in the Duke method.

ABNORMAL RESULTS

- Prolonged bleeding time may indicate disorders linked to thrombocytopenia, such as Hodgkin's disease, acute leukemia, disseminated intravascular coagulation, hemolytic disease of the newborn, Schönlein-Henoch purpura, severe hepatic disease (cirrhosis, for example), or severe deficiency of factors I, II, V, VII, VIII, IX, and XI.
- Prolonged bleeding time in a patient with a normal platelet count suggests a platelet function disorder (thrombasthenia, thrombocytopathia) and requires further investigation with clot retraction, prothrombin consumption, and platelet aggregation tests.

INTERFERING FACTORS *Anticoagulants, nonsteroidal anti-inflammatory drugs, aspirin and aspirin compounds (prolonged bleeding time)*

Blood culture

DESCRIPTION

- Involves inoculating a culture medium with a blood sample, incubating it for isolation, and identifying the causative pathogens in bacteremia and septicemia
- Identifies about 67% of pathogens within 24 hours, and up to 90% within 72 hours
- Timing of the specimen collection dependent on type of suspected bacteremia and whether drug therapy needs to restart regardless of test results

PURPOSE

- To confirm a diagnosis of bacteremia
- To identify the causative organism in bacteremia and septicemia
- To determine the cause of fever with an unknown origin

PREPARATION

- The test requires blood samples.
- No dietary restrictions are required.

Teaching points

- Explain the purpose of the test and how it's done.
- Inform the patient that he need not restrict food or fluids.
- Explain that the test requires several blood samples and that he may feel transient discomfort from the tourniquet and the needle punctures.
- Explain who will perform the test and when it'll be done.
- Tell the patient that the test usually takes less than 5 minutes.
- Tell the patient the number of samples that will be needed.

DIAGNOSTIC PROCEDURE

KEY STEPS

- Confirm the patient's identity using two patient identifiers according to facility policy.
- Clean the venipuncture site, first with an alcohol swab and then with a povidone-iodine swab, starting at the site and working outward in a circular motion.
- Wait at least 1 minute for the skin to dry.
- Perform a venipuncture, and draw 10 to 20 ml of blood for an adult, or 2 to 6 ml for a child.
- Clean the diaphragm tops of the culture bottles with alcohol or iodine, and change the needle on the syringe.
- If using broth medium, add blood to each bottle until achieving a 1:5 or 1:10 dilution. (For example, add 10 ml of blood to a 100-ml bottle.) Note that the size of the bottle may vary depending on hospital protocol.
- If using a special resin, add blood to the resin in the bottles according to facility protocol, and invert gently to mix.
- Draw the blood directly into a special collection and processing tube, if using the lysis-centrifugation technique (Isolator).
- Document the tentative diagnosis and current or recent antimicrobial therapy on the laboratory request.
- Send each sample to the laboratory immediately.
- Collect blood cultures before giving antimicrobials whenever possible, because previous or current antimicrobial therapy may give false-negative results.
- To detect most causative agents, it's best to perform the blood culture tests on 2 consecutive days.

POSTPROCEDURE CARE

- Use alcohol to remove the iodine from the venipuncture site.
- Monitor the venipuncture site for bleeding and signs of infection.

PRECAUTIONS

- Maintain standard precautions while collecting the samples.
- Send each sample to the laboratory immediately after collection.
- Collect blood cultures before giving antimicrobials, if possible.

COMPLICATIONS

- Hematoma at the venipuncture site

INTERPRETATION

NORMAL RESULTS

- Blood cultures are normally sterile.
- For negative specimens, make reports at 24 hours, 48 hours, and 1 week of incubation.

ABNORMAL RESULTS

- Positive blood cultures don't necessarily confirm pathologic septicemia.
- Mild, transient bacteremia may occur during the course of many infectious diseases or may complicate other disorders.
- Persistent, continuous, or recurrent bacteremia reliably confirms the presence of serious infection.
- Although 2% to 3% of cultured blood samples are contaminated by skin bacteria, such as *Staphylococcus epidermidis*, diphtheroids, and *Propionibacterium*, these organisms may be clinically significant when isolated from multiple cultures or from immunocompromised patients.
- Blood cultures from debilitated or immunocompromised patients may show isolates of *Candida albicans*.

⬤ **INTERFERING FACTORS** *Improper collection techniques (sample contamination)*

Blood smear

DESCRIPTION

- Provides information about drugs and disease that may affect red blood cells (RBCs) and white blood cells (WBCs)
- Identifies leukemia, infection, infestation, and other diseases
- Detects RBC, platelet, and WBC cell lines
- Able to detect five types of WBCs: neutrophils, eosinophils, basophils, lymphocytes, and monocytes
- Allows examination of WBCs for quantity, differential count, and maturity
- Allows comparison of RBCs for variations in size, shape, color, and intracellular content
- Classification of RBCs based on variations helps identify causes of anemias and other diseases
- Facilitates estimation of platelet count

PURPOSE

- To obtain information regarding RBCs, WBCs, and platelets for diagnostic purposes

PREPARATION

- The test requires a blood sample.
- No dietary restrictions are required.

Teaching points

- Tell the patient that this test looks at the components in his blood.
- Tell the patient that the test requires a blood sample and that he may experience slight discomfort from the tourniquet and needle puncture.
- Tell the patient that he need not restrict food or fluids.
- Explain who will perform the test and where it'll be done.
- Tell the patient that the test should take less than 5 minutes.

KEY STEPS

- Confirm the patient's identity using two patient identifiers according to facility policy.
- Perform a venipuncture, and collect the sample in an EDTA tube.

POSTPROCEDURE CARE

- Apply direct pressure to the venipuncture site until bleeding stops.

PRECAUTIONS

- Maintain standard precautions while collecting the sample.
- Handle the sample gently to prevent hemolysis.

COMPLICATIONS

- Hematoma at the venipuncture site

NORMAL RESULTS

- Blood smear test results show normal RBC, WBC, and platelet characteristics.

ABNORMAL RESULTS

- An increase in immature WBCs indicates leukemia or infection.
- Decreased WBCs indicates bone marrow failure to produce WBCs; this may result from fibrosis, neoplasia, or drugs.
- RBC abnormalities indicate various anemias and diseases, depending on the aspect of the RBC that's abnormal.

Blood urea nitrogen level test

DESCRIPTION

- Measures the nitrogen fraction of urea, the chief end product of protein metabolism, which is formed in the liver from ammonia and excreted by the kidneys (constitutes 40% to 50% of the blood's nonprotein nitrogen)
- Reflects protein intake and renal excretory capacity but a less reliable indicator of uremia than the serum creatinine level
- Also called *BUN*

PURPOSE

- To evaluate kidney function and aid in the diagnosis of renal disease
- To aid in the assessment of hydration

PREPARATION

- The test requires a blood sample.
- The patient should avoid a diet high in meat before the test.
- Notify the laboratory and practitioner of drugs the patient is taking that may affect test results; these drugs may need to be restricted.

Teaching points

- Explain that this test is used to evaluate kidney function.
- Inform the patient that he need not restrict food or fluids but that he should avoid a diet high in meat before the test.
- Tell the patient that the test requires a blood sample and that he may experience slight discomfort from the tourniquet and the needle puncture.
- Explain who will perform the test and where it'll be done.
- Tell the patient that the test should take less than 5 minutes.

KEY STEPS

- Confirm the patient's identity using two patient identifiers according to facility policy.
- Perform a venipuncture, and collect the sample in a 3- to 4-ml clot activator tube.

POSTPROCEDURE CARE

- Apply direct pressure to the venipuncture site until bleeding stops.
- Inform the patient that he may resume his usual medications stopped before the test.

PRECAUTIONS

- Maintain standard precautions while collecting the sample.
- Handle the sample gently to prevent hemolysis.

COMPLICATIONS

- Hematoma at the venipuncture site

NORMAL RESULTS

- BUN levels should be 8 to 20 mg/dl (SI, 2.9 to 7.5 mmol/L).

ABNORMAL RESULTS

- Elevated BUN levels may indicate renal disease, reduced renal blood flow (caused by dehydration, for example), urinary tract obstruction, or increased protein catabolism (as in burns).
- Decreased BUN levels may indicate severe hepatic damage, malnutrition, or overhydration.

Bone biopsy

DESCRIPTION
- Removal of a piece or a core of bone for histologic examination
- Performed using a special drill needle under local anesthesia (drill biopsy) or by surgical excision under general anesthesia (open biopsy)
- Excision providing a larger specimen than a drill biopsy and permitting immediate surgical treatment, if rapid histologic analysis of the specimen reveals a malignant tumor
- Indicated in patients with bone pain and tenderness for whom a bone scan, computed tomography scan, radiograph, or arteriography reveals a mass or deformity

PURPOSE
- To distinguish between benign and malignant bone tumors

PREPARATION
- Make sure the patient has signed a consent form.
- Note and report allergies.
- For a drill biopsy, food and fluid restriction isn't usually necessary.
- For an open biopsy, patient must fast after midnight the night before the test.
- Give the patient a local anesthetic before a drill biopsy.

Teaching points
- Explain the purpose of the test and how it's done.
- Explain who will perform the test and where it'll be done.
- Warn the patient that he'll experience some discomfort and pressure when the biopsy needle enters the bone during a drill biopsy.
- Tell the patient that the test should take less than 30 minutes.

DIAGNOSTIC PROCEDURE

KEY STEPS
- Confirm the patient's identity using two patient identifiers according to facility policy.

Drill biopsy
- The biopsy site is shaved and prepared. After a local anesthetic is given, a small incision (usually about 3 mm) is made.
- The biopsy needle is pushed into the bone using firm, even pressure. The needle is engaged in the bone and rotated about 180 degrees while steady pressure is maintained. When the bone core is obtained, the trocar is withdrawn by reversal of the drilling motion.
- The biopsy specimen is placed in a properly labeled container with 10% formalin solution or Zenker's solution.

Open biopsy
- After the patient is anesthetized, the biopsy site is shaved and prepared. An incision is made, and a piece of bone is removed and sent to the laboratory for immediate histologic analysis.
- The incision is closed, and a sterile dressing is applied.

POSTPROCEDURE CARE
- Apply pressure to the drill biopsy site with a sterile gauze pad until bleeding stops.
- Apply a sterile dressing to a drill or open biopsy site.
- Notify the practitioner of excessive drainage or bleeding at the biopsy site.
- Give the patient an analgesic.
- Resume the patient's usual diet after he fully recovers from anesthesia.
- Monitor the patient's vital signs, and monitor the biopsy site for signs and symptoms of infection.

WARNING *Monitor the patient for signs of bone infection for several days after the biopsy. Report such signs as fever, headache, pain on movement, and redness near the biopsy site.*

PRECAUTIONS
- Check the patient's history for hypersensitivity to the anesthetic.
- Send the specimen to the laboratory immediately.
- Perform the procedure cautiously in patients with coagulopathies.

COMPLICATIONS
- Bone fracture, damage to surrounding tissue, and infection (osteomyelitis)

INTERPRETATION

NORMAL RESULTS
- Normal bone tissue is one of two histologic types: compact or cancellous.
- Compact bone has dense, concentric layers of mineral deposits, or lamellae.
- Cancellous bone has widely spaced lamellae, with osteocytes and red and yellow marrow between them.

ABNORMAL RESULTS
- Well-circumscribed and nonmetastasizing lesions suggest benign tumors, such as osteoid osteoma, osteoblastoma, osteochondroma, unicameral bone cyst, benign giant cell tumor, and fibroma.
- Irregularly and rapidly spreading lesions suggest malignant tumors, such as multiple myeloma and osteosarcoma.

Bone densitometry

DESCRIPTION

- Noninvasive way to measure bone mass
- Uses a radiography tube and computer-analyzed images to measure bone mineral density (BMD)
- Exposes the patient to minimal radiation
- Also called *dual-energy X-ray absorptiometry*

PURPOSE

- To determine BMD
- To identify patients at risk for osteoporosis
- To evaluate clinical response to therapy aimed at reducing the rate of bone loss

PREPARATION

- Remove metal objects from the area to be scanned.

Teaching points

- Explain the purpose of the test and how it's done.
- Explain who will perform the test and where it'll be done.
- Tell the patient that the test is painless and that exposure to radiation is minimal.
- Explain that the test takes from 10 minutes to 1 hour, depending on the areas scanned.

DIAGNOSTIC PROCEDURE

KEY STEPS

- Confirm the patient's identity using two patient identifiers according to facility policy.
- The patient is positioned on a table under the scanning device, with the radiation source below him and the detector above him.
- The lumbar spine and the proximal femur, two sites at high risk for fracture, may be scanned.
- The distal forearm may be scanned (research shows a high correlation between the BMD of this area and the BMD of the spine and femur).
- Bone size, thickness, and volumetric density are calculated to determine potential resistance to mechanical stress.
- The detector measures the bone's absorption of radiation and registers a digital readout. (See *Understanding bone densitometry*.)

POSTPROCEDURE CARE

- Make sure the patient is comfortable after the test.

PRECAUTIONS

- Bone densitometry is contraindicated during pregnancy.

COMPLICATIONS

- None known

INTERPRETATION

NORMAL RESULTS

- A T-score above –1 is considered normal.

ABNORMAL RESULTS

- A T-score between –1 and –2.5 may suggest osteopenia.
- A T-score at or below –2.5 may suggest osteoporosis.

   INTERFERING FACTORS *Osteoarthritis, fractures, size of the region to be scanned and fat tissue distribution*

Understanding bone densitometry

These illustrations show the difference between normal bone and a bone with osteoporosis. The osteoporotic bone has much less density, making it less resistant to trauma.

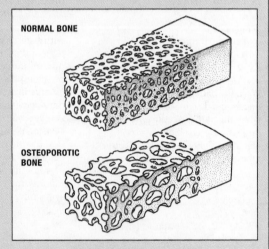

NORMAL BONE

OSTEOPOROTIC BONE

©2007 Lippincott Williams & Wilkins, courtesy of Neil O. Hardy, Westpoint, Connecticut.

Bone marrow aspiration and biopsy

OVERVIEW

DESCRIPTION
◆ Collection of a soft tissue specimen from the medullary canals of long bone and interstices of cancellous bone for histologic and hematologic examination
◆ Performed by aspiration or needle biopsy under local anesthesia
◆ Aspiration biopsy: Removal of a fluid specimen from the bone marrow
◆ Needle biopsy: Removal of a core of marrow cells
◆ Common to perform both methods at the same time, to obtain the best possible specimens

PURPOSE
◆ To diagnose thrombocytopenia, leukemias, granulomas, anemias, and primary and metastatic tumors
◆ To determine causes of infection
◆ To help stage diseases such as Hodgkin's disease
◆ To evaluate chemotherapy
◆ To monitor myelosuppression

PREPARATION
◆ Make sure the patient has signed a consent form. (See *Preparing for bone marrow aspiration and biopsy*.)
◆ Note allergies.
◆ The test requires a blood sample.
◆ Give the patient a mild sedative 1 hour before the test.

Teaching points
◆ Explain the purpose of the test and how it's done.
◆ Explain that a blood sample is required before the biopsy for laboratory testing.
◆ Explain to the patient that he'll feel pressure on insertion of the biopsy needle and a brief, pulling pain on removal of the marrow.
◆ Explain which bone site (sternum, anterior or posterior iliac crest, vertebral spinous process, rib, or tibia) will receive the test.
◆ Tell the patient that the actual test takes only 5 to 10 minutes.

DIAGNOSTIC PROCEDURE

KEY STEPS
◆ Confirm the patient's identity using two patient identifiers according to facility policy.
◆ Position the patient and instruct him to remain as still as possible.

Aspiration biopsy
◆ The biopsy site is prepared and draped, and a local anesthetic is injected. The bone marrow aspiration needle is inserted through the skin, subcutaneous tissue, and bone cortex, using a twisting motion.
◆ The stylet is removed from the aspiration needle, and a 10- to 20-ml syringe is attached. From 0.2 to 0.5 ml of bone marrow is aspirated, and the needle is withdrawn.
◆ If the aspiration specimen is inadequate, the needle may be repositioned within the bone marrow cavity or removed and reinserted in another anesthetized site. If the second attempt fails, a needle biopsy may be necessary.

Needle biopsy
◆ The biopsy site is prepared and draped. The skin is marked at the site with an indelible pencil or marking pen. A local anesthetic is injected intradermally, subcutaneously, and at the surface of the bone.
◆ The biopsy needle is inserted into the periosteum, and the needle guard is set as indicated. Rotating the inner needle alternately clockwise and counterclockwise directs the needle into the bone marrow cavity.
◆ A tissue plug is removed, and the needle assembly is withdrawn. The bone marrow is expelled into a labeled bottle containing a special fixative.

POSTPROCEDURE CARE
◆ Apply pressure to the biopsy site until bleeding stops, while the bone marrow slides are being prepared.
◆ Clean the biopsy site, and apply a sterile dressing.

◆ Monitor the patient's vital signs, and monitor the biopsy site for signs and symptoms of infection.

PRECAUTIONS
◆ Bone marrow aspiration and biopsy is contraindicated in patients with bleeding disorders.
◆ Send the tissue or specimen to the laboratory immediately.

COMPLICATIONS
◆ Hemorrhage and infection
◆ Puncture of the mediastinum (sternum)

INTERPRETATION

NORMAL RESULTS
◆ Yellow bone marrow contains fat cells and connective tissue.
◆ Red bone marrow contains hematopoietic cells, fat cells, and connective tissue.
◆ The iron stain, which measures hemosiderin (storage iron), has a +2 level.
◆ The Sudan black B stain, which shows granulocytes, is negative.
◆ The periodic acid–Schiff (PAS) stain, which detects glycogen reactions, is negative.

ABNORMAL RESULTS
◆ Decreased hemosiderin levels in an iron stain may indicate a true iron deficiency.
– A positive iron stain can differentiate acute myelogenous leukemia from acute lymphoblastic leukemia (negative stain).
– A positive iron stain may also suggest granulation in myeloblasts.
◆ Increased hemosiderin levels may suggest other types of anemias or blood disorders.
◆ A positive PAS stain may suggest acute or chronic lymphocytic leukemia, amyloidosis, thalassemia, lymphoma, infectious mononucleosis, iron deficiency anemia, or sideroblastic anemia.

(continued)

Preparing for bone marrow aspiration and biopsy

Dear Patient,

Your health care provider has ordered a bone marrow aspiration and biopsy. This test evaluates your bone marrow, which is the soft tissue inside your bone.

An aspiration biopsy involves withdrawing a fluid sample containing bone marrow particles from the marrow. A needle biopsy involves removing a core of solid cells from the marrow. Both tests take about 5 to 10 minutes.

The bone marrow sample is examined under a microscope to determine whether the marrow produces enough normal blood cells and how mature they are. You'll usually know the results in 1 or 2 days.

BEFORE THE TEST

- You may continue your usual diet and fluid intake. However, you may wish to eat lightly before the test.
- Expect to have a blood sample taken.
- You may be given a mild sedative 1 hour before the test to help you relax.

DURING THE TEST

The most common biopsy site is the back of the hip (called the *posterior superior iliac crest*). Other sites include the spine, a leg bone (epiphysis), and the breast bone.

A bone marrow sample is taken from the back of the hip while you lie on your stomach as still as you can. The skin around the site will be draped and the skin cleaned with an antiseptic solution. A local anesthetic will then be injected, which may cause brief discomfort before the area becomes numb.

For aspiration biopsy: An aspiration needle is inserted through the skin, the tissue below, and the cortex of the bone in a twisting motion until it reaches the bone marrow. Then the metal core from the needle is removed, and a bone marrow sample is drawn into the syringe.

For needle biopsy: A biopsy needle is inserted through the skin and underlying tissue and into the bone. Next, the core of the needle is removed. The needle is then advanced and rotated in both directions, forcing a tiny core of bone into the needle.

As the bone marrow sample is collected, you'll feel a pulling or grinding sensation or a brief, sharp pain. After the needle is withdrawn, pressure is applied to the biopsy site for several minutes to stop bleeding. Finally, a bandage is applied to the wound.

AFTER THE TEST

- Rest for several hours.
- Report bleeding that completely soaks the dressing or continues for more than 24 hours.
- Reinforce the dressing, if needed, but don't remove it for at least 24 hours.
- Take medication as directed, if you have discomfort.

Bone scan

OVERVIEW

DESCRIPTION
- Imaging of the skeleton with a scanning camera after I.V. injection of a radioactive tracer compound (radioactive technetium diphosphonate).
- Increased concentrations of the tracer collecting in bone tissue at sites of abnormal metabolism and appearing as hot spots (commonly detectable months before radiography reveals a lesion)
- May be performed with a gallium scan to detect lesions at an early stage
- Indicated for patients with symptoms of metastatic bone disease, patients with bone trauma, and those with known degenerative disorders that require monitoring

PURPOSE
- To detect malignant bone lesions when radiographic findings are normal but cancer is confirmed or suspected
- To rule out suspected bone lesions
- To detect occult bone trauma associated with pathologic fractures
- To monitor degenerative bone disorders
- To detect infection
- To evaluate unexplained bone pain
- To assist in staging cancer

PREPARATION
- Make sure the patient has signed an appropriate consent form, if required.
- Note allergies.
- No dietary restrictions are required.

Teaching points
- Explain the purpose of the test and how it's done.
- Inform the patient that there are no dietary restrictions.
- Instruct the patient to drink fluids to maintain hydration and to reduce the radiation dose to the bladder after the tracer injection and before scanning.
- Explain the importance of holding still during scanning.
- Explain that the scan is painless and that the radioactive isotope emits less radiation than a standard radiography machine.
- Tell the patient that he'll receive analgesics for positional discomfort.
- Tell the patient that the test will take about 1 hour.
- Explain who will perform the test and where it'll be done.

DIAGNOSTIC PROCEDURE

KEY STEPS
- Confirm the patient's identity using two patient identifiers according to facility policy.
- The I.V. tracer and imaging agent are given 3 hours before the scan.
- Encourage increased fluid intake for the next 1 to 3 hours to facilitate the renal clearance of circulating free tracer that isn't picked up by bone.
- Instruct the patient to urinate immediately before the procedure, or insert a urinary catheter to empty the bladder.
- The patient is positioned on the scanner table.
- As the scanner moves over the patient's body, it detects low-level radiation emitted by the skeleton and translates this into a two-dimensional picture.
- The scanner takes as many views as needed to cover the specified area.
- The patient may be repositioned as needed during the test to obtain adequate views.

POSTPROCEDURE CARE
- Instruct the patient to drink additional fluids and to empty his bladder frequently for the next 24 to 48 hours.
- Monitor the patient for signs and symptoms of infection at the injection site.
- Monitor intake and output.

PRECAUTIONS
- A bone scan is contraindicated during pregnancy or lactation.
- Avoid scheduling additional radionuclide tests for the next 24 to 48 hours.

COMPLICATIONS
- Infection at the injection site
- Allergic reactions to radionuclide tracer (rare)

INTERPRETATION

NORMAL RESULTS
- Uptake of the tracer is symmetrical and uniform in normal bone scan results.
- The tracer concentrates at sites of new bone formation or increased metabolism.
- The epiphyses of growing bone are normal sites of high concentration (hot spots).

ABNORMAL RESULTS
- Increased uptake of tracer where bone formation is occurring faster than in surrounding bone may suggest all types of bone cancer, infection, fracture, or additional disorders when used in conjunction with the patient's medical and surgical history, radiographic findings, and laboratory test results.

INTERFERING FACTORS *Antihypertensives; a distended bladder (may obscure pelvic detail)*

Bone turnover biochemical markers

DESCRIPTION

◆ Osteoclasts responsible for bone resorption and osteoblasts for bone formation
◆ Osteoporosis characterized by increased bone resorption and decreased bone formation
◆ Biochemical markers helpful in identifying an improvement in osteoporosis after treatment has been started (not useful in diagnosing osteoporosis due to the fluctuation in bone turnover biochemical marker levels that occur daily): N-telopeptide, osteocalcin, and pyridinium
◆ Also used to monitor the activity in Paget's disease, hyperparathyroidism, and bone metastasis
◆ N-telopeptide (NTx) (protein used in collagen and making up 90% of the bone matrix) released into the bloodstream when bone is broken down and then excreted in the urine
◆ Osteocalcin (noncollagen, vitamin-K-dependent protein made by osteoblasts) enters circulation during bone resorption and formation (a good indicator of bone metabolism)
◆ Pyridinium (PYD) crosslinks (formed when type I collagen matures during bone formation) released into the bloodstream during bone resorption

PURPOSE

◆ Monitor the effectiveness of osteoporosis treatment
◆ Monitor treatment of Paget's disease, hyperparathyroidism, and bone metastasis

PREPARATION

◆ Obtain a baseline level before beginning treatment.
◆ This test requires a urine specimen. Some laboratories require a 24-hour urine specimen.
◆ The test may require a blood sample.
◆ No dietary restrictions are required.

Teaching points

◆ Explain to the patient that this test helps determine how effective his treatment for osteoporosis, or other diseases, has been.
◆ Explain to the patient that this test requires a urine specimen; teach the patient how to collect a clean urine specimen.
◆ If the test requires a venipuncture, for osteocalcin levels, explain to the patient that he may feel slight discomfort from the tourniquet and needle puncture.
◆ Tell the patient that he need not restrict food or fluids.
◆ Explain who will perform the test and where it'll be done.

KEY STEPS

◆ Confirm the patient's identity using two patient identifiers according to facility policy.
◆ Collect a urine specimen from the patient; wait 30 to 40 minutes and collect a second specimen. This helps decrease variability in the levels.
◆ If the test requires a venipuncture, obtain 7 ml of blood in the appropriate tube.

POSTPROCEDURE CARE

◆ Apply pressure to the venipuncture site until bleeding stops.

PRECAUTIONS

◆ Maintain standard precautions while collecting the samples.
◆ Double-voided urine specimens that are collected in the morning are the best indicators of bone turnover biochemical markers.

COMPLICATIONS

◆ Hematoma at the venipuncture site

NORMAL RESULTS

◆ Urine NTx levels should be 26 to 124 nM BCE/mM creatinine for women and of 21 to 83 nM BCE/mM creatinine for men.
◆ Normal serum NTx levels are 6.2 to 19 nm BCE for women and of 5.4 to 24.2 nm BCE for men.
◆ Serum osteocalcin levels of 0.7 to 6.4 ng/ml for women and of 1.1 to 6.4 ng/ml for men are normal.
◆ Urine PYD levels of 15.3 to 33.6 nm/mm for women and of 10.3 to 33.6 nm/mm for men are normal.
◆ Normal findings indicate a balance between bone resorption and formation.

ABNORMAL RESULTS

◆ Increased levels of bone turnover biochemical markers are seen in osteoporosis, Paget's disease, bone tumors, acromegaly, hyperparathyroidism, and hyperthyroidism.
◆ Increased levels in children are associated with bone resorption and remodeling of the long bones.
◆ Decreased levels are associated with hypoparathyroidism, hypothyroidism, and cortisol therapy.

🔹 **INTERFERING FACTORS** *Estrogen, alendronate, calcitonin, and raloxifene (decreased resorption and decreased bone turnover biochemical marker levels); testosterone (lower NTx levels)*

Breast biopsy

DESCRIPTION

- Allows histologic examination of breast tissue to confirm or rule out cancer
- Needle biopsy or fine-needle biopsy: Obtains a core of tissue or a fluid aspirate; of limited diagnostic value because it may obtain small and unrepresentative specimens
- Open biopsy: Provides a complete tissue specimen, which allows sectioning of the specimen and a more accurate evaluation
- Breast tissue analysis usually including an estrogen and progesterone receptor assay to aid in selecting therapy for an identified malignancy
- Indicated in palpable masses; suspicious areas on mammography; bloody discharge from the nipples; and persistently encrusted, inflamed, or eczematoid breast lesions.

PURPOSE

- To differentiate between benign and malignant breast tumors

PREPARATION

- Make sure the patient has signed a consent form.
- Note and report allergies.
- Obtain and report abnormal results of prebiopsy studies, such as blood tests, urine tests, and chest X-rays.
- No dietary restrictions are required if the patient will undergo local anesthesia; if the patient will have general anesthesia, she should have nothing by mouth after midnight before the procedure.

Teaching points

- If the patient will undergo local anesthesia, tell her that she need not restrict food or fluids.
- If the patient will undergo general anesthesia, tell her that she is to have nothing by mouth after midnight before the procedure.
- Explain the purpose of the test and how it's done.
- Tell the patient that the test takes 15 to 30 minutes.
- Tell the patient that a breast mass doesn't always indicate cancer.
- Inform the patient that she must wear a support bra at all times after the test, until healing is complete.

DIAGNOSTIC PROCEDURE

KEY STEPS

- Confirm the patient's identity using two patient identifiers according to facility policy.

Needle biopsy

- The site is prepared and draped, and the patient is given a local anesthetic.
- The syringe is introduced into the lesion. Aspirated fluid is placed into a labeled, heparinized tube.
- The aspiration procedure is both diagnostic and therapeutic, if cyst fluid is clear yellow and the mass disappears. In this case, the aspirate is discarded.
- If cyst aspiration yields no fluid or the lesion recurs two or three times, an open biopsy is appropriate.
- The tissue is placed in a labeled specimen bottle containing normal saline solution or formalin.
- With fine-needle aspiration, a slide is made for cytology and viewed immediately under a microscope.

Open biopsy

- The site is prepared and draped, and the patient is given a local or general anesthetic.
- An incision is made in the breast to expose the mass. A portion of tissue or the entire mass is excised.
- Benign-appearing masses smaller than 2 cm in diameter are usually excised. The specimens are placed in properly labeled specimen bottles containing 10% formalin solution.
- Malignant-appearing tissue is sent for frozen section and receptor assay analysis.

POSTPROCEDURE CARE

- Apply pressure to the biopsy site until bleeding stops.
- For a needle biopsy, apply a sterile dressing.
- After an open biopsy, the site is sutured and a sterile dressing applied.
- Give the patient an analgesic.
- Apply an ice bag to the site for discomfort.
- Provide emotional support.
- Monitor the patient's vital signs and monitor the biopsy site for bleeding.
- Monitor the patient for signs and symptoms of infection at the biopsy site.

PRECAUTIONS

- Open breast biopsy is contraindicated in patients with conditions that preclude surgery.
- Send all specimens to the laboratory immediately.
- Needle biopsy should be performed only on fluid-filled cysts and advanced malignant lesions.

COMPLICATIONS

- Bleeding and infection

INTERPRETATION

NORMAL RESULTS

- Normal breast tissue consists of cellular and noncellular connective tissue, fat lobules, and various lactiferous ducts.
- Normal breast tissue is pink, more fatty than fibrous, and shows no abnormal development of cells or tissue elements.

ABNORMAL RESULTS

- Benign tumors may suggest fibrocystic disease, adenofibroma, intraductal papilloma, mammary fat necrosis, or plasma cell mastitis.
- Malignant tumors may suggest adenocarcinoma, cystosarcoma, intraductal or infiltrating carcinoma, inflammatory carcinoma, medullary or circumscribed carcinoma, colloid carcinoma, lobular carcinoma, sarcoma, or Paget's disease.

Breast cancer tumor markers

DESCRIPTION

- Used to identify patients who have a higher likelihood of breast cancer recurrence
- Tumor grade, size, histology, and hormone receptors not proven to be reliable indicators of recurrence risk; new tumor markers being sought
- Deoxyribonucleic acid (DNA) ploidy status and S-phase fraction measuring how rapidly the cells in a breast cancer tumor grow
- Cathepsin D (catabolic enzyme present in malignant breast tissue) believed to contribute to the malignant potential of a tumor (exact cutoff point still being determined)
- Levels of HER-2 protein (growth factor existing on the cell membrane) higher in malignant cancers
- *p53* (tumor suppressor gene) expressed at increased levels in aggressive breast cancer cells
- Ki67 protein expression associated with aggressive breast cancers

PURPOSE

- To determine the likelihood of breast cancer recurrence after tumor and lymph node removal
- To help determine the aggressiveness of breast cancer cells as it relates to treatment options

PREPARATION

- Explain to the patient that this test helps determine the course of treatment for her breast cancer, now and in the future.
- Explain to the patient that the specimen is obtained during a breast biopsy.
- If the patient is to undergo general anesthesia for the biopsy, instruct her not to eat or drink after midnight before the night before the test.

Teaching points

- Explain the purpose of the test and how it's done
- Explain who will perform the test and where it'll be done.

- Tell the patient whether the biopsy will be performed with a needle or as an open biopsy.
- Explain dietary restrictions that are required.
- Tell the patient that the test should take less than 1 hour and that results are usually available from the practitioner in 1 week.

DIAGNOSTIC PROCEDURE

KEY STEPS

- Confirm the patient's identity using two patient identifiers according to facility policy.
- During a breast biopsy, tumor tissue is obtained.
- When the tissue is obtained, place it on ice or in formalin and send it to the laboratory.

POSTPROCEDURE CARE

- Provide emotional support.
- Monitor the breast biopsy site for signs of infection.
- Apply an ice bag for discomfort as needed.

PRECAUTIONS

- Place the specimen on ice immediately and transport it to the laboratory.

COMPLICATIONS

- Bleeding and infection at the biopsy site

NORMAL RESULTS

- Results are classified as favorable or unfavorable; favorable results are associated with tumors with less aggressive cells and a decreased likelihood of tumor recurrence.

ABNORMAL RESULTS

- DNA ploidy stage: Aneuploid (variable number of chromosome sets) is unfavorable; diploid (one set of paired chromosomes) is favorable. As the cancer cells divide more rapidly and aggressively, the chromosome cells are seen in various stages of the mitotic phase.
- S-phase fraction: Greater than 5.5% is unfavorable; less than 5.5% is favorable. As a tumor cell increases in aggressiveness, it spends more time in the S-phase preparing for division.
- Cathepsin D: Greater than 10% is unfavorable; less than 10% is favorable.
- HER-2 protein: Moderate or strong staining in 10% of the cancer cells is unfavorable; partial staining in 10% or fewer of the cancer cells is favorable. The higher the HER-2 level, the poorer the prognosis. HER-2 cells are also a target for trastuzumab (Herceptin), and the higher the HER-2 protein levels, the more likely the tumor will respond to this drug.
- *p53*: greater than 10% is unfavorable; less than 10% is favorable.
- Ki67 protein: greater than 20% is unfavorable; 10% to 20% is borderline; and less than 20% is favorable.

⬢ **INTERFERING FACTORS** *Preoperative administration of chemotherapy (may decrease tumor marker levels)*

Bronchography

DESCRIPTION
◆ X-ray examination of the tracheo-bronchial tree after instillation of a radiopaque iodine contrast agent through a catheter into the lumens of the trachea and bronchi
◆ Contrast agent coats the bronchial tree, permitting visualization of anatomic deviations
◆ Possible to perform bronchography of a localized lung area by instilling contrast dye through a fiber-optic bronchoscope

PURPOSE
◆ To help detect bronchiectasis and map its location for surgical resection
◆ To detect bronchial obstruction, pulmonary tumors, cysts, and cavities; and to help pinpoint the cause of hemoptysis
◆ To provide permanent films of pathologic findings
◆ To guide procedures such as bronchoscopy

PREPARATION
◆ Make sure the patient has signed an informed consent form.
◆ Check the patient's history for hypersensitivity to anesthetics, iodine, or contrast media.
◆ If the patient has a productive cough, give a prescribed expectorant and perform postural drainage 1 to 3 days before the test.
◆ Just before the test, instruct the patient to remove his dentures (if present) and to void.
◆ The patient must fast for 12 hours before the test.

Teaching points
◆ Explain to the patient that bronchography helps evaluate abnormalities of the bronchial structures.
◆ Instruct the patient to fast for 12 hours before the test.
◆ Tell the patient to perform good oral hygiene the night before and the morning of the test.

◆ If the procedure involves local anesthesia, tell the patient that he'll receive a sedative to help him relax and to suppress the gag reflex. Prepare him for the unpleasant taste of the anesthetic spray.
◆ Warn the patient that he may experience some difficulty breathing during the procedure, but reassure him that his airway won't be blocked and that he'll receive enough oxygen. Tell him that the catheter or bronchoscope will pass more easily if he relaxes.
◆ If bronchography is to occur under general anesthesia, inform the patient that he'll receive a sedative before the test to help him relax.
◆ Explain who will perform the test and where it'll be done.
◆ Explain that the test should take less than 1 hour   .

KEY STEPS
◆ Confirm the patient's identity using two patient identifiers according to facility policy.
◆ After a local anesthetic is sprayed into the patient's mouth and throat, a bronchoscope or catheter is passed into the trachea, and the anesthetic and contrast medium are instilled.
◆ The patient is placed in various positions during the test to promote movement of the contrast medium into different areas of the bronchial tree.
◆ After X-rays are taken, the contrast medium is removed through postural drainage and by having the patient cough it up.

POSTPROCEDURE CARE
◆ Withhold food, fluids, and oral drugs until the gag reflex returns (usually in 2 hours). Fluid intake before the gag reflex returns may cause aspiration.
◆ Encourage gentle coughing and postural drainage to facilitate clearing of the contrast medium. A postdrainage film is usually taken in 24 to 48 hours.
◆ If the patient has a sore throat, reassure him that it's only temporary, and

provide throat lozenges or a liquid gargle when his gag reflex returns.
◆ Advise the outpatient not to resume his usual activities until the next day.

PRECAUTIONS
◆ Monitor the patient's oxygen saturation level throughout the test.
◆ Check the patient's history for allergy to iodine or contrast media.

COMPLICATIONS
◆ Laryngeal spasm (dyspnea) or edema (hoarseness, dyspnea, laryngeal stridor) because of traumatic intubation
◆ Allergic reaction to the contrast medium or anesthetic, causing itching, dyspnea, tachycardia, palpitations, excitation, hypotension, hypertension, or euphoria
◆ Chemical or secondary bacterial pneumonia (with fever, dyspnea, crackles, or rhonchi) caused by incomplete expectoration of the contrast medium
◆ Laryngeal spasm (dyspnea) because of the instillation of the contrast medium, in patients with asthma
◆ Airway occlusion secondary to the instillation of the contrast medium, in patients with chronic obstructive pulmonary disease

NORMAL RESULTS
◆ The right mainstem bronchus is shorter, wider, and more vertical than the left mainstem bronchus. Successive branches of the bronchi become smaller in diameter and are free from obstruction or lesions.

ABNORMAL RESULTS
◆ Bronchography results may identify bronchiectasis or bronchial obstruction caused by tumors, cysts, cavities, or foreign objects.

⬢ **INTERFERING FACTORS** *Presence of secretions or improper patient positioning (possible poor imaging because of inadequate filling of bronchial tree)*

Bronchoscopy

DESCRIPTION

♦ Direct visualization of the larynx, trachea, and bronchi using a rigid or fiber-optic bronchoscope
♦ Flexible, fiber-optic bronchoscope allowing a better view of the segmental and subsegmental bronchi, with less risk of trauma
– Virtual bronchoscopy becoming more prevalent (see *Virtual bronchoscopy*)

Virtual bronchoscopy

Using a computer and data from a spiral computed tomography (CT) scan, practitioners can now examine the respiratory tract noninvasively with virtual bronchoscopy. Although it is still in the early stages, researchers believe that this test can enhance screening, diagnosis, preoperative planning, surgical technique, and postoperative follow-up.

Unlike its counterpart — conventional bronchoscopy — virtual bronchoscopy is noninvasive, doesn't require sedation, and provides images for examination beyond the segmental bronchi, thus allowing for possible diagnosis of areas that may be stenosed, obstructed, or compressed from an external source. The images obtained from the CT scan include views of the airways and lung parenchyma. Anatomic structures and abnormalities can be precisely identified and, therefore, can be helpful in locating potential biopsy sites for conventional bronchoscopy and provide simulation for planning the optimal surgical approach.

Virtual bronchoscopy does have disadvantages. This technique doesn't allow for specimen collection or actual biopsies to be obtained from tissue sources. It also can't demonstrate details of the mucosal surface, such as color or texture. Moreover, if an area contains viscous secretions, such as mucus or blood, visualization becomes difficult.

More research on this technique is needed. However, researchers believe that virtual bronchoscopy may play a major role in the screening and early detection of certain cancers, thus allowing for treatment at an earlier, possibly curable, stage.

♦ Large, rigid bronchoscope removing foreign objects, excising endobronchial lesions, and controlling massive hemoptysis (requires general anesthesia)
– Possible to pass brush, biopsy forceps, or catheter through the bronchoscope to obtain specimens for cytologic or microbiologic examination

PURPOSE

♦ To allow visual examination of tumors, obstructions, secretions, and foreign bodies in the tracheobronchial tree
♦ To diagnose bronchogenic carcinoma, tuberculosis, interstitial pulmonary disease, and fungal or parasitic pulmonary infections
♦ To obtain specimens for microbiologic and cytologic examination
♦ To locate bleeding sites in the tracheobronchial tree
♦ To remove foreign bodies, malignant or benign tumors, mucous plugs, and excessive secretions from the tracheobronchial tree

PREPARATION

♦ Make sure the patient has signed an appropriate consent form.
♦ Note allergies.
♦ The patient must fast for 6 to 12 hours before the test.
♦ Obtain results of preprocedure studies; report abnormal results.
♦ Obtain baseline vital signs.
♦ An I.V. sedative may be given.
♦ Remove the patient's dentures.

Teaching points

♦ Explain the purpose of the test and how it's done. (See *Preparing for bronchoscopy,* page 90.)
♦ Instruct the patient to fast for 6 to 12 hours before the test.
♦ Explain who will perform the test and where it'll be done.
♦ Explain that the test takes 45 to 60 minutes.
♦ Inform the patient that his airway won't be blocked and that his breathing will be monitored during the test.
♦ Tell the patient that hoarseness, loss of voice, hemoptysis, and sore throat may occur.

KEY STEPS

♦ Confirm the patient's identity using two patient identifiers according to facility policy.
♦ Position the patient properly.
♦ Give the patient supplemental oxygen by nasal cannula, if ordered.
♦ Monitor the patient's pulse oximetry, vital signs, and cardiac rhythm.
♦ Local anesthetic is sprayed into the patient's mouth and throat to suppress the gag reflex.
♦ The bronchoscope is inserted through the mouth or nose; a bite block is placed in the mouth if the oral approach is used.
♦ When the bronchoscope is just above the vocal cords, about 3 to 4 ml of 2% to 4% lidocaine is flushed through the inner channel of the scope, to the vocal cords to anesthetize deeper areas.
♦ A fiber-optic camera is used to take photographs for documentation.
♦ Tissue specimens are obtained from suspect areas.
♦ A suction apparatus may remove foreign bodies or mucous plugs.
♦ Bronchoalveolar lavage may remove thickened secretions or may diagnose infectious causes of infiltrates.
♦ Specimens are prepared properly and immediately sent to the laboratory.

POSTPROCEDURE CARE

♦ Position a conscious patient in semi-Fowler's position.
♦ Position an unconscious patient on one side, with the head of the bed slightly elevated to prevent aspiration.
♦ Instruct the patient to spit out saliva rather than swallow it.
♦ Observe the patient for bleeding.
♦ Resume the patient's usual diet, beginning with sips of clear liquid or ice chips, when the gag reflex returns.
♦ Provide lozenges or a soothing liquid gargle to ease discomfort when the gag reflex returns.
♦ Check the follow-up chest X-ray for pneumothorax.

- Monitor the patient's vital signs, sputum characteristics, and respiratory status.

PRECAUTIONS
- Failure to observe dietary restrictions before the test may result in aspiration.
- Specimens should be sent to the laboratory immediately.

COMPLICATIONS
- Subcutaneous crepitus around the patient's face, neck, or chest, which may indicate tracheal or bronchial perforation or pneumothorax

  WARNING *Watch for and immediately report symptoms of respiratory difficulty associated with laryngeal edema or laryngospasm, such as laryngeal stridor and dyspnea.*
- Hypoxemia, cardiac arrhythmias, bleeding, infection, bronchospasm, and laryngeal edema

INTERPRETATION

NORMAL RESULTS
- The bronchi appear structurally similar to the trachea.
- The right bronchus is slightly larger and more vertical than the left bronchus.
- Smaller segmental bronchi branch off from the main bronchi.

ABNORMAL RESULTS
- Structural abnormalities of the bronchial wall indicate inflammation, ulceration, tumors, and enlargement of submucosal lymph nodes.
- Structural abnormalities of endotracheal origin suggest stenosis, compression, ectasia, and diverticula.
- Structural abnormalities of the trachea or bronchi suggest calculi, foreign bodies, masses, and paralyzed vocal cords.
- Tissue and cell study abnormalities suggest interstitial pulmonary disease, infection, carcinoma, and tuberculosis.

(continued)

Preparing for bronchoscopy

Dear Patient,

Here are some facts you'll want to know about the bronchoscopy your health care provider has scheduled for you.

This test permits your health care provider to examine your airway (windpipe and lungs) with a thin, flexible instrument called a bronchoscope.

By looking through the instrument's eyepiece, your health care provider can see abnormalities and obstructions. With another part of the instrument, your health care provider can obtain tiny tissue samples to help diagnose your illness or remove foreign bodies or excess mucus.

BEFORE THE TEST

Don't eat for at least 8 hours before the test, and don't drink alcoholic beverages for 24 hours beforehand. Food and alcohol can cause test complications and create problems with any sedatives you're given.

Continue to take prescribed drugs unless you're told not to.

Just before the test, you'll receive a local anesthetic to numb the back of your throat and stop you from gagging. This helps the bronchoscope slide easily inside your trachea. You'll receive a sedative to help you relax.

DURING THE TEST

The test takes 45 to 60 minutes. You'll lie on your back or sit upright. After the anesthetic takes effect, the end of the bronchoscope will be inserted through your nose or mouth.

As the instrument is advanced, small amounts of liquid anesthetic will be flushed through it to decrease any coughing and wheezing you might have. The instrument will slide through your major airways. You may experience some discomfort with breathing. Remember to stay calm. If necessary, you'll be given extra oxygen.

When the examination is over, your health care provider will remove the bronchoscope.

AFTER THE TEST

You'll lie comfortably with your head raised and be monitored closely for 1 to 2 hours. Until the anesthetic wears off and your gag reflex returns, you won't be allowed to eat, drink, or take oral medications. You may be hoarse and may have a sore throat, but this is only temporary. When your gag reflex returns, you'll be able to gargle or suck on throat lozenges.

Soon after the test, you'll have a chest X-ray to make sure that you're doing well.

Your sedative may not have worn off by the time you're ready to go home, so arrange for someone to take you home from the hospital or clinic.

Immediately report bloody mucus, difficulty breathing, wheezing, or chest pain.

B-type natriuretic peptide assay

DESCRIPTION
- A test measuring plasma levels of B-type natriuretic peptide (BNP), a neurohormone produced predominantly by the heart ventricle
- BNP released by the heart in response to blood volume expansion or pressure overload
- Plasma BNP increases with the severity of heart failure (heart is the major source of circulating BNP)

PURPOSE
- To help diagnose and determine severity of heart failure

PREPARATION
- The test requires a blood sample.
- No dietary restrictions are required.

Teaching points
- Explain that this test is used to identify the presence and severity of heart failure.
- Tell the patient that the test requires a blood sample and that he may experience slight discomfort from the tourniquet and needle puncture.
- Explain who will perform the test and where it'll be done.
- Inform the patient that he need not restrict food or fluids.
- Tell the patient that the test should take less than 5 minutes.

KEY STEPS
- Confirm the patient's identity using two patient identifiers according to facility policy.
- Perform a venipuncture, and collect the sample in a 3.5-ml EDTA tube.

POSTPROCEDURE CARE
- Apply direct pressure to the venipuncture site until bleeding stops.

PRECAUTIONS
- Maintain standard precautions while collecting the sample.
- Handle the sample gently to prevent hemolysis.

COMPLICATIONS
- Hematoma at the venipuncture site

NORMAL RESULTS
- BNP levels should be less than 100 pg/ml.

ABNORMAL RESULTS
- BNP levels greater than 100 pg/ml are an accurate predictor of heart failure.
- BNP levels are related to the severity of heart failure. The higher the level, the worse the symptoms. (See *Linking BNP levels to severity of heart failure symptoms*.)

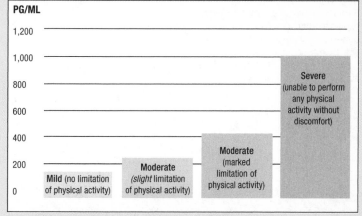

Linking BNP levels to severity of heart failure symptoms

This table shows serum B-type natriuretic peptide (BNP) levels and the correlation with symptoms of heart failure. The higher the level of BNP, the more severe the symptoms.

PG/ML

1,200

1,000

800

600

400

200

0

Mild (no limitation of physical activity)

Moderate (*slight* limitation of physical activity)

Moderate (marked limitation of physical activity)

Severe (unable to perform any physical activity without discomfort)

Adapted with permission of Biosite Diagnostics. © 2001 Biosite Diagnostics.

Calcitonin level, plasma

DESCRIPTION

◆ Radioimmunoassay that measures calcitonin levels (thyrocalcitonin) in plasma
◆ Role of calcitonin unclear; may act as antagonist to parathyroid hormone and may lower calcium levels
◆ Indicated in suspected medullary carcinoma of thyroid, which causes hypersecretion of calcitonin (without associated hypocalcemia)
◆ Provocative testing with I.V. pentagastrin or calcium needed to rule out disease

PURPOSE

◆ To aid in the diagnosis of thyroid medullary carcinoma and ectopic calcitonin-producing tumors (rare)

PREPARATION

◆ The test requires the patient to fast 12 hours the night before the test because food may interfere with calcium homeostasis and, subsequently, calcitonin levels.
◆ The test requires a blood sample.

Teaching points

◆ Explain that this test helps evaluate thyroid function.
◆ Tell the patient who will perform the test and where it will be done.
◆ Instruct the patient to fast at least 12 hours before the test.
◆ Explain to the patient that the test requires a blood sample and he may experience slight discomfort from the tourniquet and needle puncture.
◆ Inform the patient that the laboratory requires several days to complete the analysis.

KEY STEPS

◆ Confirm the patient's identity using two patient identifiers according to facility policy.
◆ Perform a venipuncture and collect the sample in a 7-ml heparinized tube.
◆ Send the sample to the laboratory immediately after collection.

POSTPROCEDURE CARE

◆ Apply direct pressure to the venipuncture site until bleeding stops.
◆ Tell the patient to resume his usual diet.

PRECAUTIONS

◆ Maintain standard precautions while collecting the sample.
◆ Handle the sample gently to prevent hemolysis.

COMPLICATIONS

◆ Hematoma at the venipuncture site

NORMAL RESULTS

◆ Serum basal calcitonin levels in men are 40 pg/ml (SI, 40 ng/L); in women, 20 pg/ml (SI, 20 ng/L).
◆ After a 4-hour calcium infusion, in men the levels rise to 190 pg/ml (SI, 190 ng/L); in women, 130 pg/ml (SI, 130 ng/L).
◆ After testing with pentagastrin infusion, in men the levels should be 110 pg/ml (SI, 110 ng/L); in women, 30 pg/ml (SI, 30 ng/L).

ABNORMAL RESULTS

◆ Elevated serum calcitonin levels in the absence of hypocalcemia usually indicate medullary carcinoma of the thyroid.
◆ Transmitted as an autosomal dominant trait, thyroid medullary carcinoma may occur as part of multiple endocrine neoplasia.
◆ Increased calcitonin levels may be caused by ectopic calcitonin production by oat cell carcinoma of the lung or by breast carcinoma.

Calcium level, ionized

DESCRIPTION
◆ Measures the fraction of serum calcium that's in the ionized form

PURPOSE
◆ To screen for or monitor diseases of the bone or calcium-regulation disorders (such as diseases of the parathyroid gland or kidneys)

PREPARATION
◆ This test requires a blood sample.
◆ A 6-hour fast is required before the test.

Teaching points
◆ Explain to the patient the purpose of the test and how it's done.
◆ Tell him who will perform the test and where it will be done.
◆ Instruct the patient to fast for at least 6 hours before the test.
◆ Inform the patient that some drugs can increase ionized calcium measurements; these include calcium salts (found in nutritional supplements or antacids), hydralazine, lithium, thiazide diuretics, and thyroxine. Tell him if the practitioner ordered any of his medications to be discontinued for the test.
◆ Tell the patient that the test should take less than 5 minutes.

KEY STEPS
◆ Confirm the patient's identity using two patient identifiers according to facility policy.
◆ Perform a venipuncture and collect 5 ml of venous blood in a gel-barrier tube.

POSTPROCEDURE CARE
◆ Apply direct pressure to the venipuncture site until bleeding stops.

PRECAUTIONS
◆ Maintain standard precautions while collecting the sample.
◆ Handle the sample gently to prevent hemolysis.

COMPLICATIONS
◆ Hematoma at the venipuncture site

NORMAL RESULTS
◆ In adults, calcium levels should range from 4.6 to 5.3 mg/dl (SI, 1.16 to 1.32 mmol/L).
◆ In children, these levels should range from 4.4 to 5.5 mg/dl (SI, 1.10 to 1.38 mmol/L).

ABNORMAL RESULTS
◆ Decreased levels (from causes such as acute pancreatitis, hypoparathyroidism, vitamin D deficiency, and multiple organ failure) may cause symptoms of neuromuscular irritability or tetany.
◆ Diarrhea, malabsorption of calcium, burns, alcoholism, and chronic renal failure may cause decreased levels of calcium.
◆ Malignant neoplasm of the bone, lung, breast, bladder, or kidney may cause increased levels of calcium.

INTERFERING FACTORS *Excessive ingestion of milk or antacids (possible increased levels of calcium)*

Calcium levels, serum and urine

DESCRIPTION
- Measures the total amount of calcium in the blood or in the urine

PURPOSE
- To evaluate endocrine function, calcium metabolism, and acid-base balance
- To guide therapy in patients with renal failure, renal transplant, endocrine disorders, malignancies, cardiac disease, and skeletal disorders

PREPARATION (SERUM)
- The test requires a blood sample.
- No dietary restrictions are required for this test.
- Notify the laboratory and practitioner of drugs the patient is taking that may affect test results; it may be necessary to restrict them.

Teaching points
- Explain that the serum calcium test determines blood calcium levels.
- Explain to the patient that the test requires a blood sample and that he may experience slight discomfort from the tourniquet and needle puncture.
- Tell the patient who will perform the test and where it will be done.
- Inform the patient that no dietary restrictions are needed.
- Tell the patient that the test takes less than 5 minutes.

PREPARATION (URINE)
- The test requires urine collection over 24 hours.
- Provide a diet that contains about 130 mg of calcium/24 hours for 3 days before the test or provide information about the diet for the patient to follow at home.
- Notify the laboratory and practitioner of drugs the patient is taking that may affect test results; it may be necessary to restrict them.

Teaching points
- Tell the patient the test requires a 24-hour urine specimen.
- Explain to the patient that this test measures the amount of calcium in the urine.
- Encourage the patient to be as active as possible before the test.
- Teach the patient how to perform a urine collection at home. Warn him not to contaminate the specimen with toilet tissue or stool.
- Tell the patient who will perform the test and where it will be done.

KEY STEPS
- Confirm the patient's identity using two patient identifiers according to facility policy.

Serum
- Perform a venipuncture (without a tourniquet if possible) and collect the sample in a 3- or 4-ml clot-activator tube.

Urine
- Collect the patient's urine for 24 hours, discarding the first specimen and retaining the last.

POSTPROCEDURE CARE
- Apply direct pressure to the venipuncture site until bleeding stops.
- Observe the patient with low urine calcium levels for tetany.
- Tell the patient to resume his usual diet, activities, and medications.

PRECAUTIONS
- Maintain standard precautions while collecting the sample.
- Handle the sample gently to avoid hemolysis.
- Keep the urine specimen on ice or in the refrigerator during the collection period.

COMPLICATIONS
- Hematoma at the venipuncture site

INTERPRETATION

NORMAL RESULTS

◆ In adults, serum calcium levels should be between 8.2 and 10.2 mg/dl (SI, 2.05 to 2.54 mmol/L).

◆ In children, these levels should be between 8.6 and 11.2 mg/dl (SI, 2.15 to 2.79 mmol/L).

◆ For a normal diet, urine calcium levels should range from 100 to 300 mg/24 hours (SI, 2.5 to 7.5 mmol/day).

ABNORMAL RESULTS

◆ Abnormally high serum calcium levels (hypercalcemia) may occur in hyperparathyroidism and parathyroid tumors, Paget's disease of the bone, multiple myeloma, metastatic carcinoma, multiple fractures, and prolonged immobilization.

◆ Elevated serum calcium levels may also result from inadequate excretion of calcium, such as adrenal insufficiency and renal disease; from excessive calcium ingestion; and from overuse of antacids such as calcium carbonate.

◆ Observe the patient with hypercalcemia for deep bone pain, flank pain caused by renal calculi, and muscle hypotonicity. Hypercalcemic crisis begins with nausea, vomiting, and dehydration, leading to stupor and coma, and can end in cardiac arrest.

◆ Low serum calcium levels (hypocalcemia) may result from hypoparathyroidism, total parathyroidectomy, and malabsorption.

◆ Low serum calcium levels may also occur with Cushing's syndrome, renal failure, acute pancreatitis, peritonitis, malnutrition with hypoalbuminemia, and blood transfusions (caused by citrate).

◆ In the patient with hypocalcemia, be alert for circumoral and peripheral numbness and tingling, muscle twitching, Chvostek's sign (facial muscle spasm), tetany, muscle cramping, Trousseau's sign (carpopedal spasm), seizures, arrhythmias, laryngospasm, decreased cardiac output, prolonged bleeding time, fractures, and prolonged QT interval.

🔷 *INTERFERING FACTORS Prolonged tourniquet application (may cause a falsely increased serum level because of venous stasis)*

◆ Many disorders can affect urine calcium levels. (See *Disorders that affect urine calcium and urine phosphorus levels.*)

Disorders that affect urine calcium and urine phosphorus levels

The table below lists some possible causes of abnormal urine calcium and phosphorus levels, along with their effect on the test results.

DISORDER	URINE CALCIUM LEVEL	URINE PHOSPHORUS LEVEL
Acute nephritis	Suppressed	Suppressed
Acute nephrosis	Suppressed	Suppressed or normal
Chronic nephrosis	Suppressed	Suppressed
Hyperparathyroidism	Elevated	Elevated
Hypoparathyroidism	Suppressed	Suppressed
Metastatic carcinoma	Elevated	Normal
Milk-alkali syndrome	Suppressed or normal	Suppressed or normal
Multiple myeloma	Elevated or normal	Elevated or normal
Osteomalacia	Suppressed	Suppressed
Paget's disease	Normal	Normal
Renal insufficiency	Suppressed	Suppressed
Renal tubular acidosis	Elevated	Elevated
Sarcoidosis	Elevated	Suppressed
Steatorrhea	Suppressed	Suppressed
Vitamin D intoxication	Elevated	Suppressed

Caloric study

DESCRIPTION
◆ Eighth cranial nerve (CN VIII)—acoustic nerve: controls hearing, equilibrium, and balance
◆ Ear stimulation with cold water: causes involuntary eye movement (rotary nystagmus) away from stimulated ear
◆ Ear stimulation with hot water: causes nystagmus toward stimulated ear

PURPOSE
◆ To help make differential diagnoses of abnormalities in the vestibular system, cerebellum, or brainstem

PREPARATION
◆ Examine the patient for the presence of nystagmus, Romberg's sign, and past-pointing to determine baseline values.
◆ Clean and examine the ear canal to allow free flow of water into the middle ear.
◆ Fasting from solid foods is required the morning of the test.

Teaching points
◆ Explain to the patient the purpose of the test and how it's done.
◆ Tell the patient who will perform the test and where it will be done.
◆ Instruct the patient to avoid solid food the morning before the test to help decrease nausea.
◆ Explain that nausea and dizziness during the test are normal.
◆ Inform the patient that the test will take about 15 minutes.

KEY STEPS
◆ Confirm the patient's identity using two patient identifiers according to facility policy.
◆ Irrigate the ear on the suspected side.
◆ Place an emesis basin under the ear and instill the solution into the auditory canal. Stop irrigating when the patient becomes dizzy or nauseated, or when nystagmus is seen.
◆ If no symptoms occur, stop irrigating after 3 minutes.
◆ Repeat the test on the same side with the other solution.
◆ Wait 5 minutes and perform the test on the other side.

POSTPROCEDURE CARE
◆ Keep the patient on bedrest until nausea and dizziness subside.

PRECAUTIONS
◆ If the patient has a perforated eardrum, use cold air instead of fluid.
◆ Don't perform the test during an acute disease process involving the labyrinth such as Ménière's syndrome.

COMPLICATIONS
◆ None

NORMAL RESULTS
◆ Nystagmus occurs with irrigation of the canal.

ABNORMAL RESULTS
◆ Nystagmus isn't induced.
◆ Abnormal results indicate that CN VIII isn't functioning properly, or a disease of the labyrinth is present.
◆ The test results indicate the presence of brainstem infarction, inflammation, or a tumor.
◆ Test results indicate the presence of an acoustic neuroma.
◆ Neuropathy or neuritis of CN VIII may be indicated by the test results.

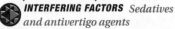 **INTERFERING FACTORS** *Sedatives and antivertigo agents*

Cancer tumor marker test

DESCRIPTION

- Detects tumor markers (CA 15-3 [27, 29]; CA 19-9; CA-125; and CA-50), substances produced and secreted by tumor cells that help determine tumor activity; found in serum of patients with cancer
- Specific test dependent on the type of cancer
- CA 15-3 antigen (breast-cystic fluid protein [BCFP]) with carcinoembryonic antigen for patients with breast cancer (CA 27, metastatic breast cancer, breast-cystic fluid protein 29, BCFP)
- CA 19-9 carbohydrate antigen for patients with pancreatic, hepatobiliary, or lung cancer
- CA-125 glycoprotein and serum carbohydrate antigens for patients with ovarian cancer
- CA-50 for patients with GI or pancreatic cancer
- Combination of markers used due to low sensitivity and specificity of markers
- Few tumor markers approved by Food and Drug Administration because of controversial role in cancer diagnosis and treatment

PURPOSE

- To assist tumor staging and identify possible metastasis
- To monitor and detect disease recurrence
- To assess the patient's response to therapy

PREPARATION

- The test requires a blood sample.
- Fasting may be required before the test.
- Identify factors that may interfere with test results and note them on the appropriate laboratory requests.
- Follow specific directions from the laboratory or cancer center for the particular test.

Teaching points

- Explain to the patient the purpose of the test, how it's done, and its helpfulness in the patient's disorder, as appropriate.
- Tell the patient who will perform the test and where it will be done.
- Advise him of any dietary or medication requirements.
- Explain to the patient that he may experience slight discomfort from the tourniquet and needle puncture.
- Inform him that the test should take less than 5 minutes.

KEY STEPS

- Confirm the patient's identity using two patient identifiers according to facility policy.
- Obtain a 10-ml venous sample in the tube specified by the laboratory or cancer center and transport the sample as directed.

POSTPROCEDURE CARE

- Apply direct pressure to the venipuncture site until bleeding stops.

PRECAUTIONS

- Maintain standard precautions while collecting the sample.

COMPLICATIONS

- Hematoma at the venipuncture site

NORMAL RESULTS

- CA 15-3 (27, 29) level is below 30 units/ml.
- CA 19-9 level is below 70 units/ml.
- CA-125 level is below 34 units/ml.
- CA-50 level is below 17 units/ml.

ABNORMAL RESULTS

- CA 15-3 (27, 29) level is greatly increased in metastatic breast cancer; it's also increased in pancreatic, lung, colorectal, ovarian, and liver cancers. Because the level decreases with therapy, an increased level after therapy indicates that the disease has progressed.
- CA 19-9 level is increased in pancreatic, hepatobiliary, and lung cancers; also, it may be mildly increased in gastric and colorectal cancers.
- CA-125 level is increased in epithelial ovary, fallopian tube, endometrium, endocervix, pancreatic, and liver cancers. It's less increased in colon, breast, lung, and GI cancers.
- CA-50 level is increased in GI and pancreatic cancers.

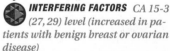 *INTERFERING FACTORS CA 15-3 (27, 29) level (increased in patients with benign breast or ovarian disease)*

CA 19-9 level (increased in patients with pancreatitis, cholecystitis, cirrhosis, gallstones, or cystic fibrosis [minimal elevations])

CA-125 level (increased during menstruation and pregnancy and in patients with endometriosis, pelvic inflammatory disease, acute and chronic hepatitis, ascites, peritonitis, pancreatitis, GI disease, Meigs syndrome, pleural effusion, or pulmonary disease)

Candida antibody test

DESCRIPTION
- *Candida albicans* normally present in the body
- Can become pathogenic when the environment favors proliferation or the host's defenses have been significantly weakened
- Usually limited to skin and mucous membranes but may cause life-threatening systemic infections
- Susceptibility to candidiasis associated with antibacterial, antimetabolic, and corticosteroid therapy
- Oral candidiasis common in children; in adults, may be early indication of acquired immunodeficiency syndrome

PURPOSE
- To identify the presence of *Candida* antibodies to diagnose systemic candidiasis

PREPARATION
- No dietary restrictions are required before the test.
- This test requires a blood sample.

Teaching points
- Explain to the patient the purpose of the test and how it's done.
- Tell him who will perform the test and where it will be done.
- Tell him that no dietary restrictions are required.
- Explain to the patient that a blood sample is needed and that he may experience slight discomfort from the tourniquet and needle puncture.
- Informhim that the test should take less than 5 minutes.

KEY STEPS
- Confirm the patient's identity using two patient identifiers according to facility policy.
- Perform a venipuncture and collect the sample in a 5-ml sterile collection tube without additives.
- Send the sample to the laboratory immediately after collection.
- Note recent antimicrobial therapy on the laboratory form.

POSTPROCEDURE CARE
- Apply pressure to the venipuncture site until bleeding stops.

PRECAUTIONS
- Maintain standard precautions while collecting the sample.
- Because the patient's immune system may be compromised, keep the venipuncture site clean and dry.

COMPLICATIONS
- Hematoma at the venipuncture site

NORMAL RESULTS
- Negative results are obtained for *Candida* antibodies.

ABNORMAL RESULTS
- The test is positive for *Candida* antibodies.
- A positive test is common in patients with disseminated candidiasis.
- There are a significant number of false-positive tests.

Capillary fragility test

DESCRIPTION
- Nonspecific method for evaluating bleeding tendencies
- Measures the ability of capillaries to remain intact under increased intra-capillary pressure
- Also called the *positive-pressure test,* the *tourniquet test,* and the *Rumpel-Leede test*

PURPOSE
- To assess the fragility of capillary walls
- To identify a platelet deficiency (thrombocytopenia)

PREPARATION
- No dietary restrictions are required for this test.

Teaching points
- Explain that the test identifies abnormal bleeding tendencies.
- Tell the patient who will perform the test and where it will be done.
- Inform the patient that no dietary restrictions are needed.
- Explain to the patient that he may feel discomfort from the pressure of the blood pressure cuff.
- Inform him that the test should take less than 10 minutes.

KEY STEPS
- Confirm the patient's identity using two patient identifiers according to facility policy.
- The patient's skin temperature and the room temperature should be normal to ensure accurate results.
- Select and mark a 2″ (5-cm) space on the patient's forearm. Ideally, the site should be free from petechiae; otherwise, record the number of petechiae before starting the test.
- Fasten the cuff around the arm and raise the pressure to a point midway between the systolic and diastolic blood pressures.
- Maintain this pressure for 5 minutes; then release the cuff.
- Count the number of petechiae that appear in the 2″ space.
- Record the test results.

POSTPROCEDURE CARE
- Encourage the patient to open and close his hand a few times to hasten the return of blood to the forearm.

PRECAUTIONS
- Don't repeat this test on the same arm within 1 week.
- The test is contraindicated in patients with disseminated intravascular coagulation (DIC) or other bleeding disorders and in those with significant petechiae already present.

COMPLICATIONS
- Excessive bleeding or bruising at the test site

NORMAL RESULTS
- A few petechiae may normally be present before the test. Fewer than 10 petechiae on the forearm 5 minutes (SI, 5 minutes) after the test are considered normal, or a negative result; more than 10 petechiae are considered a positive result.

ABNORMAL RESULTS
- A positive result (more than 10 petechiae, or a score of 2+ to 4+) indicates weakness of the capillary walls (vascular purpura) or a platelet defect. It may occur in such conditions as thrombocytopenia, thrombasthenia, purpura senilis, scurvy, DIC, von Willebrand's disease, vitamin K deficiency, dysproteinemia, polycythemia vera, and in severe deficiencies of factor VII, fibrinogen, or prothrombin. Conditions unrelated to bleeding defects, such as scarlet fever, measles, influenza, chronic renal disease, hypertension, and diabetes with coexisting vascular disease, may increase capillary fragility.
- An abnormal number of petechiae sometimes appear before menstruation and at other times in some healthy persons, especially in women over age 40.

Carboxyhemoglobin level test

DESCRIPTION
- Measures level of carboxyhemoglobin in the blood
- Carboxyhemoglobin formed when hemoglobin (Hb) combines with carbon monoxide (CO)

PURPOSE
- To detect CO poisoning

PREPARATION
- Obtain a history from the patient for possible CO exposure.
- Evaluate the patient for signs and symptoms of CO poisoning, such as headache, dizziness, malaise, or mucous membranes that appear bright red.
- No dietary or drug restrictions are required.
- The test requires a blood sample.

Teaching points
- Tell the patient that this test measures the amount of CO in his blood.
- Tell him who will perform the test and where it will be done.
- Inform him that there are no dietary restrictions.
- Explain to the patient that a blood sample is required and that he may experience slight discomfort from the tourniquet and needle puncture.
- Inform him that the test should take less than 5 minutes.

KEY STEPS
- Confirm the patient's identity using two patient identifiers according to facility policy.
- Perform a venipuncture and collect 5 ml of blood in an EDTA tube.
- Immediately place the sample on ice and send it to the laboratory.

POSTPROCEDURE CARE
- Apply pressure to the venipuncture site until bleeding stops.
- Apply high concentrations of oxygen (O_2), as ordered, to help increase O_2 in the blood and displace the CO.

PRECAUTIONS
- Maintain standard precautions while collecting the blood.
- Draw blood as soon as possible after exposure.

COMPLICATIONS
- Hematoma at the venipuncture site

NORMAL RESULTS
- In nonsmokers, CO level is 2% of total Hb.
- CO level in light smokers is 4% to 5% of total Hb.
- CO level in heavy smokers is 6% to 8% of total Hb.
- In neonates, CO level is 10% to 12% of total Hb.

ABNORMAL RESULTS
- Abnormal results indicate CO poisoning.
- If the CO level is 10% to 20% of total Hb, the patient may be asymptomatic.
- If the CO level is 20% to 30% of total Hb, the patient will have a headache, nausea, vomiting, and possible loss of judgment.
- If the CO level is 30% to 40% of total Hb, the patient will have tachycardia, hyperpnea, hypotension, and confusion.
- If the CO level is 50% to 60% of total Hb, the patient will have loss of consciousness.
- Values above 60% of the total Hb will cause seizures, respiratory arrest, and death.
- Exposure to CO occurs from smoke inhalation, exhaust fumes, fires, gas fumes (heaters and stoves), and petroleum fumes.

Carcinoembryonic antigen test

OVERVIEW

DESCRIPTION
◆ Stages and monitors treatment of certain cancers (see *Using CEA to monitor cancer treatment*)
◆ Also called *CEA*

PURPOSE
◆ To monitor the effectiveness of cancer therapy
◆ To assist in preoperative staging of colorectal cancers, to assess the adequacy of surgical resection, and to test for recurrence of colorectal cancers

PREPARATION
◆ No dietary or drug restrictions are required.
◆ The test requires a blood sample.
◆ The test may be repeated to monitor the effectiveness of therapy.

Teaching points
◆ Tell the patient that the test detects and measures a special protein that usually isn't present in adults.
◆ Inform him who will perform the test and where it will be done.
◆ Tell him that he doesn't need to restrict his diet.
◆ Explain to the patient that the test requires a blood sample and that he may experience slight discomfort from the tourniquet and needle puncture.
◆ Inform him that the test should take less than 5 minutes.

DIAGNOSTIC PROCEDURE

KEY STEPS
◆ Confirm the patient's identity using two patient identifiers according to facility policy.
◆ Perform a venipuncture; collect sample in a 7-ml tube without additives.
◆ Send the sample to the laboratory immediately after collection.

POSTPROCEDURE CARE
◆ Apply direct pressure to the venipuncture site until bleeding stops.

PRECAUTIONS
◆ Maintain standard precautions while collecting the sample.
◆ Handle the sample gently to prevent hemolysis.

COMPLICATIONS
◆ Hematoma at the venipuncture site

INTERPRETATION

NORMAL RESULTS
◆ Values are less than 5 ng/ml.

ABNORMAL RESULTS
◆ Persistent elevations suggest residual or recurrent tumor.
◆ High levels are characteristic in various malignant conditions, particularly endodermally derived neoplasms of the GI organs and lungs, and in certain nonmalignant conditions, such as benign hepatic disease, hepatic cirrhosis, alcoholic pancreatitis, and inflammatory bowel disease.
◆ Elevated levels may occur in nonendodermal carcinomas, such as breast and ovarian cancers.

Using CEA to monitor cancer treatment

Because many patients in the early stages of colorectal cancer have normal or low levels of carcinoembryonic antigen (CEA), the CEA test doesn't screen successfully for early malignancy. It's a good tool, however, for monitoring response to cancer therapy.

After a patient's serum CEA level has dropped following surgery, chemotherapy, or other treatment, an increase suggests recurrence of cancer or diminished effectiveness of treatment.

Both charts below illustrate CEA levels in patients during and after treatment for colorectal cancer. In the left chart, initial results show the usual dramatic drop in response to treatment; the subsequent rise in CEA indicates a diminishing response to chemotherapy. In the right chart, the progressive rise in CEA signals a recurrence of cancer 8 months before clinical symptoms or radiologic evidence.

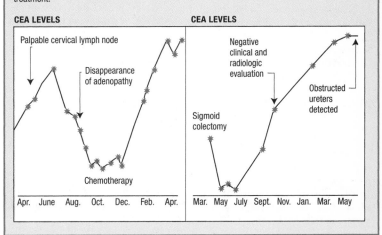

Cardiac blood pool imaging

DESCRIPTION

◆ Evaluates regional and global ventricular performance after I.V. injection of human serum albumin or red blood cells (RBCs) tagged with the isotope technetium 99m (^{99m}Tc) pertechnetate

◆ First-pass imaging: scintillation camera records radioactivity emitted by isotope as it initially passes through left ventricle

◆ Higher counts of radioactivity during diastole (more blood in ventricle); lower counts during systole

◆ May calculate portion of isotope ejected during each heartbeat to determine the ejection fraction and the presence and size of intracardiac shunts

◆ More accurate and involves less risk to the patient than left ventriculography in assessing cardiac function

PURPOSE

◆ To evaluate left ventricular function

◆ To detect aneurysms of the left ventricle and other motion abnormalities of the myocardial wall (such as areas of akinesia or dyskinesia)

◆ To detect intracardiac shunting

PREPARATION

◆ No dietary restrictions are required before the test.

◆ Make sure that the patient or a responsible family member has signed an informed consent form.

Teaching points

◆ Explain that the test allows assessment of the heart's left ventricle.

◆ Tell the patient who will perform the test and where it will be done.

◆ Inform the patient that there are no dietary restrictions.

◆ Explain to the patient that he'll receive an I.V. injection of a radioactive tracer and that a detector positioned above his chest will record the circulation of this tracer through his heart.

◆ Reassure the patient that the tracer poses no radiation hazard and rarely produces adverse effects.

◆ Inform the patient that he may experience slight discomfort from the needle puncture but that the imaging itself is painless.

◆ Instruct the patient to remain silent and motionless during imaging, unless otherwise instructed.

◆ Inform the patient that the test should take about 1½ hours.

DIAGNOSTIC PROCEDURE

KEY STEPS

◆ Confirm the patient's identity using two patient identifiers according to facility policy.

◆ The patient is placed in a supine position beneath the detector of a scintillation camera and 15 to 20 millicuries of albumin or RBCs tagged with ^{99m}Tc pertechnetate is injected I.V.

◆ For the next minute, the scintillation camera records the first pass of the isotope through the heart to locate the aortic and mitral valves.

◆ Then, using an electrocardiogram, the camera is gated for selected 60-millisecond intervals, representing end-systole and end-diastole, and 500 to 1,000 cardiac cycles are recorded on X-ray or Polaroid film.

◆ To observe septal and posterior wall motion, the patient may be assisted to a modified left anterior oblique position or he may be assisted to a right anterior oblique position and given 0.4 mg of nitroglycerin sublingually. The scintillation camera then records additional gated images to evaluate abnormal contraction in the left ventricle.

◆ The patient may be asked to exercise as the scintillation camera records gated images.

WARNING *If the patient is elderly or physically compromised, assist him to a sitting position and make sure he isn't dizzy. Then assist him in getting off the examination table.*

POSTPROCEDURE CARE

◆ Monitor the patient's vital signs and response to the testing.

◆ Answer the patient's questions.

PRECAUTIONS

◆ The test shouldn't be performed on pregnant patients.

COMPLICATIONS

◆ Reaction to the tracer (rare)

NORMAL RESULTS

◆ The left ventricle contracts symmetrically, and the isotope appears evenly distributed in the scans.

◆ Normal ejection fraction is 55% to 65%.

ABNORMAL RESULTS

◆ The patient with coronary artery disease usually has asymmetrical blood distribution to the myocardium, which produces segmental abnormalities of ventricular wall motion; such abnormalities may also result from preexisting conditions such as myocarditis.

◆ The patient with a cardiomyopathy shows globally reduced ejection fractions.

◆ In the patient with a left-to-right shunt, the recirculating radioisotope prolongs the down slope of the curve of scintigraphic data; early arrival of activity in the left ventricle or aorta signifies a right-to-left shunt.

Cardiac catheterization

DESCRIPTION

- Passage of a catheter into the right, left, or both sides of the heart
- Measures pressure in chambers of the heart; records films of the ventricles (contrast ventriculography) and arteries (coronary arteriography)
- Left-sided catheterization to check patency of coronary arteries and function of left ventricle
- Right-sided catheterization to check pulmonary artery pressures

PURPOSE

- To evaluate valvular insufficiency or stenosis, septal defects, congenital anomalies, myocardial function, myocardial blood supply, and cardiac wall motion
- To help diagnose left ventricular enlargement, aortic root enlargement, ventricular aneurysms, and intracardiac shunts

PREPARATION

- Have the patient sign a consent form.
- Stop anticoagulant as ordered to reduce complications of bleeding.
- Check patient history for sensitivity to contrast media. Mark clearly on the chart.

Teaching points

- Tell the patient the purpose of the test.
- Tell the patient who will perform the test and where it will be done.
- Instruct the patient to fast for at least 6 hours before the test. (See *Preparing for cardiac catheterization,* page 104.)
- Explain that if a mild sedative is given, the patient remains conscious.
- Warn the patient that a transient hot, flushing sensation or nausea may occur.
- Tell him that the test will take 1 to 2 hours.

DIAGNOSTIC PROCEDURE

KEY STEPS

- Confirm the patient's identity using two patient identifiers according to facility policy.
- The patient is placed in a supine position on a padded table and his heart rhythm and vital signs are monitored throughout the test.
- A local anesthetic is injected at the insertion site.
- A small incision is made into the artery or vein, depending on whether the test is for the left or right.
- In right-sided heart catheterization, the catheter is inserted into a vein and advanced through the vena cava into the right side of the heart and into the pulmonary artery.
- In left-sided heart catheterization, the catheter is inserted into an artery and advanced retrograde through the aorta into the coronary artery ostium and left ventricle.
- When the catheter is in place, contrast medium is injected to make visible the cardiac vessels and structures.
- After catheter removal, apply direct pressure to incision site until bleeding stops and apply a sterile dressing.

POSTPROCEDURE CARE

- Reinforce the dressing as needed.
- Enforce bed rest for 8 hours.
- If the femoral route was used for catheter insertion, keep the leg straight at the hip for 6 to 8 hours.
- If the antecubital fossa route was used, keep the arm straight at the elbow for at least 3 hours.
- Resume medications and give analgesics, as ordered.
- Encourage fluid intake.
- Monitor the patient's vital signs, intake and output, cardiac rhythm, neurologic and respiratory status, and peripheral vascular status distal to the puncture site.
- Check the catheter insertion site for signs and symptoms of infection.

PRECAUTIONS

- Notify practitioner of patient sensitivity to shellfish, iodine, or contrast media.
- Catheterization of both sides of the heart is contraindicated in debilitated patients and in those with coagulopathy or impaired renal function.
- Unless a temporary pacemaker is inserted to counteract induced ventricular asystole, left bundle-branch block contraindicates catheterization of the right side of the heart.
- Prophylactic antibiotics prevent endocarditis in a patient with valvular heart disease.

COMPLICATIONS

- Infective endocarditis
- *Left- or right-sided heart catheterization:* Myocardial infarction, arrhythmias, cardiac tamponade, infection, hypovolemia, pulmonary edema, hematoma, blood loss, reaction to contrast media, vasovagal response
- *Left-sided heart catheterization:* Arterial thrombus or embolism, stroke
- *Right-sided heart catheterization:* Thrombophlebitis, pulmonary embolism

INTERPRETATION

NORMAL RESULTS

- No abnormalities of heart valves, chamber size, pressures, configuration, wall motion or thickness, and blood flow are detected.
- Coronary arteries have a smooth and regular outline.

ABNORMAL RESULTS

- Coronary artery narrowing greater than 70% suggests significant coronary artery disease.
- Narrowing of the left main coronary artery and occlusion or narrowing high in the left anterior descending artery suggests the need for revascularization surgery.
- Impaired wall motion suggests myocardial incompetence.
- Retrograde flow across the valves indicates valvular incompetence.

(continued)

Preparing for cardiac catheterization

Dear Patient,

You've been scheduled for cardiac catheterization, a procedure that looks at the inside of your heart. First, a small incision is made in a blood vessel near your elbow or groin, and then a long, thin, flexible tube called a *catheter* is inserted into the vessel.

The catheter is then slowly threaded through your bloodstream into your heart. When the catheter is in place, certain tests may be performed that require the injection of a special dye. The test results will guide further treatment designed to improve the function of your heart.

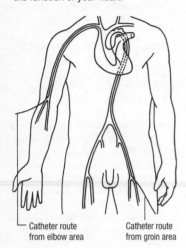

Catheter route
from elbow area

Catheter route
from groin area

BEFORE THE PROCEDURE

If your catheterization is scheduled for early morning, you probably won't be allowed to eat or drink anything after midnight the day before the test.

The area where the incision will be made may be shaved. Before you go to the catheterization laboratory, you'll be asked to urinate and then to put on a hospital gown. You will also have an I.V. line started in your arm.

When you reach the catheterization laboratory, you'll be placed on a padded table and probably be strapped to it. During the test, the table may be tilted to permit viewing of your heart from different angles. The straps will keep you from slipping out of position. Special foam pads, called *electrodes,* will be put on your chest to monitor your heartbeat.

Cardiac catheterization usually takes 1 or 2 hours. You'll be awake throughout the procedure, although you may receive medication to help you relax. Some patients even doze off. You may feel pain in your chest, flushing, or nausea during catheterization, but these sensations should pass quickly.

DURING THE PROCEDURE

First, a local anesthetic will be injected at the catheter insertion site to numb the area before the catheter is inserted. When the catheter is going in, you may feel a little pressure but no pain. You may receive nitroglycerin during the test to enlarge your heart's blood vessels and help provide a better view of your heart.

If the catheter's passage is blocked—for example, because of a narrowed blood vessel—the catheter will be removed, and a different insertion site will be used.

When the catheter enters your heart, you may feel a fluttering sensation. Report this sensation, but don't worry—this is a normal reaction. You'll probably also feel a warm sensation, some nausea, or the urge to urinate if dye is injected, but these feelings will quickly pass. Throughout the catheterization, remember to let someone know if you have chest pain. During the test, you may be given oxygen and asked to cough or to breathe deeply.

When the test is finished, the catheter will be removed, and a special bandage will be placed on your arm or groin. You may need a few stitches at the insertion site. Because the anesthetic will still be working, you shouldn't feel anything.

AFTER THE PROCEDURE

You'll be taken to a recovery area, where you'll be monitored for a short time. You'll be placed on a cardiac monitor to check your heart rhythm, and an electrocardiogram may be done. Your vital signs will be taken frequently during this time, and your bandage site will be checked for bleeding.

Your bandaged arm or leg must stay completely still for up to 8 hours. To help keep you from moving, your arm may be splinted or your leg may be weighed down with a sandbag. The site will be checked frequently for swelling and inadequate blood flow. You'll be asked to wiggle your toes or fingers once per hour or more.

As your anesthetic wears off, you'll probably feel some pain at the insertion site. Pain medication may be ordered.

As soon as the test results are available, you and your family will be informed of them. Don't hesitate to ask any questions that you may have.

Cardiac magnetic resonance imaging

DESCRIPTION

◆ Noninvasive diagnostic procedure that provides cross-sectional images of bone and delineation of fluid-filled soft tissue; produces images of organs and vessels in motion
◆ Relies on magnetic properties of hydrogen, the most abundant and magnetically sensitive of the body's atoms
◆ In cardiac magnetic resonance imaging (MRI), patient placed in a magnetic field; cross-sectional images of heart and related structures obtained in multiple planes
◆ Magnetic fields and radiofrequency (RF) energy imperceptible; no harmful effects documented
◆ Optimal magnetic fields and RF waves for investigating various tissues
◆ Also known as *MRI*

PURPOSE

◆ To identify anatomic sequelae related to myocardial infarction, such as formation of ventricular aneurysm and mural thrombus
◆ To detect and evaluate cardiomyopathy
◆ To detect and evaluate pericardial disease
◆ To identify paracardiac or intracardiac masses
◆ To detect and evaluate congenital heart disease, such as atrial or ventricular septal defects and malposition of the great vessels
◆ To identify vascular disease, such as thoracic aortic aneurysm and dissection
◆ To assess the structure of the pulmonary vasculature

PREPARATION

◆ Make sure the patient has signed an appropriate consent form.
◆ Note and report allergies.
◆ No dietary restrictions are required for this test.
◆ Have the patient remove all metal objects.

◆ Make sure the patient doesn't have a pacemaker or surgically implanted joints, pins, clips, valves, or pumps containing metal that could be attracted to the strong MRI magnet.
◆ Ask if the patient has ever worked with metals.
◆ Allow the patient to wear earplugs because the scanner makes clicking, whirring, and thumping noises as it moves.
◆ Provide reassurance to the patient that he'll be able to communicate with the technician at all times; tell him the procedure may be stopped if he feels claustrophobic.
◆ Give a sedative if ordered, especially for a claustrophobic patient.

Teaching points

◆ Tell the patient the purpose of the test and how it's done.
◆ Tell the patient who will perform the test and where it will be done.
◆ Inform the patient that no dietary restrictions are needed.
◆ Explain that MRI is painless but that remaining still inside a small space during the test may make the patient feel uncomfortable.
◆ Explain that the test takes up to 90 minutes.

KEY STEPS

◆ Confirm the patient's identity using two patient identifiers according to facility policy.
◆ Check the patient for metal objects; no metal can enter the testing area because the MRI works through a powerful magnetic field.
◆ The patient is placed in a supine position on a narrow, padded, nonmetallic bed that slides to the desired position inside the scanner.
◆ During the test the patient is asked to remain still.
◆ The patient's response to the enclosed environment is assessed; reassurance and sedation are provided if necessary.
◆ RF energy is directed at the patient's chest.

◆ Resulting images are displayed on a monitor and recorded for permanent storage.
◆ Maintain verbal contact with a conscious patient.

POSTPROCEDURE CARE

◆ No specific care is needed unless the patient received sedation.
◆ Monitor a sedated patient's hemodynamic, cardiac, respiratory, and mental status until the effects of the sedative have worn off.

PRECAUTIONS

◆ Unstable patients need an I.V. access without metal components, and all equipment must be MRI-compatible.
◆ Claustrophobic patients may experience anxiety.
◆ Monitor the cardiac patient for signs of ischemia (such as chest pressure, shortness of breath, or changes in hemodynamic status).
◆ Don't perform the test on a patient with a pacemaker or an intracranial aneurysm clip.
◆ An anesthesiologist may be needed to monitor a heavily sedated patient.
◆ A nurse or radiology technician should maintain verbal contact with the conscious patient.

COMPLICATIONS

◆ Panic attacks related to claustrophobia
◆ Adverse reactions to sedation

NORMAL RESULTS

◆ No cardiovascular abnormalities are detected.

ABNORMAL RESULTS

◆ Cardiovascular abnormalities may suggest cardiomyopathy and pericardial disease, atrial or ventricular septal defects, congenital defects, paracardiac or intracardiac masses, or pericardiac or vascular disease.

Cardiac positron emission tomography

DESCRIPTION

- Combines elements of computed tomography (CT) scanning and conventional radionuclide imaging
- Measures the particle emissions of injected radioisotopes (positrons) and converts them to tomographic images; positron emitters can be chemically tagged to biologically active molecules, such as carbon monoxide, neurotransmitters, hormones, and metabolites (particularly glucose), allowing study of their uptake and distribution in tissue
- Uses radioisotopes of biologically important elements, such as oxygen, nitrogen, carbon, and fluorine
- Radiation only 25% of that received from a CT scan
- Costly because of short half-lives of radioisotopes, which must be produced at an on-site cyclotron and attached quickly to the desired tracer molecules
- Also known as *PET scanning*

PURPOSE

- To detect coronary artery disease
- To evaluate myocardial metabolism
- To distinguish viable from infarcted cardiac tissue, especially during early stages of myocardial infarction

PREPARATION

- Make sure the patient has signed an appropriate consent form.
- Note and report allergies.
- Fasting may be needed after midnight the night before the test.
- The patient may need to avoid caffeinated beverages, alcohol, and tobacco products for 24 hours before the test.

Teaching points

- Tell the patient the purpose of the study and how it's done.
- Tell the patient who will perform the test and where it will be done.
- Assure him that the test is painless, other than minor discomfort if I.V. access is inserted.

- Tell the patient that he may have to fast after midnight the night before the test.
- Tell him that he may need to avoid caffeinated beverages, alcohol, and tobacco products for 24 hours before the test.
- Tell the patient that the test will take between 1 and 1½ hours.
- Instruct the patient to move slowly immediately after the test to avoid orthostatic hypotension.

DIAGNOSTIC PROCEDURE

KEY STEPS

- Confirm the patient's identity using two patient identifiers according to facility policy.
- The patient is placed in a supine position with his arms above his head.
- An attenuation scan, lasting about 30 minutes, is performed.
- The appropriate positron emitter is given and scanning is completed.
- A different positron emitter may be given if comparative studies are needed.

POSTPROCEDURE CARE

- After the test, encourage the patient to drink liquids to help flush the radioisotope from the bladder.

PRECAUTIONS

WARNING *Carefully screen female patients of childbearing age because the radioisotope can harm a fetus.*
- Stress the importance of remaining still during the study.

COMPLICATIONS

- Orthostatic hypotension

NORMAL RESULTS

- No areas of ischemic tissue are present.
- If the patient receives two tracers, the flow and distribution should match.

ABNORMAL RESULTS

- Reduced blood flow with increased glucose use indicates ischemia.
- Reduced blood flow with decreased glucose use indicates necrotic, scarred tissue.

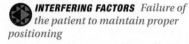 **INTERFERING FACTORS** *Failure of the patient to maintain proper positioning*

Cardiolipin antibody test

DESCRIPTION
◆ Enzyme-linked immunosorbent assay
◆ Measures serum levels of immunoglobulin (Ig) G and IgM antibodies in relation to cardiolipin

PURPOSE
◆ To aid in the diagnosis of cardiolipin antibody syndrome in patients with or without systemic lupus erythematosus (SLE) who experience recurrent episodes of spontaneous thrombosis, fetal loss, or thrombocytopenia

PREPARATION
◆ No dietary restrictions are required for this test.
◆ The test requires a blood sample.

Teaching points
◆ Tell the patient that this test helps diagnose cardiolipin antibody syndrome and SLE.
◆ Tell the patient who will perform the test and where it will be done.
◆ Inform him that there are no dietary restrictions.
◆ Explain to the patient that the test requires a blood sample and that she may experience slight discomfort from the tourniquet and needle puncture.
◆ Inform the patient that the test should take less than 5 minutes.

KEY STEPS
◆ Confirm the patient's identity using two patient identifiers according to facility policy.
◆ Perform a venipuncture and collect the sample in a 5-ml tube without additives.
◆ Send the sample to the laboratory immediately after collection.

POSTPROCEDURE CARE
◆ Apply direct pressure to the venipuncture site until bleeding stops.

PRECAUTIONS
◆ Maintain standard precautions while collecting the sample.
◆ Handle the sample gently to prevent hemolysis.

COMPLICATIONS
◆ Hematoma at the venipuncture site

NORMAL RESULTS
◆ Cardiolipin antibody results are reported as negative or positive.
◆ A positive result is titered.

ABNORMAL RESULTS
◆ A positive result along with a history of recurrent spontaneous thrombosis, fetal loss, or thrombocytopenia suggests cardiolipin antibody syndrome.
◆ A positive result may also be seen in patients with SLE whose blood contains a lupus anticoagulant.

Carotid artery duplex scanning

DESCRIPTION
- Examines the major extracranial arteries that supply blood to the brain
- Provides an image of the blood flow in the arteries; also able to provide the degree of occlusion, if present

PURPOSE
- To determine the degree of occlusion of carotid arteries after a stroke or transient ischemic attack, or in the presence of other neurologic symptoms
- To evaluate carotid arteries preoperatively

PREPARATION
- No dietary restrictions are required.
- Have the patient remove jewelry.

Teaching points
- Explain that this test determines if there's a blockage in the carotid arteries.
- Tell the patient who will perform the test and where it will be done.
- Inform the patient that the test requires no dietary restrictions.
- Tell him that gel will be applied to his neck during the procedure.
- Reassure the patient that the test is painless.
- Inform him that the test should take 30 to 60 minutes.

KEY STEPS
- Confirm the patient's identity using two patient identifiers according to facility policy.
- Have the patient lie flat on the table with his neck slightly hyperextended and turned away from the side being studied.
- Apply a water-soluble gel to the area being examined.
- Move the transducer over the area while images of the blood vessels are being made.

POSTPROCEDURE CARE
- Remove the gel from the patient.

PRECAUTIONS
- None

COMPLICATIONS
- None

NORMAL RESULTS
- Normal vascular anatomy and blood flow is noted.

ABNORMAL RESULTS
- Slowing or reversal of blood flow indicates stenosis of the artery at that point.
- Reversal of blood flow may also indicate an occlusion because of plaque.

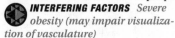 **INTERFERING FACTORS** *Severe obesity (may impair visualization of vasculature)*

Catecholamine levels, plasma

DESCRIPTION

◆ Total or fractionated analysis of plasma catecholamine levels for hypertensive patients with signs of adrenal medullary tumor or those with neural tumors affecting endocrine function

PURPOSE

◆ To rule out pheochromocytoma in patients with hypertension
◆ To help identify neuroblastoma, ganglioneuroblastoma, and ganglioneuroma
◆ To distinguish between adrenal medullary tumors through fractional analysis
◆ To help diagnose autonomic nervous system dysfunction such as idiopathic orthostatic hypotension

PREPARATION

◆ If the patient is in your facility, withhold drugs that affect catecholamine levels, such as amphetamines, phenothiazines, sympathomimetics, and tricyclic antidepressants.
◆ The test requires one or two blood samples.
◆ If possible, insert an indwelling venous catheter (heparin lock) 24 hours before the test because the stress of the venipuncture itself may significantly raise catecholamine levels.
◆ Make sure the patient is relaxed and recumbent for 45 to 60 minutes before the test.
◆ If necessary, provide blankets to keep the patient warm; low temperatures stimulate catecholamine secretion.

Teaching points

◆ Explain to the patient that this test helps determine if hypertension or other symptoms are related to improper hormonal secretion.
◆ Instruct the patient to refrain from using self-prescribed medications, especially cold and allergy remedies that may contain sympathomimetics, for 2 weeks before the test.

◆ Tell the patient who will perform the test and when it'll be done.
◆ Advise the patient to avoid amine-rich foods and beverages for 48 hours; to maintain vitamin C intake, which is necessary for formation of catecholamines; to abstain from smoking for 24 hours; and to fast for 10 to 12 hours before the test.
◆ If the patient doesn't have an indwelling venous catheter, tell him that the test requires one or two blood samples and that he may experience slight discomfort from the tourniquet and needle puncture.
◆ Inform the patient that the test should take less than 1 hour.

KEY STEPS

◆ Confirm the patient's identity using two patient identifiers according to facility policy.
◆ Perform a venipuncture between 6 a.m. and 8 a.m.
◆ Collect the sample in a 10-ml chilled EDTA tube, which can be obtained from the laboratory on request.
◆ If a second sample is requested, have the patient stand for 10 minutes and draw the sample into another tube exactly like the first.
◆ If a heparin lock is used, it may be necessary to discard the first 1 or 2 ml of blood. Check with the laboratory for the preferred diagnostic procedure.
◆ Indicate on the laboratory request whether the patient was supine or standing during the venipuncture and the time the sample was drawn.

POSTPROCEDURE CARE

◆ Apply direct pressure to the venipuncture site until bleeding stops.
◆ If the patient had an indwelling venous catheter placed for the test, remove it, as ordered.
◆ Instruct the patient to resume his usual diet and medications.

PRECAUTIONS

◆ Maintain standard precautions while collecting the sample.

◆ After collecting each sample, roll the tube slowly between your palms to distribute the EDTA without agitating the blood.
◆ Pack the tube in crushed ice to minimize deactivation of catecholamines and send it to the laboratory immediately after collection.

COMPLICATIONS

◆ Hematoma at the venipuncture site

NORMAL RESULTS

◆ In fractional analysis, catecholamine supine levels are epinephrine, undetectable to 110 pg/ml (SI, undetectable to 600 pmol/L); norepinephrine, 70 to 750 pg/ml (SI, 413 to 4,432 pmol/L).
◆ In fractional analysis, standing catecholamine levels are epinephrine, undetectable to 140 pg/ml (SI, undetectable to 764 pmol/L); norepinephrine, 200 to 1,700 pg/ml (SI, 1,182 to 10,047 pmol/L).

ABNORMAL RESULTS

◆ High catecholamine levels may indicate pheochromocytoma, neuroblastoma, ganglioneuroblastoma, ganglioneuroma, thyroid disorders, hypoglycemia, and cardiac disease; these may also result from electroconvulsive therapy, hemorrhagic shock, endotoxins, and anaphylaxis.
◆ Fractional analysis helps identify the cause of elevated catecholamine levels (for example, adrenal medullary tumors secrete epinephrine, whereas ganglioneuromas, ganglioblastomas, and neuroblastomas secrete norepinephrine).
◆ In patients with normal or low baseline catecholamine levels, failure to show an increase in the sample taken after standing suggests autonomic nervous system dysfunction.

INTERFERING FACTORS *Epinephrine, levodopa, amphetamines, phenothiazines, sympathomimetics, decongestants, and tricyclic antidepressants (increase catecholamine levels)*

Catecholamine levels, urine

DESCRIPTION

◆ Measures urine levels of the major catecholamines using spectrophoto-fluorimetry
◆ A 24-hour urine specimen preferred because catecholamine secretion fluctuates diurnally and in response to various stimuli, conditions, and drugs
◆ Random specimen useful for evaluating catecholamine levels after a hypertensive episode
◆ For complete diagnostic workup of catecholamine secretion, urine levels of metabolites measured; appear in urine in greater quantities than catecholamines

PURPOSE

◆ To aid in the diagnosis of pheochromocytoma in patients with unexplained hypertension
◆ To aid in the diagnosis of neuroblastoma, ganglioneuroma, and dysautonomia

PREPARATION

◆ The test requires collection of urine over 24 hours or a random specimen.
◆ Notify the laboratory and practitioner of medications the patient is taking that may affect test results; they may be restricted.

Teaching points

◆ Tell the patient this test evaluates his adrenal function.
◆ Explain the collection procedure to the patient.
◆ Instruct the patient to avoid chocolate, coffee, and bananas for 7 hours before the test and to avoid stressful situations and excessive physical activity during the collection period.

KEY STEPS

◆ Confirm the patient's identity using two patient identifiers according to facility policy.
◆ Collect the patient's urine over a 24-hour period. Use a bottle containing a preservative to keep the specimen acidified to a pH of 3.0 or less.
◆ If a random specimen is ordered, collect it immediately after a hypertensive episode.
◆ Send the specimen to the laboratory as soon as the collection is complete.

POSTPROCEDURE CARE

◆ Instruct the patient that he may resume his usual activities, diet, and medications.

PRECAUTIONS

◆ Refrigerate a 24-hour specimen or place it on ice during the collection period.

COMPLICATIONS

◆ None

NORMAL RESULTS

◆ Values for catecholamine fractionalization range as follows: epinephrine: 0 to 20 mcg/24 hours (SI, 0 to 109 nmol/24 hours); norepinephrine: 15 to 80 mcg/24 hours (SI, 89 to 473 nmol/24 hours); and dopamine: 65 to 400 mcg/24 hours (SI, 425 to 2,610 nmol/24 hours).

ABNORMAL RESULTS

◆ In patients with undiagnosed hypertension, elevated urine catecholamine levels after a hypertensive episode usually indicate the presence of a pheochromocytoma.
◆ If tests indicate a pheochromocytoma, the patient may undergo a test for multiple endocrine neoplasia.
◆ With the exception of homovanillic acid (HVA)—a dopamine metabolite—catecholamine metabolites may also be elevated.
◆ High HVA levels rule out a pheochromocytoma because this tumor secretes mainly epinephrine; its primary metabolite is vanillylmandelic acid, not HVA.
◆ Elevated catecholamine levels, without marked hypertension, may be caused by a neuroblastoma or a ganglioneuroma, although HVA levels reflect these conditions more accurately.
◆ Elevated levels occur in severe systemic conditions (such as burns, peritonitis, shock, and septicemia), cor pulmonale, manic-depressive disorders, or depressive neurosis.
◆ Myasthenia gravis and progressive muscular dystrophy commonly cause urine catecholamine levels to rise above normal, but use of this test is rare for diagnosing these disorders.
◆ Consistently low-normal catecholamine levels may indicate dysautonomia marked by orthostatic hypotension.

CD4/CD8 enumeration

DESCRIPTION

◆ T cells (lymphocytes): play significant role in immune function (T cells include CD4+ helper T cells and CD8+ suppressor T cells)
◆ As CD4+ T-lymphocytes decrease, increased possibility of complication from acquired immunodeficiency syndrome (AIDS)

PURPOSE

◆ To assist the diagnosis of AIDS
◆ To guide treatment for patients with AIDS
◆ To diagnose and classify malignant myeloproliferative disease
◆ To evaluate cellular competence

PREPARATION

◆ This test helps manage the patient's medical condition, as appropriate.
◆ Obtain the patient's immune system history.
◆ List medications the patient is currently taking, including herbal or alternative medications.
◆ No dietary restrictions are required.
◆ The test requires a blood sample.

Teaching points

◆ Explain to the patient the purpose of the test and how it's done.
◆ Tell the patient who will perform the test and where it will be done.
◆ Inform the patient that no dietary restrictions are required.
◆ Tell the patient when he should receive the test results.
◆ Explain to the patient that the test requires a blood sample and that he may experience slight discomfort from the tourniquet and needle puncture.
◆ Inform the patient that the test should take less than 5 minutes.

KEY STEPS

◆ Confirm the patient's identity using two patient identifiers according to facility policy.
◆ Perform a venipuncture and collect the sample in a heparinized 5-ml tube.
◆ Keep the specimen at room temperature and don't refrigerate.
◆ Send the sample to the laboratory immediately after collection.

POSTPROCEDURE CARE

◆ Apply direct pressure to the venipuncture site until bleeding stops.
◆ Provide emotional support to the patient.

PRECAUTIONS

◆ Maintain standard precautions while collecting the sample.
◆ Handle the sample gently to prevent hemolysis.

COMPLICATIONS

◆ Hematoma at the venipuncture site

NORMAL RESULTS

◆ CD4+ count is 450/µl to 1,400/µl.
◆ CD8+ count is 190/µl to 725/µl.
◆ CD4/CD8 ratio is greater than 1.

ABNORMAL RESULTS

◆ An increase will be seen in malignant myeloproliferative diseases, such as lymphoma, and lymphocytic leukemias.
◆ Decreased levels are seen in patients with AIDS, aplastic anemia, and Hodgkin's disease.
◆ Antiviral therapy should begin with a CD4+ count less than 600/µl.
◆ AIDS is expected to develop when the CD4+ count is below 100/µl.
◆ Decreased CD4+ count may also been seen in minor viral infections or after organ transplantation.
◆ A significantly decreased CD4+ count is the best indicator of imminent opportunistic infection.
◆ Prophylactic treatment for *Pneumocystis carinii* should begin when the CD4+ count is less than 300/µl.

✦ INTERFERING FACTORS *Corticosteroids (increase CD4+ count) and immunosuppressants (decrease CD4+ count)*

Celiac and mesenteric arteriography

DESCRIPTION

◆ Radiographic examination of abdominal vasculature after intra-arterial injection of a contrast medium through a catheter
◆ Catheter passed through femoral artery into abdominal aorta and positioned in celiac, superior mesenteric, or inferior mesenteric artery using fluoroscopic guidance

PURPOSE

◆ To locate the source of and to control GI bleeding when other measures fail
◆ To distinguish between benign and malignant neoplasms
◆ To evaluate cirrhosis and portal hypertension
◆ To evaluate vascular damage after abdominal trauma
◆ To detect vascular abnormalities

PREPARATION

◆ Make sure the patient has signed a consent form.
◆ Check the patient's history for hypersensitivity to iodine, shellfish, or contrast media.
◆ Obtain results of preprocedure tests and report abnormal results.
◆ Fasting is required for 8 hours before the test.
◆ Give a sedative if ordered.

Teaching points

◆ Explain the purpose of the test and how it's done.
◆ Tell the patient who will perform the test and where it will be done.
◆ Instruct the patient to fast for at least 8 hours before the test.
◆ Tell the patient that he'll receive I.V. conscious sedation and a local anesthetic.
◆ Warn him that he may feel transient burning as the contrast is injected.
◆ Tell the patient that the test can take 30 minutes to 3 hours, depending on the number of vessels studied.

DIAGNOSTIC PROCEDURE

KEY STEPS

◆ Confirm the patient's identity using two patient identifiers according to facility policy.
◆ The patient is placed in a supine position on the radiography table and an I.V. infusion is started.
◆ The puncture site, usually the right groin, is cleaned and prepared.
◆ A local anesthetic is injected.
◆ The needle is inserted into the femoral artery.
◆ A guide wire is passed through the needle into the aorta and the needle is removed.
◆ A catheter is inserted over the guide wire and advanced into the artery. The guide wire is removed.
◆ A series of films is taken as contrast is injected through the catheter.
◆ The catheter is withdrawn and firm pressure is applied.
◆ The site is cleaned and a sterile dressing is applied.

POSTPROCEDURE CARE

◆ Maintain bed rest and keep the affected leg straight for 4 to 6 hours.
◆ Raise the head of the bed 30 degrees.
◆ Assist the patient in rolling side to side.
◆ Encourage fluid intake.
◆ Monitor the patient's vital signs and intake and output.
◆ Monitor the patient's peripheral pulses, color, temperature, and sensation in the leg used for the test. Notify the practitioner immediately of changes.

⚡ **WARNING** *Check the puncture site for bleeding or expanding hematoma. If either develops, apply direct manual pressure to the site and notify the practitioner promptly.*

PRECAUTIONS

◆ The test should be performed cautiously in patients with coagulopathy.

⚡ **WARNING** *Be aware that most reactions to contrast medium occur within 30 minutes. Watch the patient carefully for cardiovascular shock or arrest, flushing, laryngeal stridor, or urticaria.*

COMPLICATIONS

◆ Reactions to the contrast medium
◆ Hemorrhage, thrombosis, and emboli
◆ Cardiac arrhythmias and infection

NORMAL RESULTS

◆ The arteries taper in size.
◆ The contrast medium spreads evenly within the sinusoids (empties from the intestine into the superior mesenteric vein and into the portal vein).

ABNORMAL RESULTS

◆ Extravasation of contrast from damaged vessels suggests GI hemorrhage.
◆ Findings suggesting abdominal neoplasm include invasion, encasement, distortion, or displacement of blood vessels; areas of necrosis appearing as puddles of contrast; a tumor blush or stain produced by contrast remaining longer in the neoplasm; and arteriovenous (AV) shunting, depending on tumor size and location.
◆ Diminished portal venous flow, dilated and tortuous collateral veins, and reversed portal venous flow suggest cirrhosis.
◆ Displaced intrasplenic arterial branches, contrast leakage from splenic arteries into splenic pulp, displaced splenic arteries and veins by enlarged spleen, and compressed intrasplenic arteries and compressed splenic pulp by an avascular mass indicating a subcapsular hematoma suggest splenic injury.
◆ Vascular distortion, displaced and stretched intrahepatic arteries by intrahepatic and subcapsular hematomas, and AV fistulas between the hepatic artery and portal vein suggest hepatic injury.
◆ Narrowed or occluded arterial lumens suggest atherosclerotic plaque, vessel spasm, or emboli.

Cerebral angiography

DESCRIPTION

- Radiographic examination of the cerebral vasculature after injection of intra-arterial contrast medium
- Performed in patients with suspected abnormalities of the cerebral vasculature (suggested by other imaging studies)

PURPOSE

- To detect cerebrovascular abnormalities, such as aneurysm or arteriovenous malformation, thrombosis, narrowing, or occlusion
- To evaluate vascular displacement caused by tumor, hematoma, edema, herniation, vasospasm, increased intracranial pressure, or hydrocephalus
- To locate clips applied to blood vessels during surgery and to evaluate the postoperative status of such vessels
- To evaluate the presence and degree of carotid artery disease

PREPARATION

- Make sure the patient has signed a consent form.
- Note and report allergies.
- Have the patient fast for 8 to 10 hours before the test.
- Initiate an I.V. access; give I.V. fluids.
- Give a sedative.

Teaching points

- Explain the purpose of the test and how it's done.
- Tell the patient who will perform the test and where it will be done.
- Tell the patient that his head will be immobilized and that he'll need to lie still.
- Explain to the patient that he'll receive a local anesthetic.
- Warn the patient that nausea, warmth, or burning may occur with the contrast injection.
- Inform the patient that the test takes about 2 to 4 hours.

KEY STEPS

- Confirm the patient's identity using two patient identifiers according to facility policy.
- The patient is placed in a supine position on a radiographic table.
- The access site is prepared and draped and a local anesthetic is injected.
- The artery is punctured with the appropriate needle and catheterized under fluoroscopic guidance.
- Catheter placement is verified by fluoroscopy and a contrast medium is injected.
- A series of radiographs is taken and reviewed.
- The patient's vital signs and neurologic status are monitored continuously.
- The catheter is removed, firm pressure is applied to the access site until bleeding stops, and a pressure dressing is applied.

POSTPROCEDURE CARE

- Enforce bed rest and apply an ice bag.
- If active bleeding or expanding hematoma occurs, apply firm pressure to the puncture site and inform the practitioner immediately.
- Ensure adequate hydration.
- Provide analgesia.
- Monitor the patient's vital signs and intake and output.
- Monitor the neurovascular status of the extremity distal to the access site.
- **WARNING** *If the femoral approach was used, keep the involved leg straight at the hip for 6 hours or longer and routinely check pulses distal to the site (dorsalis, pedis, and popliteal). Monitor the leg for temperature, color, and sensation. Thrombosis or hematoma can occlude blood flow; extravasation can also impede blood flow by exerting pressure on the artery.*
- If the carotid artery was used as the access site, watch for dysphagia or respiratory distress, which can result from hematoma or edema. Also watch for disorientation, weakness, or numbness in the extremities (signs of neurovascular compromise) and for arterial spasms, which produce symptoms of transient ischemic attacks (TIAs). Notify the practitioner promptly if abnormal signs develop.
- If the brachial artery was used, keep the arm straight at the elbow and assess distal pulses (radial and ulnar). Avoid venipuncture and blood pressures in the affected arm. Observe the extremity for changes in color, temperature, or sensation. If it becomes pale, cool, or numb, notify the practitioner at once.

PRECAUTIONS

- Check for allergy to iodine or other contrast media and notify the practitioner.
- The test is contraindicated in patients with severe renal or thyroid disease, recent anticoagulation therapy, and recent thrombotic or embolic events.

COMPLICATIONS

- Adverse reaction to contrast media
- Embolism, bleeding, hematoma, and infection
- Vasospasm, thrombosis, TIA, or stroke

NORMAL RESULTS

- The cerebral vasculature is normal.
- During the arterial phase of perfusion, the contrast medium fills and opacifies superficial and deep arteries and arterioles.
- During the venous phase, the contrast medium opacifies superficial and deep veins.

ABNORMAL RESULTS

- Changes in the caliber of vessel lumina suggest vascular disease.
- Vessel displacement suggests a possible tumor.

Cerebrospinal fluid analysis

DESCRIPTION

- Most commonly obtained by lumbar puncture (usually between the third and fourth lumbar vertebrae); rarely, by cisternal or ventricular puncture (for qualitative analysis)
- May also be obtained during other neurologic tests such as myelography

PURPOSE

- To measure cerebrospinal fluid (CSF) pressure as an aid in detecting an obstruction of CSF circulation
- To help diagnose viral or bacterial meningitis, subarachnoid or intracranial hemorrhage, tumors, and brain abscesses
- To help diagnose neurosyphilis and chronic central nervous system infections
- To check for Alzheimer's disease

PREPARATION

- No dietary restrictions are needed.
- Make sure that the patient or a responsible family member has signed an informed consent form.
- If the patient is unusually anxious, assess and report his vital signs.

Teaching points

- Explain that this test analyzes the fluid around the spinal cord.
- Tell the patient who will perform the test and where it will be done.
- Tell the patient that no dietary restrictions are required.
- Instruct the patient to remain still and breathe normally; movement and hyperventilation can alter pressure readings or cause injury.
- Advise the patient that a headache is the most common adverse effect of a lumbar puncture, but reassure him that his cooperation during the test helps minimize this effect.
- Tell the patient that when the spinal needle is inserted, he may feel slight local pain as the needle transverses the dura mater.
- Instruct the patient to report pain or sensations that differ from or continue after this expected discomfort because such sensations may indicate irritation or puncture of a nerve root, requiring needle repositioning.
- Inform the patient that the test should take less than 30 minutes.

DIAGNOSTIC PROCEDURE

KEY STEPS

- Confirm the patient's identity using two patient identifiers according to facility policy.
- During the procedure, observe closely for adverse reactions, such as elevated pulse rate, pallor, or clammy skin, and report any significant changes immediately.
- Position the patient on his side at the edge of the bed with his knees drawn up to his abdomen and his chin on his chest. Provide pillows to support the spine on a horizontal plane. This position allows full flexion of the spine and easy access to the lumbar subarachnoid space. Help him maintain this position by placing one arm around his knees and the other arm around his neck.
- If the sitting position is preferable, have the patient sit up and bend his chest and head toward his knees. Help him maintain this position throughout the procedure.
- The skin is prepared for injection and the area is draped.
- The anesthetic is injected, and the spinal needle is inserted in the midline, between the spinous processes of the vertebrae (usually between the third and fourth lumbar vertebra). At this point, initial (or opening) CSF pressure is measured and a specimen is obtained.
- After the specimen is collected, label the containers in the order in which they were filled.
- Record the collection time on the test request form. Send the labeled specimens to the laboratory immediately after collection.
- A final pressure reading is taken, and the needle is removed.
- The puncture site is cleaned with a local antiseptic, such as povidone-iodine solution, and a small adhesive bandage is applied.

POSTPROCEDURE CARE

- Check whether the patient must lie flat or if the head of his bed may be slightly elevated. In most cases, instruct the patient to keep lying flat for 8 hours after the lumbar puncture. Sometimes, a 30-degree elevation at the head of the bed is allowed. Remind the patient that although he must not raise his head, he can turn from side to side.
- Encourage the patient to drink fluids. Provide a flexible straw.
- Check the puncture site for redness, swelling, and drainage every hour for the first 4 hours, and then every 4 hours for the first 24 hours.
- If CSF pressure is elevated, assess the patient's neurologic status every 15 minutes for 4 hours. If he's stable, assess him every hour for 4 hours and then every 4 hours or according to the pretest schedule.

PRECAUTIONS

WARNING *Monitor the patient for complications of lumbar puncture, such as reaction to the anesthetic, meningitis, bleeding into the spinal canal, cerebellar tonsillar herniation, and medially compression.*

- Infection at the puncture site contraindicates removal of CSF; in patients with increased intracranial pressure, CSF should be removed with extreme caution because the rapid reduction in pressure can cause cerebellar tonsillar herniation and medullary compression.

COMPLICATIONS

- Reaction to the anesthetic, meningitis, bleeding into the spinal canal, cerebellar tonsillar herniation, and medullary compression
- Signs of meningitis, such as fever, neck rigidity, and irritability
- Signs of herniation, including decreased level of consciousness, changes in pupil size and equality, altered vital signs, and respiratory failure

NORMAL RESULTS

◆ The fluid obtained is clear and color-less.
◆ The cell count reveals no red blood cells (RBCs); 0 to 5 white blood cells (WBCs).
◆ Gram stain reveals absence of any or-ganisms.
◆ CSF pressure is between 50 and 180 mm H_2O.

ABNORMAL RESULTS

◆ The fluid obtained is cloudy, bloody, brown, orange, or yellow.
◆ There are RBCs present and in-creased WBCs.
◆ Gram stain reveals presence of Gram-positive or Gram-negative or-ganisms.
◆ Pressure is increased or decreased. (See *Findings in cerebrospinal fluid analysis.*)
◆ Presence of soluble amyloid beta protein precursor confirms diagnosis of Alzheimer's disease.

Findings in cerebrospinal fluid analysis

TEST	NORMAL	ABNORMALITY	IMPLICATIONS
Pressure	50 to 180 mm H_2O	Increase	Increased intracranial pressure
		Decrease	Spinal subarachnoid obstruction above puncture site
Appearance	Clear, colorless	Cloudy	Infection
		Xanthochromic or bloody	Subarachnoid, intracerebral, or in-traventricular hemorrhage; spinal cord obstruction; traumatic tap (usu-ally noted only in initial specimen)
		Brown, orange, or yellow	Elevated protein levels, red blood cell (RBC) breakdown (blood present for at least 3 days)
Protein	15 to 50 mg/dl (SI, 0.15 to 0.5 q/L)	Marked increase	Tumors, trauma, hemorrhage, dia-betes mellitus, polyneuritis, blood in cerebrospinal fluid (CSF)
		Marked decrease	Rapid CSF production
Gamma globulin	3% to 12% of total protein	Increase	Demyelinating disease, neu-rosyphilis, Guillain-Barré syndrome
Glucose	50 to 80 mg/dl (SI, 2.8 to 4.4 mmol/L)	Increase	Systemic hyperglycemia
		Decrease	Systemic hypoglycemia, bacterial or fungal infection, meningitis, mumps, postsubarachnoid hemorrhage
Cell count	0 to 5 white blood cells	Increase	Active disease: meningitis, acute in-fection, onset of chronic illness, tu-mor, abscess, infarction, demyelinat-ing disease
	No RBCs	RBCs	Hemorrhage or traumatic lumbar puncture
Venereal Disease Research Laboratories, test for syphilis, and other serologic tests	Nonreactive	Positive	Neurosyphilis
Chloride	118 to 130 mEq/L (SI, 118 to 130 mmol/L)	Decrease	Infected meninges
Gram stain	No organisms	Gram-positive or gram-negative organisms	Bacterial meningitis

Ceruloplasmin level test

DESCRIPTION
- Measures serum levels of ceruloplasmin, an alpha$_2$-globulin that binds about 95% of serum copper (usually in liver)
- Ceruloplasmin believed to regulate iron uptake by transferrin, making iron available to reticulocytes for heme synthesis

PURPOSE
- To help diagnose Wilson's disease, Menkes' syndrome, and copper deficiency

PREPARATION
- This test determines the copper content of blood.
- The test requires a blood sample.
- Notify the laboratory and practitioner of medications the patient is taking that may affect test results; it may be necessary to restrict them.

Teaching points
- Explain the purpose of the test and how it's done.
- Tell the patient who will perform the test and where it will be done.
- Tell the patient that no dietary restrictions are required.
- Explain to the patient that the test requires a blood sample and that he may experience slight discomfort from the tourniquet and needle puncture.
- Inform the patient that the test should take less than 5 minutes.

KEY STEPS
- Confirm the patient's identity using two patient identifiers according to facility policy.
- Perform a venipuncture and collect the sample in a 7-ml clot-activator tube.
- Send the sample to the laboratory immediately after collection.

POSTPROCEDURE CARE
- Apply direct pressure to the venipuncture site until bleeding stops.
- Instruct the patient to resume medications discontinued before the test.

PRECAUTIONS
- Maintain standard precautions while collecting the sample.

COMPLICATIONS
- Hematoma at the venipuncture site

NORMAL RESULTS
- Level is 22.9 to 43.1 g/dl (SI, 0.22 to 0.43 g/L).

ABNORMAL RESULTS
- Decreased levels usually indicate Wilson's disease.
- Decreased levels may also occur in Menkes' syndrome, nephrotic syndrome, and hypocupremia (decreased copper levels) caused by total parenteral nutrition.
- Increased levels may indicate certain hepatic diseases and infections.

Cervical punch biopsy

DESCRIPTION

◆ Involves excision by sharp forceps of a tissue specimen from the cervix for histologic examination
◆ Multiple biopsies done to obtain specimens from all areas with abnormal tissue.
◆ Performed when the cervix is least vascular (usually 1 week after menses)
◆ Site selected by direct visualization of cervix with a colposcope (most accurate method) and by Schiller's test (normal squamous epithelium stains dark mahogany, abnormal tissue doesn't change color)

PURPOSE

◆ To evaluate suspicious cervical lesions
◆ To diagnose cervical cancer

PREPARATION

◆ Make sure the patient has signed a consent form.
◆ Note and report allergies.
◆ Ask the patient to void just before the biopsy.

Teaching points

◆ Explain the purpose of the test and how it's done.
◆ Tell the patient who will perform the biopsy and where it will be done.
◆ Advise her that she may experience mild discomfort during and after the biopsy.
◆ Inform the patient that she should have someone accompany her home after the biopsy.
◆ Instruct the patient to avoid strenuous exercise for 8 to 24 hours after the test.
◆ Tell her to leave the tampon (if used) in place for 8 to 24 hours.
◆ Inform the patient that some bleeding may occur but that she should report heavy bleeding (heavier than menstrual) to the practitioner.
◆ Warn the patient to avoid using additional tampons, which can irritate the cervix and provoke bleeding, according to her practitioner's directions.
◆ Tell the patient to avoid douching.
◆ Advise her to refrain from sexual intercourse for up to 2 weeks, or as directed, if the procedure involved cryotherapy or laser treatment.
◆ Inform the patient that a foul-smelling, gray-green vaginal discharge is normal for several days after the biopsy and may persist for 3 weeks.
◆ Inform the patient that the procedure takes about 15 minutes.

KEY STEPS

◆ Confirm the patient's identity using two patient identifiers according to facility policy.
◆ Assist the patient into the lithotomy position.
◆ A nonlubricated speculum is inserted.
◆ For direct visualization, the colposcope is inserted through the speculum.
◆ The biopsy site is located, and the cervix is cleaned with a swab soaked in 3% acetic acid solution.
◆ Biopsy forceps are inserted through the speculum or the colposcope.
◆ Tissue from the lesion or selected sites is removed, starting from the posterior lip to avoid obscuring other sites with blood.
◆ Each specimen is immediately placed in 10% formalin solution in a labeled bottle.
◆ The cervix is swabbed with 5% silver nitrate solution (cautery or sutures may be used instead) to control bleeding.
◆ The examiner may insert a tampon if bleeding persists.
◆ For Schiller's test, an applicator stick saturated with iodine solution is inserted through the speculum. This stains the cervix to identify lesions for biopsy.

POSTPROCEDURE CARE

◆ If performed in the office, encourage the patient to rest briefly before leaving.

PRECAUTIONS

◆ Send the specimen to the laboratory immediately.

COMPLICATIONS

◆ Bleeding
◆ Infection

NORMAL RESULTS

◆ No dysplasia and abnormal cell growth are present.
◆ Normal cervical tissue is composed of columnar and squamous epithelial cells, loose connective tissue, and smooth-muscle fibers.

ABNORMAL RESULTS

◆ Dysplasia or abnormal cell growth on histologic examination of a cervical tissue specimen may suggest intraepithelial neoplasia or invasive cancer.

Chest radiography

DESCRIPTION
◆ Noninvasive and relatively inexpensive study
◆ Uses X-ray beams that penetrate the chest and react on specially sensitized film; air is radiolucent, so thoracic structures appear as different densities on the film
◆ Also known as *chest X-ray*

PURPOSE
◆ To establish a baseline for future comparison
◆ To detect pulmonary disorders such as pneumonia
◆ To detect mediastinal abnormalities such as tumors
◆ To verify correct placement of pulmonary artery catheters, endotracheal (ET) tubes, chest tubes, and central venous catheters
◆ To determine location of swallowed or aspirated radiopaque foreign bodies
◆ To determine location and size of lesions
◆ To evaluate response to interventions such as diuretic therapy

PREPARATION
◆ Make sure the patient has signed an appropriate consent form.
◆ No dietary restrictions are required.
◆ Move cardiac monitoring cables, oxygen tubing, I.V. tubing, pulmonary artery catheter lines, and other equipment out of the radiographic field.

Teaching points
◆ Explain the purpose of the test.
◆ Tell the patient who will perform the test and where it will be done.
◆ Tell the patient that no dietary restrictions are needed.
◆ Explain that the patient will be asked to take a deep breath and hold it momentarily during the X-ray.
◆ Inform the patient that the test takes less than 5 minutes.

DIAGNOSTIC PROCEDURE

KEY STEPS
◆ Confirm the patient's identity using two patient identifiers according to facility policy.
◆ The patient is instructed to stand or sit in front of a stationary radiography machine.
◆ Posteroanterior and left lateral views are obtained.
◆ A portable radiography machine is used at the patient's bedside if he can't travel to radiology.
◆ Because an upright chest radiograph is preferable, move the patient to the head of the bed if he can tolerate this position.
◆ Elevate the head of the bed for maximum upright positioning.

POSTPROCEDURE CARE
◆ Check that no tubes have been dislodged during positioning.

PRECAUTIONS
◆ The test is contraindicated during the first trimester of pregnancy.
◆ If possible, place a lead apron over the patient's abdomen to protect the gonads.
◆ To avoid radiation exposure, leave the area or wear lead shielding while the films are being taken.

COMPLICATIONS
◆ Potential for dislodging tubes or wires, such as the ET tube or pacemaker wires, during positioning

INTERPRETATION

NORMAL RESULTS
◆ The trachea is visible midline in the anterior mediastinal cavity, appearing translucent and tubelike.
◆ The heart is visible in the anterior left mediastinal cavity, appearing solid because of its blood content.
◆ The aortic knob is visible as water density.
◆ The mediastinum (mediastinal shadow) is visible as the space between the lungs, appearing shadowy and widened at the hilum.
◆ The ribs are visible as a thoracic cavity encasement.
◆ The spine has a visible midline in the posterior chest that's most visible on a lateral view.
◆ The clavicles are visible in the upper thorax. They're intact and equidistant in properly centered films.
◆ The hila (lung roots) are visible above the heart and exist where pulmonary vessels, bronchi, and lymph nodes join the lungs. They appear as small, white, bilateral branching densities.
◆ The mainstem bronchus is visible as part of the hila. It has a translucent, tubelike appearance.
◆ The bronchi aren't usually visible.
◆ The lung fields aren't usually visible, except for blood vessels.
◆ The hemidiaphragm is rounded and visible. The right side is $3/8''$ to $3/4''$ (1 to 2 cm) higher than the left side.

ABNORMAL RESULTS
◆ Deviation of the trachea from midline suggests possible tension pneumothorax or pleural effusion.
◆ Right side of the heart hypertrophy suggests possible cor pulmonale or heart failure.
◆ A tortuous aortic knob suggests atherosclerosis.
◆ Gross widening of the mediastinum suggests neoplasm or aortic aneurysm.
◆ A break or misalignment of bones suggests fracture.
◆ Visible bronchi suggest bronchial pneumonia.
◆ Flattening of the diaphragm suggests emphysema or asthma.
◆ Irregular, patchy infiltrates in the lung fields suggest pneumonia.

INTERFERING FACTORS *Inability to take a full inspiration (results in a decreased quality of the view)*

Chlamydia culture

DESCRIPTION
- Cultivation in the laboratory to identify parasite
- *Chlamydia*-infected cells detected by fluorescein isothiocyanate-conjugated monoclonal antibodies or by iodine stain
- Detection of *C. psittaci* and *C. pneumoniae* in cell cultures: requires specific technical manipulations and reagents; deoxyribonucleic acid detection may be seen in women susceptible to infections, irrespective of symptoms.
- Detection method of choice, although rapid noncultural (antigen detection) procedures also available

PURPOSE
- To confirm infections caused by *C. trachomatis*

PREPARATION
- Ensure patient privacy during specimen collection.

Teaching points
- Explain the purpose of the test.
- Tell the patient who will perform the test and where it will be done.
- Describe the procedure for collecting a specimen for culture.
- If the specimen will be collected from the patient's genital tract, instruct him not to urinate for 3 to 4 hours before the specimen is taken.
- Tell a female patient not to douche for 24 hours before the test.
- Tell a male patient that he may experience some burning and pressure during the collection process but that the discomfort will subside after a few minutes.
- Inform the patient that the test takes less than 30 minutes.
- Advise the patient to avoid all sexual contact until after the test results are known.

DIAGNOSTIC PROCEDURE

KEY STEPS
- Confirm the patient's identity using two patient identifiers according to facility policy.
- Obtain a specimen of the epithelial cells from the infected site. In adults, these sites may include the eye, urethra (rather than from the purulent exudate that may be present), endocervix, and rectum.
- Obtain a urethral specimen by inserting a cotton-tipped applicator ¾″ to 2″ (2 to 5 cm) into the urethra.
- To collect a specimen from the endocervix, use a microbiologic transport swab or Cytobrush.
- Extract the specimen into an appropriate transport medium.
- Extract the specimens from the throat, eye, and nasopharynx, and aspirates from infants into an appropriate transport medium. Send the specimens to the laboratory at 39.2° F (4° C).
- If the anticipated time between specimen collection and inoculation into cell culture is more than 24 hours, freeze the transport medium and send it to the laboratory with dry ice.

WARNING *In the patient suspected of being sexually abused, be sure to process the specimen by culture rather than by antigen detection methods.*

- After collecting the specimens, carefully dispose of gloves, swabs, and speculum to prevent staff exposure.

POSTPROCEDURE CARE
- Answer the patient's questions about testing.
- Monitor the patient for adverse effects.
- If the culture confirms infection, provide counseling for the patient regarding treatment of sexual partners.

PRECAUTIONS
- Assist the male patient into a supine position to prevent him from falling if vasovagal syncope occurs when the cotton swab or wire loop enters the urethra. Observe him for profound hypotension, bradycardia, pallor, and sweating.
- Wear gloves when performing the procedure and handling the specimens.
- Collect a urethral specimen at least 1 hour after the patient has voided to prevent loss of urethral secretions.

COMPLICATIONS
- Hypotension
- Bradycardia
- Pallor
- Diaphoresis

INTERPRETATION

NORMAL RESULTS
- No *C. trachomatis* is identified in the culture.

ABNORMAL RESULTS
- A positive culture confirms *C. trachomatis* infection.

Chloride level, serum

OVERVIEW

DESCRIPTION
- Measures the serum levels of chloride, the major extracellular fluid anion
- Chloride: helps maintain osmotic pressure of blood and, therefore, helps regulate blood volume and arterial pressure; affects the acid-base balance; absorbed in the intestines and excreted primarily by the kidneys

PURPOSE
- To detect acid-base imbalance (acidosis or alkalosis) and to help evaluate fluid status and extracellular cation-anion balance

PREPARATION
- The test evaluates the chloride content of blood.
- This test requires a blood sample.
- No dietary restrictions are required.
- Notify the laboratory and practitioner of drugs the patient is taking that may affect test results; it may be necessary to restrict them.

Teaching points
- Explain the purpose of the test and how it's done.
- Tell the patient who will perform the test and where it will be done.
- Tell the patient that no dietary restrictions are needed.
- Explain to the patient that the test requires a blood sample and that he may experience slight discomfort from the tourniquet and needle puncture.
- Inform the patient that the test takes less than 5 minutes.

DIAGNOSTIC PROCEDURE

KEY STEPS
- Confirm the patient's identity using two patient identifiers according to facility policy.
- Perform a venipuncture and collect the sample in a 3- or 4-ml clot-activator tube.

POSTPROCEDURE CARE
- Apply direct pressure to the venipuncture site until bleeding stops.
- Instruct the patient that he may resume his medications.

PRECAUTIONS
- Maintain standard precautions while collecting the sample.
- Handle the sample gently to prevent hemolysis.

COMPLICATIONS
- Hematoma at the venipuncture site
- Hypertonicity of muscles, tetany, depressed respirations, and decreased blood pressure with dehydration, indicating hypochloremia
- Stupor, rapid deep breathing, and weakness, which may lead to coma, indicating hyperchloremia

INTERPRETATION

NORMAL RESULTS
- In adults, chloride levels range from 100 to 108 mEq/L (SI, 100 to 108 mmol/L).

ABNORMAL RESULTS
- Chloride levels are inversely related to bicarbonate levels, reflecting acid-base balance.
- Excessive loss of gastric juices or other secretions containing chloride may cause hypochloremic metabolic alkalosis; excessive chloride retention or ingestion may lead to hyperchloremic metabolic acidosis.
- An increase in chloride levels may be evident in severe dehydration, complete renal shutdown, head injury (producing neurogenic hyperventilation), and primary aldosteronism.
- Decreased levels of chloride may result from low sodium and potassium levels due to prolonged vomiting, gastric suctioning, intestinal fistula, chronic renal failure, and Addison's disease. Heart failure or edema resulting in excess extracellular fluid can cause dilutional hypochloremia.

Chloride level, urine

DESCRIPTION
- Measures urine chloride level, evaluates renal conservation of this electrolyte, and confirms serum chloride values

PURPOSE
- To help evaluate fluid and electrolyte imbalance
- To help evaluate renal and adrenal disorders

PREPARATION
- This test helps determine the balance of salt and water in the body.
- No dietary restrictions are needed.
- The test requires urine collection over a 24-hour period.
- Notify the laboratory and practitioner of the medications the patient is taking that may affect test results; the medications may need to be restricted.

Teaching points
- Explain the purpose of the test and how it's done.
- If the patient will be collecting the specimen at home, teach him the proper collection technique.
- Tell the patient not to contaminate the specimen with toilet tissue or stool.
- Instruct the patient not to use a metallic bedpan for specimen collection.
- Tell the patient that no dietary restrictions are needed.

KEY STEPS
- Confirm the patient's identity using two patient identifiers according to facility policy.
- Collect the patient's urine during a 24-hour period, discarding the first specimen and retaining the last.

POSTPROCEDURE CARE
- Instruct the patient to resume his usual medications.

PRECAUTIONS
- Keep the specimen on ice or refrigerated during the collection period.

COMPLICATIONS
- None

NORMAL RESULTS
- In adults, chloride levels are 110 to 250 nmol/24 hours (SI, 110 to 250 mmol/day).
- In children, they are 15 to 40 nmol/24 hours (SI, 15 to 40 mmol/day).
- In infants, the level ranges from 2 to 10 mmol/24 hours (SI, 2 to 10 mmol/day).

ABNORMAL RESULTS
- High urine chloride levels may result from water-deficient dehydration, salicylate toxicity, diabetic ketoacidosis, adrenocortical insufficiency (Addison's disease), or salt-losing renal disease.
- Low urine chloride levels may result from excessive diaphoresis, heart failure, hypochloremic metabolic alkalosis, or prolonged vomiting or gastric suctioning.

Cholangiography, postoperative

OVERVIEW

DESCRIPTION

- Radiographic and fluoroscopic examination of the biliary ducts after injection of a contrast medium
- Performed through a T-shaped rubber tube inserted into the common bile duct, immediately after cholecystectomy or common bile duct exploration, to facilitate drainage
- Also known as *T-tube cholangiography*

PURPOSE

- To assess size and patency of the biliary ducts
- To detect obstructions overlooked during surgery
- To detect calculi, strictures, neoplasms, and fistulae in the biliary ducts

PREPARATION

- Make sure the patient has signed an appropriate consent form.
- Check the patient's history for hypersensitivity to iodine, seafood, or contrast media.
- Note and report allergies.
- Clamp the T-tube the day before the procedure if ordered.
- Withhold the meal preceding the test.
- Give an enema about 1 hour before the procedure if ordered.

Teaching points

- Explain the purpose of the test and how it's done.
- Tell the patient who will perform the test and where it will be done.
- Warn the patient that he may feel a bloating sensation in the right upper quadrant during injection of the contrast medium.
- Inform the patient that the test takes about 15 minutes.

DIAGNOSTIC PROCEDURE

KEY STEPS

- Confirm the patient's identity using two patient identifiers according to facility policy.
- The patient is placed in a supine position on the radiograph table.
- The injection area of the T tube is cleaned.
- A needle attached to a long transparent catheter is inserted into the end of the T tube.
- Injecting air into the biliary tree is avoided because air bubbles may affect the clarity of the radiograph films.
- A contrast medium is injected under fluoroscopic guidance.
- A series of radiographs is taken.
- The T tube is clamped and additional films are taken in the erect position (to distinguish air bubbles from calculi).
- Final films are taken to record emptying of contrast-laden bile into the duodenum.

POSTPROCEDURE CARE

- Reattach the T tube to the drainage system.
- Tell the patient to resume his usual diet.
- Monitor the patient's vital signs, intake and output, and T-tube drainage.

PRECAUTIONS

- The test is contraindicated in patients who are hypersensitive to iodine, seafood, or contrast media.

COMPLICATIONS

- Adverse reaction to the contrast medium
- Infection

INTERPRETATION

NORMAL RESULTS

- Filling of the bile ducts with contrast medium is homogeneous.
- The diameter of the biliary ducts is normal.
- The flow of contrast into the duodenum is unimpeded.

ABNORMAL RESULTS

- Biliary duct filling defects, associated with dilation, suggest calculi or neoplasms.
- Abnormal channels of contrast medium from biliary ducts suggest possible fistulae.

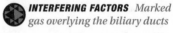 **INTERFERING FACTORS** *Marked gas overlying the biliary ducts*

Chorionic villi sampling

OVERVIEW

DESCRIPTION
◆ Prenatal test for quick detection of fetal chromosomal and biochemical disorders
◆ Performed during first trimester

PURPOSE
◆ To analyze for fetal abnormalities

PREPARATION
◆ No dietary or activity restrictions are required.
◆ Samples are best obtained between the 8th and 10th week of pregnancy.

Teaching points
◆ Explain the purpose of the test and how it's done.
◆ Explain to the patient that samples are best obtained between the 8th and 10th week of pregnancy.
◆ Tell the patient who will perform the test and where it will be done.
◆ Tell the patient that no dietary restrictions are required.
◆ Inform the patient that the test takes less than 15 minutes.

DIAGNOSTIC PROCEDURE

KEY STEPS
◆ Confirm the patient's identity using two patient identifiers according to facility policy.
◆ Assist the patient into the lithotomy position.
◆ The practitioner checks placement of the patient's uterus bimanually and then inserts a Graves speculum and swabs the cervix with an antiseptic solution.
◆ If necessary, a tenaculum is used to straighten an acutely flexed uterus, permitting cannula insertion.
◆ Guided by ultrasound and possibly endoscopy, the catheter is directed through the cannula to the villi.
◆ Suction is applied to the catheter to remove about 30 mg of tissue from the villi.

◆ A specimen is withdrawn and placed in a Petri dish. It's examined with a dissecting microscope. Part of the specimen is then cultured for further testing. (See *Chorionic villi sampling.*)

POSTPROCEDURE CARE
◆ Monitor the patient closely for adverse effects.

PRECAUTIONS
◆ If the patient experiences vaginal bleeding or abdominal cramps, call the practitioner immediately

COMPLICATIONS
◆ Slight risk of spontaneous abortion, cramps, infection, and bleeding

INTERPRETATION

NORMAL RESULTS
◆ No abnormalities are found.

ABNORMAL RESULTS
◆ The test can detect about 200 diseases prenatally, including chromosome disorders, hemoglobinopathies, and Tay-Sachs disease.

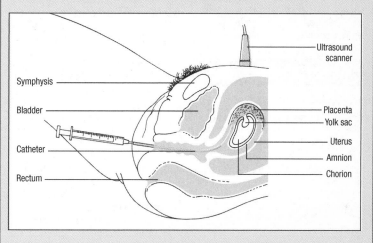

Chorionic villi sampling

Chorionic villi sampling is a prenatal test for quick detection of fetal chromosomal and biochemical disorders that's performed during the first trimester of pregnancy.

Chromosome analysis

DESCRIPTION

◆ Studies the relationship between the microscopic appearance of chromosomes and an individual's phenotype—the expression of genes in physical, biochemical, or physiologic traits
◆ Specimen (blood, bone marrow, amniotic fluid, skin, or placental tissue) and specific procedure determined by reason for test
◆ May involve umbilical cord sampling

PURPOSE

◆ To identify chromosomal abnormalities, such as hypoploidy or hyperploidy, as the underlying cause of malformation, maldevelopment, or disease

PREPARATION

◆ If necessary, have the patient or responsible family member sign an informed consent form.

Teaching points

◆ Explain to the patient or parents, if appropriate, the purpose of the chromosome analysis.
◆ Tell the patient who will perform the test and the type of specimen required.
◆ Advise the patient of any dietary restrictions required.
◆ Inform the patient when results will be available, according to the specimen required.

DIAGNOSTIC PROCEDURE

KEY STEPS

◆ Confirm the patient's identity using two patient identifiers according to facility policy.
◆ Collect a blood sample (in a 5- to 10-ml heparinized tube), a tissue specimen, 1 ml of bone marrow, or at least 20 ml of amniotic fluid.

◆ To facilitate interpretation of test results, send the sample and specimen to the laboratory immediately after collection, with a brief patient history and the indication for the test.
◆ Refrigerate the specimen if transport is delayed, but never freeze it.

POSTPROCEDURE CARE

◆ Provide appropriate care after the test, depending on the type of procedure.
◆ Recommend appropriate genetic or other counseling and follow-up care if necessary, such as an infant stimulation program for a patient with Down syndrome.
◆ Explain to the patient, or parents if appropriate, the test results and their implications if a chromosomal abnormality exists.

PRECAUTIONS

◆ Keep all specimens sterile, especially those that require a tissue culture.

⚡ **WARNING** *Before a skin biopsy, make sure the povidone-iodine solution is thoroughly removed with alcohol. This solution could prevent cell growth.*

COMPLICATIONS

◆ None

INTERPRETATION

NORMAL RESULTS

◆ There are 46 chromosomes present: 22 pairs of nonsex chromosomes (autosomes) and 1 pair of sex chromosomes (Y for the male-determining chromosome, X for the female-determining chromosome). On a karyotype, chromosomes are arranged according to size and the location of their primary constrictions, or centromeres.
◆ The centromere may be medial (metacentric), slightly to one end of the chromosome (submetacentric), or entirely to one end (acrocentric).
◆ The largest chromosomes are displayed first; the others are arranged in order of decreasing size, with the two sex chromosomes traditionally

placed last. By convention, the centromere is always placed at the top in a karyotype. If the two pairs of chromosomal arms are of unequal length, the arm above the centromere will be shorter. The letter "p" designates the short arm; the letter "q" the long arm.
◆ Special stains identify individual chromosomes and locate and enumerate portions of chromosomes.

ABNORMAL RESULTS

◆ Chromosomal abnormalities may be numerical or structural.
◆ Any numerical deviation from the norm of 46 chromosomes is called aneuploidy.
◆ Fewer than 46 chromosomes is called hypoploidy; more than 46, hyperploidy.
◆ Special designations exist for whole multiples of the haploid number 23; for example, diploidy for the normal somatic number of 46, triploidy for 69, and tetraploidy for 92.
◆ Aneuploidy usually follows failure of the chromosomal pair to separate (nondisjunction) in anaphase.
◆ If nondisjunction or anaphase lag occurs during meiosis, the cells of the zygote will all be the same.
◆ Errors in mitotic division after zygote formation will produce more than one cell line (mosaicism).
◆ Structural chromosomal abnormalities result from chromosome breakage.
◆ Intrachromosomal rearrangement occurs within a single chromosome in deletion (loss of an end [terminal] or middle [interstitial] portion of a chromosome); inversion (end-to-end reversal of a chromosome segment); ring chromosome formation (breakage of both ends of a chromosome and reunion of the ends); or isochromosome formation (abnormal splitting of the centromere in a transverse rather than a longitudinal plane); interchromosomal rearrangements also occur.

Clostridial toxin assay

DESCRIPTION
- *Clostridium difficile:* opportunistic infection occurring in patients taking broad-spectrum antibiotics that suppress normal flora of the bowel; releases toxin that causes colonic epithelial necrosis
- Toxin usually found in stool
- Can also test colonic-rectal tissue for presence of toxin

PURPOSE
- To determine the presence of *C. difficile* and diagnose clostridial enterocolitis

PREPARATION
- No dietary restrictions are required.

Teaching points
- Explain that this test helps determine the cause of the patient's diarrhea, as applicable.
- Inform the patient who will collect the stool specimen and when.
- Explain the method of stool collection to the patient.
- If the patient will be collecting the stool specimen himself, instruct him to collect it in a clean container. A rectal swab can't be used because it won't collect an adequate sample for testing.
- Tell the patient that no dietary restrictions are required.

KEY STEPS
- Confirm the patient's identity using two patient identifiers according to facility policy.
- If you'll be collecting the stool sample, collect it in a clean container.
- Send the specimen to the laboratory immediately after collection to prevent breakdown of the toxin.

POSTPROCEDURE CARE
- Instruct the patient to continue any precautions to prevent transmission of the bacteria.

PRECAUTIONS
- Maintain contact precautions while handling the specimen and during contact with the patient.
- Refrigerate the specimen if it isn't going directly to the laboratory.

COMPLICATIONS
- None

NORMAL RESULTS
- No *Clostridium* toxin is identified.

ABNORMAL RESULTS
- The presence of *Clostridium* toxin is confirmed.

Coagulation factor test

DESCRIPTION

- Clotting process initiated when injury occurs to blood vessel
- Involves protein fibrinogens, also known as *coagulation factors,* and intrinsic and extrinsic pathways and factors that keep coagulation process and hemostasis process in balance
- Factor I (fibrinogen): involved in intrinsic and extrinsic clotting pathways; one of the most highly consumed clotting factors
- Factor II (prothrombin): production depends on presence of vitamin K in liver
- Factor V (proaccelerin): used during the clotting process
- Factor VII (proconvertin): also vitamin K dependent
- Factor VIII (antihemophilic factor): highly consumed; has two factors—one involved in hemostatic process and related to hemophilia A, other plays role in platelet adhesion and aggregation and is related to von Willebrand's disease
- Factor IX (plasma thromboplastic component or Christmas factor): vitamin K dependent
- Factor X (Stuart-Prower factor): vitamin K dependent
- Factor XI: plasma thromboplastin antecedent; activated in body by collagen
- Factor XII (Hageman factor): activated by collagen; associated with myocardial infarction and venous thrombosis
- Factor XIII (fibrin-stabilizing factor): another highly consumed clotting factor
- Identification of factor or factors involved in coagulation deficiencies helps determine treatment

PURPOSE

- To identify the presence of congenital or inherited bleeding disorders
- To identify clotting factor excess or deficiency

PREPARATION

- This test measures the clotting factors in the blood.
- Ask the patient if he is aware of a clotting disorder.
- Ask the patient if he takes any medication for clotting.
- No dietary restrictions are needed.

Teaching points

- Explain the purpose of the test and how it's done.
- Tell the patient who will perform the test and where it will be done.
- Tell the patient that no dietary restrictions are required.
- Explain to the patient that the test requires a blood sample and that he may experience slight discomfort from the tourniquet and needle puncture.
- Inform the patient that the test takes less than 10 minutes.

KEY STEPS

- Confirm the patient's identity using two patient identifiers according to facility policy.
- Perform a venipuncture and collect 7 ml of blood in a metal and heparin free tube.

POSTPROCEDURE CARE

- Apply pressure to the venipuncture site until bleeding stops. Note that in some patients, this may be as long as 15 minutes.

PRECAUTIONS

- Maintain standard precautions while collecting the sample.
- If the patient has a known or suspected clotting deficiency, monitor the venipuncture site for hematoma formation.

COMPLICATIONS

- Hematoma at venipuncture site

Clotting factors and causes of abnormal results

Results for most clotting factors are reported using percentages of established normals.

CLOTTING FACTOR	REFERENCE VALUES	CAUSES OF INCREASED VALUES	CAUSES OF DECREASED VALUES
I	200 to 400 mg/dl (2 to 4 g/L)	◆ Acute inflammatory reaction ◆ Coronary artery disease ◆ Trauma	◆ Liver deficiency ◆ Disseminated intravascular coagulation (DIC) ◆ Impaired intake or synthesis of vitamin K
II	80% to 120% of normal	None identified	◆ Impaired synthesis of vitamin K ◆ Liver disease ◆ Warfarin
V	50% to 150% of normal	None identified	◆ Liver deficiency ◆ DIC ◆ Myeloproliferative disorders ◆ Streptokinase

Clotting factors and causes of abnormal results *(continued)*

CLOTTING FACTOR	REFERENCE VALUES	CAUSES OF INCREASED VALUES	CAUSES OF DECREASED VALUES
VII	65% to 140% of normal	None identified	◆ Autosomal recessive inherited disorder (hypoproconvertinemia) ◆ Liver disease ◆ Kwashiorkor ◆ Warfarin
VIII	55% to 145% of normal	◆ Acute inflammation ◆ Stress ◆ Thromboembolic conditions ◆ Late stages of pregnancy	◆ Autosomal inherited disorder ◆ Depending on component of factor involved, hemophilia A or von Willebrand's disease ◆ DIC ◆ Myeloproliferative disorders
IX	60% to 140% of normal	◆ Oral contraceptives	◆ Sex-linked recessive ◆ Hemophilia B or Christmas disease ◆ Liver disease ◆ Nephrotic syndrome ◆ DIC ◆ Vitamin K deficiency ◆ Warfarin
X	45% to 155% of normal	None identified	◆ Vitamin K deficiency ◆ Liver disease ◆ Amyloidosis ◆ DIC ◆ Warfarin ◆ Oral contraceptives
XI	65% to 135% of normal	None identified	◆ Autosomal dominant ◆ Hemophilia C (occurs predominantly in the Jewish population) ◆ Liver disease ◆ DIC ◆ Intestinal malabsorption of vitamin K ◆ Low levels are normal in infants under age 6 months
XII	50% to 150% of normal	None identified	◆ Nephrotic syndrome ◆ Vitamin K deficiency ◆ Liver disease ◆ DIC ◆ Chronic granulocytic leukemia
XIII	45% to 185% of normal	None identified	◆ Liver disease ◆ Obstetric complications ◆ DIC ◆ Acute myelogenous leukemia

NORMAL RESULTS
See *Clotting factors and causes of abnormal results.*

ABNORMAL RESULTS
◆ Decreased or increased level of factors indicates a clotting abnormality.
◆ Any factor may be decreased in an inherited disorder.
◆ Any value less than 10% of normal is a critical value.

Cold agglutinins test

DESCRIPTION

- Cold agglutinins: antibodies, usually of immunoglobulin M type, that cause red blood cells (RBCs) to aggregate at low temperatures
- May occur in small amounts in healthy people
- Transient elevations of antibodies during certain infectious diseases, such as primary atypical pneumonia
- Reliably detects such pneumonia within 1 or 2 weeks after its onset
- High titers, such as in patients with primary atypical pneumonia: may lead to acute transient hemolytic anemia after repeated exposure to cold; persistent high titers may result in chronic hemolytic anemia

PURPOSE

- To help confirm primary atypical pneumonia
- To provide additional diagnostic evidence for cold agglutinin disease associated with many viral infections and lymphoreticular cancer
- To detect cold agglutinins in patients with suspected cold agglutinin disease

PREPARATION

- This test detects antibodies in the blood that attack RBCs after exposure to low temperatures.
- The test may be repeated to monitor the patient's response to therapy, if appropriate.
- No dietary restrictions are required.
- The test requires a blood sample.
- If the patient is receiving antimicrobial drugs, note this on the laboratory request because the use of such drugs may interfere with the development of cold agglutinins.

Teaching points

- Explain the purpose of the test and how it's done.
- Tell the patient who will perform the test and where it will be done.
- Tell the patient that he doesn't have to restrict his diet.

- Explain to the patient that the test requires a blood sample and that he may experience slight discomfort from the tourniquet and needle puncture.
- Inform the patient that the test should take less than 5 minutes.

DIAGNOSTIC PROCEDURE

KEY STEPS

- Confirm the patient's identity using two patient identifiers according to facility policy.
- Perform a venipuncture and collect the sample in a 7-ml tube without additives that has been prewarmed to 98.6° F (37° C).

POSTPROCEDURE CARE

- If cold agglutinin disease is suspected, keep the patient warm. If he's exposed to low temperatures, agglutination may occur within peripheral vessels, possibly leading to frostbite, anemia, Raynaud's phenomenon and, rarely, focal gangrene.
- Watch for signs of vascular abnormalities, such as mottled skin, purpura, jaundice, pallor, pain or swelling of extremities, and cramping of fingers and toes. Hemoglobinuria may result from severe intravascular hemolysis on exposure to severe cold.
- Apply direct pressure to the venipuncture site until bleeding stops.

PRECAUTIONS

- Handle the sample gently to prevent hemolysis.
- Send it to the laboratory immediately after collection.

  WARNING *Don't refrigerate the sample; cold agglutinins will coat the RBCs, leaving none in the serum for testing.*

COMPLICATIONS

- Hematoma at the venipuncture site

INTERPRETATION

NORMAL RESULTS

- Results are reported as negative or positive.
- A positive result, indicating the presence of cold agglutinin, is titered.
- A normal titer is less than 1:64.

ABNORMAL RESULTS

- High titers may occur as primary phenomena or secondary to infections or lymphoreticular cancer.
- High titers may be present in infectious mononucleosis, cytomegalovirus infection, hemolytic anemia, multiple myeloma, scleroderma, malaria, cirrhosis of the liver, congenital syphilis, peripheral vascular disease, pulmonary embolism, trypanosomiasis, tonsillitis, staphylococcemia, scarlatina, influenza and, occasionally, pregnancy.
- Chronically elevated titers are most commonly associated with pneumonia and lymphoreticular cancer; an acute transient elevation typically accompanies many viral infections.
- In primary atypical pneumonia, cold agglutinins appear in serum in one-half to two-thirds of all patients during the first week of acute infection, even before antimycoplasmal antibodies are detectable by complement fixation or metabolic inhibition tests. Titers usually become positive at 7 days, peak above 1:32 in 4 weeks, and disappear rapidly after 6 weeks. Sequential titers verifying this pattern and symptoms of pneumonia confirm the diagnosis.
- Titers exceeding 1:2,000 can occur with idiopathic cold agglutinin disease that precedes lymphoma. Patients with titers this high are susceptible to intravascular agglutination.

Cold stimulation test

DESCRIPTION

◆ Records temperature changes in patient's fingers before and after submersion in ice water

PURPOSE

◆ To detect Raynaud's disease

PREPARATION

◆ No dietary restrictions are required.
◆ Have the patient remove his watch and other jewelry and encourage him to relax.
◆ To minimize extraneous environmental stimuli; make sure the test room is neither too warm nor too cold.
◆ Precede test with digital blood pressure recording or examination of the arteries in arm and palmar arch to rule out arterial occlusive disease.

Teaching points

◆ Explain that this test detects vascular disorders.
◆ Tell the patient who will perform the test and where it will be done.
◆ Tell the patient that no dietary restrictions are required.
◆ Explain to the patient that he may experience discomfort when his hands are briefly immersed in ice water.
◆ Inform the patient that the test should take about 30 minutes.

KEY STEPS

◆ Confirm the patient's identity using two patient identifiers according to facility policy.
◆ Tape a thermistor to each of the patient's fingers and record the temperature.
◆ Have the patient submerge his hands in an ice-water bath for 20 seconds.
◆ When the patient removes his hands from the water, record the temperature of his fingers immediately and every 5 minutes thereafter until it returns to the baseline temperature.

POSTPROCEDURE CARE

◆ Monitor the circulation in the patient's extremities.

PRECAUTIONS

◆ Make sure the water that the patient is to put his hands into is significantly colder than the environment.
◆ The test is contraindicated in patients with gangrenous fingers or open, infected wounds.

COMPLICATIONS

◆ None

NORMAL RESULTS

◆ The digital temperature returns to the baseline levels within 15 minutes.

ABNORMAL RESULTS

◆ If digital temperature takes longer than 20 minutes to return to the baseline level, Raynaud's disease is indicated.
◆ Its benign form requires no specific treatment and has no serious sequelae.
◆ Its more serious form, Raynaud's phenomenon, involves connective tissue disorders that may not be clinically apparent for several years, such as scleroderma, systemic lupus erythematosus, and rheumatoid arthritis. Distinguishing between Raynaud's phenomenon and Raynaud's disease is difficult.

Colonoscopy

DESCRIPTION

◆ Visual examination of the lining of the large intestine with a flexible fiber-optic video endoscope
◆ Indicated in patients with history of constipation or diarrhea, persistent rectal bleeding, and lower abdominal pain when results of proctosigmoidoscopy and barium enema test are negative or inconclusive

PURPOSE

◆ To detect or evaluate inflammatory and ulcerative bowel disease
◆ To locate the origin of lower GI bleeding
◆ To help diagnose colonic strictures and benign or malignant lesions
◆ To evaluate postoperatively for recurrence of polyps and malignant lesions

PREPARATION

◆ Make sure the patient has signed an appropriate consent form.
◆ Check the patient's medical history for allergies, medications, and information pertinent to the current complaint.
◆ Insert an I.V. line and administer sedation, as ordered.

Teaching points

◆ Explain the purpose of the test and how it's done.
◆ Tell the patient who will perform the test and where it will be done.
◆ Tell the patient to maintain a clear liquid diet for 24 to 48 hours before the test and to take nothing by mouth after midnight the night before the test.
◆ Instruct the patient regarding the appropriate bowel preparation.
◆ Inform him that he'll receive an I.V. line and I.V. sedation before the procedure.
◆ Tell the patient that the colonoscope is well lubricated to ease insertion and that it will initially feel cool.

◆ Advise the patient that he may feel an urge to defecate when the colonoscope is inserted and advanced into this body.
◆ Inform him that air may be introduced through the colonoscope to distend the intestinal wall and to facilitate viewing the lining and advancing the instrument.
◆ Inform the patient that the test will take about 30 to 60 minutes.

KEY STEPS

◆ Confirm the patient's identity using two patient identifiers according to facility policy.
◆ The patient is assisted onto his left side with knees flexed. Cover him with a drape.
◆ Baseline vital signs are obtained; vital signs and electrocardiogram are monitored during the procedure.
◆ Continuous or periodic pulse oximetry is advisable.
◆ The physician palpates the mucosa of the anus and rectum and inserts the lubricated colonoscope through the patient's anus into the sigmoid colon under direct vision.
◆ A small amount of air is insufflated to locate the bowel lumen and then advance the scope through the rectum.
◆ Abdominal palpation or fluoroscopy may be used to help guide the colonoscope through the large intestine.
◆ Suction may be used to remove blood and secretions that obscure vision.
◆ Biopsy forceps or a cytology brush may be passed through the colonoscope to obtain specimens for histologic or cytologic examination; an electrocautery snare may be used to remove polyps.
◆ Tissue specimens are immediately placed in a specimen bottle containing 10% formalin and cytology smears in a Coplin jar containing 95% ethyl alcohol.
◆ Specimens are sent to the laboratory immediately after collection.

POSTPROCEDURE CARE

◆ The patient is observed closely for signs of bowel perforation.
◆ Check the patient's vital signs and document them accordingly.
◆ After recovery from sedation, the patient may resume his usual diet unless the practitioner orders otherwise.

- The patient may pass large amounts of flatus after insufflation.
- After polyp removal, the stool may contain some blood. Report excessive bleeding immediately.
- If a polyp is removed, but not retrieved, give the patient an enema and strain the stools to retrieve it.

PRECAUTIONS
- The test is contraindicated in pregnant women near term, in patients who have had recent abdominal surgery, and in those with peritonitis, colitis, or a perforated viscus. These patients may benefit from a virtual colonoscopy. (See *Virtual colonoscopy.*)

⚡ **WARNING** *Monitor the patient closely for adverse effects from the sedative. Have emergency resuscitation equipment and an opioid antagonist available.*

COMPLICATIONS
- Perforation of the large intestine
- Excessive bleeding
- Retroperitoneal emphysema

NORMAL RESULTS
- The mucosa of the large intestine beyond the sigmoid colon appears light pink-orange and is marked by semilunar folds and deep tubular pits.
- Blood vessels are visible beneath the intestinal mucosa.

ABNORMAL RESULTS
- Results may indicate proctitis, granulomatous or ulcerative colitis, Crohn's disease, and malignant or benign lesions.
- Findings may suggest diverticular disease or lower GI bleeding.

Virtual colonoscopy

Virtual colonoscopy combines computed tomography (CT) scanning and X-ray images with sophisticated image processing computers to generate three-dimensional (3-D) images of the patient's colon. These images are interpreted by a skilled radiologist to recreate and evaluate the colon's inner surface. Although this procedure isn't as accurate as a routine colonoscopy, it's less invasive and is useful in screening the patient with small polyps. The colon must be free from residue and fecal material. Bowel preparation consists of following a clear-liquid diet for 24 hours before the procedure; also, the patient performs GoLYTELY bowel preparation the evening before and takes a rectal suppository on the morning of the test.

Before performing the CT scan, a thin, red rectal tube is placed, and air is introduced into the colon to distend the bowel. This insertion may produce mild cramping. The CT scan is done with the patient in the supine position and again while prone. The scans are then shipped over a network to a 3-D image processing computer, and a radiologist evaluates the images obtained. If polyps are identified, a colonoscopy may be scheduled to remove them.

Colposcopy

DESCRIPTION
◆ Visual examination of the cervix and vagina with a colposcope, an instrument with a magnifying lens and light source

PURPOSE
◆ To confirm cervical intraepithelial neoplasia or invasive carcinoma after an abnormal Papanicolaou (Pap) test
◆ To evaluate vaginal or cervical lesions
◆ To monitor conservatively treated cervical intraepithelial neoplasia
◆ To monitor patients whose mothers received diethylstilbestrol during pregnancy

PREPARATION
◆ Make sure the patient has signed an appropriate consent form.
◆ Note and report allergies.
◆ No dietary restrictions are required.

Teaching points
◆ Explain that the procedure is similar to a routine pelvic examination, except the practitioner looks through the colposcope.
◆ Tell the patient who will perform the procedure and where it will be done.
◆ Instruct her not to douche, to use tampons or vaginal medication, or to have sexual intercourse for 2 days before the procedure.
◆ Explain that the procedure is safe and painless and takes about 10 to 15 minutes.
◆ Advise the patient that she may experience minimal bleeding and mild cramping with biopsy and endocervical curettage, if performed.
◆ Instruct the patient to avoid inserting anything into the vagina (such as a tampon) until the biopsy site has healed.
◆ Tell the patient to expect a watery vaginal discharge, which is normal during healing.

KEY STEPS
◆ Confirm the patient's identity using two patient identifiers according to facility policy.
◆ Assist the patient into the lithotomy position.
◆ A speculum is inserted into the vagina.
◆ A Pap test is performed, if indicated.
◆ A small amount of dilute vinegar solution is applied to the cervix to aid in differentiating the cell types; it makes abnormal areas more readily visible.
◆ The cervix and vagina are visually examined.
◆ A biopsy is performed on areas that appear abnormal.
◆ Endocervical curettage to sample the cells just inside the cervical canal is then performed.
◆ Bleeding is controlled by applying pressure or hemostatic solutions or by cautery.

POSTPROCEDURE CARE
◆ After a biopsy, instruct the patient to abstain from sexual intercourse until the biopsy site heals (about 10 days).

PRECAUTIONS
◆ Make sure the cervix is clean for adequate visualization.

COMPLICATIONS
◆ Bleeding (especially in pregnant patients)
◆ Infection

NORMAL RESULTS
◆ The surface contour of the cervical vessels is smooth and pink.
◆ The columnar epithelium appears grapelike.
◆ Different tissue types are sharply demarcated.

ABNORMAL RESULTS
◆ White epithelium or punctuation and mosaic patterns may indicate underlying cervical intraepithelial neoplasia.
◆ Keratinization in the transformation zone may indicate cervical intraepithelial neoplasia or invasive carcinoma.
◆ Atypical vessels may indicate invasive carcinoma.
◆ Inflammatory changes suggest possible infection.
◆ Condyloma suggests human papillomavirus.

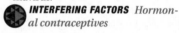 **INTERFERING FACTORS** *Hormonal contraceptives*

Complement assays

DESCRIPTION

- Evaluate and measure total complement and its components; include hemolytic assay, laser nephelometry, and radial immunodiffusion
- Complement deficiency: increases susceptibility to infection and predisposes patient to other diseases
- Complement components designated C1 to C9; three subcomponents of C1: C1q, C1r, and C1s (constitute 3% to 4% of total serum globulins and play key role in antibody-mediated immune reactions)
- Assays performed in patients with immune-mediated disease or in those who have repeatedly abnormal response to infection
- Results considered with serum immunoglobulin and autoantibody tests for definitive diagnosis of immune-mediated disease or abnormal response to infection

PURPOSE

- To help detect immune-mediated disease and genetic complement deficiency
- To monitor the effectiveness of therapy

PREPARATION

- No dietary restrictions are required.
- The test requires a blood sample.
- If the patient is scheduled for a C1q assay, check his history for recent heparin therapy and report such therapy to the laboratory.

Teaching points

- Explain that this test measures a group of proteins that fight infection.
- Tell the patient who will perform the test and where it will be done.
- Advise the patient that no dietary restrictions are required.
- Explain to the patient that the test requires a blood sample and that he may experience slight discomfort from the tourniquet and needle puncture.
- Inform the patient that the test should take less than 5 minutes.

KEY STEPS

- Confirm the patient's identity using two patient identifiers according to facility policy.
- Perform a venipuncture and collect the sample in a 7-ml tube without additives.
- Send the sample to the laboratory immediately after collection because the complement is heat labile and deteriorates rapidly.

POSTPROCEDURE CARE

- Apply direct pressure to the venipuncture site until bleeding stops.

PRECAUTIONS

- Maintain standard precautions while collecting the sample.
- Handle the sample gently to prevent hemolysis.
- Because many patients with complement defects have a compromised immune system, keep the venipuncture site clean and dry.

COMPLICATIONS

- Hematoma at the venipuncture site

NORMAL RESULTS

- The total complement level is 25 to 110 units/ml (SI, 0.25 to 1.1 g/L).
- C3 level is 70 to 150 mg/dl (SI, 0.7 to 1.5 g/L).
- C4 level is 15 to 45 mg/dl (SI, 0.15 to 0.45 g/L).

ABNORMAL RESULTS

- Complement abnormalities may be genetic or acquired (most common).
- Depressed total complement levels (which are clinically more significant than elevations) may result from excessive formation of antigen-antibody complexes, insufficient complement synthesis, inhibitor formation, or increased complement catabolism and are characteristic in such conditions as systemic lupus erythematosus (SLE), acute poststreptococcal glomerulonephritis, and acute serum sickness.
- Low levels may also occur in some patients with advanced cirrhosis of the liver, multiple myeloma, hypogammaglobulinemia, or rapidly rejecting allografts.
- Elevated total complement may occur in obstructive jaundice, thyroiditis, acute rheumatic fever, rheumatoid arthritis, acute myocardial infarction, ulcerative colitis, and diabetes.
- C1 esterase inhibitor deficiency is characteristic in hereditary angioedema, the most common genetic abnormality associated with complement.
- C3 deficiency is characteristic in recurrent pyogenic infection and disease activation in SLE.
- C4 deficiency is characteristic in SLE and rheumatoid arthritis. C4 is increased in autoimmune hemolytic anemia.

Computed tomography scanning, abdomen and pelvis

OVERVIEW

DESCRIPTION
◆ Combines radiologic and computer technology to produce cross-sectional images of various layers of tissue
◆ Computed tomography (CT) scan of abdomen: includes area between dome of diaphragm and iliac crests; may be performed with or without a CT scan of the pelvis
◆ CT scan of pelvis: includes area between iliac crests and perineum; in men, includes bladder and prostate, in women, includes bladder and adnexa
◆ May also involve spiral CT scans of the abdomen and pelvis

PURPOSE
◆ To evaluate soft tissue and organs of the abdomen, pelvis, and retroperitoneal space
◆ To evaluate inflammatory disease
◆ To aid staging of neoplasms
◆ To evaluate trauma
◆ To detect tumors, cysts, hemorrhage, or edema
◆ To evaluate response to chemotherapy

PREPARATION
◆ Make sure the patient has signed an appropriate consent form.
◆ Note and report allergies.
◆ CT scanning of the abdomen and pelvis usually isn't recommended during pregnancy because of potential risk to the fetus.
◆ Check the patient's history for hypersensitivity to shellfish, iodine, or iodinated contrast media and document such reactions on the patient's chart.
◆ There are dietary restrictions if a contrast medium is to be used.

Teaching points
◆ Explain the purpose of the test and how it's done.
◆ Tell the patient who will perform the test and where it will be done.
◆ Inform the practitioner of any sensitivity so that prophylactic medications may be ordered; the practitioner may choose not to use the contrast.
◆ If the patient won't receive a contrast medium, tell him that he doesn't need to restrict food and fluids.
◆ If the patient will receive a contrast medium, instruct him to fast for 4 hours before the test.
◆ Stress the need to remain still during testing because movement can limit accuracy. Tell the patient that he may experience minimal discomfort because of lying still.
◆ Warn the patient about transient discomfort from the needle puncture and a warm or flushed feeling or metallic taste if an I.V. contrast medium is used.
◆ Inform the patient that he'll hear clacking sounds as the table moves into the scanner.
◆ Inform the patient that the test takes about 35 to 40 minutes.

DIAGNOSTIC PROCEDURE

KEY STEPS
◆ Confirm the patient's identity using two patient identifiers according to facility policy.
◆ The test usually requires oral contrast material to outline the intestines.
◆ Assist the patient into a supine position with his arms above his head.
◆ I.V. contrast agent may be injected into a vein to help define certain tissues.
◆ The table will advance slightly between each scan.
◆ Cross-sectional images are obtained and reviewed.

POSTPROCEDURE CARE
◆ Instruct the patient to resume his normal diet and activities unless ordered otherwise.

PRECAUTIONS
⚡ **WARNING** *Tell the patient to immediately report feelings of nausea, vomiting, dizziness, headache, itching, or hives. Check the patient's history for hypersensitivity to iodine or contrast media used in other diagnostic tests.*
◆ The test is contraindicated during pregnancy due to potential risk to the fetus.

COMPLICATIONS
◆ Adverse reaction to iodinated contrast medium

INTERPRETATION

NORMAL RESULTS
◆ The organs are normal in size and position.
◆ There are no masses or other abnormalities.

ABNORMAL RESULTS
◆ Well-circumscribed or poorly defined areas of slightly lower density than normal parenchyma suggest possible primary and metastatic neoplasms.
◆ Relatively low-density, homogeneous areas, usually with well-defined borders suggest possible abscesses.
◆ Sharply defined round or oval structures, with densities less than that of abscesses and neoplasms, suggest cysts.
◆ Dilatation of the biliary ducts suggests obstructive disease from a tumor or calculi.

Computed tomography scanning, bone

DESCRIPTION

- Series of tomograms, translated by a computer and displayed on a monitor, representing cross-sectional images of various layers (or slices) of bone
- Can reconstruct cross-sectional, horizontal, sagittal, and coronal plane images
- By taking collimated (parallel) radiographs, increases the number of radiation density calculations the computer makes and improves the degree of resolution, specificity, and accuracy
- Combines hundreds of thousands of readings of radiation levels absorbed by tissues to depict anatomic slices of varying thicknesses

PURPOSE

- To determine the existence and extent of primary bone tumors, skeletal metastases, soft-tissue tumors, injuries to ligaments or tendons, and fractures
- To diagnose joint abnormalities that are difficult to detect by other methods

PREPARATION

- Dietary restrictions apply if a contrast medium is to be used.
- Check the patient's history for hypersensitivity reactions to iodine, shellfish, or contrast media. Mark such reactions in the chart and notify the practitioner.
- If the patient appears restless or apprehensive about the procedure, a mild sedative may be prescribed.
- Give analgesics to the patient with significant bone or joint pain so that he can lie comfortably during the scan.

Teaching points

- Explain the purpose of the test and how it's done.
- Tell the patient who will perform the test and where it will be done.

- If the patient won't receive a contrast medium, tell him that he need not restrict food and fluids.
- If the patient receive a contrast medium, instruct him to fast for 4 hours before the test.
- Explain to the patient that he'll lie on an X-ray table inside a CT scanner and be asked to lie still; the computer-controlled scanner will revolve around him taking multiple scans.
- If the patient is to receive a contrast medium, tell him that he may feel flushed and warm and may experience a transient headache, a salty or metallic taste, and nausea or vomiting after receving the injection.
- Instruct the patient to remove all metal objects and jewelry in the X-ray field.
- Stress the need to remain as still as possible during the test.
- Inform the patient that the test takes about 35 to 40 minutes.

KEY STEPS

- Confirm the patient's identity using two patient identifiers according to facility policy.
- Assist the patient into a supine position on an X-ray table and ask him to lie as still as possible.
- The table is slid into the circular opening of the CT scanner. The scanner revolves around the patient, taking radiographs at preselected intervals.
- After the first set of scans is taken, the patient is removed from the scanner and a contrast medium is given, if necessary.
- Observe the patient for signs and symptoms of a hypersensitivity reaction, including pruritus, rash, and respiratory difficulty, for 30 minutes after injection of the contrast medium.
- After the contrast medium I.V. injection, the patient is moved back into the scanner and another series of scans is taken. The images obtained from the scan are displayed on a monitor during the diagnostic proce-

dure and stored on magnetic tape to create a permanent record for subsequent study.

POSTPROCEDURE CARE

- If contrast medium is used, observe the patient for a delayed allergic reaction and treat as necessary.
- Encourage fluids to assist in eliminating the contrast medium.
- Provide comfort measures and pain medication because of prolonged positioning on the table.
- Tell the patient to resume his usual diet and activities, if appropriate.

PRECAUTIONS

⚡ **WARNING** *Tell the patient to immediately report feelings of nausea, vomiting, dizziness, headache, itching, or hives. Check the patient's history for hypersensitivity to iodine or contrast media used in other diagnostic tests.*

- The test is contraindicated during pregnancy due to potential risk to the fetus.

COMPLICATIONS

- Strong feelings of claustrophobia or anxiety (when inside the CT body scanner)

NORMAL RESULTS

- No abnormal pathology in the bones or joints is noted.
- Bone or joint structures appear as crisp images and surrounding structures are blurred or lack detail.

ABNORMAL RESULTS

- Differentiation of tissues is visible on images, showing primary bone tumors, soft-tissue tumors, and skeletal metastasis.
- Details of bone fractures are visible.
- Different characteristics of tissues and organs are noted, revealing other abnormalities.
- Joint abnormalities are revealed (hard to detect by other methods).

Computed tomography scanning, brain

DESCRIPTION

- Series of tomograms, translated by a computer and displayed on an oscilloscope screen, usually using a contrast medium
- Provides layers of cross-sectional images of the brain
- Reconstructs cross-sectional, horizontal, sagittal, and coronal-plane images
- Also known as *intracranial computed tomography scan*

PURPOSE

- To diagnose intracranial lesions and abnormalities
- To monitor the effects of surgery, radiotherapy, or chemotherapy in treatment of intracranial tumors
- To guide cranial surgery
- To assess focal neurologic abnormalities
- To evaluate suspected head injury such as subdural hematoma

PREPARATION

- Make sure the patient has signed an appropriate consent form.
- Note and report allergies.
- There are dietary restrictions if a contrast medium is to be used.

Teaching points

- Explain the purpose of the test and how it's done.
- Tell the patient who will perform the test and where it will be done.
- If the patient won't receive a contrast medium, tell him that he need not restrict food and fluid intake before the test.
- If the patient will receive a contrast medium, instruct him to fast for 4 hours before the test.
- Advise the patient that he may experience transient discomfort from the needle puncture and a warm or flushed feeling if an I.V. contrast medium is used.
- Stress the need to remain still during the test because movement can limit accuracy of the test.

- Warn the patient that he may experience minimal discomfort because of lying still and immobilizing his head.
- Caution that the patient will hear clacking sounds as the head of the table moves into the scanner, which rotates around his head.
- Inform the patient that the test takes about 30 minutes.

DIAGNOSTIC PROCEDURE

KEY STEPS

- Confirm the patient's identity using two patient identifiers according to facility policy.
- Assist the patient into a supine position on a radiographic table.
- The patient's head is immobilized with straps and he's asked to lie still.
- The head of the table is moved into the scanner, which rotates around the patient's head, taking radiographs.
- When the initial series of radiographs is complete, the contrast enhancement is given if ordered.
- Usually, 50 to 100 ml of contrast medium is injected by I.V. bolus or infusion.
- Observe the patient for hypersensitivity reactions.
- Another series of scans is taken.
- Selected views are taken for further study.

POSTPROCEDURE CARE

- If the patient received a contrast medium, watch for delayed adverse reactions.
- Instruct the patient to resume his usual diet and medications unless ordered otherwise.

PRECAUTIONS

WARNING *Tell the patient to immediately report feelings of nausea, vomiting, dizziness, headache, itching, or hives. Check the patient's history for hypersensitivity to iodine or contrast media used in other diagnostic tests.*

- The test is contraindicated during pregnancy due to potential risk to the fetus.

COMPLICATIONS

- Adverse reaction to iodinated contrast medium

NORMAL RESULTS

- Brain matter appears in shades of gray.
- Ventricular and subarachnoid cerebrospinal fluid appears black.

ABNORMAL RESULTS

- Enlarged ventricles with large sulci suggest cerebral atrophy.
- In children, enlargement of the fourth ventricle usually indicates hydrocephalus.
- Areas of marked generalized lucency suggest cerebral edema.
- Cerebral vessels appearing with slightly increased density suggest possible arteriovenous malformation.
- Areas of altered density or displaced vasculature or other structures may indicate intracranial tumors, intracranial hematoma, cerebral atrophy, infarction, edema, and congenital anomalies such as hydrocephalus.

Computed tomography scanning, cardiac scoring

DESCRIPTION
- Series of tomograms, translated by a computer and displayed on an oscilloscope screen, usually using a contrast medium
- Provides layers of cross-sectional images of the heart
- Reconstructs cross-sectional, horizontal, sagittal, and coronal-plane images

PURPOSE
- To diagnose coronary artery calcium content
- To screen for coronary artery calcium content in high-risk patients and patients with chest pain of unknown origin

PREPARATION
- Make sure the patient has signed an appropriate consent form.
- Note and report allergies.
- No dietary restrictions are required.

Teaching points
- Explain the purpose of the test and how it's done.
- Tell the patient who will perform the test and where it will be done.
- Reassure the patient that he won't receive contrast media for this test.
- Stress to the patient that he must remain still during the test because movement can limit accuracy of the test.
- Tell the patient that he may be asked to hold his breath at times during the test.
- Warn the patient that he may experience minimal discomfort because of lying still.
- Advise the patient that he'll hear clacking sounds as the head of the table moves into the scanner, which rotates around him.
- Inform the patient that the test takes about 10 minutes.

KEY STEPS
- Confirm the patient's identity using two patient identifiers according to facility policy.
- The patient is assisted into the supine position on an X-ray table and asked to lie as still as possible.
- The table slides into the circular opening of the computed tomography scanner and the scanner revolves around the patient, taking radiographs at preselected intervals.

POSTPROCEDURE CARE
- Instruct the patient to resume his usual diet and medications unless ordered otherwise.

PRECAUTIONS
- The test is contraindicated during pregnancy due to potential risk to the fetus.

COMPLICATIONS
- None

NORMAL RESULTS
- Calcium score for each vessel is 100 or less.
- Findings indicate that the risk of significant coronary artery disease is minimal.
- It's unlikely the patient has a narrowing of the arteries.

ABNORMAL RESULTS
- A score between 101 and 400 indicates a significant amount of calcified plaque in the arteries.
- This score indicates an increased risk of myocardial infarction in the future and further testing is suggested.
- A score greater than 400 signifies extensive calcification, and that the patient may have a critical narrowing of the arteries due to plaque. Further assessment is required immediately.

INTERFERING FACTORS *Presence of coronary stents (may impair picture quality)*

Computed tomography scanning, ear

DESCRIPTION

◆ Combines radiologic and computer technology to produce cross-sectional images of various layers of tissue
◆ Uses high-resolution computed tomography (HRCT) scanning to evaluate patients for cochlear implants, differentiate osseous changes involving the external auditory canal and middle ear, differentiate the osseous structures of the temporal bone and petrous bone, and provide differential diagnoses for middle ear and inner ear problems
◆ Evaluates cholesteatomas, establishes surgical and other therapeutic approaches for the patient, and evaluates the postsurgical management of a patient with a middle or inner ear disorder

PURPOSE

◆ To investigate the cause of bilateral hearing loss
◆ To confirm cochlear abnormalities
◆ To differentiate chronic inflammation from cholesteatoma
◆ To evaluate ossification of the cochlea coils before cochlear implantation
◆ To depict osseous changes involving the temporal and petrous bone contained in the inner ear
◆ To accurately define appropriate surgical and therapeutic approaches for patients with middle ear and inner ear disorders
◆ To assess postsurgical management of patients with middle ear and inner ear disorders

PREPARATION

◆ Check the patient for allergies to iodine products if a contrast medium is to be used. Tell him that he'll receive the contrast medium I.V.
◆ A contrast medium isn't required for evaluating ossification of the cochlea coils or studying the petrous portion of the temporal bone.
◆ Ask the patient about feelings of claustrophobia because he may require preprocedure medication to alleviate his fears.

Teaching points

◆ Describe the procedure to the patient. Tell him to remove any metal objects such as jewelry.
◆ Explain to the patient that he'll be secured to the scanner table to eliminate movement.
◆ Inform the patient that his body and head will be moved into the scanner, which is an air-conditioned chamber that resembles a giant doughnut. The technician will remain present and communicate with the patient during the test.
◆ Tell the patient who will perform the test and where it will be done.
◆ Tell the patient that he need not restrict food and fluids.
◆ Advise the patient that he'll hear a clacking sound while the machine records the images.
◆ Inform the patient that the test takes about 15 to 20 minutes.

KEY STEPS

◆ Confirm the patient's identity using two patient identifiers according to facility policy.
◆ The protocol for each HRCT scan depends on the purpose of the test, with most HRCT studies focused on the axial and coronal planes.
◆ In the radiology department, the patient is placed on the scanner table with his head toward the machine. The mobile scanner table allows for easy transfer and accurate positioning in the machine.
◆ A trained technician conducts the study under the supervision of a radiologist.
◆ The technician explains the details of the diagnostic procedure to the patient to reassure him and gain his cooperation.
◆ Numerous low-dose X-ray beams pass through the patient's body at different angles for a fraction of a second as the scanner rotates around him.

◆ Detectors in the scanner record the number of X-rays absorbed by different tissues, and a computer transforms these data into an image, which is interpreted by the radiologist.
◆ The temporal bones are imaged separately in the axial and coronal planes. Because contrast already exists between bone, air, and soft tissue, the use of a contrast medium isn't necessary in most cases.

POSTPROCEDURE CARE

◆ Instruct the patient to resume his normal diet and activities unless ordered otherwise.

PRECAUTIONS

WARNING *Tell the patient to immediately report feelings of nausea, vomiting, dizziness, headache, itching, or hives. Check the patient's history for hypersensitivity to iodine or contrast media used in other diagnostic tests.*
◆ The test is contraindicated during pregnancy due to potential risk to the fetus.

COMPLICATIONS

◆ None

NORMAL RESULTS

◆ Normal anatomic structures are easily identified.

ABNORMAL RESULTS

◆ Tympanosclerosis and osseous changes of the external auditory canal and middle and inner ear structures are noted.
◆ Cochlear abnormalities may be revealed.

Computed tomography scanning, kidneys

OVERVIEW

DESCRIPTION

- Combines radiologic and computer technology to produce cross-sectional images of layers of tissue
- Reveals masses and other lesions by measuring the amount of radiation the kidney tissue absorbs
- Highly accurate test to investigate diseases found by other tests such as excretory urography

PURPOSE

- To detect and evaluate renal abnormalities, such as tumor, obstruction, calculi, polycystic disease, congenital anomalies, and abnormal fluid accumulation
- To evaluate the retroperitoneum

PREPARATION

- Make sure the patient has signed an appropriate consent form.
- Check the patient's history for hypersensitivity to shellfish, iodine, or contrast media.
- Have the patient put on a gown and remove any metallic objects that could interfere with the scan.
- Give the patient any prescribed sedatives.

Teaching points

- Tell the patient that this computed tomography (CT) scan will examine his kidneys.
- Inform the patient that he'll lie on an X-ray table and that he'll need to be secured to the table with straps while a scanner takes films of his kidneys.
- Tell the patient who will perform the test and where it will be done.
- If the patient will receive a contrast medium, instruct him to fast for 4 hours before the test.
- Advise the patient that the scanner may make loud clacking sounds as it rotates around his body.
- Tell the patient that flushing, metallic taste, and headache may occur after the contrast medium is injected.
- Inform the patient that the test takes about 30 minutes.

DIAGNOSTIC PROCEDURE

KEY STEPS

- Confirm the patient's identity using two patient identifiers according to facility policy.
- Assist the patient into the supine position on the X-ray table and secure him with straps.
- The scanner rotates around the patient, taking multiple images at different angles within each cross-sectional slice.
- When one series of tomograms is complete, the I.V. contrast enhancement may be performed. Another series of tomograms is then taken.
- After the I.V. contrast medium is given, the patient is monitored for signs and symptoms of an allergic reaction, such as respiratory difficulty, urticaria, or skin eruptions.

POSTPROCEDURE CARE

- If the procedure used contrast enhancement, watch for hypersensitivity to the contrast medium.
- If calculi are present, strain the urine, hydrate the patient, and discuss nutritional adaptations.
- Support the patient and his family if surgery is indicated for a neoplasm.
- Monitor the patient's vital signs if he received a sedative.
- After the test, instruct the patient to resume his usual diet, as ordered.

PRECAUTIONS

WARNING *Tell the patient to immediately report feelings of nausea, vomiting, dizziness, headache, itching, or hives. Check the patient's history for hypersensitivity to iodine or contrast media used in other diagnostic tests.*

- The test is contraindicated during pregnancy due to potential risk to the fetus.

COMPLICATIONS

- Hypersensitivity to contrast medium

INTERPRETATION

NORMAL RESULTS

- Renal parenchyma appears denser than hepatic but less than bone, which appears white on a CT scan.
- The density of the collecting system is generally low (black), unless a contrast medium enhances it to a higher density (whiter).
- Evaluating kidney position depends on the surrounding structures; counting cuts between the superior and inferior poles and following the contour of the kidneys' outline gives size and shape.

ABNORMAL RESULTS

- Renal masses appear as areas of different density than normal parenchyma, possibly altering the shape of the kidneys or projecting beyond their margins.
- Renal cysts appear as smooth, sharply defined masses with thin walls and a lower density than normal parenchyma.
- Tumors such as renal cell carcinoma usually aren't well delineated; they have thick walls and nonuniform density.
- With contrast enhancement, solid tumors appear denser than renal cysts but less dense than normal parenchyma.
- Tumors with hemorrhage, calcification, or necrosis appear denser.
- Vascular tumors are more clearly defined with contrast enhancement.
- Adrenal tumors are confined masses, usually detached from kidneys and from other retroperitoneal organs.
- Obstructions, calculi, polycystic kidney disease, congenital anomalies, and abnormal accumulations of fluid around the kidneys, such as hematomas, lymphoceles, and abscesses can also be identified.
- The kidney may be abnormally large or small, may appear damaged, or may be infected.
- After nephrectomy, scanning can detect abnormal masses such as recurrent tumors in a renal fossa that should be empty.

Computed tomography scanning, liver and biliary tract

DESCRIPTION

- Combines radiologic and computer technology to produce cross-sectional images of various layers of tissue
- Penetrates the upper abdomen with multiple X-rays, while a detector records the differences in tissue thickness, displayed as an image on a screen
- Distinguishes the biliary tract and the liver, if the ducts are large, through a series of cross-sectional views
- Performed in obese patients and in those with livers positioned high under the rib cage because excessive fat and bone hinder ultrasound transmission

PURPOSE

- To distinguish between obstructive and nonobstructive jaundice
- To detect intrahepatic tumors and abscesses, subphrenic and subhepatic abscesses, cysts, and hematomas

PREPARATION

- Check the patient's history for hypersensitivity to iodine, seafood, or the contrast media used in other diagnostic tests.
- Give the patient the oral contrast medium supplied by the radiology department. The patient should drink the contrast medium and fast until after the examination.
- Describe possible adverse reactions to the medium, such as nausea, vomiting, dizziness, headache, and hives, and tell him to report these symptoms.

Teaching points

- Explain to the patient that computed tomography (CT) scanning helps detect biliary tract and liver disease.
- Tell the patient who will perform the test and where it will be done.
- If the patient is to receive an oral contrast medium, tell him to drink it and then fast until after the examination.

- If the test involves an I.V. contrast medium, tell the patient that he may experience transient discomfort from the needle puncture and a localized feeling of warmth on injection, as well as a salty or metallic taste.
- Inform the patient that he'll lie on an adjustable table inside a scanning gantry.
- Tell the patient that he'll need to remain still during the test and periodically hold his breath. Stress the importance of remaining still during the test because movement can cause artifacts, thereby prolonging the test and limiting its accuracy.
- Inform the patient that the test takes about 30 minutes.

KEY STEPS

- Confirm the patient's identity using two patient identifiers according to facility policy.
- The patient is placed in the supine position on an X-ray table, and the table is positioned within the opening in the scanning gantry.
- A series of transverse X-rays is taken and recorded on magnetic tape.
- This information is reconstructed by a computer and appears as images on a television screen.
- When the first series of X-rays is completed, the images are reviewed.
- If contrast enhancement is ordered, the contrast medium is injected. A second series of X-rays is taken. The patient is observed carefully for an allergic reaction.

POSTPROCEDURE CARE

- Monitor the patient for adverse effects to the contrast medium.

PRECAUTIONS

⚡ **WARNING** *Tell the patient to immediately report feelings of nausea, vomiting, dizziness, headache, itching, or hives. Check the patient's history for hypersensitivity to iodine or contrast media used in other diagnostic tests.*

- The test is contraindicated during pregnancy due to potential risk to the fetus.

COMPLICATIONS

- Adverse effects from contrast medium

INTERPRETATION

NORMAL RESULTS

- The liver has a uniform density that's slightly greater than that of the pancreas, kidneys, and spleen.
- Linear and circular areas of slightly lower density, representing hepatic vascular structures, may interrupt this uniform appearance.
- The portal vein is usually visible; the hepatic artery usually isn't.
- I.V. contrast medium enhances the isodensity of vascular structures and liver parenchyma.
- Intrahepatic biliary radicles aren't visible, but the common hepatic and bile ducts may be visible as low-density structures.
- Because bile has the same density as water, use of an I.V. contrast medium improves demarcation of the biliary tract by enhancing the surrounding parenchyma and vascular structures.
- Like the biliary ducts, the gallbladder is visible as a round or elliptic low-density structure.

ABNORMAL RESULTS

- Most focal hepatic defects appear less dense than the normal parenchyma, and CT scans can detect small lesions.
- Use of rapid-sequence scanning with an I.V. contrast medium helps distinguish between the two because the normal parenchyma shows greater enhancement than focal defects.
- Primary and metastatic neoplasms may appear as well-circumscribed or poorly defined areas of slightly lower density than the normal parenchyma.
- Some lesions have the same density as the liver parenchyma and may be undetectable.
- Especially large neoplasms may distort the liver's contour.
- Hepatic abscesses appear as relatively low-density, homogeneous areas, usually with well-defined borders.
- Hepatic cysts appear as sharply defined round or oval structures and have a density lower than abscesses and neoplasms.

- Density of a hepatic hematoma varies with its age.
- Subcapsular hematomas are usually crescent-shaped and compress the liver away from the capsule.
- Absence of dilation indicates nonobstructive jaundice.
- Biliary duct dilation indicates obstructive jaundice.
- Dilated intrahepatic bile ducts appear as low-density linear and circular branching structures.
- Dilation of the common hepatic duct, common bile duct, and gallbladder may also be apparent, depending on the site and severity of obstruction.
- Usually, CT scanning can identify the cause of obstruction.

Computed tomography scanning, pancreas

DESCRIPTION

- Combines radiologic and computer technology to produce cross-sectional images of various layers of tissue
- Penetrates the upper abdomen with multiple X-rays, while a detector records the differences in tissue thickness, displayed as an image on a screen
- Provides a detailed look at the pancreas through a series of cross-sectional views
- Accurately distinguishes the pancreas and surrounding organs and vessels if enough fat is present between the structures
- More accurate than ultrasonography; shows general swelling that accompanies acute inflammation of the gland (in retroperitoneal disorders, specifically when pancreatitis is suspected)
- Easily detects calcium deposits commonly missed by simple radiography, particularly in obese patients (in chronic cases)

PURPOSE

- To detect pancreatic carcinoma or pseudocysts
- To detect or evaluate pancreatitis
- To distinguish between pancreatic disorders and disorders of the retroperitoneum

PREPARATION

- Check the patient's history for recent barium studies and for hypersensitivity to iodine, seafood, or contrast media used in previous tests.
- The test may require an I.V. or oral contrast medium, or both, to enhance visualization of the pancreas.
- Give the oral contrast medium if ordered.
- Describe possible adverse reactions to the medium, such as nausea, flushing, dizziness, and sweating, and tell him to report these symptoms.

Teaching points

- Explain to the patient that computed tomography scanning helps detect disorders of the pancreas.
- Tell the patient who will perform the test and where it will be done.
- Tell the patient that he may receive an I.V. or oral contrast medium, or both, to enhance visualization of the pancreas.
- Instruct the patient to fast after receiving the oral contrast medium.
- If the patient is to receive I.V. contrast, tell him to fast for 4 hours before the test.
- Tell the patient that he'll lie on an adjustable table that's positioned inside a scanning gantry. Assure him that the procedure is painless.
- Explain to the patient that he'll need to remain still during the test and periodically hold his breath.
- Inform the patient that the test takes about 20 minutes.

KEY STEPS

- Confirm the patient's identity using two patient identifiers according to facility policy.
- The patient is helped into the supine position on the X-ray table and the table is positioned within the opening in the scanning gantry.
- A series of transverse X-rays is taken and recorded on magnetic tape. The images are studied, and selected ones are photographed.
- After the first series of X-rays is complete, the images are reviewed. Contrast enhancement may be ordered.
- After the contrast medium is given, another series of X-rays is taken. The patient is observed for an allergic reaction, such as itching, hypotension, hypertension, diaphoresis, or dyspnea.

POSTPROCEDURE CARE

- Instruct the patient to resume his usual diet, as ordered.

PRECAUTIONS

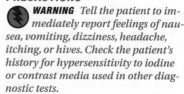 **WARNING** *Tell the patient to immediately report feelings of nausea, vomiting, dizziness, headache, itching, or hives. Check the patient's history for hypersensitivity to iodine or contrast media used in other diagnostic tests.*

- The test is contraindicated during pregnancy due to potential risk to the fetus.

COMPLICATIONS

- Delayed allergic reaction to the contrast dye, such as urticaria, headache, and vomiting

NORMAL RESULTS

- The pancreatic parenchyma displays a uniform density, especially when an I.V. contrast medium is used.
- The gland thickens from tail to head and has a smooth surface.

ABNORMAL RESULTS

- Because the tissue density of pancreatic carcinoma resembles that of the normal parenchyma, changes in pancreatic size and shape help demonstrate carcinoma and pseudocysts.
- Usually, a carcinoma first appears as a localized swelling of the head, body, or tail of the pancreas and may spread to obliterate the fat plane, dilate the main pancreatic duct and common bile duct by obstructing them, and produce low-density focal lesions in the liver from metastasis.
- Use of an I.V. contrast medium helps detect metastases by opacifying the pancreatic and hepatic parenchyma.
- Adenocarcinoma and islet cell tumors are the most common carcinomas of the pancreas.
- Cystadenoma and cystadenocarcinoma, usually multilocular, occur most frequently in the body and tail of the pancreas and can appear as low-density focal lesions marked by internal septa.
- Acute pancreatitis, either edematous (interstitial) or necrotizing (hemorrhagic), produces diffuse enlargement of the pancreas.
- In acute edematous pancreatitis, parenchyma density is uniformly decreased.
- In acute necrotizing pancreatitis, the density is nonuniform because of the presence of necrosis and hemorrhage. The areas of tissue necrosis have diminished density.
- In acute pancreatitis, inflammation typically spreads into the peripancreatic fat, causes stranding in the mesenteric fat, and blurs the gland margin.
- Abscesses, within or outside the pancreas, appear as low-density areas and are most readily detected when they contain gas.
- Pseudocysts, which may be unifocal or multifocal, appear as sharply circumscribed, low-density areas that may contain debris.
- Ascites and pleural effusion may also be apparent in acute pancreatitis.
- In chronic pancreatitis, the pancreas may appear normal, enlarged, or atrophic, depending on disease severity.

Computed tomography scanning, spine

DESCRIPTION

- Provides detailed high-resolution images in the cross-sectional, longitudinal, sagittal, and lateral planes
- Multiple X-ray beams from computerized body scanner directed at spine from different angles; beams pass through body and strike radiation detectors, producing electrical impulses that computer converts into three-dimensional image on monitor
- Allows electronic recreation and manipulation of the image, creating a permanent record that enables reexamination without repeating the procedure
- Helps define lesions causing spinal cord compression and diagnose conditions such as metastatic disease and discogenic disease with osteophyte formation and calcification

PURPOSE

- To diagnose spinal lesions and abnormalities
- To monitor the effects of spinal surgery or therapy

PREPARATION

- Have the patient wear a radiologic examining gown and remove all metal objects and jewelry.
- Check the patient's history for hypersensitivity reactions to iodine, shellfish, or contrast media. Note them in the chart and notify the practitioner who may order prophylactic medications or choose not to use contrast enhancement.
- There are dietary restrictions if a contrast medium is to be used.
- If the patient appears restless or apprehensive about the procedure, a mild sedative may be prescribed.
- For the patient with significant back pain, give prescribed analgesics before the scan.

Teaching points

- Explain that spinal CT scanning allows imaging of the spine.
- Tell the patient who will perform the test and where it will be done.
- If the patient will receive a contrast medium, instruct him to fast for 4 hours before the test.
- If the patient won't receive a contrast medium, tell him that he need not fast.
- Explain to the patient that he'll lie on an X-ray table inside a CT body scanning unit and be asked to lie still because movement during the procedure may cause distorted images.
- Tell the patient that the computer-controlled scanner will revolve around him, taking multiple scans.
- If the patient will receive a contrast medium, tell him that he may feel flushed and warm and may experience a transient headache, a salty taste, and nausea or vomiting after the injection. Reassure him that these reactions are normal.
- Inform the patient that the test takes about 30 minutes.

KEY STEPS

- Confirm the patient's identity using two patient identifiers according to facility policy.
- The patient is assisted into the supine position on an X-ray table and asked to lie as still as possible.
- If the patient becomes claustrophobic or anxious inside the CT body scanner, give him a mild sedative to help relieve these symptoms.
- The table slides into the circular opening of the CT scanner and the scanner revolves around the patient, taking radiographs at preselected intervals.
- After the first set of scans is taken, the patient is removed from the scanner. Contrast medium may be given.
- Observe the patient for signs and symptoms of a hypersensitivity reaction, including pruritus, rash, and respiratory difficulty, for 30 minutes after injection of the contrast medium.
- After the contrast medium is injected, the patient is moved back into the scanner, and another series of scans is taken.

POSTPROCEDURE CARE

- Observe the patient for residual effects, such as headache, nausea, and vomiting.
- Instruct the patient to resume his usual diet, as ordered.

PRECAUTIONS

WARNING *Tell the patient to immediately report feelings of nausea, vomiting, dizziness, headache, itching, or hives. Check the patient's history for hypersensitivity to iodine or contrast media used in other diagnostic tests.*

- The test is contraindicated during pregnancy due to potential risk to the fetus.

COMPLICATIONS

- Claustrophobia or anxiety (when inside the CT body scanner)

INTERPRETATION

NORMAL RESULTS

◆ The spinal tissue appears white, black, or gray, depending on its density.

◆ Vertebrae, the densest tissues, appear white; cerebrospinal fluid is black; soft tissues appear in shades of gray.

ABNORMAL RESULTS

◆ Spinal lesions and other abnormalities are visualized on the scan.

◆ Tumors appear as masses varying in density. Measuring this density and noting the configuration and location relative to the spinal cord can usually identify the type of tumor. For example, a neurinoma (schwannoma) appears as a spherical mass dorsal to the cord. A darker, wider mass lying more lateral or ventral to the cord may be a meningioma.

◆ Degenerative processes and structural changes show in detail.

◆ A herniated nucleus pulposus shows as an obvious herniation of disk material with unilateral or bilateral nerve root compression; if the herniation is midline, spinal cord compression will be evident.

◆ Cervical spondylosis shows as cervical cord compression; lumbar stenosis, as hypertrophy of the lumbar vertebrae.

◆ Facet disorders show as soft-tissue changes, bony overgrowth, and spurring of the vertebrae.

◆ Fluid-filled arachnoidal and other paraspinal cysts show as dark masses displacing the spinal cord.

◆ Vascular malformations, evident after contrast, show as masses or clusters, usually on the dorsal aspect of the spinal cord.

◆ Congenital spinal malformations show as abnormally large, dark gaps between the white vertebrae.

Computed tomography scanning, thorax

DESCRIPTION

+ Provides cross-sectional views of the chest by passing an X-ray beam from a computerized scanner through the body at different angles
+ Provides a three-dimensional image and is especially useful in detecting small differences in tissue density
+ May replace mediastinoscopy in diagnosing mediastinal masses and Hodgkin's disease; proven value in evaluating pulmonary pathology

PURPOSE

+ To locate suspected neoplasms (such as in Hodgkin's disease), especially with mediastinal involvement
+ To differentiate coin-sized calcified lesions (indicating tuberculosis) from tumors
+ To differentiate emphysema or bronchopleural fistula from lung abscess
+ To distinguish tumors adjacent to the aorta from aortic aneurysms
+ To detect the invasion of a neck mass in the thorax
+ To evaluate primary malignancy that may metastasize to the lungs, especially in patients with a primary bone tumor, soft-tissue sarcoma, or melanoma
+ To evaluate the mediastinal lymph nodes
+ To evaluate the severity of lung disease such as emphysema
+ To detect a dissection or leak of an aortic aneurysm or aortic arch aneurysm
+ To plan radiation treatment

PREPARATION

+ Ask the patient to remove all jewelry and metallic objects in the X-ray field.
+ Check the patient's history for hypersensitivity to iodine, shellfish, or contrast media.
+ There are dietary restrictions if a contrast medium is to be used.
+ Make sure that the patient or a responsible family member has signed an informed consent form, if required.

Teaching points

+ Explain that the thoracic computed tomography (CT) scan provides cross-sectional views of the chest and distinguishes small differences in tissue density.
+ Tell the patient who will perform the test and where it will be done.
+ If the patient will receive a contrast medium, instruct him to fast for 4 hours before the test.
+ If the patient won't receive a contrast medium, tell him that he need not fast.
+ Inform the patient that a contrast medium may be injected into a vein in his arm and that he may experience nausea, warmth, flushing of the face, and a salty or metallic taste. Reassure him that these symptoms are normal and that radiation exposure is minimal.
+ Inform the patient that he'll lie on an X-ray table that moves into the center of a large ring-shaped piece of X-ray equipment and that the equipment may be noisy.
+ Tell the patient that he must remain still during the test, breathing normally until told to follow specific breathing instructions.
+ Inform the patient that the test takes about 30 minutes.

KEY STEPS

+ Confirm the patient's identity using two patient identifiers according to facility policy.
+ The patient is assisted into the supine position on the X-ray table and the contrast medium is injected. The machine scans the patient at different angles while the computer calculates small differences in densities of various tissues, water, fat, bone, and air.
+ Information is displayed as a printout of numerical values and a projection on a monitor. Images may be recorded for further study.

POSTPROCEDURE CARE

+ Watch the patient for signs of delayed hypersensitivity to the contrast medium (itching, hypotension or hypertension, or respiratory distress).
+ Encourage the patient to drink lots of fluids.

PRECAUTIONS

WARNING *Tell the patient to immediately report feelings of nausea, vomiting, dizziness, headache, itching, or hives. Check the patient's history for hypersensitivity to iodine or contrast media used in other diagnostic tests.*

+ The test is contraindicated during pregnancy due to potential risk to the fetus.

COMPLICATIONS

+ Adverse effects from contrast medium

NORMAL RESULTS

+ Black and white areas on a thoracic CT scan refer, respectively, to air and bone densities.
+ Shades of gray correspond to water, fat, and soft-tissue densities.

ABNORMAL RESULTS

+ Tumors, nodules, cysts, aortic aneurysms, enlarged lymph nodes, pleural effusion, and accumulations of blood, fluid, or fat may be found.

Concentration and dilution tests

DESCRIPTION

- Evaluates renal capacity to concentrate urine in response to fluid deprivation or to dilute it in response to fluid overload
- Also known as the *water loading test* or *water deprivation test*

PURPOSE

- To evaluate renal tubular function
- To detect renal impairment
- To diagnose disorders such as diabetes insipidus

PREPARATION

- The test evaluates kidney function.
- Multiple urine specimens are required.
- Withhold diuretics as needed.
- For a concentration test, limit the patient's salt intake during the evening meal to prevent excessive thirst.
- For the dilution test, preparation is the same as for the concentration test. If it's performed alone, withhold breakfast.

Teaching points

- Explain the purpose of the test and how it's done.
- Tell the patient who will perform the test and where it will be done.
- Because the test requires multiple urine specimens, explain how many specimens will be collected and at what intervals.
- Instruct the patient to discard urine voided for a specific time, according to laboratory protocol, such as urine collected during the night.
- Instruct the patient to eat a high-protein meal and only 200 ml of fluid the night before the test. Then tell him to fast for at least 14 hours before the test.

KEY STEPS

- Confirm the patient's identity using two patient identifiers according to facility policy.
- For the concentration test, collect urine specimens at 6 a.m., 8 a.m., and 10 a.m.
- For the dilution test, instruct the patient to void and discard the first urine sample. Give the patient 1,500 ml of water to drink within a 30-minute period. Collect urine specimens every half hour or every hour for 4 hours thereafter.
- Provide the patient with a clean bedpan, urinal, or toilet specimen pan if he's unable to urinate into the specimen containers.
- Send each specimen to the laboratory immediately after collection.

POSTPROCEDURE CARE

- For both tests provide a balanced meal or a snack after collecting the final specimen. Make sure the patient voids within 8 hours after the catheter is removed.

PRECAUTIONS

- The test is contraindicated in patients with advanced renal disease or cardiac dysfunction.
- If the patient is catheterized, empty the drainage bag before the test. Obtain the specimens from the catheter and clamp the catheter between collections.

COMPLICATIONS

- None

NORMAL RESULTS

- Specific gravity ranges from 1.005 to 1.035; osmolality normally ranges from 300 to 900 mOsm/kg.
- In the concentration test, specific gravity ranges from 1.025 to 1.032, and osmolality rises above 800 mOsm/kg of water (SI, greater than 800 mmol/kg) in patients with normal renal function.
- In the dilution test, specific gravity falls below 1.003 and osmolality below 100 mOsm/kg for at least one specimen; 80% or more of the ingested water is eliminated in 4 hours.

ABNORMAL RESULTS

- Decreased renal capacity to concentrate urine in response to fluid deprivation, or to dilute urine in response to fluid overload, may indicate tubular epithelial damage, decreased renal blood flow, loss of functional nephrons, or pituitary or cardiac dysfunction.
- In elderly patients, depressed values may indicate normal renal function.

Contraction stress test

DESCRIPTION

- Measures fetal heart rate in response to uterine contractions; usually, the heart rate of a healthy fetus won't slow down when contractions begin and after they end
- May be performed weekly until delivery

PURPOSE

- To measure fetal heart rate in response to contractions

PREPARATION

- Make sure the patient has signed an appropriate consent form

Teaching points

- Explain the purpose of the test and how it's done.
- Tell the patient who will perform the test and where it will be done.
- Advise the patient of dietary restrictions associated with the test, as ordered.
- If the patient smokes, tell her not to smoke for 2 hours before the test.
- Explain that the test generally lasts for 30 to 40 minutes.

KEY STEPS

- Confirm the patient's identity using two patient identifiers according to facility policy.
- After the patient lies down, place two belts around the abdomen with transducers positioned over the fetal heartbeat and over the uterus for contractions.
- Connect the belts to an external fetal monitor.
- Record the fetal heart rate and contractions on the monitor and on a paper printout.
- If the patient isn't having contractions, ask her to stimulate one of her nipples for a brief time, until contractions begin.
- In some cases, oxytocin is given I.V. to stimulate contractions.
- Give a diluted solution of oxytocin at a rate of 1 mU/minute, increasing the oxytocin rate until the patient experiences three contractions within 10 minutes, each lasting longer than 45 seconds.
- If no decelerations occur during three contractions, the patient may be discharged. Late decelerations during any of the contractions require notification of the practitioner and further tests.

POSTPROCEDURE CARE

- Monitor the patient closely.

PRECAUTIONS

- Monitor the patient receiving oxytocin carefully for tetanic contractions

COMPLICATIONS

- None

NORMAL RESULTS

- Three contractions occur in a 10-minute period with no slowing (or late decelerations) of the fetal heart rate in response to contractions.

ABNORMAL RESULTS

- Late decelerations of the fetal heart rate occur in response to the contractions, indicating a problem that requires further testing or delivery.

Coombs' test, direct

DESCRIPTION
◆ Detects the presence of immuno-globulins (antibodies) on the surface of red blood cells (RBCs), which happens when they're sensitized to antigens (such as Rh factor)

PURPOSE
◆ To diagnose hemolytic disease of the newborn
◆ To investigate hemolytic transfusion reactions
◆ To aid in the differential diagnosis of hemolytic anemias, which may be congenital or may result from an autoimmune reaction or use of certain drugs

PREPARATION
◆ The test helps determine whether the condition results from an abnormality of the body's immune system, the use of certain drugs, or an unknown cause.
◆ The test helps diagnose hemolytic disease of the newborn.
◆ No dietary restrictions are required.
◆ Withhold medications that may interfere with test results, including quinidine, methyldopa, cephalosporins, sulfonamides, chlorpromazine, diphenylhydantoin, ethosuximide, hydralazine, levodopa, mefenamic acid, melphalan, penicillin, procainamide, rifampin, streptomycin, tetracyclines, and isoniazid, as ordered.

Teaching points
◆ Explain the purpose of the test and how it's done.
◆ Tell the patient who will perform the venipuncture and where it will be done.
◆ Tell the patient that no dietary restrictions are needed.
◆ Explain to the patient that the test requires a blood sample and that he may experience slight discomfort from the tourniquet and needle puncture.
◆ Give the patient a list of medications to stop, as ordered

KEY STEPS
◆ Confirm the patient's identity using two patient identifiers according to facility policy.
◆ Perform a venipuncture and collect two 5-ml EDTA tubes.

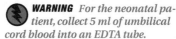 **WARNING** *For the neonatal patient, collect 5 ml of umbilical cord blood into an EDTA tube.*

POSTPROCEDURE CARE
◆ Apply direct pressure to the venipuncture site until bleeding stops.
◆ Instruct the patient to resume any medications.

PRECAUTIONS
◆ Maintain standard precautions while collecting the samples.
◆ Handle the sample gently to avoid hemolysis.
◆ Send the sample to the laboratory immediately after collection.

COMPLICATIONS
◆ Hematoma at the venipuncture site

NORMAL RESULTS
◆ A negative test, in which neither antibodies nor complements appears on the RBCs.

ABNORMAL RESULTS
◆ A positive test in the neonate indicates that maternal antibodies have crossed the placental barrier and coated the fetal RBCs, causing hemolytic disease of the neonate.
◆ In other patients, a positive test result may indicate hemolytic anemia, and may help differentiate between autoimmune and secondary hemolytic anemia.
◆ A positive test may also indicate sepsis.
◆ A weakly positive test may indicate a transfusion reaction where the patient's antibodies reacted with transfused RBCs that contained the corresponding antigen.

Coombs' test, indirect

DESCRIPTION
- Detects unexpected circulating anti-bodies
- Detects 95% to 99% of circulating antibodies

PURPOSE
- To detect unexpected circulating antibodies to red blood cell (RBC) antigens in the recipient's or donor's serum before transfusion
- To determine the presence of anti-D antibody in maternal blood
- To evaluate the need for $Rh_o(D)$ immune globulin
- To help diagnose acquired hemolytic anemia

PREPARATION
- This test helps evaluate the possibility of a transfusion reaction or determines whether fetal antibodies are in the patient's blood and whether treatment is needed.
- If the test is for a patient who's anemic, explain that it helps identify the type of anemia present.
- No dietary restrictions are required.
- The test requires a blood sample.
- Check the patient's history for recent administration of blood, dextran, or I.V. contrast media.

Teaching points
- Explain the purpose of the test and how it's done.
- Tell the patient who will perform the venipuncture and where it will be done.
- Tell the patient that no dietary restrictions are needed.
- Explain to the patient that the test requires a blood sample and that he may experience slight discomfort from the tourniquet and needle puncture.
- Inform the patient that the test should take less than 5 minutes.

KEY STEPS
- Confirm the patient's identity using two patient identifiers according to facility policy.
- Perform a venipuncture and collect the sample in two 10-ml tubes. If the antibody screen is positive, antibody identification is performed on the blood.
- Label the sample with the patient's name, the hospital or blood bank number, the date, and the phlebotomist's initials. Be sure to include on the laboratory request the patient's diagnosis and pregnancy status, history of transfusions, and current drug therapy.
- Send the sample to the laboratory immediately after collection.

POSTPROCEDURE CARE
- Apply direct pressure to the venipuncture site until bleeding stops.

PRECAUTIONS
- Maintain standard precautions while collecting the sample.
- Handle the sample gently to prevent hemolysis.

COMPLICATIONS
- Hematoma at the venipuncture site

NORMAL RESULTS
- Agglutination doesn't occur, indicating that the patient's serum contains no circulating antibodies other than anti-A or anti-B.

ABNORMAL RESULTS
- A positive result indicates the presence of unexpected circulating antibodies to RBC antigens, which demonstrates donor and recipient incompatibility.
- A positive result in a pregnant patient with Rh-negative blood may indicate the presence of antibodies to the Rh factor from an earlier transfusion with incompatible blood or from a previous pregnancy with an Rh-positive fetus.
- A positive result indicates that the fetus may develop hemolytic disease of the newborn. Repeated testing during pregnancy is needed to evaluate the development of circulating antibody levels.

Corticotropin level, plasma

OVERVIEW

DESCRIPTION

- Measures the plasma levels of corticotropin by radioimmunoassay; levels vary diurnally; peak between 6 a.m. and 8 a.m. and ebb between 6 p.m. and 11 p.m.
- Secretion stimulated by emotional and physical stress (such as pain, surgery, insulin-induced hypoglycemia); may override effects of plasma cortisol levels
- May be performed in patients with signs of adrenal hypofunction (insufficiency) or hyperfunction (Cushing's syndrome)
- Corticotropin suppression or stimulation testing needed to confirm diagnosis

PURPOSE

- To facilitate a differential diagnosis of primary and secondary adrenal hypofunction
- To aid a differential diagnosis of Cushing's syndrome

PREPARATION

- This test helps determine if the patient's hormonal secretion is normal.
- The patient must fast and limit physical activity for 10 to 12 hours before the test.
- The test requires a blood sample.
- Check the patient's history for medications that may affect the accuracy of the test results. Withhold these medications for 48 hours or longer before the test. If the patient must continue them, note this on the laboratory request.

Teaching points

- Explain the purpose of the test and how it's done.
- Tell the patient who will perform the test and where it will be done.
- Tell the patient what time the sample needs to be drawn.
- Instruct the patient to fast for at least 10 hours before the test.
- Advise the patient to restrict physical activity for at least 10 hours before the test.
- Explain to the patient that the test requires a blood sample and that he may experience slight discomfort from the tourniquet and needle puncture.
- Inform the patient that the test should take less than 5 minutes.

DIAGNOSTIC PROCEDURE

KEY STEPS

- Confirm the patient's identity using two patient identifiers according to facility policy.
- For a patient with suspected adrenal hypofunction, perform the venipuncture for a baseline level between 6 a.m. and 8 a.m. (peak secretion).
- For a patient with suspected Cushing's syndrome, perform the venipuncture between 6 p.m. and 11 p.m. (low secretion).
- Collect the sample in a plastic EDTA tube (corticotropin may adhere to glass). The tube must be full because excess anticoagulant affects results.
- Pack the sample in ice and send it to the laboratory immediately after collection, where plasma must be rapidly separated from blood cells at 39.2° F (4° C). The collection technique may vary, depending on the laboratory.

POSTPROCEDURE CARE

- Apply direct pressure to the venipuncture site until bleeding stops.
- Tell the patient to resume his usual diet, activities, and medications.

PRECAUTIONS

- Maintain standard precautions while collecting the sample.
- Make sure to collect the sample at the right time of day, depending on if the patient has suspected adrenal hypofunction or hyperfunction.
- Be sure to collect a full tube and place it on ice immediately after collection.

COMPLICATIONS

- Hematoma at the venipuncture site

INTERPRETATION

NORMAL RESULTS

- Mayo Medical Laboratories sets baseline values at less than 120 pg/ml (SI, less than 26.4 pmol/L at 6 a.m. to 8 a.m.), but these may vary with each laboratory.

ABNORMAL RESULTS

- A higher-than-normal corticotropin level may indicate primary adrenal hypofunction (Addison's disease), in which the pituitary gland attempts to compensate for the unresponsiveness of the target organ by releasing excessive corticotropin.
- The underlying cause of adrenocortical hypofunction may be idiopathic atrophy of the adrenal cortex or partial destruction of the gland by granuloma, neoplasm, amyloidosis, or inflammatory necrosis.
- A low-normal corticotropin level suggests secondary adrenal hypofunction resulting from pituitary or hypothalamic dysfunction.
- The primary determinant may be panhypopituitarism, absence of corticotropin-releasing hormone in the hypothalamus, or chronic blunting of corticotropin levels by long-term corticosteroid therapy.
- In suspected Cushing's syndrome, an elevated corticotropin level suggests Cushing's disease, in which pituitary dysfunction (from adenoma) causes continuous hypersecretion of corticotropin and, consequently, continuously elevated cortisol levels without diurnal variations.
- Moderately elevated corticotropin levels suggest pituitary-dependent adrenal hyperplasia and nonadrenal tumors such as oat cell carcinoma of the lungs.
- A low-normal corticotropin level implies adrenal hyperfunction due to adrenocortical tumor or hyperplasia.

◆ **INTERFERING FACTORS** *Corticosteroids (may cause decreased values)*

Cortisol levels, plasma and urine

DESCRIPTION

- Quantitative analysis of plasma cortisol levels for patients with signs of adrenal dysfunction
- Involves dynamic tests, suppression tests for hyperfunction, and stimulation tests for hypofunction to confirm diagnosis
- Cortisol: helps metabolize nutrients, mediate physiologic stress, and regulate the immune system; levels rise in morning, peak at about 8 a.m., and decline in evening and during sleep (see *Diurnal variations in cortisol secretion*)
- Intense heat or cold, infection, trauma, exercise, obesity, and debilitating disease influence cortisol secretion

PURPOSE

- To help diagnose Cushing's disease, Cushing's syndrome, Addison's disease, and secondary adrenal insufficiency
- To evaluate adrenocortical function

PREPARATION

- This test helps determine if the patient's symptoms are caused by improper hormonal secretion.
- Review dietary and activity restrictions with the patient.
- Withhold all drugs that may interfere with plasma cortisol levels, such as estrogens, androgens, and phenytoin, for 48 hours before the test.

Plasma

- The test requires a blood sample.
- If the patient is receiving replacement therapy and is dependent on exogenous corticosteroids for survival, note this on the laboratory request along with other drugs that he must continue.
- Make sure the patient is relaxed and recumbent for at least 30 minutes before the test.

Urine

- The test involves a urine collection for 24 hours.

Teaching points

- Explain the purpose of the test and how it's done.
- Tell the patient who will perform the test and where it will be done.
- Explain to the patient that the test requires a blood sample and that he may experience slight discomfort from the tourniquet and needle puncture.
- If the patient is doing an at home urine cortisol test, teach the patient how to collect and store the urine.
- Tell the patient to maintain a normal salt diet (2 to 3 g/day) for 3 days before the test and to fast and limit his physical activity for 10 to 12 hours before the test.

Diurnal variations in cortisol secretion

Cortisol secretion rises in the early morning, peaking after the patient awakens. Levels decline sharply in the evening and during the early phase of sleep. They rise again during the night and peak by the next morning.

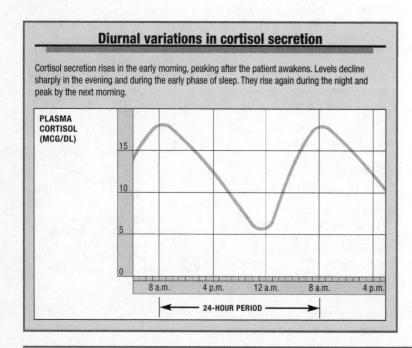

DIAGNOSTIC PROCEDURE

KEY STEPS
◆ Confirm the patient's identity using two patient identifiers according to facility policy.

Plasma
◆ Perform a venipuncture between 6 a.m. and 8 a.m.
◆ Collect the sample in a 7-ml heparinized tube, label it appropriately, and send it to the laboratory immediately after collection.
◆ For diurnal variation testing, draw another sample between 4 p.m. and 6 p.m.
◆ Collect the second sample in a 7-ml heparinized tube, label it appropriately, and send it to the laboratory immediately after collection.
◆ Record the collection time on the laboratory request.

Urine
◆ Collect the patient's urine during a 24-hour period, discarding the first specimen and retaining the last.
◆ Use a bottle containing a preservative to keep the specimen at a pH of 4.0 to 4.5.

POSTPROCEDURE CARE
◆ Apply direct pressure to the venipuncture site until bleeding stops, as applicable.
◆ Tell the patient to resume his usual diet, activities, and medications.

PRECAUTIONS
◆ Handle the blood sample gently to prevent hemolysis.
◆ Refrigerate the urine specimen or place on ice during the collection period.

COMPLICATIONS
◆ Hematoma at the venipuncture site

INTERPRETATION

NORMAL RESULTS
◆ Values are 9 to 35 mcg/dl (SI, 250 to 690 nmol/L) in the morning; 3 to 12 mcg/dl (SI, 80 to 330 nmol/L) in the afternoon.

ABNORMAL RESULTS
◆ High plasma cortisol levels may indicate adrenocortical hyperfunction in Cushing's disease (a rare disease caused by basophilic adenoma of the pituitary gland) or Cushing's syndrome (glucocorticoid excess from any cause); hepatic disease; or obesity.
◆ In most patients with Cushing's syndrome, the adrenal cortex secretes independently of a natural rhythm; absence of diurnal variation in cortisol secretion is a significant finding in these patients.
◆ Diurnal variations may also be absent in otherwise healthy people who are under considerable emotional or physical stress.
◆ Low plasma cortisol levels may indicate primary adrenal hypofunction (Addison's disease), usually caused by idiopathic glandular atrophy (a presumed autoimmune process).
◆ Adrenocortical destruction can result from tuberculosis, fungal invasion, and hemorrhage.
◆ Low plasma cortisol levels resulting from secondary adrenal insufficiency may occur in conditions of impaired corticotropin secretion, such as hypophysectomy, postpartum pituitary necrosis, craniopharyngioma, and chromophobe adenoma.
◆ High urine cortisol levels may indicate Cushing's syndrome caused by adrenal hyperplasia, adrenal or pituitary tumor, or ectopic corticotropin production.

Cortisol stimulation test

DESCRIPTION

- Performed on patients with an adrenal insufficiency
- Cortisol-like drug given, and plasma cortisol level measured
- Cortisol: helps metabolize nutrients, mediate physiologic stress, and regulate the immune system; levels rise in the morning, peak around 8 a.m., and decline in the evening and during sleep
- Also called the *adrenocorticotropic hormone (ACTH) stimulation test*

PURPOSE

- To determine if the cause of adrenal insufficiency is primary (Addison's disease) or secondary (hypopituitarism)
- To evaluate patients with Cushing's syndrome

PREPARATION

- The test helps determine the cause of the patient's adrenal insufficiency.
- The test requires fasting for at least 8 hours before the test.
- The test requires several blood samples.

Teaching points

- Explain the purpose of the test and how it's done.
- Tell the patient who will perform the test and where it will be done.
- Tell the patient to fast for at least 8 hours before the test.
- Explain to the patient that the test requires several blood samples and that he may experience slight discomfort from the tourniquet and needle puncture.
- Inform the patient that the test will take about 1 hour.

KEY STEPS

- Confirm the patient's identity using two patient identifiers according to facility policy.
- Perform a venipuncture and obtain a baseline cortisol level.
- Administer an I.V. injection of cosyntropin (ACTH-like drug) over 2 minutes.
- Perform a venipuncture and collect cortisol levels at 30 minutes and 60 minutes after the administration of the drug.

POSTPROCEDURE CARE

- Apply pressure to the venipuncture site until bleeding stops.

PRECAUTIONS

- Maintain standard precautions while collecting the sample.
- Collect the baseline cortisol level within 30 minutes of drug administration.
- Collect the 30 minute and 60 minute samples at the appropriate times.

COMPLICATIONS

- Hematoma at the venipuncture site

NORMAL RESULTS

- An increase in cortisol level after stimulation by ACTH is normal; level should be greater than 20 mcg/dl.

ABNORMAL RESULTS

- Cortisol level less than 7 mcg/dl over baseline indicates primary adrenal insufficiency.
- Cortisol level greater than 7 mcg/dl over baseline indicates secondary adrenal insufficiency, due to inadequate stimulation of the adrenal gland from the pituitary gland.

C-peptide test

DESCRIPTION

◆ Measures biologically inactive chain formed during proteolytic conversion of proinsulin to insulin in pancreatic beta cells

PURPOSE

◆ To determine the cause of hypoglycemia
◆ To indirectly measure insulin secretion in the presence of circulating insulin antibodies
◆ To detect residual tissue after total pancreatectomy for carcinoma
◆ To determine beta-cell function in the patient with diabetes mellitus

PREPARATION

◆ This test helps to evaluate pancreatic function and to determine the cause of hypoglycemia.
◆ The test requires fasting for 8 to 12 hours before testing, but no restrictions on water intake.
◆ The test requires a blood sample.
◆ If the patient is to receive radioisotope testing, it should take place after blood is drawn for C-peptide levels.
◆ Blood glucose levels are usually drawn at the same time as C-peptide levels.
◆ If the patient receives a C-peptide stimulation test, give I.V. glucagon after a baseline blood sample is drawn.
◆ Withhold medications that may interfere with test results. If the patient must continue them, note this on the laboratory request.

Teaching points

◆ Explain the purpose of the test and how it's done.
◆ Tell the patient who will perform the test and where it will be done.
◆ Instruct the patient to fast for at least 8 hours before the test.

◆ Explain to the patient that the test requires a blood sample and that he may experience slight discomfort from the tourniquet and needle puncture.
◆ Advise the patient that the test should take less than 5 minutes.

DIAGNOSTIC PROCEDURE

KEY STEPS

◆ Confirm the patient's identity using two patient identifiers according to facility policy.
◆ Perform a venipuncture and collect a 1-ml sample in a chilled clot-activator tube. The blood is separated and frozen to be tested later.
◆ Collect a sample for testing glucose level in a tube with sodium fluoride and potassium oxalate, if ordered.
◆ Pack the sample in ice and send it immediately after collection, with the glucose sample, to the laboratory.

POSTPROCEDURE CARE

◆ Apply direct pressure to the venipuncture site until bleeding stops.
◆ Tell the patient to resume his usual activities, diet, and medications, as ordered.

PRECAUTIONS

◆ Maintain standard precautions while collecting the sample.
◆ Handle the samples gently to prevent hemolysis.

COMPLICATIONS

◆ Hematoma at the venipuncture site

INTERPRETATION

NORMAL RESULTS

◆ Serum C-peptide levels generally parallel those of insulin.
◆ Normal fasting values range between 0.78 and 1.89 ng/ml (SI, 0.26 to 0.63 mmol/L).
◆ An insulin:C-peptide ratio may be calculated to differentiate insulinoma from factitious hypoglycemia.
◆ A ratio of 1.0 or less indicates increased, endogenous insulin secretion; a ratio of 1.0 or more indicates exogenous insulin.

ABNORMAL RESULTS

◆ Elevated levels may indicate endogenous hyperinsulinism (insulinemia), oral hypoglycemic drug ingestion, pancreas or B-cell transplantation, renal failure, or type 2 diabetes mellitus.
◆ Decreased levels may indicate factitious hypoglycemia (surreptitious insulin administration), radical pancreatectomy, or type 1 diabetes.

C-reactive protein test

DESCRIPTION

- C-reactive protein (CRP) present in blood during inflammatory process; not present in healthy people
- Mainly synthesized in liver and found in body fluids
- Appears in blood 18 to 24 hours after onset of tissue damage; levels increase up to 1,000 fold and then decline when inflammatory process regresses
- Rises before antibody titers and erythrocyte sedimentation rates
- After a myocardial infarction (MI), levels correlated with CK-MB levels, but peaking 1 to 3 days after CK-MB
- If CRP remains elevated, ongoing myocardial tissue damage suggested

PURPOSE

- To evaluate the inflammatory disease course and severity in conditions that include tissue necrosis
- To monitor acute inflammatory phases of rheumatoid arthritis (RA) and rheumatic fever for early initiation of treatment
- To monitor the patient's response to treatment or determine if the acute phase is declining
- To help interpret the erythrocyte sedimentation rate
- To monitor the wound-healing process of internal incisions, burns, and organ transplantation

PREPARATION

- This test identifies inflammation or monitors treatment.
- All fluids except water should be restricted for 8 to 12 hours before the test.
- The test requires a blood sample.
- Notify the laboratory and practitioner of medications that the patient is taking that may affect test results.

Teaching points

- Explain the purpose of the test and how it's done.
- Tell the patient who will perform the test and where it will be done.
- Tell the patient not to drink any fluids except water for at least 8 hours before the test.
- Explain to the patient that the test requires a blood sample and that he may experience slight discomfort from the tourniquet and needle puncture.
- Inform the patient that the test should take less than 5 minutes.

DIAGNOSTIC PROCEDURE

KEY STEPS

- Confirm the patient's identity using two patient identifiers according to facility policy.
- Perform a venipuncture and collect the sample in a 5-ml clot activator tube.

POSTPROCEDURE CARE

- Apply pressure to the venipuncture site until bleeding stops.
- Tell the patient that he may resume his usual diet, as ordered.

PRECAUTIONS

- Maintain standard precautions while collecting the sample.
- Keep the blood sample away from heat.

COMPLICATIONS

- Hematoma at the venipuncture site

INTERPRETATION

NORMAL RESULTS

- CRP is less than 0.8 mg/dl (SI, < 8 mg/L).

ABNORMAL RESULTS

- CRP may be present in patients with RA, rheumatic fever, MI, cancer, acute bacterial and viral infections, inflammatory bowel disease, Hodgkin's disease, or systemic lupus erythematosus and for the first three days postoperatively.
- Value may be increased in the third trimester of pregnancy.

INTERFERING FACTORS *Corticosteroids (false normal levels); hormonal contraceptives (may cause false increased levels)*

Creatine kinase and isoform tests

DESCRIPTION

- Fractionates and measures three distinct creatine kinase (CK) isoenzymes — CK-BB, CK-MB, and CK-MM — to accurately localize site of increased tissue destruction
- CK-BB: occurs in brain tissue
- CK-MM and CK-MB: found in skeletal and heart muscle
- May increase test sensitivity by assaying subunits of CK-MB and CK-MM (*isoforms* or *isoenzymes*)

PURPOSE

- To detect and diagnose acute myocardial infarction (MI)
- To evaluate possible causes of chest pain and to monitor the severity of myocardial ischemia
- To detect early dermatomyositis and musculoskeletal disorders that aren't neurogenic in origin

PREPARATION

- If the test is for musculoskeletal disorders, the patient should avoid exercising for 24 hours before the test.
- Notify the laboratory and practitioner of drugs the patient is taking that may affect test results; it may be necessary to restrict them.

Teaching points

- Explain the purpose of the test and how it's done.
- Tell the patient who will perform the test and where it will be done.
- Advise the patient that there are no dietary restrictions.
- If the test is for musculoskeletal disorders, instruct the patient to restrict physical activity for 24 hours before the test.
- Explain to the patient that the test requires a blood sample and that he may experience slight discomfort from the tourniquet and needle puncture.
- Inform the patient that the test should take less than 5 minutes.

DIAGNOSTIC PROCEDURE

KEY STEPS

- Confirm the patient's identity using two patient identifiers according to facility policy.
- Perform a venipuncture and collect the sample in a 4-ml tube without additives.
- Note on the laboratory request the time the sample was drawn.
- Send the sample to the laboratory immediately after collection because CK activity diminishes significantly after 2 hours at room temperature.

POSTPROCEDURE CARE

- Apply direct pressure to the venipuncture site until bleeding stops.
- Tell the patient that he may resume activity and medications, as ordered.

PRECAUTIONS

- Maintain standard precautions while collecting the sample.
- Handle the sample gently to prevent hemolysis.
- Draw the sample before giving I.M. injections or 1 hour after giving them because muscle trauma increases the total CK level.

COMPLICATIONS

- Hematoma at the venipuncture site

INTERPRETATION

NORMAL RESULTS

- Total CK values determined by ultraviolet or kinetic measurement range from 55 to 170 units/L (SI, 0.94 to 2.89 µkat/L) for men; for women, 30 to 135 units/L (SI, 0.51 to 2.3 µkat/L).
- CK levels may be significantly higher in muscular people.
- Infants up to age 1 have levels two to four times higher than adult levels, possibly reflecting birth trauma and striated muscle development.
- Ranges for isoenzyme levels are CK-BB, undetectable; CK-MB, less than 5% (SI, less than 0.05); and CK-MM, 90% to 100% (SI, 0.9 to 1.0).

ABNORMAL RESULTS

- Without confirming brain tissue injury, detectable CK-BB isoenzyme may suggest widespread malignant tumors, severe shock, or renal failure.
- CK-MB levels greater than 5% of the total CK level indicate an MI, especially if the lactate dehydrogenase (LD) isoenzyme ratio is more than 1 (flipped LD).
- In acute MI and after cardiac surgery, CK-MB begins to increase within 2 to 4 hours, peaks within 12 to 24 hours, and usually returns to normal within 24 to 48 hours; persistent elevations and increasing levels indicate ongoing myocardial damage. Total CK follows similar pattern increases slightly later.
- Serious skeletal muscle injury that occurs in certain muscular dystrophies, polymyositis, and severe myoglobinuria may produce a mild CK-MB increase because a small amount of this isoenzyme exists in some skeletal muscles.
- Increasing CK-MM values follow skeletal muscle damage from trauma, such as surgery and I.M. injections, and from diseases, such as dermatomyositis and muscular dystrophy.
- Moderately increasing CK-MM levels develop in a patient with hypothyroidism; sharp increases occur with muscle activity caused by agitation such as during an acute psychotic episode.
- Total CK levels may increase in patients with severe hypokalemia, carbon monoxide poisoning, malignant hyperthermia, alcoholic cardiomyopathy, after seizures, and in patients who have suffered pulmonary or cerebral infarctions.

Creatinine level, serum

OVERVIEW

DESCRIPTION
- Provides a more sensitive measure of renal damage than blood urea nitrogen levels
- Creatinine: nonprotein end product of creatine metabolism appearing in serum proportional to body's muscle mass

PURPOSE
- To assess glomerular filtration
- To screen for renal damage

PREPARATION
- This test evaluates kidney function.
- The test requires a blood sample.
- No dietary restrictions are required.
- Notify the laboratory and practitioner of drugs the patient is taking that may affect test results; it may be necessary to restrict them.

Teaching points
- Explain the purpose of the test and how it's done.
- Tell the patient who will perform the test and where it will be done.
- Advise the patient that there are no dietary restrictions.
- Explain to the patient that the test requires a blood sample and that he may experience slight discomfort from the tourniquet and needle puncture.
- Inform the patient that the test should take less than 5 minutes.

DIAGNOSTIC PROCEDURE

KEY STEPS
- Confirm the patient's identity using two patient identifiers according to facility policy.
- Perform a venipuncture and collect the sample in a 3- or 4-ml clot-activator tube.
- Send the sample to the laboratory immediately after collection.

POSTPROCEDURE CARE
- Apply direct pressure to the venipuncture site until bleeding stops.
- Tell the patient that he may resume his usual medications, as ordered.

PRECAUTIONS
- Maintain standard precautions while collecting the sample.
- Handle the sample gently to prevent hemolysis.

COMPLICATIONS
- Hematoma at the venipuncture site

INTERPRETATION

NORMAL RESULTS
- In men, 0.8 to 1.2 mg/dl (SI, 62 to 115 µmol/L).
- In women, 0.6 to 0.9 mg/dl (SI, 53 to 97 µmol/L).

ABNORMAL RESULTS
- Elevated levels usually indicate renal disease that has seriously damaged 50% or more of the nephrons.
- Elevated levels may also indicate gigantism and acromegaly.

INTERFERING FACTORS *Exceptionally large muscle mass, such as that found in athletes (possible increase despite normal renal function)*

Creatinine level, urine

DESCRIPTION

- Measures urine levels of creatinine, the chief metabolite of creatine
- Standard method for determining urine creatinine levels based on Jaffe's reaction, in which creatinine treated with alkaline picrate solution yields bright orange-red complex
- Amount of creatinine produced proportional to total body muscle mass; removed from plasma by glomerular filtration and excreted in urine
- Not recycled by body; relatively high, constant clearance rate; efficient indicator of renal function
- Creatinine clearance test a more precise index than this test

PURPOSE

- To help assess glomerular filtration
- To check the accuracy of 24-hour urine collection, based on the relatively constant levels of creatinine excretion

PREPARATION

- This test helps evaluate kidney function.
- The test usually requires urine collection during a 24-hour period; teach the patient the proper collection technique.
- Notify the laboratory and practitioner of drugs the patient is taking that may affect test results; it may be necessary to restrict them.

Teaching points

- Explain the purpose of the test and how it's done.
- Teach the patient how to collect a 24-hour urine specimen at home.
- Inform the patient that he need not restrict fluids, but that he shouldn't eat an excessive amount of meat before the test.
- Advise the patient to avoid strenuous physical exercise during the collection period.

KEY STEPS

- Confirm the patient's identity using two patient identifiers according to facility policy.
- Collect the patient's urine during a 24-hour period, discarding the first specimen and retaining the last. Use a specimen bottle that contains a preservative to prevent creatinine degradation.
- Send the specimen to the laboratory immediately after the collection is complete.

POSTPROCEDURE CARE

- Tell the patient that he may resume his usual activities, diet, and medications, as ordered.

PRECAUTIONS

- Refrigerate the specimen or keep it on ice during the collection period.

COMPLICATIONS

- None

NORMAL RESULTS

- In males, 14 to 26 mg/kg body weight/24 hours (SI, 124 to 230 μmol/kg body weight/day).
- In females, 11 to 20 mg/kg body weight/24 hours (SI, 97 to 177 μmol/kg body weight/day).

ABNORMAL RESULTS

- Decreased urine creatinine levels may result from impaired renal perfusion (for example, associated with shock) or from renal disease due to urinary tract obstruction.
- Chronic bilateral pyelonephritis, acute or chronic glomerulonephritis, and polycystic kidney disease may also depress creatinine levels.
- Increased levels generally have little diagnostic significance.

Creatinine clearance test

DESCRIPTION

◆ Excellent diagnostic indicator of renal function; determines how efficiently kidneys are clearing creatinine from the blood
◆ Rate of clearance expressed as volume of blood (in milliliters) that can be cleared of creatinine in 1 minute
◆ Creatinine levels abnormal when more than 50% of nephrons are damaged

PURPOSE

◆ To assess renal function (primarily glomerular filtration)
◆ To monitor progression of renal insufficiency

PREPARATION

◆ This test assesses kidney function.
◆ The patient should avoid meat, poultry, fish, tea, or coffee for 6 hours before the test.
◆ The patient should avoid strenuous physical exercise during the collection period.
◆ The test requires a timed urine specimen and at least one blood sample.
◆ Notify the laboratory and practitioner of drugs the patient is taking that may affect test results; they may be restricted.

Teaching points

◆ Explain the purpose of the test and how it's done.
◆ Tell the patient how the urine specimen will be collected.
◆ Inform him who will perform the venipuncture when and where it will be done.
◆ Tell him that he may feel slight discomfort from the tourniquet and needle puncture.
◆ Explain that more than one venipuncture may be necessary.
◆ Inform the patient that he may need to avoid meat, poultry, fish, tea, or coffee for 6 hours before the test.
◆ Advise the patient to avoid strenuous physical exercise during the collection period.

KEY STEPS

◆ Confirm the patient's identity using two patient identifiers according to facility policy.
◆ Collect a timed urine specimen at 2, 6, 12, or 24 hours in a bottle containing a preservative to prevent creatinine degradation.
◆ Perform a venipuncture anytime during the collection period and collect the sample in a 7-ml tube without additives.

POSTPROCEDURE CARE

◆ Apply direct pressure to the venipuncture site until bleeding stops.
◆ Tell the patient that he may resume his usual activities, diet, and medications, as ordered.

PRECAUTIONS

◆ Maintain standard precautions while collecting the samples.
◆ Refrigerate the urine specimen or keep it on ice during the collection period.
◆ Send the specimen to the laboratory as soon as the collection is complete.

COMPLICATIONS

◆ Hematoma at the venipuncture site

NORMAL RESULTS

◆ Results vary with age: in males, it ranges from 94 to 140 ml/minute/1.73 m^2 (SI, 0.91 to 1.35 ml/s/m^2); in females, 72 to 110 ml/minute/1.73 m^2 (SI, 0.69 to 1.06 ml/s/m^2).

ABNORMAL RESULTS

◆ Low creatinine clearance may result from reduced renal blood flow (associated with shock or renal artery obstruction), acute tubular necrosis, acute or chronic glomerulonephritis, advanced bilateral chronic pyelonephritis, advanced bilateral renal lesions (which may occur in polycystic kidney disease, renal tuberculosis, and cancer), nephrosclerosis, heart failure, or severe dehydration.
◆ High creatinine clearance can suggest poor hydration.

Crossmatching

DESCRIPTION

- Establishes compatibility or incompatibility of donor's and recipient's blood
- Best antibody detection test available for avoiding lethal transfusion reactions
- After donor's and recipient's ABO and Rh-factor type determined: major crossmatching determines compatibility between donor's red blood cells (RBCs) and recipient's serum
- Minor crossmatching: determines compatibility between donor's serum and recipient's RBCs (because all blood donors routinely receive the antibody-screening test, minor crossmatching omitted)
- Complete crossmatch: may take 45 minutes to 2 hours
- Incomplete (10-minute) crossmatch: may be done in emergency such as severe blood loss due to trauma
- In emergency: transfusion can begin with limited amounts of group O packed RBCs until crossmatching completed
- Incomplete typing and crossmatching: increase risk of complications
- After crossmatching, compatible units of blood labeled and compatibility record completed
- Also known as *compatibility testing*

PURPOSE

- To serve as the final check for compatibility between a donor's and a recipient's blood

PREPARATION

- This test ensures that the blood the patient receives matches his own to prevent a transfusion reaction.
- There are no dietary restrictions.
- The test requires a blood sample.
- Check the patient's history for recent administration of blood, dextran, or I.V. contrast media.
- If more than 72 hours have elapsed since an earlier transfusion, previously crossmatched donor blood must be crossmatched again with a new recipient serum sample to detect newly acquired incompatibilities.
- If the patient is scheduled for surgery and has received blood during the past three months, be aware that his blood needs to be crossmatched again if his surgery is rescheduled to detect recently acquired incompatibilities.

Teaching points

- Explain the purpose of the test and how it's done.
- Tell the patient who will perform the test and where it will be done.
- Advise the patient that no dietary restrictions are needed.
- Explain to the patient that the test requires a blood sample and that he may experience slight discomfort from the tourniquet and needle puncture.
- Inform the patient that the test should take less than 5 minutes.

KEY STEPS

- Confirm the patient's identity using two patient identifiers according to facility policy.
- Perform a venipuncture and collect the sample in a 10-ml tube without additives or EDTA. ABO typing, Rh typing, and crossmatching all occur together.
- Label the sample with the patient's name, the hospital or blood bank number, the date, and the phlebotomist's initials.
- Indicate on the laboratory request the amount and type of blood component needed.
- Send the sample to the laboratory immediately after collection.

POSTPROCEDURE CARE

- Apply direct pressure to the venipuncture site until bleeding stops.

PRECAUTIONS

- Maintain standard precautions while collecting the sample.
- Make sure to put all appropriate information on the blood slip, per facility policy.
- Handle the sample gently to prevent hemolysis, which can mask hemolysis of the donor's RBCs.

COMPLICATIONS

- Hematoma at the venipuncture site

NORMAL RESULTS

- Absence of agglutination indicates compatibility between the donor's and the recipient's blood, which means that the transfusion of donor blood can proceed. Note that this doesn't guarantee a safe transfusion.

ABNORMAL RESULTS

- A positive crossmatch indicates incompatibility between the donor's blood and the recipient's blood, which means that the donor's blood can't be transfused to the recipient.
- The sign of a positive crossmatch is agglutination, or clumping, when the donor's RBCs and the recipient's serum are correctly mixed and incubated. Agglutination indicates an undesirable antigen-antibody reaction.
- The donor's blood must be withheld and the crossmatch continued to determine the cause of the incompatibility and identify the antibody.

Cryoglobulin level test

DESCRIPTION

- Measures cryoglobulins in blood (cryoglobulinemia), indicating immunologic disease; cryoglobulins can also occur without known immunopathology (see *Diseases associated with cryoglobulinemia*)
- If patients with cryoglobulinemia subjected to cold, may experience Raynaud-like symptoms (such as pain, cyanosis, and cold fingers and toes), which usually result from cryoglobulin precipitation in cooler parts of body
- Involves refrigerating a serum sample at 33.8° F (1° C) for 24 hours and observing it for formation of a heat-reversible precipitate
- Further study by immunoelectrophoresis or double diffusion required to identify cryoglobulin components

PURPOSE

- To detect cryoglobulinemia in the patient with Raynaud-like vascular symptoms

PREPARATION

- This test detects antibodies in blood that may cause sensitivity to low temperatures.
- The patient should fast for 4 to 6 hours before the test.
- The test requires a blood sample.

Teaching points

- Explain the purpose of the test and how it's done.
- Tell the patient who will perform the test and where it will be done.
- Advise the patient not to take any food or fluids for at least 4 hours before the test.
- Explain to the patient that the test requires a blood sample and that he may experience slight discomfort from the tourniquet and needle puncture.
- Inform the patient that the test should take less than 5 minutes.

DIAGNOSTIC PROCEDURE

KEY STEPS

- Confirm the patient's identity using two patient identifiers according to facility policy.
- Perform a venipuncture and collect the sample in a prewarmed 10-ml tube without additives.
- Send the sample to the laboratory immediately after collection.

POSTPROCEDURE CARE

- Apply direct pressure to the venipuncture site until bleeding stops.
- Tell the patient to resume his usual diet.
- Tell him to avoid cold temperatures or contact with cold objects if the test is positive for cryoglobulins.

PRECAUTIONS

- Maintain standard precautions while collecting the sample.
- Warm the syringe and collection tube to 98.6° F (37° C) before venipuncture and keep the tube at that temperature to prevent cryoglobulin loss.

COMPLICATIONS

- Hematoma at the venipuncture site
- Intravascular coagulation, with such signs as decreased color and temperature in fingers and toes and increased pain

INTERPRETATION

NORMAL RESULTS

- Serum is negative for cryoglobulins.
- Positive results are reported as a percentage based on the amount of sample cryoprecipitation.

ABNORMAL RESULTS

- The presence of cryoglobulins in the blood confirms cryoglobulinemia. This finding doesn't always indicate the presence of clinical disease.

Diseases associated with cryoglobulinemia

TYPE OF CRYOGLOBULIN	SERUM LEVEL	ASSOCIATED DISEASES
Type I		
Monoclonal cryoglobulin	> 5 mg/ml	◆ Myeloma ◆ Waldenström's macroglobulinemia ◆ Chronic lymphocytic leukemia
Type II		
Mixed cryoglobulin	> 1 mg/ml	◆ Rheumatoid arthritis ◆ Sjögren's syndrome ◆ Mixed essential cryoglobulinemia ◆ Human immunodeficiency virus-1 infection
Type III		
Mixed polyclonal cryoglobin	< 1 mg/ml (50% below 80 mcg/ml)	◆ Systemic lupus erythematosus ◆ Rheumatoid arthritis ◆ Sjögren's syndrome ◆ Infectious mononucleosis ◆ Cytomegalovirus infection ◆ Acute viral hepatitis ◆ Chronic active hepatitis ◆ Primary biliary cirrhosis ◆ Poststreptococcal glomerulonephritis ◆ Infective endocarditis ◆ Leprosy ◆ Kala-azar ◆ Tropical splenomegaly syndrome

Cyclic adenosine monophosphate test

DESCRIPTION
◆ Nucleotide cyclic adenosine monophosphate (cAMP): influences protein synthesis rate within cells
◆ Measures urinary excretion of cAMP after I.V. infusion of parathyroid hormone (PTH); may show renal tubular resistance in patients with hypoparathyroid symptoms and high PTH levels, suggesting type I pseudohypoparathyroidism, a rare inherited disorder
◆ In type II pseudohypoparathyroidism: urinary cAMP levels are normal because this defect is beyond the level of cAMP production

PURPOSE
◆ To help in the differential diagnosis of hypoparathyroidism and pseudohypoparathyroidism

PREPARATION
◆ This test evaluates parathyroid function.
◆ The test requires a 15-minute I.V. infusion of PTH and a 3- to 4-hour urine specimen collection.
◆ Perform a skin test to detect an allergy to PTH; keep epinephrine or a histamine-1 receptor antagonist, such as diphenhydramine or glucocorticoids (methylprednisolone), readily available in case of an adverse reaction.

Teaching points
◆ Explain the purpose of the test and how it's done.
◆ Tell the patient who will perform the test and where it will be done.
◆ Advise the patient that no dietary restrictions are needed.
◆ Just before performing the procedure, instruct the patient not to touch the I.V. line or exert pressure on the arm receiving the infusion.
◆ Tell the patient that he may experience discomfort from the tourniquet and needle puncture. Ask him to notify you if he feels severe burning or if the site becomes inflamed or swollen.
◆ Tell the patient to avoid contaminating the urine specimen with toilet tissue or stool.
◆ Inform the patient that the test will take several hours to complete.

DIAGNOSTIC PROCEDURE

KEY STEPS
◆ Confirm the patient's identity using two patient identifiers according to facility policy.
◆ Instruct the patient to empty his bladder.
◆ If the patient has an indwelling urinary catheter in place, replace the collection apparatus with an unused one.
◆ Send this specimen to the laboratory if ordered; otherwise, discard it.
◆ Prepare the PTH for infusion, as directed, using sterile water for dilution.
◆ Start the infusion with dextrose 5% in water, and infuse the PTH over 15 minutes. Record the start of the infusion as time zero.
◆ Collect a urine specimen 3 to 4 hours after the infusion.
◆ Stop the I.V. infusion.
◆ Send the specimen to the laboratory immediately after the collection is completed; if transport is delayed, refrigerate the specimen.

POSTPROCEDURE CARE
◆ Observe the patient for symptoms of hypercalcemia, including lethargy, anorexia, nausea, vomiting, vertigo, and abdominal cramps.

PRECAUTIONS
◆ Maintain standard precautions while collecting the samples.
◆ Keep the collection bag on ice if the patient has a catheter in place.
◆ The test is contraindicated in patients with a positive PTH test result and in those with high calcium levels.
◆ The test should be done cautiously in patients receiving a cardiac glycoside and in those with sarcoidosis or renal or cardiac disease.

COMPLICATIONS
◆ Hematoma or irritation at the venipuncture site

INTERPRETATION

NORMAL RESULTS
◆ Levels of cAMP are normally 0.3 to 3.6 mg/day (SI, 100 to 723 nmol/day) or 0.29 to 2.1 mg/g creatinine (SI, 100 to 723 nmol/day creatinine).

ABNORMAL RESULTS
◆ Failure to respond to PTH, indicated by normal urinary excretion of cAMP, suggests type I pseudohypoparathyroidism.

Cystometry

DESCRIPTION

◆ Measures pressure and volume of fluid in the bladder during filling, storing, and voiding
◆ Assesses neuromuscular function of the bladder

PURPOSE

◆ To evaluate detrusor muscle function and tonicity
◆ To determine the cause of bladder dysfunction
◆ To measure bladder reaction to thermal stimulation
◆ To detect the cause of involuntary bladder contractions and incontinence

PREPARATION

◆ Note and report any allergies.
◆ Check the medication history for medications that may affect test results such as antihistamines.
◆ Have the patient void before the test.
◆ Assess for signs and symptoms of urinary tract infection (UTI).

Teaching points

◆ Explain the purpose of the test and how it's done.
◆ Tell the patient who will perform the test and where it will be done.
◆ Tell the patient he may feel a strong urge to urinate during the test.
◆ Warn the patient that the procedure may cause embarrassment and be uncomfortable.
◆ Inform the patient that the test takes about 40 minutes.

DIAGNOSTIC PROCEDURE

KEY STEPS

◆ Confirm the patient's identity using two patient identifiers according to facility policy.
◆ Assist the patient into the supine position on an examination table.
◆ A catheter is passed into the bladder to measure residual urine.
◆ To test the response to thermal sensation, 30 ml of room-temperature normal saline solution or sterile water is instilled into the bladder.
◆ An equal volume of warm fluid (110° to 115° F [43.3° to 46.1° C]) is then instilled.
◆ Fluid is drained from the bladder and the catheter is connected to the cystometer.
◆ Normal saline solution, sterile water, or gas (usually carbon dioxide) is slowly introduced into the bladder.
◆ When the bladder reaches its full capacity, the patient is asked to void.
◆ Related pressures and volumes are automatically plotted on a graph.
◆ The bladder is drained.
◆ If abnormal bladder function is the result of muscle incompetence or disrupted innervation, anticholinergic or cholinergic medication may be injected and the study repeated in 20 to 30 minutes.

POSTPROCEDURE CARE

◆ Give a sitz bath or warm tub bath for discomfort.
◆ Encourage oral fluid intake (unless contraindicated) to relieve dysuria.
◆ Notify the practitioner if hematuria persists after the third voiding.
◆ Give the patient a prescribed antibiotic.
◆ Monitor the patient's vital signs, intake and output, and signs of infection.

PRECAUTIONS

◆ The test is contraindicated in patients with acute UTIs.
◆ Tell the patient not to strain at voiding as it could cause ambiguous readings.

COMPLICATIONS

◆ Infection
◆ Bleeding

INTERPRETATION

NORMAL RESULTS

◆ The patient is able to start and stop micturition and there's no residual urine.
◆ The patient demonstrates positive vesical sensation.
◆ The patient's first urge to void is at 150 to 200 ml.
◆ The bladder capacity is 400 to 500 ml.
◆ There are no bladder contractions and the intravesical pressure is low.
◆ The patient shows a positive bulbocavernosus reflex and positive saddle sensation test.
◆ The patient shows a positive ice water test and positive anal reflex.
◆ Heat sensation and pain are present.

ABNORMAL RESULTS

◆ Inability to stop micturition, early first urge to void, decreased bladder capacity, bladder contractions, increased intravesical pressure, and positive bethanechol sensitivity test suggest inhibited neurogenic bladder.
◆ Inability to start and stop micturition, residual urine, absent vesical sensation, absent first urge to void, decreased bladder capacity, bladder contractions, increased intravesical pressure, increased bulbocavernosus reflex, negative saddle sensation test, and absent heat sensation and pain suggest reflex neurogenic bladder.
◆ Inability to start and stop micturition, residual urine, absent vesical sensation, increased bladder capacity, decreased intravesical pressure, absent bulbocavernosus reflex, negative saddle sensation test, negative ice water test, absent anal reflex and heat sensation, and pain, suggest autonomous neurogenic bladder.
◆ Residual urine, absent vesical sensation, delayed first urge to void, increased bladder capacity, decreased intravesical pressure, negative ice water test, variable anal reflex, and absent heat sensation and pain suggest sensory paralytic bladder.
◆ Inability to start and stop micturition, residual urine, negative ice water test, and variable anal reflex suggest motor paralytic bladder.

Cystourethroscopy

DESCRIPTION

- Allows visual examination of the bladder, urethra, ureter orifice, ureters, and prostate in males
- Combines two endoscopic techniques, namely cystoscopy and urethroscopy
- Cystoscopy: examines the bladder
- Urethroscopy or panendoscopy: examines bladder neck and urethra
- Access for cystoscope and urethroscope through a common sheath inserted into the urethra to obtain the desired view
- Usually preceded by kidney-ureter-bladder radiography, excretory urography, and the bladder tumor antigen urine test

PURPOSE

- To diagnose and evaluate urinary tract disorders by direct visualization of urinary structures
- To facilitate biopsy, lesion resection, removal of calculi, dilatation of a constricted urethra, and catheterization of the renal pelvis for pyelography

PREPARATION

- Make sure the patient has signed a consent form.
- Note and report allergies.
- Give a sedative if ordered.
- Have the patient void before the test.
- Fasting isn't needed unless general anesthesia is to be used.

Teaching points

- Explain the purpose of the test and how it's done.
- Tell the patient who will perform the test and where it will be done.
- If only local anesthesia is used, inform the patient that he'll feel a burning sensation when the instrument enters the urethra and an urgent need to urinate as the bladder fills with irrigating solution.
- Inform the patient that the test takes about 20 to 30 minutes.
- Advise the patient that he may experience some discomfort after the procedure, including a slight burning during voiding.

KEY STEPS

- Confirm the patient's identity using two patient identifiers according to facility policy.
- General or regional anesthesia is given.
- The patient is assisted into the lithotomy position on a cystoscopic table.
- The genitalia are cleaned with an antiseptic solution and the patient is draped.
- The urethra is examined with a urethroscope.
- The urethroscope is removed and a cystoscope is inserted into the bladder.
- The bladder is filled with irrigating solution and the entire bladder surface wall and ureteral orifices are examined.
- The cystoscope is removed and the urethroscope reinserted.
- The bladder neck and various portions of the urethra, including the internal and external sphincters, are examined as the urethroscope is withdrawn.
- A urine specimen is taken from the bladder for culture and sensitivity testing.
- Residual urine volume is measured.
- Urine is taken for a cytologic examination if a tumor is suspected.
- If a tumor is found, it may be necessary to perform a biopsy.
- If a urethral stricture is present, urethral dilatation may be necessary before cystourethroscopy.

POSTPROCEDURE CARE

- Give postoperative general anesthesia care.
- Encourage oral fluid intake and give I.V. fluids.
- Give the patient analgesics.
- Give the patient antibiotics, as ordered.
- Instruct the patient to abstain from alcohol for 48 hours.
- Report flank or abdominal pain, chills, fever, an elevated white blood cell count, or low urine output to the practitioner immediately.
- Notify the practitioner if the patient doesn't void within 8 hours after the test or if bright red blood persists after three voidings.
- Apply heat to the lower abdomen to relieve pain and muscle spasm (if ordered).
- Give a warm sitz bath.
- Monitor the patient's vital signs, intake and output, and bleeding.
- Monitor the patient for hematuria and signs and symptoms of infection.
- Watch for bladder distention.

PRECAUTIONS

- The test is contraindicated in acute forms of urethritis, prostatitis or cystitis.
- The test is contraindicated in bleeding disorders.

COMPLICATIONS

- Sepsis
- Infection
- Bleeding

NORMAL RESULTS

- Urethra, bladder, and ureteral orifices appear normal in size, shape, and position.
- Mucosal lining of the lower urinary tract appears smooth and shiny.
- Erythema, cysts, or other abnormalities aren't noted.
- There are no obstructions, tumors, or calculi in the bladder.

ABNORMAL RESULTS

- Structural abnormalities suggest various disorders, including enlarged prostate gland in older men, urethral strictures, calculi, tumors, diverticula, ulcers and polyps.

Cytomegalovirus antibody screening

DESCRIPTION

- Detects antibodies to cytomegalovirus (CMV) with passive hemagglutination, latex agglutination, enzyme immunoassay, and indirect immunofluorescence
- Complement fixation test only 60% sensitive compared with other assays; shouldn't be used to screen for CMV antibodies
- Qualitative; detects presence of antibody at single low dilution (in quantitative methods, several dilutions of the serum sample are tested to indicate acute CMV infection)

PURPOSE

- To detect CMV infection in donors and recipients of organs and blood and in immunocompromised patients
- To screen for CMV infection in infants who require blood transfusions or tissue transplants

PREPARATION

- The test requires a blood sample.

Teaching points

- Explain the purpose of the test to the patient or the parents of an infant, as appropriate.
- Tell the patient who will perform the test and where it will be done.
- Advise the patient that no dietary restrictions are needed.
- Explain to the patient that the test requires a blood sample and he may experience slight discomfort from the tourniquet and needle puncture.
- Inform the patient that the test should take less than 5 minutes.

KEY STEPS

- Confirm the patient's identity using two patient identifiers according to facility policy.
- Perform a venipuncture and collect the sample in a 5-ml tube designated by the laboratory.
- Allow the blood to clot for at least 1 hour at room temperature.
- Transfer the serum to a sterile tube or vial and send it to the laboratory.
- If transfer must be delayed, store the serum at 39.2° F (4° C) for 1 or 2 days or at -4° F (-20° C) for longer periods to avoid contamination.

POSTPROCEDURE CARE

- Apply direct pressure to the venipuncture site until bleeding stops.
- Because the patient may have a compromised immune system, keep the venipuncture site clean and dry.

PRECAUTIONS

- Handle the sample gently to prevent hemolysis.

COMPLICATIONS

- Hematoma at the venipuncture site

NORMAL RESULTS

- The patient who has never been infected with CMV has no detectable antibodies to the virus.
- Immunoglobulin (Ig) G and IgM are normally negative.

ABNORMAL RESULTS

- A serum sample collected early during the acute phase or late in the convalescent stage may not contain detectable IgG or IgM antibodies to CMV. Therefore, a negative result doesn't preclude recent infection. More than a single sample is needed to ensure accurate results.
- A serum sample that tests positive for antibodies at this single dilution indicates that the patient has been infected with CMV and that his white blood cells contain latent virus capable of being reactivated in an immunocompromised host.
- An immunosuppressed patient lacking CMV antibodies should receive blood products or organ transplants from a donor who is also seronegative.
- A patient with CMV antibodies doesn't need seronegative blood products.

ᴅ-dimer test

DESCRIPTION

- ᴅ-dimer: asymmetrical carbon compound fragment formed after thrombin converts fibrinogen to fibrin
- Stabilized by factor XIIIa into a clot; plasma acts on cross-linked, or clotted, fibrin
- Specific for fibrinolysis because test confirms presence of fibrin-split products

PURPOSE

- To diagnose disseminated intravascular coagulation (DIC)
- To differentiate subarachnoid hemorrhage from a traumatic lumbar puncture in spinal fluid analysis

PREPARATION

- Obtain the patient's history of hematologic diseases, recent surgery, and the results of other tests.
- The test requires a blood sample.

Teaching points

- This test determines whether blood is clotting normally.
- Tell the patient who will perform the test and where it'll be done.
- Advise the patient that no dietary restrictions are needed.
- Explain to the patient that a blood sample is required and that he may feel slight discomfort from the tourniquet and needle puncture.
- Inform the patient that the test should take less than 5 minutes.

KEY STEPS

- Confirm the patient's identity using two patient identifiers according to facility policy.
- Perform a venipuncture and collect the sample in a 4.5-ml tube with sodium citrate added.
- For a spinal fluid analysis, the sample is collected during a lumbar puncture and placed in a plastic vial.

POSTPROCEDURE CARE

- Apply pressure to the venipuncture site for 5 minutes or until bleeding stops.

PRECAUTIONS

- Completely fill the collection tube, invert it gently several times, and send it to the laboratory immediately after collection.
- For a patient with coagulation problems, apply additional pressure at the venipuncture site, as needed, to control bleeding.

COMPLICATIONS

- Hematoma at the venipuncture site

NORMAL RESULTS

- Collection yields less than 250 mcg/L (SI, less than 1.37 nmol/L).

ABNORMAL RESULTS

- A level greater than 250 mcg/L (SI, greater than 1.37 nmol/L) may indicate DIC, pulmonary embolism, arterial or venous thrombosis, neoplastic disease, pregnancy (late and postpartum), surgery occurring up to 2 days before testing, subarachnoid hemorrhage (spinal fluid only), or secondary fibrinolysis.

Delayed-type hypersensitivity skin tests

DESCRIPTION

- Evaluates T-cell mediated immune response; tests for delayed-type hypersensitivity (DTH)
- Assesses status of a patient's immune system in severe infection, cancer, pretransplantation, and malnutrition
- Previous exposure to antigen and intact immune system required for accurate response
- Most commonly used recall antigen: *Mycobacterium tuberculosis* (purified protein derivative Mantoux test)
- Other antigens: *Candida, Trichophyton,* and mumps (antigens previously used for DTH testing, such as fungi and streptococci, no longer available or recommended)
- Limited value in infants because of their immature immune system and lack of previous sensitization
- Involves applying antigenic material to the skin; helps confirm allergic contact sensitization and isolate the causative agent

PURPOSE

- To assess for exposure to or activation of certain diseases, most commonly tuberculosis (TB)
- To assess the status of a patient's immune system during illness
- To evaluate sensitivity to environmental antigens in patients with persistent symptoms

PREPARATION

- The testing takes a few minutes for each antigen; reactions are evaluated after 48 to 72 hours.
- If the first result is negative, the test may be repeated in 2 to 3 weeks. The first test "reminds" the body that it was previously exposed to the antigen, and a response is noted on retesting. This is called a "two-step test" and is commonly used for testing TB.
- Ask the patient about sensitivity to the test antigens, whether he has had previous skin testing, and what the outcomes of that testing were.
- Ask the patient if he has had TB or been exposed to it and if he has had bacille Calmette-Guérin vaccination.

Teaching points

- Explain to the patient that a small amount of antigenic material will be injected superficially or applied to the skin.
- Tell the patient who will perform the test and where it'll be done.
- Tell him he doesn't need to restrict his diet.
- Inform the patient that the test should take less than 5 minutes, but will need to be repeated over several weeks.
- Tell the patient who experiences hypersensitivity that corticosteroids will control the reaction; skin lesions may persist for 10 to 14 days after the test.

KEY STEPS

- Confirm the patient's identity using two patient identifiers according to facility policy.
- Inject each antigen being tested intradermally, using a separate tuberculin syringe, on the patient's forearm. (See *Administering test antigens.*)
- Inject the control allergy diluent on the other forearm.
- Inspect the injection sites for reactivity after 48 to 72 hours.
- Record induration and erythema in millimeters.
- Confirm a negative test result at the first concentration of antigen by using a higher concentration.

POSTPROCEDURE CARE

WARNING *Watch closely for severe local reactions that may occur at the test site, such as pain, blistering, swelling, induration, itching, and ulceration. Scarring or hyperpigmentation may also result.*

- Watch for swelling and tenderness in lymph nodes at elbow or axillary region. Check for tachycardia and fever; these rarely occur. Symptoms typically appear in 15 to 30 minutes.
- If signs or symptoms of anaphylactic shock develop, give epinephrine and notify the practitioner immediately.
- After the test, advise the patient to avoid scratching the affected area.

PRECAUTIONS

- If appropriate, store antigens in lyophilized (freeze-dried) form at 39.2° F (4° C) and protect from light. Reconstitute shortly before use and check expiration dates. If the patient may be hypersensitive to the antigens, apply them initially in low concentrations.
- If the patient's forearms aren't free of disease (for example, if he has atopic dermatitis), use other sites such as the back.

COMPLICATIONS

- Anaphylactic shock

INTERPRETATION

NORMAL RESULTS

◆ The test result is positive (at least 5 mm of induration at the test site, appearing 48 hours after injection).
◆ Positive reactions don't indicate protection against antigen

ABNORMAL RESULTS

◆ Diminished DTH is demonstrated by a positive response to fewer than two of the test antigens, a persistent unresponsiveness to intradermal injection of higher-strength antigens, or a generalized diminished reaction (causing 10 mm combined induration).
◆ Diminished DTH can result from Hodgkin's disease; sarcoidosis; liver disease; congenital immunodeficiency disease, such as ataxia-telangiectasia, DiGeorge's syndrome, and Wiskott-Aldrich syndrome; uremia; acute leukemia; viral diseases, such as influenza, infectious mononucleosis, measles, mumps, and rubella; fungal diseases, such as coccidioidomycosis and cryptococcosis; bacterial diseases, such as leprosy and TB; terminal cancer; and immunosuppressive or steroid therapy or viral vaccination.

Administering test antigens

This illustration shows the arm of a patient undergoing a recall antigen test, which determines whether he has previously been exposed to certain antigens. A sample panel of four test antigens has been injected into his forearm, and the test site has been marked and labeled for each antigen.

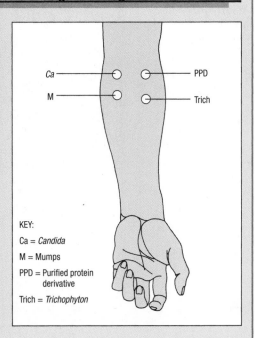

Ca
M
PPD
Trich

KEY:

Ca = Candida

M = Mumps

PPD = Purified protein derivative

Trich = Trichophyton

Delta-aminolevulinic acid level, urine

DESCRIPTION

- Using colorimetric technique for quantitative analysis, determines urine delta-aminolevulinic acid (ALA) levels, to help diagnose porphyrias, hepatic disease, and lead poisoning
- In emergency, performed by simple qualitative screening test
- ALA, basic precursor of porphyrins, converts to porphobilinogen during heme synthesis
- Impaired conversion occurs in porphyrias and lead poisoning; causes increased urine ALA levels before other chemical or hematologic changes

PURPOSE

- To screen for lead poisoning
- To help diagnose porphyrias and certain hepatic disorders, such as hepatitis and hepatic carcinoma

PREPARATION

- This test detects the amount of delta-ALA in the urine.
- Notify the laboratory and practitioner of medications the patient is taking that may affect test results; they may need to be restricted.
- Inform the patient or parents that there are no dietary restrictions.
- The test requires urine collection for a 24-hour period.

Teaching points

- Explain the purpose of the test and how it's done.
- Tell the patient who will perform the test and where it'll be done.
- If lead poisoning is suspected, tell the patient (or parents, as appropriate) that the test helps detect the presence of too much lead in the body.
- Advise the patient that there are no dietary restrictions.
- Teach the patient or parents how to do a 24-hour urine collection at home.

KEY STEPS

- Confirm the patient's identity using two patient identifiers according to facility policy.
- Collect the patient's urine over a 24-hour period, discarding the first specimen and retaining the last.
- Use a light-resistant bottle containing a preservative (usually glacial acetic acid) to prevent ALA degradation.
- Refrigerate the specimen or keep it on ice during the collection period.
- Insert the drainage bag in a dark plastic bag if the patient has an indwelling urinary catheter in place.
- Send the specimen to the laboratory when the collection is complete.

POSTPROCEDURE CARE

- Tell the patient to resume his usual medications.

PRECAUTIONS

- Be sure to protect the specimen from light.

COMPLICATIONS

- None

NORMAL RESULTS

- Level ranges from 1.3 to 7 mg/24 hours (SI, 10 to 53 µmol/day).

ABNORMAL RESULTS

- Increased levels may occur in patients with lead poisoning, hereditary tyrosinemia, acute porphyria, hepatic carcinoma, or hepatitis.

Dexamethasone suppression test

DESCRIPTION
◆ Requires administration of dexamethasone, an oral steroid
◆ Suppresses levels of circulating adrenal steroid hormones in healthy people but fails to suppress them in patients with Cushing's syndrome and certain forms of clinical depression

PURPOSE
◆ To diagnose Cushing's syndrome
◆ To help diagnose clinical depression

PREPARATION
◆ Restrict food and fluids for 10 to 12 hours before the test.
◆ The test requires two blood samples drawn after the patient receives dexamethasone.

Teaching points
◆ Explain to the patient the purpose of the dexamethasone suppression test.
◆ Tell the patient who will perform the test and where it'll be done.
◆ Advise the patient to avoid food or fluids for at least 10 hours before the test.
◆ Explain to the patient that a blood sample is required and that he may feel slight discomfort from the tourniquet and needle puncture.

KEY STEPS
◆ Confirm the patient's identity using two patient identifiers according to facility policy.
◆ On the first day, give the patient 1 mg of dexamethasone at 11 p.m.
◆ On the next day, collect blood samples at 4 p.m. and 11 p.m.

POSTPROCEDURE CARE
◆ Apply pressure to venipuncture site.
◆ Observe the site for complications.

PRECAUTIONS
◆ Check the patient's medication history and have the patient withhold medications for 24 to 48 hours if possible.

COMPLICATIONS
◆ Hematoma at the venipuncture site

NORMAL RESULTS
◆ Failure of dexamethasone suppression is indicated by a cortisol level of 5 g/dl (140 nmol/L) or greater.
◆ A normal test result doesn't rule out major depression.

ABNORMAL RESULTS
◆ If test result isn't normal, abnormal secretion of cortisol is likely (Cushing's syndrome).
◆ An abnormal test result strengthens a clinically based diagnosis of major depression.

INTERFERING FACTORS *Many drugs, including corticosteroids, hormonal contraceptives, lithium, methadone, aspirin, diuretics, morphine, and monoamine oxidase inhibitors*

Digital subtraction angiography, cerebral

OVERVIEW

DESCRIPTION
◆ Sophisticated radiographic technique using video equipment and computer-assisted image enhancement to provide a high-contrast view of blood vessels without interfering images or shadows of bone and soft tissue
◆ Superior image quality and I.V., rather than intra-arterial, administration of contrast media
◆ Used to study peripheral and renal vascular disease but is most useful to evaluate cerebrovascular disorders

PURPOSE
◆ To show extracranial and intracranial cerebral blood flow
◆ To detect and evaluate cerebrovascular abnormalities
◆ To aid postoperative evaluation of cerebrovascular surgery

PREPARATION
◆ Make sure the patient has signed an appropriate consent form.
◆ Note previous hypersensitivity on the patient's medical record and notify the practitioner.

Teaching points
◆ Explain the purpose of the test and how it's done.
◆ Tell the patient who will perform the test and where it'll be done.
◆ Instruct the patient to fast for 4 hours before the test. Tell him that he need not restrict fluids.
◆ Stress the importance of lying still during the procedure; even swallowing can interfere with imaging. Tell the patient that he will need to hold his breath for 10-second intervals at various times during the test.
◆ Warn the patient that he may experience warmth, headache, metallic taste, nausea, or vomiting after injection of the contrast medium.
◆ Inform the patient that the test may take 1 or 2 hours.

DIAGNOSTIC PROCEDURE

KEY STEPS
◆ Confirm the patient's identity using two patient identifiers according to facility policy.
◆ The patient is assisted into the supine position on a radiography table with his arms at his sides.
◆ An initial series of fluoroscopic pictures (mask images) is taken.
◆ The access site is shaved and prepared (a vein or artery may be used).
◆ The patient is given a local anesthetic.
◆ The patient is given an I.V. sedative.
◆ The vessel is cannulated and a catheter is inserted and advanced to the area to be studied.
◆ The contrast medium is injected and films are taken in various views.
◆ Monitor the patient's vital signs and neurologic status. Observe him for signs of a hypersensitivity reaction, such as urticaria, pruritus, and respiratory distress.

POSTPROCEDURE CARE
◆ Have the patient drink at least 1 qt (1 L) of fluid on the day of the procedure because the contrast medium acts as a diuretic. Extra fluid intake also aids excretion of the contrast medium.
◆ Monitor vital signs, intake and output, puncture site, neurologic status, and signs and symptoms of infection.
◆ Monitor the patient for a delayed hypersensitivity reaction to the contrast medium and thrombotic events.
◆ If bleeding occurs, apply firm pressure to the puncture site and notify the practitioner promptly.
◆ Tell the patient to resume his normal diet.

PRECAUTIONS
◆ Check the patient's history for any allergies, including hypersensitivity to iodine, iodine-containing substances such as shellfish, and contrast media.
◆ Contraindicated in patients with poor cardiac function, renal, hepatic, or thyroid disease, severe diabetes, or multiple myeloma.

COMPLICATIONS
◆ Infection
◆ Thrombotic and embolic events
◆ Bleeding

INTERPRETATION

NORMAL RESULTS
◆ The contrast medium fills and opacifies all superficial and deep arteries, arterioles, and veins.

ABNORMAL RESULTS
◆ Vascular filling defects may indicate arteriovenous occlusion or stenosis.
◆ Outpouchings in vessel lumina may reflect aneurysms.
◆ Vessel displacement or vascular masses may indicate a tumor.

Doppler ultrasonography

OVERVIEW

DESCRIPTION
- Noninvasive test to evaluate blood flow in major veins and arteries of arms, legs, and extracranial cerebrovascular system
- High-frequency sound waves directed by handheld transducer to artery or vein; sound waves amplified to permit direct listening and graphic recording of blood flow
- Measures systolic pressure to help detect peripheral arterial occlusive disease

PURPOSE
- To help diagnose venous insufficiency, superficial and deep vein thromboses, and peripheral artery disease and arterial occlusion
- To monitor arterial reconstruction and bypass graft patients
- To detect abnormalities of carotid artery blood flow
- To evaluate arterial trauma

PREPARATION
- Make sure patient has signed a consent form.
- Note and report any allergies.

Teaching points
- Explain the purpose of the test and how it's done.
- Tell the patient who will perform the test and where it'll be done.
- Tell him the test takes 20 minutes.

DIAGNOSTIC PROCEDURE

KEY STEPS
- Confirm the patient's identity using two patient identifiers according to facility policy.
- Doppler ultrasonography is performed bilaterally.
- The patient is assisted into the supine position on the examination table with his arms at his sides.

Peripheral arterial evaluation
- For peripheral arterial evaluation in the leg, the usual test sites are the common and superficial femoral, popliteal, posterior tibial, and dorsalis pedis arteries.
- For peripheral arterial evaluation in the arm, the usual test sites are the subclavian, brachial, radial, and ulnar arteries.
- Brachial blood pressure is measured, and the transducer is placed at various points along the test arteries.
- The signals are monitored and waveforms recorded for later analysis.
- The blood flow velocity is monitored and recorded over the test artery.
- Segmental limb blood pressures are obtained to localize arterial occlusive disease.

Peripheral venous evaluation
- For peripheral venous evaluation in the leg, the usual test sites are the popliteal, superficial and common femoral, and posterior tibial veins.
- For extracranial cerebrovascular evaluation, usual test sites are the supraorbital artery; the common, external, and internal carotid arteries; the vertebral arteries; and the brachial, axillary, subclavian, and jugular veins.
- The transducer is placed over the appropriate vessel, waveforms are recorded, and respiratory modulations are noted.
- Proximal limb compression maneuvers are performed.
- Augmentation after release of compression is noted to evaluate venous valve competency.
- For tests involving legs and feet, patient is asked to perform Valsalva's maneuver and venous blood flow is recorded.

POSTPROCEDURE CARE
- Remove the conductive jelly from the patient's skin.

PRECAUTIONS
- Don't place the Doppler probe over an open or draining lesion.

COMPLICATIONS
- Bradyarrhythmia (if probe placed near carotid sinus)

INTERPRETATION

NORMAL RESULTS
- Arterial waveforms of the arms and legs are multiphasic, with a prominent systolic component and one or more diastolic sounds.
- Arm pressure is unchanged despite postural changes.
- Proximal thigh pressure is 20 to 30 mm Hg greater than arm pressure.
- Venous blood flow velocity is phasic with respiration, with a lower pitch than arterial flow.
- Blood flow velocity increases with distal compression or release of proximal limb compression.
- Valsalva's maneuver interrupts venous flow velocity.
- In cerebrovascular testing, a strong velocity signal is present.
- In the common carotid artery, blood flow velocity increases in diastole.
- Periorbital arterial flow is normally anterograde out of the orbit.
- Ankle-brachial index (ABI) is 0.9.

ABNORMAL RESULTS
- Reduced blood flow velocity signal implies arterial stenosis or occlusion.
- Absent velocity signal suggests complete occlusion and lack of collateral circulation.
- ABI of 0.5 to 0.9 shows claudication; ABI, 0.5, resting ischemic pain; and ABI, 0.2, gangrenous foot or leg.
- Venous blood flow velocity unchanged by respirations, compression, or Valsalva's maneuver or absent indicates venous thrombosis.
- Reversed flow velocity signal suggests chronic venous insufficiency and varicose veins.
- Absent Doppler signals during cerebrovascular examination implies total arterial occlusion.

Ductal lavage of breast tissue

OVERVIEW

DESCRIPTION

- Minimally invasive method for assessing risk for development of breast cancer
- Uses a collection of cells from inside the milk ducts
- Most cancers begin in cells lining milk ducts
- Cells may take 8 to 10 years to develop into tumor visible on mammogram or palpated by breast examination
- Indicated only in women who are at high risk for developing breast cancer based on personal and family factors

PURPOSE

- To identify a woman's risk for developing breast cancer

PREPARATION

- Describe the procedure and explain that ductal lavage of the breast tissue help identify cells that have the potential to become cancerous.
- No dietary restrictions are required.
- Check the patient's history for hypersensitivity to local anesthetics.

Teaching points

- Explain the purpose of the test and how it's done.
- Tell the patient who will perform the test and where it'll be done.
- Advise the patient that no dietary restrictions are needed.
- Warn the patient that she may feel tingling, pinching, or a sensation of breast fullness similar to lactation.
- Inform the patient that the test takes about 2 hours.

DIAGNOSTIC PROCEDURE

KEY STEPS

- Confirm the patient's identity using two patient identifiers according to facility policy.
- Apply a topical anesthetic agent, if appropriate, about 30 minutes to 1 hour before the test.

- Have the patient apply warmth to the breast and massage if indicated.
- The physician places a syringe-like aspirator device on the breast at the nipple area and gently pulls back on the syringe to expel fluid from the ducts. Typically only one or two ducts produce extremely minute amounts of fluid.
- When the fluid producing ducts are identified, the physician inserts a microcatheter into these ducts and instills an anesthetic followed by saline to rinse the ducts.
- The breasts are massaged gently to move the fluid toward the nipple.
- The physician aspirates the fluid into the syringe and then transfers the fluid to specialized vials, which are sent to the laboratory for analysis.
- The procedure is repeated for other ducts that produced fluid. (See *Understanding breast ductal lavage.*)

POSTPROCEDURE CARE

- Offer emotional support and assure the patient that evidence of atypical cells doesn't indicate cancer.

PRECAUTIONS

WARNING *Fluid production suggests a higher risk for breast cancer development. If no fluid is aspirated, the lavage isn't performed.*

COMPLICATIONS

- None

INTERPRETATION

NORMAL RESULTS

- No atypical or malignant cells are noted.

ABNORMAL RESULTS

- The presence of atypical cells suggests a significant increase in the risk for developing breast cancer.
- Evidence of atypical cells doesn't positively indicate that breast cancer will develop.
- Although rare, malignant cells may be found.

Understanding breast ductal lavage

1. A syringe-like aspirator is placed over the breast at the nipple area. Suction is applied to the aspirator to draw out small amounts of fluid from the ducts to the nipple surface. Usually only 1 or 2 ducts produce fluid.

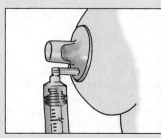

2. A microcatheter is then inserted into the ducts from which fluid was obtained.

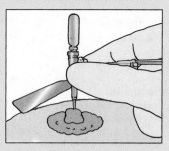

3. A small amount of anesthetic may be instilled followed by a small amount of saline. The breast is massaged and then fluid is withdrawn into the catheter which is attached to a syringe. The sample is then placed in a preservative and sent to the laboratory for analysis.

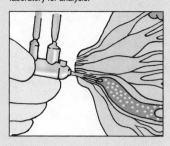

Duodenal contents culture

DESCRIPTION

◆ Duodenal tube insertion, aspiration of duodenal contents, and cultivation of microbes to isolate and identify pathogens that may cause duodenitis, cholecystitis, and cholangitis
◆ Specimen obtained during surgery
◆ Duodenal contents (pancreatic and duodenal enzymes and bile) normally almost sterile; subject to infection by such pathogens as *Escherichia coli, Staphylococcus aureus,* and *Salmonella;* result in duodenitis, cholecystitis, or cholangitis

PURPOSE

◆ To detect bacterial infection of the biliary tract and duodenum
◆ To differentiate between infection and gallstones
◆ To rule out bacterial infection as the cause of persistent GI symptoms (epigastric pain, nausea, vomiting, and diarrhea)

PREPARATION

◆ This test determines the cause of the patient's symptoms.
◆ Fasting for 12 hours before the test is required.
◆ Describe the insertion procedure to the patient. Assure him that although this procedure is uncomfortable, it isn't dangerous; tell him that passage of the tube may cause gagging, but that by following the practitioner's instructions about proper positioning, breathing, swallowing, and relaxing his discomfort will be minimized.
◆ Have the patient empty his bladder before the procedure to increase his general comfort.

Teaching points

◆ Explain the purpose of the test and how it's done.
◆ Tell the patient who will perform the test and where it'll be done.
◆ Advise the patient to fast for 12 hours before the test.
◆ Inform the patient that the test takes about 2 hours.

DIAGNOSTIC PROCEDURE

KEY STEPS

◆ Confirm the patient's identity using two patient identifiers according to facility policy.
◆ After the nasoenteric tube is inserted, place the patient in a left lateral decubitus position with his feet elevated to allow peristalsis to move the tube into the duodenum.
◆ Determine the pH of a small amount of aspirated fluid to ascertain the tube position. If the tube is in the stomach, pH is lower than 7.0; if the tube is in the duodenum, pH is higher than 7. The position of the tube can also be confirmed by fluoroscopy.
◆ Aspirate duodenal contents.
◆ Occasionally, a specimen for culture of duodenal contents is obtained during duodenoscopy.
◆ Transfer the specimen to a sterile container and label it with the patient's name, the practitioner's name, the date and time of collection, and the collector's initials.
◆ Send the specimen to the laboratory immediately after collection.

POSTPROCEDURE CARE

◆ After duodenal tube placement or duodenoscopy, observe the patient carefully for signs of perforation, such as dysphagia, epigastric or shoulder pain, dyspnea, and fever.
◆ After duodenoscopy, monitor the patient's vital signs until he's stable; keep the side rails up and enforce bed rest until he's fully alert.
◆ Slowly withdraw the tube at a rate of 6″ to 8″ (15 to 20 cm) every 10 minutes until it reaches the esophagus; then clamp the tube and remove it quickly. If you can't withdraw the tube easily, report the problem; never force the tube.
◆ Tell the patient to resume his usual diet.

PRECAUTIONS

◆ Wear gloves when assisting with this procedure and handling the specimen.

◆ Collect the specimen for culture before antimicrobial therapy begins.
◆ The test is contraindicated during pregnancy and in patients with acute pancreatitis or cholecystitis; esophageal varices, stenosis, and diverticular malignant neoplasms; recent severe gastric hemorrhage; aortic aneurysm; heart failure; and myocardial infarction

COMPLICATIONS

◆ Perforation

INTERPRETATION

NORMAL RESULTS

◆ Small amounts of polymorphonuclear leukocytes and epithelial cells with no pathogens are present; the bacterial count is usually below 100,000/ml of body fluid.

ABNORMAL RESULTS

◆ Bacterial counts of 100,000/ml or more or the presence of pathogens in any number indicates infection. Susceptibility testing may be needed.
◆ Numerous polymorphonuclear leukocytes, copious mucus, and bile-stained epithelial cells in the bile fluid suggest inflammation of the biliary tract; many segmented neutrophils and exfoliated epithelial cells suggest pancreatic, duodenal, or bile duct inflammation.
◆ The presence of bile sand indicates cholelithiasis or calculi in the biliary tract. Differential diagnosis requires further testing.

D-xylose absorption test

DESCRIPTION

- Evaluates patients with symptoms of malabsorption, such as weight loss and generalized malnutrition, weakness, and diarrhea
- D-xylose: pentose sugar that's absorbed in small intestine without pancreatic enzymes; passes through the liver without being metabolized and excreted in urine
- Measures D-xylose in urine and blood, indicating absorptive capacity of small intestine

PURPOSE

- To aid in the differential diagnosis of malabsorption
- To determine the cause of malabsorption syndrome

PREPARATION

- Fasting overnight before the test is required.
- The test requires several blood samples.
- Withhold drugs that alter test results, such as aspirin and indomethacin. Record any drugs the patient is taking on the laboratory request.

Teaching points

- Explain that this test helps evaluate digestive function by analyzing blood samples and urine specimens after ingestion of a sugar solution.
- Tell the patient who will perform the test and where it'll be done.
- If the patient will be collecting urine at home, teach the patient how to perform a urine collection.
- Inform the patient that all of his urine will be collected for either a 5-hour or a 24-hour period.
- Tell the patient not to contaminate the urine specimens with toilet tissue or feces.
- Explain to the patient that several blood samples are also required and that he may feel slight discomfort from the tourniquet and needle punctures.

- Instruct the patient to fast overnight before the test and to fast and remain in bed during the test.
- Inform the patient that the test takes up to 24 hours.

DIAGNOSTIC PROCEDURE

KEY STEPS

- Confirm the patient's identity using two patient identifiers according to facility policy.
- Perform a venipuncture, and collect the sample in a 10-ml tube without additives. Collect a first-voided morning urine specimen. Label these specimens and send them to the laboratory immediately after collection to serve as a baseline.
- Give the patient 25 g of d-xylose dissolved in 8 ounces (240 ml) of water, followed by an additional 8 ounces of water. If the patient is a child, give 0.5 g of D-xylose per pound of body weight, up to 25 g. Record the time of D-xylose ingestion.
- For an adult, draw a blood sample 2 hours after D-xylose ingestion; for a child, 1 hour after ingestion. Collect the sample in a 10-ml tube without additives. Occasionally, a 5-hour sample may be drawn to support the findings of the 1- or 2-hour sample.
- Collect and pool all urine during the 5 hours or 24 hours after D-xylose ingestion.

WARNING *Because patients age 65 and older and those with borderline or elevated creatinine levels tend to have low 5-hour urine levels but normal 24-hour levels, the practitioner must establish the length of the collection period.*

POSTPROCEDURE CARE

- Observe the patient for abdominal discomfort or mild diarrhea caused by D-xylose ingestion.
- Tell the patient to resume his usual diet and medications.

PRECAUTIONS

- Maintain bed rest and withhold food and fluids (other than D-xylose) during the test period.

- Be sure to collect all urine and refrigerate the specimen during the collection period.
- Handle the sample gently to prevent hemolysis.

COMPLICATIONS

- Hematoma at the venipuncture site

INTERPRETATION

NORMAL RESULTS

- In children, blood concentration is greater than 30 mg/dl within 1 hour; 16% to 33% of ingested D-xylose is excreted in the urine within 5 hours.
- In adults, blood concentration ranges from 25 to 40 mg/dl in 2 hours; 3.5 g is excreted in the urine within 5 hours (age 65 or older, more than 5 g is excreted within 24 hours).

ABNORMAL RESULTS

- Depressed blood and urine D-xylose levels most commonly result from malabsorption disorders that affect the proximal small intestine, such as sprue and celiac disease.
- Depressed levels may also result from regional enteritis involving the jejunum, Whipple's disease, multiple jejunal diverticula, myxedema, diabetic neuropathic diarrhea, rheumatoid arthritis, alcoholism, severe heart failure, and ascites.

Echocardiography

DESCRIPTION

- Noninvasive test to examine the size, shape, and motion of cardiac structures
- Ultra-high-frequency sound waves directed by transducer toward cardiac structures, which reflect these waves; echoes picked up, converted to electrical impulses, and displayed on an echocardiography machine
- M-mode (motion-mode) echocardiography: single, pencil-like ultrasound beam strikes the heart and produces a vertical view (records motion and dimensions of intracardiac structures)
- Two-dimensional echocardiography: cross-sectional view of cardiac structures records lateral motion and spatial relationship between structures

PURPOSE

- To diagnose and evaluate valvular abnormalities
- To measure and evaluate the size of the heart's chambers and valves
- To help diagnose cardiomyopathies and atrial tumors
- To evaluate cardiac function or wall motion after a myocardial infarction
- To detect pericardial effusion or mural thrombi

PREPARATION

- No dietary restrictions are needed.

Teaching points

- Explain the purpose of the test and how it's done.
- Tell the patient who will perform the test and where it will be done.
- Inform the patient that he may be asked to breathe in and out slowly, to hold his breath, or to inhale a gas with a slightly sweet odor (amyl nitrite) while changes in heart function are recorded.
- Warn the patient about the possible adverse effects of amyl nitrite (dizziness, flushing, tachycardia); reassure him that such effects quickly subside.
- Stress the need to remain still during the test to avoid distorting results.

- Tell the patient that the test takes 15 to 30 minutes. (See *Preparing for an echocardiogram*, page 178.)

KEY STEPS

- Confirm the patient's identity using two patient identifiers according to facility policy.
- The patient is placed into a supine position and conductive gel is applied to the third or fourth intercostal space to the left of the sternum. The transducer is placed directly over it.
- The transducer is systematically angled to direct ultrasonic waves at specific parts of the patient's heart.
- During the test, the oscilloscope screen is observed; findings are recorded.
- For a left lateral view, the patient is placed on his left side.
- Doppler echocardiography may also be used: color flow simulates red blood cell flow through the heart valves. The sound of blood flow may also be used to assess heart sounds and murmurs.

POSTPROCEDURE CARE

- Remove the conductive gel from the patient's skin.

PRECAUTIONS

- None

COMPLICATIONS

- None

NORMAL RESULTS

- For the mitral valve, anterior and posterior mitral valve leaflets separate in early diastole and attain maximum excursion rapidly and then move toward each other during ventricular diastole; after atrial contraction, the mitral valve leaflets come together and remain together during ventricular systole.

- For the aortic valve, aortic valve cusps move anteriorly during systole and posteriorly during diastole.
- For the tricuspid valve, motion resembles that of the mitral valve.
- For the pulmonic valve, movement is posterior during atrial and ventricular systole. In right ventricular ejection, the cusp moves anteriorly, attaining its most anterior position during diastole.
- For the ventricular cavities, the left ventricular cavity appears as an echo-free space between the interventricular septum and the posterior left ventricular wall.
- The right ventricular cavity appears as an echo-free space between the anterior chest wall and the interventricular septum.

ABNORMAL RESULTS

- In mitral stenosis, the valve narrows because of the leaflets' thickening and disordered motion; during diastole, both leaflets move anteriorly instead of posteriorly.
- In mitral valve prolapse, one or both leaflets balloon into the left atrium during systole.
- In aortic insufficiency, leaflets of the aortic valve flutter during diastole.
- In aortic stenosis, the aortic valve thickens and generates more echoes.
- In bacterial endocarditis, valve motion is disrupted and fuzzy echoes usually appear on or near the valve.
- A large chamber may indicate cardiomyopathy, valvular disorders, or heart failure.
- A small chamber may indicate restrictive pericarditis.
- Hypertrophic cardiomyopathy can be identified by systolic anterior motion of the mitral valve and asymmetrical septal hypertrophy.
- Myocardial ischemia or infarction may cause absent or paradoxical motion in ventricular walls.
- Pericardial effusion is suggested when fluid accumulates in the pericardial space, causing an abnormal echo-free space to appear.
- In large effusions, pressure exerted by excess fluid can restrict pericardial motion.

(continued)

Preparing for an echocardiogram

Dear Patient,

You've been ordered a test called echocardiography to learn about your heart's size, shape, movement, and surrounding structures. The test doesn't hurt. It takes 30 minutes or less to perform, and you don't have to do anything special to prepare for it.

WHAT HAPPENS FIRST

When you reach the test location — usually the echocardiography laboratory, but elsewhere if the hospital has portable equipment — you'll undress and put on a hospital gown or cover yourself with a large, sheetlike drape. Most likely, you'll see an examining table, some machines, and a TV screen. The laboratory may be darkened to help the technician view the TV screen.

WHAT HAPPENS NEXT

A technician will ask you to lie on the table, either on your back or on your side. Then gel will be applied to your chest and an instrument called a transducer will be positioned over your heart. Disk-shaped electrodes will then be applied to your chest and arms. These electrodes will record the electrical activity coming from your heart. (This procedure is called *electrocardiography.*)

HOW THE TEST WORKS

Because the echocardiography machine generates high-pitched sound waves, you won't be able to hear them, but the transducer will transmit them toward your heart. The sound waves will bounce off your heart walls, valves, and surrounding structures and will be received by the same transducer that transmitted them.

Then these echoes will be translated electronically into an image of your heart and its structures that can be seen on the TV screen (or read on special paper).

Simultaneous electrocardiogram tracings will be used to interpret the echocardiogram.

TEST VARIATIONS

The technician may obtain a series of heart images by positioning the transducer at different angles to observe different parts of your heart.

You may be asked to breathe in and out slowly, to hold your breath, or to inhale a sweet-smelling gas (amyl nitrite). Changes in the way your heart functions during each task will be noted.

You may experience some dizziness, flushing, or rapid heartbeats from the gas, but these will subside quickly.

Remember to stay still during the test because movement can distort results.

TEST RESULTS

The technician will remove the transducer and electrodes and wipe the gel off your chest. The test results will be interpreted by a cardiologist.

Echocardiography, dobutamine stress

OVERVIEW

DESCRIPTION
- Detects changes in regional cardiac wall motion
- Increases myocardial contractility and stroke volume, permits study of heart under stress conditions without need for the patient to exercise
- Imaging done during infusion of increasing amounts of dobutamine until maximum predicted heart rate reached

PURPOSE
- To identify causes of anginal symptoms
- To measure chambers of the heart and determine functional capacity
- To help set limits for an exercise program
- To diagnose and evaluate valvular and wall motion abnormalities
- To detect atrial tumors, mural thrombi, vegetative growth on valve leaflets, and pericardial effusions
- To evaluate myocardial perfusion, coronary artery disease and obstruction, and the extent of myocardial damage after a myocardial infarction (MI)

PREPARATION
- Make sure that the patient has signed an appropriate consent form.
- Note and report all allergies.
- Withhold drugs the patient is currently taking before the test begins.
- Make sure the patient has a patent I.V. line.
- Withhold food and fluid for at least 4 hours before the test.

Teaching points
- Explain the purpose of the test and how it's done.
- Tell the patient who will perform the test and where it will be done.
- Instruct the patient to refrain from eating, smoking, or drinking alcoholic or caffeinated beverages for at least 4 hours before the test or as directed by the practitioner.
- Warn the patient that when the dobutamine infusion begins, he may feel palpitations, some mild shortness of breath, and some fatigue.
- Instruct the patient to report all symptoms experienced during the study.
- Tell the patient that the test should take 60 to 90 minutes.

DIAGNOSTIC PROCEDURE

KEY STEPS
- Confirm the patient's identity using two patient identifiers according to facility policy.
- The patient is placed in the supine position and an echocardiogram is obtained.
- An initial electrocardiogram (ECG) is obtained.
- ECG rhythm and blood pressure are monitored during the procedure.
- After I.V. access is obtained, a dobutamine infusion is given in increasing amounts, usually up to a maximum of 30 mcg/kg/minute.
- The infusion is continued until the patient reaches his maximum predicted heart rate or becomes symptomatic.
- If the maximum predicted heart rate isn't reached with maximum dobutamine, I.V. atropine may be given.
- As the maximum predicted heart rate is achieved, a second (stress) echocardiogram is obtained.
- After the dobutamine infusion is completed, a third (recovery) echocardiogram is obtained.

WARNING *Stop the test if significant ECG changes, hypertension, hypotension, angina, dyspnea, or syncope occurs or critical symptoms develop.*

POSTPROCEDURE CARE
- Give an I.V. beta-adrenergic blocker if the heart rate doesn't return to baseline or if the patient becomes symptomatic.
- Remove the electrodes and conductive gel from the patient's chest.
- Monitor the patient's vital signs, ECG tracing, heart sounds, anginal symptoms, and respiratory status.

PRECAUTIONS
WARNING *The procedure should be performed only by a physician, with emergency resuscitation equipment readily available.*
- The procedure is contraindicated in patients who have had an MI within 10 days of testing and in those with acute myocarditis or pericarditis, ventricular or atrial arrhythmias, severe aortic or mitral stenosis, hyperthyroidism, severe anemia, ventricular or dissecting aortic aneurysms, clinical heart failure, or acute severe infections.

COMPLICATIONS
- Angina
- Dyspnea
- Hypertension
- Hypotension
- Significant ECG changes
- Syncope

INTERPRETATION

NORMAL RESULTS
- Ventricular wall contractility is increased.

ABNORMAL RESULTS
- Abnormal regional wall motion may indicate cardiac ischemia or infarction.

Echocardiography, exercise

DESCRIPTION

- Detects changes in cardiac wall motion
- Collects images before and after exercise stress testing
- Specificity and sensitivity adjunct to results obtained in exercise electrocardiography

PURPOSE

- To identify the causes of chest pain
- To determine chamber size and functional capacity of the heart
- To screen for cardiac disease that's producing no symptoms
- To set limits for an exercise program
- To diagnose and evaluate valvular and wall motion abnormalities
- To detect atrial tumors, mural thrombi, vegetative growth on valve leaflets, and pericardial effusions
- To evaluate myocardial perfusion, coronary artery disease (CAD) and obstructions, and the extent of myocardial damage after a myocardial infarction (MI)

PREPARATION

- Make sure that the patient has signed a consent form.
- Note and report all allergies.
- Withhold drugs the patient is currently taking before the test.
- Withhold food and fluid for at least 4 hours before the test.

Teaching points

- Explain the purpose of the test and how it's done.
- Tell him who will perform the test and where it will be done.
- Instruct the patient to refrain from eating, smoking, or drinking alcoholic or caffeinated beverages for at least 4 hours before the test.
- Warn the patient that he might feel tired, sweaty, and slightly short of breath. Reassure him that if symptoms become severe or if chest pain develops, the test will be stopped.
- Tell the patient that the test takes about 60 minutes.

DIAGNOSTIC PROCEDURE

KEY STEPS

- Confirm the patient's identity using two patient identifiers according to facility policy.
- The patient is placed in the supine position and a baseline echocardiogram is obtained.
- An initial baseline electrocardiogram (ECG) and an initial blood pressure reading are obtained.
- The patient is placed on the treadmill at slow speed until he becomes acclimated to it.
- The work rate is increased every 3 minutes as tolerated (increasing the speed of the machine slightly and increasing the degree of incline by 3% each time).
- The cardiac monitor is observed continuously for changes, and blood pressure is monitored at predetermined intervals.
- The rhythm strip is checked at preset intervals for arrhythmias, premature ventricular contractions, ST-segment changes, and T-wave changes.
- The test level and the amount of time it took to reach that level are noted on each strip.
- Common responses to maximal exercise include dizziness, lightheadedness, leg fatigue, dyspnea, diaphoresis, and a slightly ataxic gait. If symptoms become severe, the test is stopped.
- The test is stopped if the patient has significant ECG changes, arrhythmias, or symptoms that include hypertension, hypotension, or angina.
- After the patient has reached the maximum predicted heart rate, the treadmill is slowed.
- While the patient's heart rate is still elevated, he's helped off the treadmill and placed on a litter for a second echocardiogram.

POSTPROCEDURE CARE

- Remove the electrodes and conductive gel.
- Monitor the patient's vital signs, ECG tracing, and heart sounds.

PRECAUTIONS

WARNING *The procedure should be performed only by a physician, with emergency resuscitation equipment readily available.*

- The test is contraindicated in patients with ventricular or dissecting aortic aneurysms, uncontrolled arrhythmias, pericarditis, myocarditis, severe anemia, uncontrolled hypertension, unstable angina, and heart failure.

COMPLICATIONS

- Cardiac arrhythmias
- Angina
- Myocardial ischemia or MI
- Cardiac arrest
- Death

INTERPRETATION

NORMAL RESULTS

- Contractility of the ventricular walls increases and results in hyperkinesis linked to sympathetic and catecholamine stimulation.
- The heart rate increases in direct proportion to the workload and metabolic oxygen demand. Systolic blood pressure also increases as the workload increases.
- The patient attains the endurance level appropriate for his age and exercise limits.

ABNORMAL RESULTS

- Exercise-induced myocardial ischemia suggests disease in the coronary artery supplying the involved area of myocardium.
- Hypokinesis or akinesis of the myocardium indicates significant CAD.
- Exercise-induced hypotension, ST-segment depression of 2 mm or more, or downsloping ST segments appearing within the first 3 minutes of exercise and lasting 8 minutes after the test ends may indicate multivessel or left CAD.
- ST-segment elevation may indicate critical myocardial ischemia or injury.

Electrocardiography

DESCRIPTION

◆ Graphically records the electrical current generated by the heart and measured by electrodes connected to an amplifier and strip chart recorder
◆ Measures the electrical potential from 12 different leads: the standard limb leads (I, II, III), the augmented limb leads (aV_F, aV_L, aV_R), and the precordial, or chest, leads (V_1 through V_6)
◆ Displays P wave, QRS complex, and T wave
◆ Also known as *ECG*

PURPOSE

◆ To identify conduction abnormalities, cardiac arrhythmias, and myocardial ischemia or myocardial infarction (MI)
◆ To monitor recovery from an MI
◆ To document pacemaker performance

PREPARATION

◆ Note current cardiac drug therapy on the test request form and other pertinent clinical information, such as chest pain or pacemaker placement.

Teaching points

◆ Explain the purpose of the procedure and how it's done.
◆ Tell the patient who will perform the test and where it will be done.
◆ Tell the patient that no dietary restrictions are required.
◆ Instruct the patient to lie still, relax, and breathe normally during the procedure.
◆ Inform the patient that the test is painless and takes 5 to 10 minutes. (See *Learning about an electrocardiogram*, page 182.)

KEY STEPS

◆ Confirm the patient's identity using two patient identifiers according to facility policy.
◆ Place the patient in a supine or semi-Fowler's position.
◆ Expose the chest, ankles, and wrists.
◆ Place the electrodes on the inner aspect of the wrists, on the medial aspect of the lower legs, and on the chest.
◆ After all the electrodes are in place, connect the lead wires.
◆ Press the START button and input any required information.
◆ Make sure that all leads are represented in the tracing. If not, determine which electrode has come loose, reattach it, and restart the tracing.

POSTPROCEDURE CARE

◆ Disconnect the equipment, remove the electrodes, and remove the gel with a moist cloth towel.
◆ If the patient is having recurrent chest pain or if serial ECGs are ordered, leave the electrode patches in place.

PRECAUTIONS

◆ Make sure that all recording and other nearby electrical equipment are properly grounded.
◆ Make sure that the electrodes are firmly attached.

COMPLICATIONS

◆ Skin sensitivity to the electrodes

NORMAL RESULTS

◆ The heart rate is 60 to 100 beats/minute.
◆ Cardiac rhythm is a normal sinus rhythm.
◆ A P wave precedes each QRS complex.
◆ The PR interval lasts 0.12 to 0.20 second.
◆ The QRS complex lasts 0.06 to 0.10 second.
◆ The ST segment isn't more than 0.1 mV.
◆ The T wave is rounded and smooth and is positive in leads I, II, V_3, V_4, V_5, and V_6.
◆ The QT interval duration varies but usually lasts 0.36 to 0.44 second. (See *Normal ECG waveforms*, page 183.)

ABNORMAL RESULTS

◆ A heart rate below 60 beats/minute indicates bradycardia.
◆ A heart rate above 100 beats/minute suggests tachycardia.
◆ Missing P waves may indicate atrioventricular (AV) block, atrial arrhythmia, or junctional rhythm.
◆ A short PR interval may indicate a junctional arrhythmia; a prolonged PR interval may indicate an AV block.
◆ A prolonged QRS complex may indicate intraventricular conduction defects; missing QRS complexes may indicate an AV block or ventricular asystole.
◆ ST-segment elevation of 0.2 mV or more above the baseline may indicate myocardial injury; ST-segment depression may indicate myocardial ischemia or injury.
◆ T wave inversion in leads I, II, and V_3 to V_6 may indicate myocardial ischemia; peaked T waves may indicate hyperkalemia or myocardial ischemia; and variations in T wave amplitude may indicate electrolyte imbalances.
◆ A prolonged QT interval may suggest life-threatening ventricular arrhythmias. (See *Abnormal ECG waveforms*, page 183.)

(continued)

Learning about an electrocardiogram

Dear Patient:

An electrocardiogram (ECG) has been ordered for you. This test tells how well your heart works.

Your heart is a pump that has a built-in pacemaker. This pacemaker is actually a group of special cells in the upper right part of the heart.

About every second, this natural pacemaker releases an electrical impulse that travels down a path of muscle fibers and spreads throughout your heart.

This impulse makes your heart contract and pump blood through its chambers and into the rest of the body through the blood vessels.

HOW AN ECG WORKS

An ECG records the electrical impulses that travel through your heart. The ECG machine then converts these impulses to pencil-like tracings that print on long strips of graph paper. By looking at these tracings, your health care provider can tell whether your heart is healthy or has a problem.

BEFORE THE TEST

You'll be asked to lie on your back, with the skin of your chest, arms, and legs exposed. Lie perfectly still and relax. (Don't even talk.) The test is painless and only takes a few minutes.

DURING THE TEST

Electrodes, which resemble small stickers, will be placed on your chest, arms, and legs. Wires attached to the ECG machine will then be connected to the electrodes, and the machine will be prompted to record.

AFTER THE TEST

When the test is over, the electrodes will be removed. You'll be able to resume your usual activities. Your health care provider will inform you of the test results.

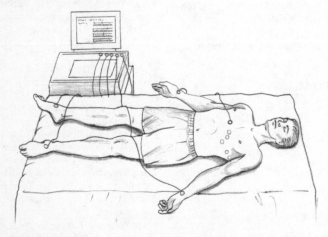

Normal ECG waveforms

Because each lead takes a different view of heart activity, it generates a characteristic tracing on an electrocardiogram (ECG). The traces shown here are representative of each of the 12 leads. Leads aV_R, V_1, V_2, V_3, and V_4 normally show strong negative deflections. Negative deflections indicate that the current is moving away from the positive electrode; positive deflections, that the current is moving toward the positive electrode.

Lead I

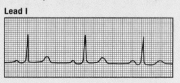

Lead aV$_F$

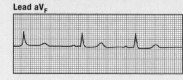

Lead V$_3$

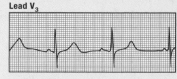

Lead II

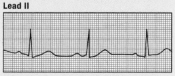

Lead aV$_L$

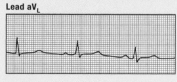

Lead V$_4$

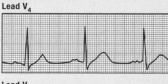

Lead III

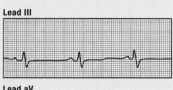

Lead V$_1$

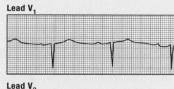

Lead V$_5$

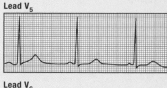

Lead aV$_R$

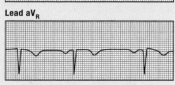

Lead V$_2$

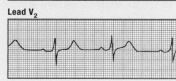

Lead V$_6$

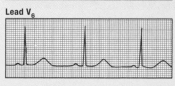

Abnormal ECG waveforms

Premature ventricular contractions (PVCs) originate in an ectopic focus of the ventricular wall. They can be unifocal (having the same single focus), as shown in this electrocardiogram (ECG) tracing from lead V_1, or multifocal (arising from more than one ectopic focus). In PVCs, the P wave is absent and the QRS complex shows considerable distortion, usually deflecting in the opposite direction from the patient's normal QRS complex. The T wave also deflects in the opposite direction from the QRS complex, and the PVC usually precedes a compensatory pause. Some examples of abnormalities causing PVCs include electrolyte imbalances (especially hypokalemia), myocardial infarction (MI), reperfusion of a new MI or injury, hypoxia, and drug toxicity (cardiac glycosides, beta-adrenergic blockers).

First-degree heart block, the most common conduction disturbance, occurs in healthy hearts as well as diseased hearts and usually is clinically insignificant. It's typically characteristic in elderly patients with chronic degeneration of the cardiac conduction system, and it occasionally occurs in patients receiving cardiac glycosides or antiarrhythmic drugs, such as procainamide and quinidine. In children, first-degree heart block may be the earliest sign of acute rheumatic fever. In this lead V_1 tracing, the interval between the P wave and the QRS complex (the PR interval) exceeds 0.20 second.

Hypokalemia is a common electrolyte imbalance that's caused by low serum potassium levels and affects the electrical activity of the myocardium. Mild hypokalemia may cause only muscle weakness, fatigue and, possibly, atrial or ventricular irritability; a severe imbalance causes pronounced muscle weakness, paralysis, atrial tachycardia with varying degrees of block, and PVCs that may progress to ventricular tachycardia and ventricular fibrillation.

Early signs of hypokalemia, as shown on this lead V_1 tracing, include prominent U waves, a prolonged QT interval, and flat or inverted T waves. Usually, T waves don't flatten or invert until potassium depletion becomes severe.

PVC — Lead V$_1$

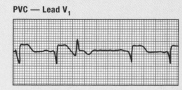

First-degree heart block — Lead V$_1$

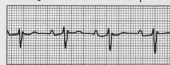

Hypokalemia — Lead V$_1$

Electrocardiography, exercise

DESCRIPTION

- Monitors electrocardiogram (ECG) and blood pressure while the patient walks on a treadmill or pedals a stationary bicycle; notes response to a constant or increasing workload
- Evaluates the heart during physical stress
- Also known as an *exercise stress test*

PURPOSE

- To diagnose the cause of chest pain
- To determine the functional capacity of the heart
- To screen for coronary artery disease (CAD) that's causing no symptoms
- To help set limitations for an exercise program
- To identify cardiac arrhythmias that develop during physical exercise
- To evaluate the effectiveness of antiarrhythmic or antianginal therapy
- To evaluate myocardial perfusion

PREPARATION

- Make sure that the patient has signed an appropriate consent form.
- Note and report all allergies.
- Check the patient's history for a recent physical examination (within 1 week) and for baseline 12-lead ECG results.
- Continue drugs the patient is currently taking unless the practitioner directs otherwise.

Teaching points

- Explain the purpose of the test and how it's done.
- Tell the patient who will perform the test and where it will be done.
- Instruct the patient not to eat, smoke, or drink alcoholic or caffeinated beverages before the test.
- Warn the patient that he might feel fatigued, slightly breathless, and sweaty during the test.
- Reassure the patient that testing will stop if he experiences significant symptoms such as chest pain.
- Instruct the patient to wear comfortable socks and shoes and loose, lightweight shorts or slacks during the procedure.
- Inform the patient that the test takes about 30 minutes.

DIAGNOSTIC PROCEDURE

KEY STEPS

- Confirm the patient's identity using two patient identifiers according to facility policy.
- Baseline ECG and blood pressure readings are taken.
- ECG and blood pressure readings are taken while the patient walks on a treadmill or pedals a stationary bicycle.
- Unless complications develop, the test continues until the patient reaches the target heart rate, determined by an established protocol (usually 85% of the maximum predicted heart rate for the patient's age and gender).
- The cardiac monitor is observed continuously for changes in the heart's electrical activity.
- The rhythm strip is checked at preset intervals for arrhythmias, premature ventricular contractions (PVCs), ST-segment changes, and T-wave changes.
- Blood pressure is monitored at predetermined intervals (usually at the end of each test level).
- The test is stopped when the patient reaches the target heart rate or if symptoms become severe.
- The test is stopped immediately if the ECG shows significant arrhythmias or an increase in ectopy, if systolic blood pressure falls below the resting level, if the heart rate falls 10 beats/minute or more below the resting level, or if the patient becomes exhausted or experiences severe symptoms such as chest pain.

POSTPROCEDURE CARE

- Assist the patient to a chair and continue monitoring his heart rate and blood pressure for 10 to 15 minutes or until the ECG returns to the baseline.
- Remove the electrodes and clean the application sites.
- Monitor the patient's vital signs, ECG tracing, heart sounds, and anginal symptoms.
- Have the patient resume his normal diet and activities.

PRECAUTIONS

WARNING *Stop the test if the patient has persistent ST-segment elevation, possibly indicating myocardial injury.*

WARNING *Stop the test if the patient experiences a new bundle-branch block, an ST-segment depression greater then 1.5 mm, frequent or multifocal PVCs, blood pressure failing to rise above the resting level, systolic pressure above 220 mm Hg, or angina.*

COMPLICATIONS

- Cardiac arrhythmias
- Angina
- Myocardial ischemia or infarction

NORMAL RESULTS

- The heart rate increases in direct proportion to the workload and metabolic oxygen demand.
- Systolic blood pressure increases as workload increases.
- The patient attains the endurance levels appropriate for his age and the exercise protocol.

ABNORMAL RESULTS

- T-wave inversion or ST-segment depression may signify ischemia.
- Exercise-induced hypotension, an ST-segment depression of 2 mm or more, and downsloping ST segments may indicate significant CAD.
- ST-segment elevation may indicate myocardial injury.

Electrocardiography, signal-averaged

DESCRIPTION

- Amplifies, averages, and filters an electrocardiogram (ECG) signal recorded on the body surface
- Detects high-frequency, low-amplitude cardiac electrical signals in the last part of the QRS complex and in the ST segment

PURPOSE

- To detect destructive signals called *late potentials* that may represent delayed, disorganized activity (in patients who have survived an acute myocardial infarction)
- To evaluate the risk of life-threatening arrhythmias

PREPARATION

- Make sure that the patient has signed an appropriate consent form.
- Note and report all allergies.
- Record the use of antiarrhythmics on the patient's chart.
- No dietary restrictions are needed.

Teaching points

- Explain the purpose of the test and how it's done.
- Tell the patient who will perform the test and where it will be done.
- Tell the patient that he doesn't need to restrict his diet.
- Inform the patient that electrodes will be attached to his arms, legs, and chest and that the procedure is painless.
- Instruct the patient to lie still and breathe normally during the procedure.
- Tell him that the test takes about 30 minutes.

DIAGNOSTIC PROCEDURE

KEY STEPS

- Confirm the patient's identity using two patient identifiers according to facility policy.
- The patient is placed in the supine position (or semi-Fowler's position if the patient can't tolerate lying supine).
- Electrodes are attached to the patient's chest, ankles, and wrists. (See *Electrode placement for a signal-averaged ECG.*)
- Multiple inputs are obtained from standard orthogonal bipolar X, Y, and Z leads over a series of ECG cycles.
- The average is taken over a large number of beats, typically 100 or more.

POSTPROCEDURE CARE

- Wash conductive gel from the skin.

PRECAUTIONS

- Electrical equipment should be properly grounded to prevent electrical interference.
- Poor tissue electrode contact produces artifact.

COMPLICATIONS

- Skin sensitivity to the electrodes

INTERPRETATION

NORMAL RESULTS

- QRS complexes lack low potentials that would indicate disorganized activity.

ABNORMAL RESULTS

- Late potentials after the QRS complex indicate a risk of ventricular arrhythmias.

Electrode placement for a signal-averaged ECG

Positioning electrodes for a signal-averaged ECG is much different than for a 12-lead ECG. Here's one method:

- Place the positive X electrode at the left fourth intercostal space, midaxillary line.
- Place the negative X electrode at the right fourth intercostal space, midaxillary line.
- Place the positive Y electrode at the left iliac crest.
- Place the negative Y electrode at the superior aspect of the manubrium of the sternum.
- Place the positive Z electrode at the fourth intercostal space, left of the sternum.
- Place the ground (G) on the lower right at the eighth rib.
- Reposition the patient on his side, or have him sit forward. Then place the negative Z electrode on his back (not shown), directly posterior to the positive Z electrode.
- Attach all the leads to the electrodes, being careful not to dislodge the posterior lead. Now, you can obtain the tracing.

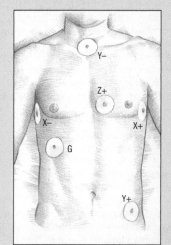

Electroencephalography

OVERVIEW

DESCRIPTION

- Records a portion of the brain's electrical activity through electrodes attached to the scalp
- Electrical impulses transmitted, magnified, and recorded as brain waves
- Intracranial electrodes sometimes surgically implanted to record electroencephalographic changes to locate seizure focus
- Also called *EEG*

PURPOSE

- To determine the presence and type of seizures
- To help diagnose intracranial lesions
- To evaluate brain activity in metabolic disease, head injury, meningitis, encephalitis, and psychological disorders
- To help confirm brain death

PREPARATION

- Make sure that the patient has signed a consent form.
- Note and report all allergies.
- Wash and dry the patient's hair to remove hairsprays, creams, or oils.
- Withhold tranquilizers, barbiturates, and other sedatives for 24 to 48 hours before the test.
- Stimulants, such as caffeinated beverages, chocolate, and tobacco, should be avoided for 8 hours before the test.
- The test requires minimal sleep (4 to 5 hours) the night before the study.
- If a sleep EEG is ordered, give a sedative to promote sleep during the test.
- Very young children may require sedation to prevent crying and restlessness; however, these drugs may alter test results.

Teaching points

- Explain the purpose of the test and how it's done.
- Tell the patient who will perform the test and where it will be done.
- Instruct him to avoid stimulants, such as caffeinated beverages, chocolate, and tobacco, for 8 hours before the test.
- Advise him to sleep only 4 to 5 hours the night before the test.
- Reassure him that the electrodes won't shock him.
- If the test involves needle electrodes, warn the patient that he might feel pricking sensations during insertion.
- Inform the patient that the test takes about 1 hour.

DIAGNOSTIC PROCEDURE

KEY STEPS

- Confirm the patient's identity using two patient identifiers according to facility policy.
- The patient is positioned and electrodes are attached to the scalp.
- During recording, the patient is carefully observed and movements, such as blinking, swallowing, or talking, are noted; these movements can cause artifacts.
- The patient may undergo testing in various stress situations, including hyperventilation and photic stimulation to elicit abnormal patterns not obvious in the resting stage.

POSTPROCEDURE CARE

- Provide a safe environment.
- Monitor the patient for seizures and maintain seizure precautions.
- Help the patient remove the electrode paste from his hair.
- Tell the patient that he may resume drug therapy.
- If brain death is confirmed, provide emotional support for the family.

PRECAUTIONS

- Skipping the meal before the test can cause hypoglycemia and alter brain wave patterns.

COMPLICATIONS

- Adverse effects of sedation, if used
- Possible seizure activity

INTERPRETATION

NORMAL RESULTS

- Alpha waves (8 to 13 cycles/second) follow a regular rhythm.
- Alpha waves occur only in the waking state when the patient's eyes are closed but he's mentally alert and usually disappear with visual activity or mental concentration.
- Alpha waves are decreased by apprehension or anxiety and are most prominent in the occipital leads.
- Beta waves (13 to 30 cycles/second) occur when the patient is alert with eyes open and are seen most readily in the frontal and central regions of the brain.
- Theta waves (4 to 7 cycles/second) are most common in children and young adults. They appear primarily in the parietal and temporal regions and indicate drowsiness or emotional stress in adults.
- Delta waves (fewer than 4 cycles/second) are visible in deep sleep stages and in serious brain dysfunction.

ABNORMAL RESULTS

- Spikes and waves at 3 cycles/second suggest absence seizures.
- Multiple, high-voltage, spiked waves in both hemispheres suggest generalized tonic-clonic seizures.
- Spiked waves in the affected temporal region suggest temporal lobe epilepsy.
- Localized, spiked discharges suggest focal seizures.
- Slow waves (usually delta waves but possibly unilateral beta waves) suggest intracranial lesions.
- Focal abnormalities in the injured area suggest vascular lesions.
- Generalized, diffuse, and slow brain waves suggest metabolic or inflammatory disorders or increased intracranial pressure.
- An absent EEG pattern or a flat tracing (except for artifacts) may indicate brain death.

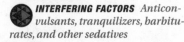 ***INTERFERING FACTORS*** *Anticonvulsants, tranquilizers, barbiturates, and other sedatives*

Electromyography

DESCRIPTION

- Records the electrical activity of selected skeletal muscle groups at rest and during voluntary contraction
- Measures nerve conduction time (see *Nerve conduction studies*)

PURPOSE

- To differentiate between primary muscle disorders, such as muscular dystrophies, and certain metabolic disorders
- To identify diseases characterized by central neuronal degeneration such as amyotrophic lateral sclerosis (ALS)
- To help diagnose neuromuscular disorders such as myasthenia gravis
- To help diagnose radiculomyopathies

PREPARATION

- Make sure that the patient has signed an appropriate consent form.
- Note and report all allergies.
- Check for and note drugs that may interfere with test results (such as cholinergics, anticholinergics, anticoagulants, and skeletal muscle relaxants).
- Smoking, coffee, tea, and cola must be restricted for 2 to 3 hours before the test.

Teaching points

- Explain the purpose of the test and how it's done.
- Tell the patient who will perform the test and where it will be done.
- Instruct the patient to avoid smoking, coffee, tea, and cola for 2 to 3 hours before the test.
- Warn the patient that he might experience some discomfort when a needle is inserted into certain muscles.
- Inform the patient that the test takes at least 1 hour.

KEY STEPS

- Confirm the patient's identity using two patient identifiers according to facility policy.
- The patient is positioned in a way that relaxes the muscle to be tested.
- Needle electrodes are quickly inserted into the selected muscle.
- A metal plate lies under the patient to serve as a reference electrode.
- The resulting electrical signal is recorded during rest and contraction, amplified 1 million times, and displayed on an oscilloscope or computer screen.
- Lead wires are usually attached to an audio-amplifier so that voltage fluctuations within the muscle are audible.

POSTPROCEDURE CARE

- Apply warm compresses and give analgesics for discomfort.
- Monitor the patient for signs and symptoms of infection.
- Monitor the patient's pain level and response to the analgesics.
- Tell the patient to resume drugs that were withheld.

PRECAUTIONS

- The procedure is contraindicated in patients with bleeding disorders.

COMPLICATIONS

- Infection at the insertion site
- Pain

NORMAL RESULTS

- At rest, the muscle exhibits minimal electrical activity.
- During voluntary contraction, electrical activity markedly increases.
- A sustained contraction, or one of increasing strength, produces a rapid "train" of motor unit potentials.

ABNORMAL RESULTS

- Short (low-amplitude) motor unit potentials, with frequent, irregular discharges suggest possible primary muscle disease such as muscular dystrophies.
- Isolated and irregular motor unit potentials with increased amplitude and duration suggest possible disorders, such as ALS and peripheral nerve disorders.
- Initially normal motor unit potentials that progressively diminish in amplitude with continuing contractions suggest possible myasthenia gravis.

Nerve conduction studies

Nerve conduction studies help diagnose peripheral nerve injuries and diseases affecting the peripheral nervous system such as peripheral neuropathies. To measure nerve conduction time, a nerve is stimulated electrically through the skin and underlying tissues. The patient experiences a mild electric shock with each stimulation. At a known distance from the point of stimulation, a recording electrode detects the response from the stimulated nerve.

The time between stimulation of the nerve and the detected response is measured on an oscilloscope. The speed of conduction along the nerve is then calculated by dividing the distance between the point of stimulation and the recording electrode by the time between stimulus and response. In peripheral nerve injuries and diseases, such as peripheral neuropathies, nerve conduction time is abnormal.

Electromyography of the external sphincter

OVERVIEW

DESCRIPTION
- Measures electrical activity of the external urinary sphincter
- Measures activity by skin electrodes (most commonly used), by needle electrodes inserted in perineal or periurethral tissues, or by electrodes in an anal plug
- Commonly used with cystometry and voiding urethrography as part of a full urodynamic study

PURPOSE
- To evaluate incontinence
- To assess neuromuscular function of the external urinary sphincter
- To assess the functional balance between bladder and sphincter muscle activity

PREPARATION
- Make sure that the patient has signed a consent form.
- Note and report all allergies.
- If the patient is taking cholinergic or anticholinergic drugs, notify the practitioner and stop the drugs.
- Provide reassurance that there's no danger of electric shock.
- No dietary restrictions are needed.

Teaching points
- Explain the purpose of the test and how it's done.
- Tell the patient who will perform the test and where it will be done.
- Instruct him which of his medications to stop, as ordered by the practitioner.
- Tell him he doesn't have to restrict his diet.
- If the patient is to receive needle electrodes, warn him that he may feel discomfort during insertion.
- If the patient is to receive an anal plug, assure him that only the tip of the plug will be inserted into the rectum — he may feel fullness but no discomfort.
- Tell the female patient that slight bleeding may occur with the first voiding after the procedure.

- Inform the patient that the test takes 30 to 60 minutes.

DIAGNOSTIC PROCEDURE

KEY STEPS
- Confirm the patient's identity using two patient identifiers according to facility policy.
- The patient is placed in the lithotomy position for electrode placement; he may then lie in a supine position.
- Electrode paste is applied to the ground plate, which is taped to the thigh and grounded. Electrodes are applied and connected to electrode adapters.
- For the female patient, skin electrodes are placed in the periurethral area; for a male, the perineal area beneath the scrotum is used.
- For the female patient, needle electrodes are inserted in the periurethral area; for a male, they are inserted through the perineal skin toward the apex of the prostate.
- The electrodes are connected to adapters inserted into the preamplifier and recording begins.
- The patient is asked alternately to relax and tighten the sphincter.
- He's asked to bear down and exhale while the anal plug and needle electrodes are removed.
- Cystometrography may be done with electromyography for a thorough evaluation of detrusor and sphincter coordination.

POSTPROCEDURE CARE
- Clean and dry the area.
- Report hematuria after the first voiding in the female patient tested with needle electrodes.
- Report signs and symptoms of mild urethral irritation, including dysuria, hematuria, and urinary frequency.
- Advise the patient to use warm sitz baths and increase oral fluids to 2 to 3 qt (2 to 3 L)/day, unless contraindicated.

PRECAUTIONS
- None

COMPLICATIONS
- Bleeding
- Infection

INTERPRETATION

NORMAL RESULTS
- Muscle activity increases when the external urinary sphincter is tightened.
- Muscle activity decreases when the external urinary sphincter is relaxed.
- If electromyography and cystometrography are done together, a comparison of results shows muscle activity of the sphincter that increases as the bladder fills, as the patient voids, and as the bladder contracts and muscle activity that decreases as the sphincter relaxes.

ABNORMAL RESULTS
- Failure of the sphincter to relax or increased muscle activity during voiding indicates detrusor-sphincter dyssynergia.

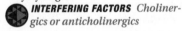 **INTERFERING FACTORS** *Cholinergics or anticholinergics*

Electroneurography

DESCRIPTION

- Electrical impulse stimulated at a proximal nerve site; measures time taken to travel a distal site along the same nerve
- Usually done with electromyography

PURPOSE

- To detect the location of peripheral nerve injury or disease

PREPARATION

- No dietary restrictions are needed.

Teaching points

- Explain that this test will help locate the nerve injury.
- Tell the patient who will perform the test and where it will be done.
- Inform him that he may feel a slight shock when the nerve impulse is delivered.
- Tell him that he doesn't have to restrict his diet.
- Inform the patient that the test takes about 15 minutes.

KEY STEPS

- Confirm the patient's identity using two patient identifiers according to facility policy.
- Position the patient so the area with suspected nerve damage is easily accessible.
- Place a recording electrode on the patient's skin over a muscle that's innervated solely by the nerve suspected to be damaged.
- Place a second electrode, a reference electrode, close to the first electrode.
- Stimulate the nerve by using an appropriate device.
- An EMG machine will measure the time between the nerve impulse and muscular contraction, known as *distal latency.*
- A second impulse is generated and transmitted to a location proximal to the suspected injury or disease.
- The time from nerve stimulation to muscle contraction is measured again, and this is known as total latency.
- Record the distance between the stimulation site and the recording electrode in centimeters.
- Conduction velocity of the nerve is determined by the equation: distance (in meters)/(total latency – distal latency).

POSTPROCEDURE CARE

- Remove the electrodes and gel from the patient's skin.

PRECAUTIONS

- Make sure you correctly place the electrodes over the nerve that's believed to be injured.

COMPLICATIONS

- None

NORMAL RESULTS

- Normal conduction velocity is 50 to 60 m/second.

ABNORMAL RESULTS

- Increased conduction has no pathologic meaning.
- Slowed conduction is seen in neuropathies, neurologic disorders, and nerve disease.
- Diseases that have slow nerve conduction include carpal tunnel syndrome, herniated discs, poliomyelitis, myasthenia gravis, diabetic neuropathy, and Guillain-Barré syndrome.
- Further testing is needed to determine the cause of nerve injury or disease.

Electronystagmography and video nystagmography

DESCRIPTION

- Evaluate interactions of vestibular system and muscles controlling eye movement
- Vestibulo-ocular reflex: reflex that causes nystagmus — involuntary back-and-forth eye movements; maintains vision when the head moves (see *Understanding eye movement patterns*)
- Traditional electronystagmography (ENG): records nystagmus; electrodes detect and chart corneoretinal potential
- Video nystagmography (VNG): eye movements recorded by infrared camera
- Help determine the origin of the disorder (peripheral or central nervous system [CNS])

PURPOSE

- To help identify the cause of dizziness and vertigo
- To confirm the presence and location of a lesion
- To assess neurologic disorders

PREPARATION

- Make sure that the patient's ear canals are free from cerumen and that he doesn't have a tympanic membrane perforation.
- Reassure the patient that the test isn't painful and that someone will be present to ensure that he doesn't fall. Fasting is needed for at least 4 hours before the test because portions of the test may briefly make him dizzy.
- Find out about the progression of the patient's symptoms by asking him to describe the dizziness in words other than "dizzy."
- Suggest that someone accompany the patient to the test because he may not feel well enough to drive afterward.

Teaching points

- Explain the purpose of the test and how it's done.
- Tell the patient who will perform the test and where it will be done.
- Inform the patient that tympanometry will occur before caloric testing to ensure tympanic membrane integrity.
- Tell the patient that his dizziness will be assessed by recording his eye movements.
- Instruct the patient to fast for at least 4 hours before the test.
- Encourage the patient to wear comfortable clothing.
- If testing will involve traditional ENG with attachment of recording electrodes, instruct the patient not to use make-up or facial creams on the day of the test.
- Advise the patient not to wear mascara because it can affect VNG testing.
- Instruct the patient not to smoke or drink caffeinated beverages the day of the test and to refrain from taking nonessential medication for 48 hours before the test.
- If the patient wears glasses, tell him to bring them to the test. Also, tell the patient who wears contact lenses to bring eyeglasses to the test, if possible.
- Tell the patient that the audiologist will ask him to describe the dizziness, including when it began and what situations create it or make it worse.
- Inform the patient that the test takes about 45 minutes.

KEY STEPS

- Confirm the patient's identity using two patient identifiers according to facility policy.
- After the device is set up, light bars are connected to the equipment.
- The patient is positioned a calibrated distance from the light source and asked to follow the movement of the lights using eye movement only. These movements are recorded and graphed.

Understanding eye movement patterns

There are several types of eye movement patterns to look for during electronystagmography testing. Here are some patterns along with their definitions.

- Bilateral weakness — reduced nystagmus (slow-phase velocity) after the caloric irrigation of both ears.
- Conjugate deviation — drawing of the eyes to one side in unison.
- Directional preponderance — difference in beat intensity in one direction as opposed to the other direction during caloric testing; commonly associated with existing spontaneous nystagmus.
- Nystagmus — involuntary, rhythmic, back-and-forth movement of the eyes, usually composed of a slow deviation in one direction and a rapid return in the other. Types of nystagmus include:
  - fast phase of nystagmus — quick, jerky component of nystagmus controlled by the central nervous system
  - horizontal nystagmus — nystagmus in the horizontal plane, either left- or right-beating
  - inverted nystagmus — nystagmus beating in the direction opposite to that anticipated

  - positional nystagmus — persistent nystagmus appearing while in a particular head position
  - positioning nystagmus — transient nystagmus occurring immediately after a change in head position
  - rotary nystagmus — nystagmus that rotates about the axis of the eye
  - slow phase of nystagmus — the vestibular phase of nystagmus or the slow deviation of the eyes from the midline
  - spontaneous nystagmus — occurring in the absence of stimuli
  - vertical nystagmus — occurring in the vertical plane, either up- or down-beating.
- Saccades — rapid, involuntary, jerky movements that occur simultaneously in both eyes when they change their fixation to a new point.
- Unilateral weakness — reduced nystagmus (slow-phase velocity) after one ear is exposed to cold and warm irrigations (averaged), and then those results are compared with the other ear's results.

Saccade test

+ The patient watches the movement of a dot on the light bar. The accuracy and velocity of eye tracking is measured. The traces are analyzed to determine if there's symmetrical eye movement or dysmetria. Glissades — a slowing of the eye movement as it approaches a target — is also ruled out.

Gaze nystagmus test

+ The patient looks at the light on the light bar and holds the gaze steady. Gaze is directed left, right, up, and down.
+ The patient closes his eyes and retains the gaze direction in traditional ENG testing. When VNG recordings are made, goggles exclude light, and the recordings are made with the eyes open.

Smooth pursuit (sinusoidal) tracking test

+ The patient watches the dot on the light bar as it moves back and forth at varying rates. Tracings are analyzed for left/right symmetry and smoothness of the eye's tracking of the target.

Optokinetics test

+ The patient looks at the light bar as a series of dots moves across the screen, first in one direction and then in the other. The patient's eyes rapidly move back to center and track another dot. This creates a tracing that looks like nystagmus.
+ This test assesses CNS ability to control rapid eye movement and is affected by an existing nystagmus.

Positional and positioning test

+ The patient's eye movements are recorded as he's moved into various body positions and as he remains in them.
+ Recordings note whether nystagmus is present and, if so, which positions elicit them and have diagnostic significance.

Dix-Hallpike test

+ This test helps diagnose benign paroxysmal positional vertigo.

+ The patient is seated, and then he's rapidly moved into a supine, head-hanging position, with the head deviated to the side and then returned to a sitting position.

Caloric test

+ The patient lies supine with his head elevated 30 degrees so that the horizontal semicircular canals are perpendicular to the floor. The patient's ear is irrigated with water or air for about 60 seconds per irrigation. Four irrigations are completed.
+ Fluid in the semicircular canal or middle ear moves when the temperature of the fluid is changed, eliciting nystagmus.
+ The patient is instructed to open his eyes during one portion of each recording. Visual fixation reduces nystagmus if the CNS is normal. The symmetry of the nystagmus elicited by irrigation of each ear is assessed. Symmetry of the left beating nystagmus and the right beating nystagmus is analyzed.
+ If the patient fails to respond to standard caloric stimulation, a small quantity of ice water or cold air is introduced into the ear canal to determine if there's residual functioning of that ear's vestibular system.

POSTPROCEDURE CARE

+ The audiologist monitors the patient's status and advises him to remain in a position that reduces dizziness, if present.
+ Advise the patient not to drive until dizziness subsides.

PRECAUTIONS

+ Find out if the patient has a history of back or neck problems that would be worsened by head or neck movement.
+ Water caloric testing can't be safely used if the patient has a perforated tympanic membrane.

COMPLICATIONS

+ Dizziness

INTERPRETATION

NORMAL RESULTS

+ Nystagmus accompanies a head turn.
+ In saccadic pursuit testing, square wave patterns of different amplitudes are seen along with good accuracy of eye movements.
+ In gaze testing, no nystagmus occurs with the eyes open or closed.
+ In smooth pursuit, the patient shows volitional smooth tracking of the target, accurate for age norms.
+ In optokinetic tests, eye movement follows a stimulus at speeds of up to 30 degrees per second; triangular wave pattern is clear, and the pattern is similar for stimuli traveling in both directions.
+ In positional and positioning testing, no nystagmus occurs with the eyes open, eyes closed, or with light-excluding goggles; no more than weak nystagmus occurs in one or more positions.
+ In caloric testing, with the eyes closed, nystagmus occurs in all conditions; suppressed by visual fixation with cold stimuli, nystagmus beats to the opposite ear; with warm stimuli, it beats to the same ear. The acronym COWS is used to remember cold, opposite; warm, same.

ABNORMAL RESULTS

+ Nystagmus is prolonged after a head turn or occurs when the patient isn't turning his head.
+ ENG or VNG results are reported as normal, vestibular (peripheral), CNS, or multifactorial.
+ A peripheral lesion may involve the end organ or the vestibular branch of the eighth cranial nerve and may result from such conditions as Ménière's disease, multiple sclerosis, ischemic damage to the cochlea, autoimmune disease, and vestibular ototoxicity and eighth nerve tumors.
+ A central lesion may involve the brain stem, cerebellum, cerebrum, or the connecting structures and may result from demyelinating diseases, tumors, or circulatory disorders.

Electrophysiology studies

DESCRIPTION
- Measure discrete conduction intervals
- Record electrical conduction during the slow withdrawal of an electrode catheter from the right ventricle through the bundle of His to the sinoatrial node
- Also known as *EPS* or *bundle of His electrography*

PURPOSE
- To diagnose arrhythmias and conduction anomalies
- To determine the need for an implanted pacemaker, internal cardioverter-defibrillator, and cardioactive drugs
- To locate the site of a bundle-branch block, especially in asymptomatic patients with conduction disturbances
- To determine the presence and location of accessory conducting pathways

PREPARATION
- Make sure that the patient has signed an appropriate consent form.
- Note and report all allergies.
- Fasting is required for at least 6 hours before the test.
- Provide reassurance to the patient that he'll remain conscious during the test.

Teaching points
- Explain the purpose of the test and how it's done.
- Tell the patient who will perform the test and where it will be done.
- Instruct the patient to fast for at least 6 hours before the test.
- Instruct the patient to report discomfort or pain during the test.
- Inform the patient that the test usually takes 1 to 3 hours, but may take longer.

DIAGNOSTIC PROCEDURE

KEY STEPS
- Confirm the patient's identity using two patient identifiers according to facility policy.
- The patient is placed in the supine position on a special table.
- Electrocardiogram (ECG) monitoring starts.
- The insertion site (usually the groin or antecubital fossa) is shaved and prepared.
- A local anesthetic is injected. A catheter is inserted intravenously, using fluoroscopic guidance.
- The catheter is advanced into the right ventricle and then slowly withdrawn.
- Recordings of conduction intervals are taken from each pole of the catheter, either simultaneously or sequentially.
- After recordings and measurements are complete, the catheter is removed.
- The insertion site is cleaned and a sterile dressing is applied.

POSTPROCEDURE CARE
- Monitor the patient's vital signs.
- Enforce bed rest.
- Obtain a 12-lead resting ECG.
- Monitor the insertion site and watch for bleeding.
- Monitor the patient for signs and symptoms of infection.
- Monitor the patient for cardiac arrhythmias and symptoms of angina.
- Watch him for signs and symptoms of embolism.
- Monitor ECG changes.
- Have the patient resume his usual diet.

PRECAUTIONS
- **WARNING** *Emergency resuscitation equipment should be readily available in case arrhythmias occur during the test.*
- The test is contraindicated in patients with severe uncorrected coagulopathy, recent thrombophlebitis, and acute pulmonary embolism.

COMPLICATIONS
- Arrhythmias
- Pulmonary emboli and thromboemboli
- Hemorrhage
- Infection

INTERPRETATION

NORMAL RESULTS
- The conduction time from the bundle of His to the Purkinje fibers (HV interval) is 35 to 55 msec.
- The conduction time from the atrioventricular node to the bundle of His (AH interval) is 45 to 150 msec.
- The intra-atrial conduction time (PA interval) is 20 to 40 msec.

ABNORMAL RESULTS
- A prolonged HV interval suggests possible acute or chronic disease.
- AH interval delays suggest atrial pacing, chronic conduction system disease, carotid sinus pressure, recent myocardial infarction, and the use of certain drugs.
- PA interval delays suggest possible acquired, surgically induced, or congenital atrial disease and atrial pacing.

Endoscopic retrograde cholangiopancreatography

DESCRIPTION

◆ X-ray of the pancreatic ducts and hepatobiliary tree after injection of a contrast medium into the duodenal papilla
◆ Also known as *ERCP*

PURPOSE

◆ To evaluate obstructive jaundice
◆ To diagnose cancer of the duodenal papilla, pancreas, and biliary ducts
◆ To locate calculi and stenosis in the pancreatic ducts and hepatobiliary tree

PREPARATION

◆ Make sure that the patient has signed a consent form.
◆ Note and report all allergies.
◆ Inform the practitioner about the patient's hypersensitivity to iodine, seafood, or iodinated contrast media.
◆ Give the patient a sedative.
◆ A local anesthetic spray may be used to suppress the gag reflex and a mouth guard may be used to protect the teeth.
◆ Provide reassurance that oral insertion of the endoscope doesn't obstruct breathing and that the patient will remain conscious during the procedure.

Teaching points

◆ Explain the purpose of the test and how it's done.
◆ Tell the patient who will perform the test and where it will be done.
◆ Instruct the patient to fast after midnight before the test.
◆ Explain that he may have a sore throat for 3 to 4 days after the test.
◆ Tell the patient to avoid alcohol and driving for 24 hours after the test.
◆ Inform the patient that the test takes at least 1 hour. (See *Preparing for ERCP,* page 194.)

DIAGNOSTIC PROCEDURE

KEY STEPS

◆ Confirm the patient's identity using two patient identifiers according to facility policy.
◆ An I.V. infusion is started.
◆ The patient is given a local anesthetic and I.V. sedation.
◆ The patient's vital signs, cardiac rhythm, and pulse oximetry are continuously monitored.
◆ The patient is placed in a left lateral position.
◆ The endoscope is inserted into the mouth and advanced, using fluoroscopic guidance, into the stomach and duodenum.
◆ The patient is helped into the prone position.
◆ An I.V. anticholinergic or glucagon may be given to decrease GI motility.
◆ A cannula is passed through the biopsy channel of the endoscope, into the duodenal papilla, and into the ampulla of Vater; contrast medium is injected.
◆ The pancreatic duct and hepatobiliary tree become visible.
◆ Rapid-sequence X-rays are taken after each contrast injection.
◆ A tissue specimen or fluid may be aspirated for histologic and cytologic examination.
◆ Therapeutic measures (sphincterectomy, stent placement, stone removal, or balloon dilatation) may be performed before endoscope withdrawal, as indicated.
◆ After the films are reviewed, the cannula is removed.

POSTPROCEDURE CARE

◆ Withhold food and fluids until the gag reflex returns, and then have the patient resume his usual diet, as ordered.
◆ Provide soothing lozenges and warm saline gargles for sore throat.
◆ Monitor the patient's vital signs, cardiac rhythm, and pulse oximetry.
◆ Observe the patient's level of consciousness.
◆ Monitor the patient for abdominal distention and bowel sounds.

◆ Watch the patient for adverse drug reactions.
◆ Monitor the patient for complications.

PRECAUTIONS

◆ Inform the practitioner if the patient is hypersensitive to iodine, seafood, or iodinated contrast media.

   WARNING *Emergency resuscitation equipment and a benzodiazepine and opioid antagonist should be readily available during and after the test.*

COMPLICATIONS

◆ Ascending cholangitis
◆ Pancreatitis
◆ Adverse drug reactions
◆ Cardiac arrhythmias
◆ Perforation of the bowel
◆ Respiratory depression
◆ Urine retention

INTERPRETATION

NORMAL RESULTS

◆ A duodenal papilla appears as a small red or pale erosion protruding into the lumen.
◆ Pancreatic and hepatobiliary ducts usually join and empty through the duodenal papilla; separate orifices are sometimes present.
◆ Contrast medium uniformly fills the pancreatic duct, hepatobiliary tree, and gallbladder.

ABNORMAL RESULTS

◆ Hepatobiliary tree filling defects, strictures, or irregular deviations suggest possible biliary cirrhosis, primary sclerosing cholangitis, calculi, or cancer of the bile ducts.
◆ Filling defects, strictures, and irregular deviations of the pancreatic duct suggest possible pancreatic cysts and pseudocysts, pancreatic tumors, chronic pancreatitis, pancreatic fibrosis, calculi, or papillary stenosis.

(continued)

Preparing for ERCP

Dear Patient,

You're about to undergo endoscopic retrograde cholangiopancreatography —
called *ERCP* for short. This procedure uses a dyelike substance, a flexible tube
called an *endoscope,* and X-rays to outline your gallbladder and pancreatic
structures.

ERCP is performed in the radiology department and may take up to 1 hour to
complete. Read the information below to help you prepare.

BEFORE THE TEST

The day before ERCP, you can eat and
drink as usual. After midnight before
the procedure, don't eat or drink
anything unless your health care
provider directs otherwise. He may tell
you to continue taking certain
medications. Before you enter the test
room, be sure to urinate because an
ERCP can cause you to retain urine.

DURING THE TEST

You'll lie on an X-ray table for this test.
The nurse will take your temperature,
blood pressure, and pulse rate. An I.V.
line will be inserted into your hand or
arm to administer medication. You'll
receive a sedative to relax you and to
ease the discomfort of the procedure.

The health care provider will spray
your throat with a bitter-tasting
anesthetic, which will make your
mouth and throat feel swollen and
numb. Because you'll have difficulty
swallowing, you may be given a device
to suction your saliva.

Next, a mouthguard will be placed in
your mouth to keep your mouth open
and to protect your teeth during ERCP.
You'll be unable to talk but won't have
trouble breathing. When the health care
provider passes the endoscope down
your throat, you may gag a little, but
this reflex is normal.

As the tube reaches the duodenum
(small intestine), the health care
provider may inject air through the
tube. You'll also receive medication
through your I.V. line to relax the
duodenum. Next, the health care
provider will thread a thinner tube
through the endoscope to the biliary
structures and the duodenum.

When the second tube is in place,
dye will be injected and X-ray images
will be taken quickly from several
angles. After the images are viewed
and a tissue sample obtained, the
endoscope, tube, and mouthguard will
be gently removed.

AFTER THE TEST

The nurse will check your blood
pressure, pulse rate, and temperature
frequently for several hours.

When you regain feeling in your
throat and your gag reflex returns,
you'll be allowed to have a light meal
and liquids. You can resume your
regular diet the next day.

Expect to have a sore throat for a
few days. Call the health care provider
if you can't urinate or if you experience
chills, abdominal pain, nausea, or
vomiting.

Endoscopic ultrasonography

DESCRIPTION
- Uses ultrasonography and endoscopy to show the GI wall and adjacent structures
- Allows ultrasound imaging with high resolution

PURPOSE
- To evaluate or stage lesions of the esophagus, stomach, duodenum, pancreas, ampulla, biliary ducts, and rectum
- To evaluate submucosal tumors

PREPARATION
- Make sure that the patient has signed an appropriate consent form.
- Note and report all allergies.
- Fasting is required for 6 to 8 hours before the test.
- An I.V. sedative may be given to help the patient relax before the endoscope insertion.

Teaching points
- Explain the purpose of the test and how it's done.
- Tell the patient who will perform the test and where it will be done.
- Instruct the patient to fast for 6 to 8 hours before the test.
- For sigmoid endoscopic ultrasonography (EUS), inform the patient that the scope is inserted through the anus. He may have to take a laxative the evening before and may feel an urge to defecate during the study.
- Inform the patient that the test takes 30 to 90 minutes.
- If the patient received I.V. sedation, tell him to avoid alcohol and driving for 24 hours after the test.

KEY STEPS
- Confirm the patient's identity using two patient identifiers according to facility policy.
- Monitor the patient's vital signs during the procedure.
- Monitor oxygen saturation and cardiac rhythm if the patient receives I.V. sedation.
- Follow the procedures for esophagogastroduodenoscopy or sigmoidoscopy, depending on which type of EUS is to be performed.

POSTPROCEDURE CARE
- Monitor the patient's vital signs, level of consciousness, and cardiac rhythm.
- Monitor the patient for bleeding and signs and symptoms of perforation.
- Tell the patient to resume his usual diet and activity, as ordered.

PRECAUTIONS
- Esophageal stricture hinders passage of the endoscope.

COMPLICATIONS
- Perforation
- Bleeding

NORMAL RESULTS
- Anatomy is normal, with no evidence of tumor.

ABNORMAL RESULTS
- Results may show evidence of acute or chronic ulcers, benign or malignant tumors, or inflammatory disease.

Endoscopy

DESCRIPTION
- Shows the lining of a hollow viscus
- Mechanism: cablelike cluster of glass fibers in the endoscope transmits light into the viscus; image reflected to the scope's optical head or video monitor

PURPOSE
- To diagnose inflammatory, ulcerative, and infectious diseases
- To diagnose benign and malignant tumors and other mucosal lesions

PREPARATION
- Make sure that the patient has signed a consent form.
- Note and report all allergies.
- Give the patient an I.V. sedative to help him relax before the endoscope insertion.
- For the patient taking an anticoagulant, it may be necessary to adjust his drug dosage.

Teaching points
- Explain the purpose of the test and how it's done.
- Tell the patient who will perform the test and where it will be done.
- Advise the patient of any dietary and medication restrictions as ordered.
- Inform the patient that the test takes about 1 hour.

KEY STEPS
- Confirm the patient's identity using two patient identifiers according to facility policy.
- Start an I.V. line, if indicated.
- Monitor the patient's vital signs, pulse oximetry, and cardiac rhythm during the procedure.
- Follow the procedure for the specific endoscopy to be performed (such as arthroscopy, bronchoscopy, colonoscopy, colposcopy, cystourethroscopy, endoscopic retrograde cholangiopancreatography, esophagogastroduodenoscopy, hysteroscopy, laparoscopy, laryngoscopy, mediastinoscopy, proctosigmoidoscopy, sigmoidoscopy, or thoracoscopy).

POSTPROCEDURE CARE
- Provide a safe environment.
- Withhold food and fluids until the gag reflex returns.
- Monitor the patient's vital signs.
- Monitor the patient's respiratory and neurologic status.
- Monitor the patient's cardiac rhythm.
- Tell the patient to resume his usual medications and diet, as ordered.

PRECAUTIONS
- For high-risk procedures, stop warfarin for 3 to 5 days before the test; low-molecular-weight heparin may be ordered.
- Stop aspirin or nonsteroidal anti-inflammatory drugs 3 to 7 days before the study.

COMPLICATIONS
- Adverse reaction to sedation
- Cardiac arrhythmias
- Respiratory depression
- Bleeding

NORMAL RESULTS
- Refer to the specific endoscopy procedure.

ABNORMAL RESULTS
- Refer to the specific endoscopy procedure.

Enteroclysis

DESCRIPTION
◆ Fluoroscopic examination of the small bowel using a contrast medium
◆ Also called a *small-bowel enema*

PURPOSE
◆ To diagnose and evaluate Crohn's disease
◆ To diagnose Meckel's diverticulum
◆ To help diagnose small-bowel obstruction
◆ To detect tumors

PREPARATION
◆ Make sure that the patient has signed an appropriate consent form.
◆ Note and report all allergies.
◆ Give the patient a laxative the afternoon before the examination.
◆ Give the patient an I.V. sedative to help him relax.

Teaching points
◆ Explain the purpose of the test and how it's done.
◆ Tell the patient who will perform the test and where it will be done.
◆ Instruct the patient not to use peristalsis-inhibiting drugs (such as Demerol or Percodan) on the day of the test.
◆ Instruct the patient to restrict food and fluids, as instructed by the practitioner.
◆ Inform the patient that he'll be asked to change position frequently during the test.
◆ Inform the patient that the test takes about 45 minutes.

KEY STEPS
◆ Confirm the patient's identity using two patient identifiers according to facility policy.
◆ The patient is given a local anesthetic. A small-lumen catheter is then inserted through the nose or mouth.
◆ The catheter passes through the stomach and into the distal duodenum or jejunum.
◆ A contrast medium is instilled to distend and opacify the bowel loops.
◆ The patient may receive metoclopramide to facilitate peristalsis.
◆ Fluoroscopy and spot films are obtained.
◆ After the films are reviewed, the catheter is removed.

POSTPROCEDURE CARE
◆ Assist the patient to the bathroom to expel the barium.
◆ Monitor the patient's vital signs, intake and output, and feces.

PRECAUTIONS
◆ This test is contraindicated during pregnancy.
◆ Complete gastric or duodenal obstruction may interfere with accurate testing.

COMPLICATIONS
◆ Constipation
◆ Adverse reactions to sedation, if used

NORMAL RESULTS
◆ The size and contours of the small intestine are unremarkable.
◆ Contrast travels through the bowel at a normal rate without any sign of obstruction.
◆ Bowel loops and walls are visible and free from tumors, ulcers, and constrictions.

ABNORMAL RESULTS
◆ Anatomic abnormalities of the bowel loops, diameter, and wall thickness may indicate Crohn's disease, tumors, partial or complete bowel obstruction, Meckel's diverticula, or congenital disorders.

Epstein-Barr virus antibodies test

DESCRIPTION

- Two tests that detect antibodies to virus that causes heterophil-positive infectious mononucleosis, Burkitt's lymphoma, and nasopharyngeal carcinoma but doesn't replicate in standard cell cultures
- Monospot test: confirms most infections; tests serum for heterophil antibodies, which appear within the first 3 weeks of illness and then rapidly decline
- Negative monospot test results despite primary Epstein-Barr virus (EBV) infection in 10% of adults and a larger percentage of children
- EBV linked to lymphoproliferative processes in immunosuppressed patients, which occur with reactivated EBV infections and are also monospot-negative
- Indirect immunofluorescence: accurately measures specific EBV antibodies

PURPOSE

- To provide a laboratory diagnosis of heterophil — or monospot — negative cases of infectious mononucleosis
- To determine the antibody status to EBV of immunosuppressed patients with lymphoproliferative processes

PREPARATION

- No dietary restrictions are needed for the test.
- The test requires a blood sample.

Teaching points

- Explain the purpose of the test and how it's done.
- Tell the patient who will perform the test and where it will be done.
- Tell the patient that the test requires a blood sample.
- Explain that he may experience slight discomfort from the tourniquet and needle puncture.
- Tell the patient that no dietary restrictions are needed.
- Inform the patient that the test should take less than 5 minutes.

KEY STEPS

- Confirm the patient's identity using two patient identifiers according to facility policy.
- Perform a venipuncture and collect 5 ml of sterile blood in a clot-activator tube.
- Allow the blood to clot for at least 1 hour at room temperature.
- Transfer the serum to a sterile tube or vial and send it to the laboratory immediately.

POSTPROCEDURE CARE

- Apply direct pressure to the venipuncture site until bleeding stops.

PRECAUTIONS

- Maintain standard precautions while collecting the sample.
- Handle the sample gently to prevent hemolysis.
- If transfer can't occur immediately, store the serum at 39.2° F (4° C) for 1 or 2 days, or at –4° F (–20° C) for longer periods to prevent contamination.

COMPLICATIONS

- Hematoma at the venipuncture site

NORMAL RESULTS

- Sera from patients who have never been infected with EBV have no detectable antibodies to the virus, as measured by either the monospot test or the indirect immunofluorescence test.
- The monospot test result is positive only during the acute phase of infection with EBV; the indirect immunofluorescence test detects and discriminates between acute and past infection.

ABNORMAL RESULTS

- EBV infection can be ruled out if no antibodies to EBV antigens are detected in the indirect immunofluorescence test.
- A positive monospot test result or an indirect immunofluorescence test result that's positive for immunoglobulin (Ig) M or negative for Epstein-Barr nuclear antigen (EBNA) indicates acute EBV infection.
- A monospot-negative result doesn't necessarily rule out acute or past infection with EBV. Conversely, an IgG class antibody to viral capsid antigen and EBNA antigens (IgM-negative) indicates remote (more than 2 months) infection with EBV.
- Most cases of monospot-negative infectious mononucleosis are caused by cytomegalovirus infections.

Erythrocyte sedimentation rate test

DESCRIPTION
- Measures the degree of erythrocyte settling in a blood sample during a specified period
- Sensitive but nonspecific; commonly the earliest indicator of disease when other chemical or physical signs are normal
- Usually increases significantly in widespread inflammatory disorders; prolonged elevations may exist in localized inflammation and malignant disease

PURPOSE
- To monitor inflammatory or malignant disease
- To help detect and diagnose occult disease, such as tuberculosis, tissue necrosis, or connective tissue disease

PREPARATION
- This test requires a blood sample.
- No dietary restrictions are needed.

Teaching points
- Explain that the test evaluates the condition of red blood cells.
- Tell him who will perform the test and where it will be done.
- Tell him that the test requires a blood sample.
- Explain that he may feel slight discomfort from the tourniquet and needle puncture.
- Inform the patient that he need not restrict food and fluids.
- Tell him that the test should take less than 5 minutes.

KEY STEPS
- Confirm the patient's identity using two patient identifiers according to facility policy.
- Perform a venipuncture and collect the sample in a 4.5-ml tube with EDTA added or in a tube with sodium citrate added. (Check with the laboratory to determine its preference.)
- Completely fill the collection tube and invert it gently several times to thoroughly mix the sample and anticoagulant.
- Because prolonged standing decreases the erythrocyte sedimentation rate (ESR), examine the sample for clots or clumps and send it to the laboratory immediately. It must be tested within 2 to 4 hours.

POSTPROCEDURE CARE
- Make sure that subdermal bleeding has stopped before removing pressure.
- For a large hematoma at the venipuncture site, monitor pulses distal to the phlebotomy site.

PRECAUTIONS
- Maintain standard precautions while collecting the sample.
- Handle the sample gently to prevent hemolysis.

COMPLICATIONS
- Hematoma at the venipuncture site

NORMAL RESULTS
- In men, ESR is 0 to 10 mm/hour (SI, 0 to 10 mm/hour); in women, 0 to 20 mm/hour (SI, 0 to 20 mm/hour).
- The ESR gradually increases with age.

ABNORMAL RESULTS
- The ESR rises in pregnancy, anemia, acute or chronic inflammation, tuberculosis, paraproteinemias (especially multiple myeloma and Waldenström's macroglobulinemia), rheumatic fever, rheumatoid arthritis, and some cancers.
- Polycythemia, sickle cell anemia, hyperviscosity, and low plasma fibrinogen or globulin levels tend to lower the ESR.

Erythropoietin level test

OVERVIEW

DESCRIPTION
- Immunoassay that measures erythropoietin (EPO) to assess renal hormone production
- EPO secreted by liver in fetus, by kidney in adult
- EPO action: acts on stem cells in the bone marrow to stimulate production of red blood cells (RBCs); regulated by a feedback loop involving red cell volume and oxygen saturation of the blood, especially in the brain

PURPOSE
- To help diagnose anemia and polycythemia
- To help diagnose kidney tumors
- To detect EPO abuse by athletes

PREPARATION
- The patient must fast for 8 to 10 hours before the test.
- This test requires a blood sample.
- Keep the patient relaxed and recumbent for 30 minutes before the test.

Teaching points
- Explain that this test determines if hormonal secretion is causing changes in his RBCs.
- Tell him who will perform the test and where it will be done.
- Instruct the patient to fast for at least 8 hours before the test.
- Tell him that the test requires a blood sample.
- Explain that he may experience slight discomfort from the tourniquet and needle puncture.
- Inform him that the test takes about 45 minutes.

DIAGNOSTIC PROCEDURE

KEY STEPS
- Confirm the patient's identity using two patient identifiers according to facility policy.
- Perform a venipuncture and collect the sample in a 5-ml clot-activator tube.
- If requested, draw a hematocrit at the same time by collecting an additional sample in a 2-ml EDTA tube.

POSTPROCEDURE CARE
- Apply direct pressure to the venipuncture site until bleeding stops.

PRECAUTIONS
- Maintain standard precautions while collecting the sample.
- Handle the sample gently to prevent hemolysis.

COMPLICATIONS
- Hematoma at the venipuncture site

INTERPRETATION

NORMAL RESULTS
- EPO levels are 5 to 36 milliunits/ml (SI, 5 to 36 International Units/L).

ABNORMAL RESULTS
- Low levels of EPO appear in the patient with anemia who has inadequate or absent hormone production.
- Congenital absence of EPO can occur.
- Severe renal disease may decrease EPO production.
- Elevated EPO levels occur in anemias as a compensatory mechanism in the reestablishment of homeostasis.
- Inappropriate elevations (when the hematocrit is normal to high) occur in polycythemia and EPO-secreting tumors.
- Some athletes use EPO to enhance performance. The increased RBC volume conveys additional oxygen-carrying capacity to the blood. Adverse reactions include clotting abnormalities, headache, seizures, hypertension, nausea, vomiting, diarrhea, and rash. An elevated blood EPO level is highly suspicious of EPO abuse. A urine EPO test is the only method available to test for recombinant EPO and determine if an athlete is using EPO illegally.

Esophageal acidity test

DESCRIPTION
- Sensitive indicator of gastric reflux
- Indicated for patients who complain of persistent heartburn with or without regurgitation
- Measures esophageal sphincter pressure
- Newer method being developed (see *Monitoring pH with the Bravo system*)

PURPOSE
- To evaluate the competence of the lower esophageal sphincter
- To measure intraesophageal pH

PREPARATION
- Make sure that the patient has signed an appropriate consent form.
- Note and report all allergies.
- Withhold antacids, anticholinergics, cholinergics, adrenergic-receptor blockers, alcohol, corticosteroids, histamine-2 receptor antagonists, proton pump inhibitors, and reserpine for 24 hours before the test.

Teaching points
- Explain the purpose of the test and how it's done.
- Tell the patient who will perform the test and where it will be done.
- Instruct the patient to fast and avoid smoking after midnight before the test.
- Tell him which, if any, medications he should withhold before the test.
- Warn the patient that he might experience slight discomfort and may cough or gag during the passage of a tube through his mouth and into the stomach.
- Inform the patient that the test takes about 45 minutes.

KEY STEPS
- Confirm the patient's identity using two patient identifiers according to facility policy.
- The patient is placed in high Fowler's position.
- A catheter, with a pH electrode, is inserted into the mouth and advanced to the lower esophageal sphincter.
- The patient performs Valsalva's maneuver or lifts his legs to stimulate reflux.
- The intraesophageal pH is determined.

POSTPROCEDURE CARE
- Provide soothing lozenges for sore throat.
- Clamp the catheter before removing it to prevent aspiration.
- Tell the patient to resume his diet and medications, as ordered.

PRECAUTIONS
WARNING *During insertion, the catheter may enter the trachea; if respiratory distress or paroxysmal coughing occurs, clamp the catheter and remove it immediately.*

COMPLICATIONS
- Aspiration of gastric contents
- Respiratory distress

NORMAL RESULTS
- Esophageal pH is greater than 5.0.

ABNORMAL RESULTS
- An intra-esophageal pH of 1.5 to 2.0 indicates gastric acid reflux caused by incompetence of the lower esophageal sphincter.

Monitoring pH with the Bravo system

Traditional testing for esophageal acid levels typically uses an esophageal catheter that's inserted for a 24-hour period. Recently, a new technique called the *Bravo pH monitoring system* was developed to measure acid levels in the esophagus via a capsule (about the size of a gel cap). The capsule is temporarily attached to the patient's esophageal wall using an endoscope and collects pH data, which are transmitted to a pager-sized receiver that the patient wears. Data are collected for 48 hours, downloaded from the receiver, and analyzed with special software.

The Bravo method is more accurate than catheter methods because the patient can eat normally and maintain regular activities during testing. The additional 24 hours also provides more information for diagnosing certain esophageal disorders.

In 7 to 10 days, the capsule spontaneously detaches from the esophageal wall and is passed through the patient's digestive system.

Esophagogastroduodenoscopy

DESCRIPTION
◆ Visual examination of the lining of the esophagus, stomach, and upper duodenum using a flexible fiber-optic endoscope

PURPOSE
◆ To detect small or surface lesions missed by radiography
◆ To diagnose inflammatory disease, tumors, ulcers, and structural abnormalities
◆ To evaluate the stomach and duodenum postoperatively
◆ To obtain specimens for laboratory evaluation
◆ To allow for the removal of foreign bodies by suction, snare, or forceps

PREPARATION
◆ Note and report all allergies.
◆ Fasting is required for 6 to 12 hours before the test.
◆ Remove the patient's dentures.
◆ Insert a mouth guard to protect the patient's teeth from the endoscope.
◆ Make sure the patient has a patent I.V. line.

Teaching points
◆ Explain the purpose of the test and how it's done.
◆ Tell the patient who will perform the test and where it will be done.
◆ Instruct the patient to fast for 6 to 12 hours before the test.
◆ Tell him that a flexible tube will be inserted through his mouth.
◆ Explain that a bitter-tasting local anesthetic will be sprayed into the mouth and throat to suppress the gag reflex.
◆ Tell the patient that he'll receive an I.V. line to allow administration of a sedative or I.V. fluids.
◆ Explain that he'll remain conscious during the procedure.
◆ Inform the patient that the test takes about 30 minutes.

DIAGNOSTIC PROCEDURE

KEY STEPS
◆ Confirm the patient's identity using two patient identifiers according to facility policy.
◆ Monitor the patient's vital signs, cardiac rhythm, and pulse oximetry during the procedure.
◆ When emergency esophagogastroduodenoscopy (EGD) is performed, the stomach contents are first aspirated through a nasogastric tube.
◆ Assist the patient into a left lateral position.
◆ The endoscope is inserted into the mouth and advanced under direct vision to examine the esophagus and cardiac sphincter, the stomach, and the duodenum.
◆ Air may be instilled to open the bowel lumen and flatten tissue folds.
◆ The endoscope is slowly withdrawn and suspicious areas are reexamined.
◆ Tissue specimens are sent to the laboratory for analysis.

POSTPROCEDURE CARE
◆ Provide a safe environment until the patient has recovered from sedation.
◆ Withhold food and fluids until the gag reflex returns.
◆ Provide throat lozenges and warm saline gargles for sore throat.
◆ Monitor the patient's vital signs, cardiac rhythm, and intake and output.
◆ Instruct the patient not to consume alcohol, operate machinery, or drive for 24 hours after I.V. sedation.
◆ Tell him to report persistent difficult swallowing, pain, fever, black feces, or bloody vomitus.
◆ Explain that belching of insufflated air after the test is normal, as is a sore throat for 3 to 4 days.

PRECAUTIONS
◆ The procedure is contraindicated in patients with Zenker's diverticulum, a large aortic aneurysm, a recent ulcer perforation, known or suspected viscus perforation, or an unstable cardiac or pulmonary condition.

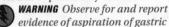 **WARNING** *Observe for and report evidence of aspiration of gastric*

contents, which could precipitate aspiration pneumonia.

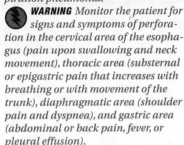 **WARNING** *Monitor the patient for signs and symptoms of perforation in the cervical area of the esophagus (pain upon swallowing and neck movement), thoracic area (substernal or epigastric pain that increases with breathing or with movement of the trunk), diaphragmatic area (shoulder pain and dyspnea), and gastric area (abdominal or back pain, fever, or pleural effusion).*
◆ Observe patient closely for adverse reactions to drugs; have emergency resuscitation equipment handy.
◆ EGD shouldn't be performed within 2 days after an upper GI series; barium can obscure visual examination.

COMPLICATIONS
◆ Adverse reaction to sedation
◆ Aspiration of gastric contents
◆ Aspiration pneumonia
◆ Perforation of the esophagus, stomach, or duodenum

INTERPRETATION

NORMAL RESULTS
◆ The esophageal mucosa is smooth and yellow-pink with fine vascular markings.
◆ The gastric mucosa is orange-red beginning at the Z line, slightly above the esophagogastric junction.
◆ Rugae are present in the stomach.
◆ The duodenal bulb mucosa is reddish and marked by a few shallow longitudinal folds.
◆ The distal duodenum has prominent circular folds lined with villi.

ABNORMAL RESULTS
◆ Anatomic abnormalities of the stomach and duodenum suggest acute or chronic ulcers, benign or malignant tumors, or diverticula.
◆ Inflammatory changes suggest esophagitis, gastritis, and duodenitis.
◆ Anatomic abnormalities of the esophagus suggest tumors, varices, Mallory-Weiss syndrome, esophageal hiatal hernia, and stenoses.

Estrogen test

DESCRIPTION

◆ Radioimmunoassay that measures estradiol, estrone, and estriol levels (only estrogens appearing in serum in measurable amounts)
◆ Diagnosis confirmed by tests of hypothalamic-pituitary function
◆ Hormone secreted by ovaries; influenced by pituitary gonadotropins, follicle-stimulating hormone (FSH), and luteinizing hormone (LH)
◆ Interacts with hypothalamic-pituitary axis through negative and positive feedback mechanisms (slowly rising or sustained high levels inhibit secretion of FSH and LH [negative feedback], but a rapid rise in estrogen just before ovulation seems to stimulate LH secretion [positive feedback])
◆ Responsible for development of secondary sexual characteristics in women and for normal menstruation; levels undetectable in children
◆ Secreted by ovarian follicular cells during the first half of the menstrual cycle and by the corpus luteum during the luteal phase and during pregnancy
◆ Constant low-level secretion in menopause

PURPOSE

◆ To determine sexual maturation and fertility
◆ To help diagnose gonadal dysfunction, such as precocious or delayed puberty, menstrual disorders (especially amenorrhea), and infertility
◆ To determine fetal well-being
◆ To help diagnose tumors known to secrete estrogen

PREPARATION

◆ No dietary restrictions are needed.
◆ This test requires a blood sample.
◆ Withhold all steroid and pituitary-based hormones. Note on the laboratory request form if the patient must continue them.

Teaching points

◆ Explain that this test helps determine whether secretion of female hormones is normal and that it may repeated during the various phases of the menstrual cycle.
◆ Tell the patient who will perform the test and where it will be done.
◆ Tell her that no dietary restrictions are needed.
◆ Tell her that the test requires a blood sample.
◆ Explain that she may experience slight discomfort from the tourniquet and needle puncture.
◆ Inform the patient that the test should take less than 5 minutes.

KEY STEPS

◆ Confirm the patient's identity using two patient identifiers according to facility policy.
◆ Perform a venipuncture and collect the sample in a 10-ml clot-activator tube.
◆ If the patient is premenopausal, indicate the phase of her menstrual cycle on the laboratory request.
◆ Send the sample to the laboratory immediately.

POSTPROCEDURE CARE

◆ Apply direct pressure to the venipuncture site until bleeding stops.
◆ Instruct the patient that she may resume her medications.

PRECAUTIONS

◆ Handle the sample gently to prevent hemolysis.
◆ Maintain standard precautions while collecting the sample.

COMPLICATIONS

◆ Hematoma at the venipuncture site

NORMAL RESULTS

◆ For premenopausal women, the estrogen level is 26 to 149 pg/ml (SI, 90 to 550 pmol/L).
◆ For postmenopausal women, the level is 0 to 34 pg/ml (SI, 0 to 125 pmol/L).
◆ In men, the estrogen level is 12 to 34 pg/ml (SI, 40 to 125 pmol/L).
◆ In children younger than age 6, the level is 3 to 10 pg/ml (SI, 10 to 36 pmol/L).
◆ In pregnant women, the estriol level is 2 ng/ml (SI, 7 nmol/L) by 30 weeks' gestation to 30 ng/ml (SI, 105 nmol/L) by week 40.

ABNORMAL RESULTS

◆ Decreased levels may indicate primary hypogonadism, or ovarian failure, such as in Turner's syndrome or ovarian agenesis; secondary hypogonadism, such as in hypopituitarism; or menopause.
◆ Increased levels may occur with estrogen-producing tumors; in precocious puberty; in severe hepatic disease, such as cirrhosis; and in congenital adrenal hyperplasia.

⬢ **INTERFERING FACTORS** *Pregnancy and pretest use of estrogens, such as hormonal contraceptives, may increase values.*

Ethanol level test

DESCRIPTION

◆ By-product after alcohol ingestion; occurs in the blood, urine, and saliva
◆ Amount in blood dependent on sex, weight, and the time since the last drink (see *Blood alcohol chart*)
◆ Can cause depression of the central nervous system (CNS) and lead to coma and death
◆ Testing sample of choice: blood
◆ Can also test urine or gastric contents or use breath analysis

PURPOSE

◆ To evaluate suspected alcohol-impaired driving
◆ To determine a possible cause of unknown coma
◆ To screen for alcoholism
◆ To monitor ethanol treatment of methanol intoxication

PREPARATION

◆ Follow your facility's policy if the specimen is to be used for legal purposes.
◆ Have the patient sign a consent form, if required.
◆ The test requires a blood sample.
◆ Clean the site with a non–alcohol-based solution such as povidone-iodine.

Teaching points

◆ Explain to the patient that this test will measure the alcohol level in his blood.
◆ Tell the patient who will perform the test and where it will be done.
◆ Tell the patient that no dietary restrictions are needed.
◆ Inform the patient that he may experience slight discomfort from the tourniquet and needle puncture.
◆ Inform the patient that the test should take less than 5 minutes.

Blood alcohol chart

The following charts show the relationship among the number of alcoholic drinks, the person's weight, and his probable level of impairment.

MALES
Approximate blood alcohol percentage

Drinks*	BODY WEIGHT IN POUNDS								Effect on person
	100	120	140	160	180	200	220	240	
0	.00	.00	.00	.00	.00	.00	.00	.00	Only safe driving limit
1	.04	.03	.03	.02	.02	.02	.02	.02	Impairment begins.
2	.08	.06	.05	.05	.04	.04	.03	.03	
3	.11	.09	.08	.07	.06	.06	.05	.05	Driving skills significantly affected.
4	.15	.12	.11	.09	.08	.08	.07	.06	
5	.19	.16	.13	.12	.11	.09	.09	.08	**Criminal penalties in most states
6	.23	.19	.16	.14	.13	.11	.10	.09	
7	.26	.22	.19	.16	.15	.13	.12	.11	Legally intoxicated.
8	.30	.25	.21	.19	.17	.15	.14	.13	Criminal penalties in ALL states
9	.34	.28	.24	.21	.19	.17	.15	.14	
10	.38	.31	.27	.23	.21	.19	.17	.16	

FEMALES
Approximate blood alcohol percentage

Drinks*	BODY WEIGHT IN POUNDS									Effect on person
	90	100	120	140	160	180	200	220	240	
0	.00	.00	.00	.00	.00	.00	.00	.00	.00	Only safe driving limit
1	.05	.05	.04	.03	.03	.03	.02	.02	.02	Impairment begins.
2	.10	.09	.08	.07	.06	.05	.05	.04	.04	
3	.15	.14	.11	.11	.09	.08	.07	.06	.06	Driving skills significantly affected.
4	.20	.18	.15	.13	.11	.10	.09	.08	.08	
5	.25	.23	.19	.16	.14	.13	.11	.10	.09	**Criminal penalties in most states
6	.30	.27	.23	.19	.17	.15	.14	.12	.11	Legally intoxicated.
7	.35	.32	.27	.23	.20	.18	.16	.14	.13	
8	.40	.36	.30	.26	.23	.20	.18	.17	.15	Criminal penalties in ALL states
9	.45	.41	.34	.29	.26	.23	.20	.19	.17	
10	.51	.45	.38	.32	.28	.25	.23	.21	.19	

Subtract 0.01% for each 40 minutes of drinking.

*One drink is equal to 1¼ oz of 80-proof liquor, 12 oz of beer, or 4 oz of table wine.

Source: *www.ou.edu/oupd/bac.htm*

DIAGNOSTIC PROCEDURE

KEY STEPS
◆ Confirm the patient's identity using two patient identifiers according to facility policy.
◆ Perform a venipuncture and collect 5 ml of blood in a sodium fluoride tube.
◆ Carefully label the tube with your initials and the date and time of collection.

POSTPROCEDURE CARE
◆ Apply pressure to the venipuncture site until bleeding stops.
◆ Obtain the signature of a witness, if required by your facility or for legal purposes.

PRECAUTIONS
◆ Carefully follow all legal and facility policies during specimen collection.

COMPLICATIONS
◆ Hematoma at the venipuncture site

INTERPRETATION

NORMAL RESULTS
◆ A negative result is a level below 10 mg/dl (SI, < 2 mmol/L).
◆ The U.S. Department of Transportation considers levels below 20 mg/dl (SI, < 4.34 mmol/L) as negative.
◆ Signs of intoxication with normal results may indicate a serious medical problem and should be evaluated immediately.

ABNORMAL RESULTS
◆ A positive result is a level over 40 mg/dl (SI, 8.68 mmol/L).
◆ Most states' drunk driving laws consider a positive result to be a level over 80 mg/dl (SI, > 17.4 mmol/L).
◆ Flushing, decreased reflexes, and impaired visual acuity occur in patients with ethanol levels of 50 to 100 mg/dl (SI, 10.8 to 21.7 mmol/L).
◆ CNS depression is noted with levels over 100 mg/dl (SI, > 21.7 mmol/L).
◆ Coma usually occurs when levels exceed 300 mg/dl (SI, > 64.8 mmol/L).
◆ Death may occur when levels exceed 400 mg/dl (SI, > 86.4 mmol/L).

Evoked potential studies

DESCRIPTION

◆ Measures the brain's electrical response to stimulation of the sensory organs or peripheral nerves
◆ Evaluates visual, somatosensory, and auditory nerve pathways
◆ Involves electronic impulses detected and recorded by electrodes attached to the scalp and skin over various peripheral sensory nerves
◆ Low-amplitude impulses extracted by computer from background brain wave activity; signals averaged from repeated stimuli (see *Visual evoked potentials*)
◆ Can be used during therapeutic coma and in patients with traumatic brain injury

PURPOSE

◆ To help diagnose nervous system lesions and abnormalities
◆ To monitor spinal cord function during spinal surgery
◆ To assess neurologic function
◆ To evaluate neurologic function in infants
◆ To monitor comatose or anesthetized patients

PREPARATION

◆ Make sure that the patient or responsible family member has signed a consent form.
◆ Note and report all allergies.
◆ Provide reassurance to the patient that the electrodes won't hurt, but that he may feel a small shock when somatosensory evoked responses occur.
◆ Encourage the patient to relax because tension can affect the test results.

Teaching points

◆ Explain the purpose of the test and how it's done.
◆ Tell the patient who will perform the test and where it will be done.
◆ Inform the patient that the test takes about 45 to 60 minutes.

Visual evoked potentials

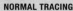

VISUAL (PATTERN-SHIFT) EVOKED POTENTIALS

In the visual (pattern-shift) evoked potentials test, visual neural impulses are recorded as they travel along the pathway from the eye to the occipital cortex. Wave P100 is the most significant component of the resultant waveform. Normal P100 latency is about 100 msec after the application of a visual stimulus, as shown in the top diagram. Increased P100 latency, shown in the bottom diagram, is an abnormal finding, indicating a lesion along the visual pathway.

NORMAL TRACING

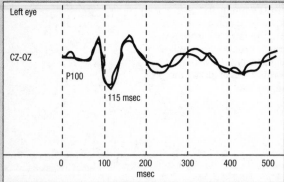

TRACING IN MULTIPLE SCLEROSIS

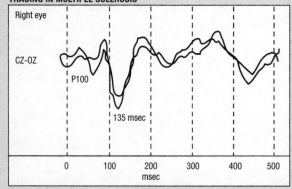

Key: CZ = vertex; OZ = midocciput

KEY STEPS

- Confirm the patient's identity using two patient identifiers according to facility policy.
- The patient is positioned in a reclining or straight-backed chair or on a bed.
- The patient is asked to relax and remain still.
- Depending on the specific type of evoked potential study, electrodes may be attached.
- Visual evoked potentials, produced by exposing the eye to a rapidly reversing checkerboard pattern, help evaluate demyelinating disease (such as multiple sclerosis), traumatic injury, and puzzling visual complaints.
- Somatosensory evoked potentials, produced by electrically stimulating a peripheral sensory nerve, help diagnose peripheral nerve disease and locate brain and spinal cord lesions.
- Auditory brain stem evoked potentials, produced by delivering clicks to the ear, are used in locating auditory lesions and evaluating brain stem integrity when cranial nerve testing is inconclusive or can't be performed.
- A computer amplifies and averages the brain's response to each stimulus and plots the results as a waveform.

POSTPROCEDURE CARE

- Monitor the patient's response to testing.

PRECAUTIONS

- None

COMPLICATIONS

- None

NORMAL RESULTS

- In visual evoked potential testing, the most significant wave on the waveform is P100, a positive wave appearing about 100 msec after the pattern-shift stimulus is applied.
- Normal results vary greatly among laboratories and patients.
- In somatosensory evoked potential testing, the waveforms vary, depending on locations of the stimulating and recording electrodes.

ABNORMAL RESULTS

- In visual evoked potential testing, abnormal (extended) P100 latencies confined to one eye suggest a visual pathway lesion anterior to the optic chiasm; bilateral abnormal P100 latencies suggest multiple sclerosis.
- In somatosensory evoked potential testing, changes in the electrical waveforms may indicate damaged or degenerated nerve pathways to the brain from the eyes, ears, or limbs. Absence of activity in a pathway may mean complete loss of nerve function in that pathway.
- Other changes may provide evidence of the type and location of nerve damage.
- Abnormal upper-limb interwave latencies suggest possible cervical spondylosis, intracerebral lesions, or sensorimotor neuropathies.
- Abnormalities in the lower limb suggest peripheral nerve and root lesions such as those in Guillain-Barré syndrome.

Excretory urography

OVERVIEW

DESCRIPTION
- Allows imaging of the renal parenchyma, calyces, and pelvis as well as the ureters, bladder, and sometimes the urethra after I.V. administration of a contrast medium
- Also known as *intravenous pyelography*

PURPOSE
- To evaluate the structure and excretory function of the kidneys, ureters, and bladder
- To support a differential diagnosis of renovascular hypertension

PREPARATION
- Make sure that the patient has signed an appropriate consent form.
- Note and report all allergies.
- Check the patient's history for hypersensitivity to iodine, iodine-containing foods, or iodinated contrast media.
- Fasting is required for 8 hours before the test.
- Give a laxative, if necessary, the night before the test.
- Obtain and report any abnormal results of renal function testing, such as blood urea nitrogen and creatinine.

Teaching points
- Explain the purpose of the test and how it's done.
- Tell the patient who will perform the test and where it will be done.
- Instruct the patient to fast for at least 8 hours before the test.
- Warn the patient that he might experience a transient burning sensation and metallic taste with injection of the contrast agent.
- Inform him that the test takes 30 to 45 minutes.

DIAGNOSTIC PROCEDURE

KEY STEPS
- Confirm the patient's identity using two patient identifiers according to facility policy.
- The patient is assisted into a supine position.
- A kidney-ureter-bladder X-ray is performed.
- I.V. contrast medium is injected.
- X-rays are obtained at regular intervals.
- Ureteral compression is performed after the 5-minute film to facilitate retention of the contrast medium by the upper urinary tract.
- After the 10-minute film, ureteral compression is released.
- Another film is taken of the lower halves of both ureters and bladder.
- The patient is asked to void and final films are taken immediately to show residual bladder contents or mucosal abnormalities of the bladder or urethra.

POSTPROCEDURE CARE
- Observe the patient for delayed reactions to the contrast medium.
- Continue I.V. fluids or provide oral fluids to promote hydration.
- If the patient has pyelonephritis, he may have to take antibiotics.

PRECAUTIONS
- The test is contraindicated in patients with abnormal renal function and in children and the elderly with actual or potential dehydration.

COMPLICATIONS
- Adverse reaction to the contrast medium
- Dehydration
- Impaired renal function

INTERPRETATION

NORMAL RESULTS
- Kidneys, ureters, and bladder show no gross evidence of soft- or hard-tissue lesions.
- Visualization of the contrast medium in the kidneys occurs promptly.
- Bilateral renal parenchyma and pelvicaliceal systems have normal conformity.
- There's no postvoiding mucosal abnormality and little residual urine.

ABNORMAL RESULTS
- Anatomic abnormalities may suggest renal and ureteral calculi; supernumerary or absent kidney; polycystic kidney disease; redundant pelvis or ureter; space-occupying lesions or tumors; renal, bladder, or ureteral hematoma, laceration, or trauma; or hydronephrosis.

External fetal monitoring

DESCRIPTION

♦ Uses an electronic transducer and a cardiotachometer to amplify and record fetal heart rate (FHR) while a pressure-sensitive transducer (tocodynamometer) records uterine contractions (see *Understanding fetal monitoring terminology*)
♦ Records baseline FHR (average FHR over two contraction cycles or 10 minutes), periodic fluctuations in the baseline FHR, and beat-to-beat heart rate variability
♦ Also used during other tests of fetal health, notably the nonstress test and the contraction stress test (CST)

PURPOSE

♦ To measure FHR and the frequency of uterine contractions
♦ To evaluate antepartum and intrapartum fetal health during stress and nonstress situations
♦ To detect fetal distress
♦ To determine the necessity for internal fetal monitoring

Understanding fetal monitoring terminology

♦ Baseline fetal heart rate (FHR): Average FHR over two contraction cycles or 10 minutes
♦ Baseline changes: Fluctuations in FHR unrelated to uterine contractions
♦ Periodic changes: Fluctuations in FHR related to uterine contractions
♦ Amplitude: Difference in beats per minute between baseline readings and fluctuation in FHR
♦ Recovery time: Difference between the end of the contraction and the return to the baseline FHR
♦ Acceleration: Transient rise in FHR lasting longer than 15 seconds and related to a uterine contraction
♦ Deceleration: Transient fall in FHR related to a uterine contraction
♦ Lag time: Difference between the peak of the contraction and the lowest point of deceleration

---

PREPARATION

♦ If the monitoring is to be done antepartum, give the patient a meal just before the test.

Teaching points

♦ Explain that external fetal monitoring assesses fetal health.
♦ Explain the procedure to the patient and answer her questions. Assure her that external fetal monitoring is painless and won't hurt the fetus or interfere with normal labor.
♦ Tell the patient who will perform the test and where it will be done.
♦ If monitoring is to occur antepartum, instruct the patient to eat a meal just before the test to increase fetal activity, which decreases the test time.
♦ If the patient is still smoking, advise her to abstain for 2 hours before testing because smoking decreases fetal activity.
♦ Explain that she may have to restrict movement during baseline readings but that she may change position between the readings.
♦ Inform the patient that the test takes about 1 hour.

KEY STEPS

♦ Confirm the patient's identity using two patient identifiers according to facility policy.
♦ Place the patient in the semi-Fowler or left lateral position with her abdomen exposed. Cover the ultrasound transducer receiver crystal with ultrasound transmission jelly.
♦ Palpate the patient's abdomen to identify the fetal chest area and locate the most distinct fetal heart sounds; secure the ultrasound transducer over the area with the elastic band, stockinette, or abdominal strap.
♦ Check the recording equipment to ensure an adequate printout and verify the alarm boundaries of the fetal monitor.
♦ During monitoring, check the elastic band, stockinette, or abdominal strap to make sure that the fit is comfortable yet tight enough to produce a good tracing.
♦ As labor progresses, reposition the pressure transducer as necessary so that it remains on the fundal portion of the uterus.
♦ Reposition the ultrasound transducer whenever fetal or maternal position changes.

For antepartum monitoring with nonstress tests

♦ Ask the patient to hold the pressure transducer in her hand and to push it each time she feels the fetus move.
♦ Within a 20-minute period, monitor baseline FHR until you record two fetal movements that last longer than 15 seconds each and cause heart rate accelerations of more than 15 beats/minute from the baseline. If you can't obtain two FHR accelerations within 30 minutes, gently shake the patient's abdomen to stimulate the fetus and repeat the test.

For antepartum monitoring with a CST

♦ Induce contractions by oxytocin infusion or nipple stimulation (endogenous oxytocin).
♦ When giving oxytocin, infuse a dilute solution at 1 milliunit/minute, increasing the oxytocin rate until the patient experiences three contractions within 10 minutes, each lasting longer than 45 seconds.
♦ When using nipple stimulation, tell the patient to stimulate one nipple by hand until contractions begin. If a second contraction doesn't occur in 2 minutes, have her stimulate the nipple again. Stimulate both nipples if contractions don't occur in 15 minutes. Continue the test until contractions occur in 10 minutes.
♦ If no decelerations occur during three contractions, the patient may be discharged. Late decelerations during any of the contractions require the practitioner to be notified and further testing.
♦ Repeat antepartum monitoring weekly as long as indications, such as pregnancy over 42 weeks' gestation or fetal growth retardation, persist.

(continued)

For intrapartum monitoring

♦ Secure the pressure transducer with an elastic band, a stockinette, or an abdominal strap over the area of greatest uterine electrical activity during contractions (usually the fundus).
♦ Adjust the machine to record 0 to 10 mm Hg of pressure between palpable contractions.
♦ Reposition the ultrasound and pressure transducers as necessary to ensure continuous accurate readings. Review the tracings frequently for baseline abnormalities, periodic changes, variability of changes, and uterine contraction abnormalities.
♦ Record maternal movement, administration of drugs, and procedures performed directly on the tracing to assist in the evaluation of changes in the tracing.
♦ Report abnormalities immediately.

POSTPROCEDURE CARE

♦ Answer the patient's questions about the test.

PRECAUTIONS

♦ Properly ground all electrical equipment to prevent interference.

COMPLICATIONS

♦ Fetal distress with oxytocin infusion or nipple stimulation

INTERPRETATION

NORMAL RESULTS

♦ FHR may range from 120 to 160 beats/minute, with a variability of 5 to 25 beats/minute.
♦ *Antepartum nonstress test:* If two fetal movements cause a heart rate acceleration of more than 15 beats/minute from baseline in a 20-minute period, then the fetus is considered healthy and should remain so for another week .
♦ *Nonstress test:* A normal, healthy fetus usually has three rises in FHR within 10 to 15 minutes, but fetuses may sleep up to 45 minutes at a time. If there's no change in FHR in a 10-minute period, consider shaking the patient's abdomen gently, clapping loudly, or having the patient drink ice water or apple juice. If the FHR remains unchanged, a contraction stress test or biophysical profile test should be ordered. The fetus is assessed by watching fetal movements, muscle tone, fetal breathing, and the amniotic fluid index.
♦ *CST:* The fetus is assumed to be healthy and should remain so for another week if three contractions occur during a 10-minute period, with no late decelerations.

ABNORMAL RESULTS

♦ Bradycardia (FHR less than 120 beats/minute) may indicate fetal heart block, malposition, or hypoxia. Fetal bradycardia may also be drug induced.
♦ Tachycardia (FHR greater than 160 beats/minute) may result from maternal fever, tachycardia, hyperthyroidism, or use of vagolytic drugs or opioids; early fetal hypoxia; or fetal infection or arrhythmia.
♦ Decreased variability (a fluctuation of less than 5 beats/minute in the FHR) may indicate fetal arrhythmia or heart block; fetal hypoxia, central nervous system malformation, or infections; or vagolytic drugs.

♦ FHR accelerations may result from early hypoxia. They may precede or follow variable decelerations and may indicate that the fetus is in a breech position.
♦ *Antepartum nonstress test:* A positive result (fewer than two accelerations of FHR that last longer than 15 seconds each, with a heart rate acceleration of over 15 beats/minute) indicates an increased risk of perinatal morbidity and mortality and usually requires a CST.
♦ *CST:* Persistent late decelerations during two or more contractions may indicate an increased risk of fetal morbidity or mortality.
♦ Hyperstimulation (long or frequent uterine contractions) or suspicious results require biophysical profile assessment.
♦ If findings are unsatisfactory, cesarean delivery may be indicated.

Extractable nuclear antigen antibodies test

DESCRIPTION

- Extractable nuclear antigen: a complex of at least four antigens
- Ribonucleoprotein (RNP), degraded by ribonuclease
- Smith (Sm) antigen, an acidic nuclear protein that resists RNP degradation
- Sjögren's syndrome A (SS-A) antigen and Sjögren's syndrome B (SS-B) antigen, which form a precipitate when antibody is present
- Associated with certain autoimmune disorders
- RNP antibodies: associated with systemic lupus erythematous (SLE), progressive systemic sclerosis, and other rheumatic disorders
- Anti-Sm antibodies: specific markers for SLE
- Sjögren's antibodies: produced in Sjögren's syndrome

PURPOSE

- To aid in the differential diagnosis of autoimmune diseases
- To distinguish between anti-RNP and anti-Sm antibodies
- To screen for anti-RNP antibodies
- To screen for anti-Sm antibodies
- To support the diagnosis of collagen vascular autoimmune diseases
- To monitor the patient's response to therapy

PREPARATION

- No dietary restrictions are needed for the test.
- This test requires a blood sample.

Teaching points

- Explain that this test helps detect certain antibodies and will help determine a diagnosis and treatment.
- Tell the patient who will perform the test and where it will be done.
- Tell the patient that no dietary restrictions are needed.
- Inform the patient that the test requires a blood sample.
- Explain that he may experience slight discomfort from the tourniquet and needle puncture.
- Inform the patient that the test should take less than 5 minutes.

KEY STEPS

- Confirm the patient's identity using two patient identifiers according to facility policy.
- Perform a venipuncture and collect the sample in a 7-ml tube without additives.

POSTPROCEDURE CARE

- Apply direct pressure to the venipuncture site until bleeding stops.
- Because a patient with an autoimmune disease has a compromised immune system, check the venipuncture site for infection and report changes immediately.
- Keep a clean, dry bandage over the site for at least 24 hours.

PRECAUTIONS

- Maintain standard precautions while collecting the sample.
- Send the sample to the laboratory immediately.

COMPLICATIONS

- Hematoma at the venipuncture site

NORMAL RESULTS

- Serum should be negative for anti-RNP, anti-Sm, and SS-B antibodies.

ABNORMAL RESULTS

- Anti-RNP antibodies are elevated in SLE and in mixed connective tissue diseases.
- Anti-Sm antibodies are specific for SLE.
- Anti-SS-A and anti-SS-B antibodies are elevated in Sjögren's syndrome.
- Anti-SS-B antibodies are also elevated in SLE.

Fasting plasma glucose level test

OVERVIEW

DESCRIPTION
◆ Measures plasma glucose levels after a 12- to 14-hour fast
◆ With absence or deficiency of insulin glucose levels persistently high in patients with diabetes mellitus

PURPOSE
◆ To screen for diabetes mellitus
◆ To monitor drug or diet therapy in patients with diabetes mellitus

PREPARATION
◆ The patient must fast for 12 to 14 hours before the test.
◆ This test requires a blood sample.
◆ Notify the laboratory and practitioner of medications the patient is taking that may affect test results; it may be necessary to restrict them.

Teaching points
◆ Explain that this test detects disorders of glucose metabolism and helps diagnose diabetes.
◆ Tell the patient who will perform the test and where it will be done.
◆ Instruct him to fast for at least 12 hours before the test.
◆ Tell the patient that the test requires a blood sample.
◆ Explain that he may experience slight discomfort from the tourniquet and needle puncture.
◆ Alert him to the symptoms of hypoglycemia (weakness, restlessness, nervousness, hunger, sweating) and tell him to report such symptoms immediately.
◆ Inform the patient that the test should take less than 5 minutes.

DIAGNOSTIC PROCEDURE

KEY STEPS
◆ Confirm the patient's identity using two patient identifiers according to facility policy.
◆ Perform a venipuncture and collect the sample in a 5-ml clot-activator tube.
◆ Note on the laboratory request when the patient last ate, when the sample was collected, and when the patient received the last pretest dose of insulin or oral antidiabetic drug (if applicable).

POSTPROCEDURE CARE
◆ Apply direct pressure to the venipuncture site until bleeding stops.
◆ Provide a balanced meal or a snack.
◆ Tell the patient to resume his usual medications that were stopped.

PRECAUTIONS
◆ Maintain standard precautions while collecting the sample.
◆ Send the sample to the laboratory immediately.

COMPLICATIONS
◆ Hematoma at the venipuncture site

INTERPRETATION

NORMAL RESULTS
◆ Results vary according to the laboratory procedure.
◆ After at least an 8-hour fast, 70 to 100 mg of true glucose per deciliter of blood (SI, 3.9 to 5.6 mmol/L).

ABNORMAL RESULTS
◆ Levels of 126 mg/dl (SI, 7 mmol/L) or more, obtained on two or more occasions, confirm diabetes mellitus.
◆ Borderline or transient increased levels require a 2 hour after-meal plasma glucose test or oral glucose tolerance test to confirm the diagnosis of diabetes.
◆ Increased levels may indicate pancreatitis, recent acute illness (myocardial infarction), Cushing's syndrome, acromegaly, and pheochromocytoma.
◆ Increased fasting plasma glucose levels may also stem from hyperlipoproteinemia (especially types III, IV, or V), chronic hepatic disease, nephrotic syndrome, brain tumor, sepsis, or gastrectomy with dumping syndrome and is typical in eclampsia, anoxia, and seizure disorders.
◆ Low levels may result from hyperinsulinism, insulinoma, von Gierke's disease, functional and reactive hypoglycemia, myxedema, adrenal insufficiency, congenital adrenal hyperplasia, hypopituitarism, malabsorption syndrome, and hepatic insufficiency.

Febrile agglutination test

DESCRIPTION
- Provides diagnostic information in patients with fever of undetermined origin, infection, or with conditions in which isolation of microorganisms from blood or excreta is difficult
- Includes Weil-Felix test for rickettsial disease, Widal's test for *Salmonella,* and tests for brucellosis and tularemia

Weil-Felix test
- Establishes rickettsial antibody titers, using three forms of *Proteus* antigens (OX-19, OX-2, and OX-K) that cross-react with strains of rickettsiae
- Antibodies to certain rickettsial strains reacting with more than one *Proteus* antigen; antibodies to other strains not reacting with any *Proteus* antigens

Widal's test
- Establishes titers for flagellar (H) and somatic (O) antigens, which may indicate *Salmonella* gastroenteritis and extraintestinal focal infections caused by *S. enteritidis,* or enteric (typhoid) fever, caused by *S. typhosa*
- Vi (or envelope) antigen indicating typhoid carrier status; tests negative for H and O antigens

Slide agglutination and tube dilution tests
- Uses killed suspensions of disease organisms as antigens
- Establishes titers for the gram-negative coccobacilli *Brucella* and *Francisella tularensis,* which cause brucellosis and tularemia, respectively

PURPOSE
- To support clinical findings in the diagnosis of disorders caused by *Rickettsia, Salmonella, Brucella,* and *F. tularensis* organisms
- To identify the cause of a fever of undetermined origin

PREPARATION
- No dietary restrictions are needed.
- The test requires a blood sample.
- Note on the laboratory request when antimicrobial therapy began, if appropriate.

Teaching points
- Explain that this test detects and quantifies microorganisms that may cause fever and other symptoms.
- Tell the patient that this test requires a series of blood samples to detect a pattern of titers characteristic of the suspected disorder, if appropriate. Reassure him that a positive result only suggests a disorder.
- Tell the patient who will perform the test and where it will be done.
- Tell him that no dietary restrictions are needed.
- Explain to the patient that he may experience slight discomfort from the tourniquet and needle puncture.
- Inform him that the test should take less than 5 minutes.

KEY STEPS
- Confirm the patient's identity using two patient identifiers according to facility policy.
- Perform a venipuncture and collect the sample in a 7-ml clot-activator tube.

POSTPROCEDURE CARE
- Apply pressure to the venipuncture site until bleeding stops.
- In a fever of undetermined origin and suspected infection, contact the facility's infection control department. Isolation may be required.

PRECAUTIONS
- Maintain appropriate precautions while collecting the sample.

COMPLICATIONS
- Hematoma at the venipuncture site

NORMAL RESULTS
- Dilutions for rickettsial antibody are below 1:40, *Salmonella* antibody, below 1:80, brucellosis antibody, below 1:80, and tularemia antibody, below 1:40.

ABNORMAL RESULTS
- Observing the rise and fall of titers is crucial for detecting active infection. If this isn't possible, certain titer levels can suggest the disorder.
- For all febrile agglutinins, a fourfold increase in titers is evidence of infection.
- The Weil-Felix test result is positive for rickettsiae with antibodies to *Proteus* occurring 6 to 12 days after infection; titers peak in 1 month and usually drop to negative in 5 to 6 months. This test can't diagnose rickettsialpox or Q fever because the antibodies of these diseases don't cross-react with *Proteus* antigens; the test shows positive titers in *Proteus* infections and, in such cases, is non-specific for rickettsiae.
- In *Salmonella* infection, H and O agglutinins usually appear in serum after 1 week, and titers rise for 3 to 6 weeks. O agglutinins usually fall to insignificant levels in 6 to 12 months. Agglutinin titers may remain increased for years.
- Although the absence of *Brucella* agglutinins doesn't rule out brucellosis, titers usually rise after 2 to 3 weeks and peak in 4 to 8 weeks.
- In tularemia, titers usually become positive during the second week of infection, exceed 1:320 by the third week, peak within 4 to 7 weeks, and usually decline gradually 1 year after recovery.

Fecal lipid level test

DESCRIPTION

◆ Measures levels of monoglycerides, diglycerides, triglycerides, phospholipids, glycolipids, soaps (fatty acids and fatty acid salts), sterols, and cholesterol esters in stool
◆ Excessive excretion (steatorrhea) common in several malabsorption syndromes
◆ Detects steatorrhea in cases of malabsorption (such as weight loss, abdominal distention, and scaly skin)
◆ Qualitative test: involves staining fecal specimen with Sudan III dye and examining microscopically for malabsorption (such as undigested muscle fibers and various fats)
◆ Quantitative test: involves drying and weighing 72-hour specimen and then using a solvent to extract the lipids, which are subsequently evaporated and weighed; confirms steatorrhea

PURPOSE

◆ To confirm steatorrhea

PREPARATION

◆ The test requires a 72-hour fecal collection.
◆ Notify the laboratory and practitioner of drugs the patient is taking that may affect test results; they may be restricted.

Teaching points

◆ Explain to the patient that the fecal lipid test evaluates fat digestion.
◆ Tell the patient who will perform the test and where it will be done.
◆ Instruct the patient to abstain from alcohol and to maintain a high-fat diet (100 g/day) for 3 days before the test and during the collection period.
◆ Advise the patient of any medication restrictions.
◆ Teach to the patient how to collect a timed fecal specimen and provide him with the necessary equipment.
◆ Tell the patient to avoid contaminating the fecal specimen with toilet tissue or urine.

◆ Inform the patient that the laboratory requires 1 or 2 days to complete the analysis.

KEY STEPS

◆ Confirm the patient's identity using two patient identifiers according to facility policy.
◆ Collect a 72-hour fecal specimen.

POSTPROCEDURE CARE

◆ Answer the patient's questions about the test.
◆ After the test, tell the patient to resume his usual diet and medications, as ordered.

PRECAUTIONS

◆ Don't use a waxed collection container because the wax may become incorporated in the feces and interfere with accurate testing.
◆ Refrigerate the collection container and keep it tightly covered.

COMPLICATIONS

◆ None

NORMAL RESULTS

◆ Analysis reveals less than 20% of excreted solids, with excretion more than 7 g/24 hours.

ABNORMAL RESULTS

◆ Digestive disorders may affect the production and release of pancreatic lipase or bile; absorptive disorders may affect the intestine's integrity, causing steatorrhea.
◆ In pancreatic insufficiency, impaired lipid digestion may result from insufficient lipase production.
◆ Pancreatic resection, cystic fibrosis, chronic pancreatitis, or ductal obstruction by stone or tumor may prevent the normal release or action of lipase.
◆ In impaired hepatic function, faulty lipid digestion may result from inadequate bile salt production.
◆ Biliary obstruction may prevent the normal release of bile salts into the duodenum.
◆ Extensive small-bowel resection or bypass may also interrupt normal enterohepatic bile salt circulation.
◆ Diseases of the intestinal mucosa affect the normal absorption of lipids.
◆ Regional ileitis and atrophy caused by malnutrition cause gross structural changes in the intestinal wall; celiac disease and tropical sprue produce mucosal abnormalities.
◆ Scleroderma, radiation enteritis, fistulas, intestinal tuberculosis, small intestine diverticula, and altered intestinal flora may also cause steatorrhea.
◆ Whipple's disease and lymphomas cause lymphatic obstruction that may inhibit fat absorption.

Fecal occult blood test

DESCRIPTION

- Test to detect hemoglobin in the stool by microscopic analysis or chemical tests such as the guaiac test
- Detects quantities of blood greater than 2 to 2.5 ml/day
- Indicated when clinical symptoms and preliminary blood studies suggest GI bleeding
- Additional tests needed to identify the origin of bleeding (see *Common sites and causes of GI blood loss*)

PURPOSE

- To detect GI bleeding
- To help in the early diagnosis of colorectal cancer

PREPARATION

- Notify the laboratory and practitioner of drugs the patient is taking that may affect test results; they may be restricted. If the patient must continue using these drugs, note this on the laboratory request.

Teaching points

- Explain that this test detects abnormal GI bleeding.
- Tell the patient who will perform the test and where it will be done.
- Instruct him to maintain a high-fiber diet and to refrain from eating red meat, turnips, and horseradish for 48 to 72 hours before the test as well as during the collection period.
- Tell the patient that the test usually requires three fecal specimens but that sometimes only one sample is needed.
- Teach the patient how to collect a fecal sample.
- Instruct him to avoid contaminating the fecal specimen with toilet tissue or urine.
- Advise him of any dietary or medication restrictions needed.

DIAGNOSTIC PROCEDURE

KEY STEPS

- Confirm the patient's identity using two patient identifiers according to facility policy.
- Collect three fecal specimens or a random fecal specimen.
- Obtain specimens from two different areas of each fecal specimen.

Hematest

- Use a wooden applicator to smear a bit of the fecal specimen on the filter paper supplied with the kit. Or, after performing a digital rectal examination, wipe the finger you used for the examination on a square of the filter paper. Place the filter paper with the fecal smear on a glass plate.
- Remove a reagent tablet from the bottle and immediately replace the cap tightly. Place the tablet in the center of the fecal smear on the filter paper. Add 1 drop of water to the tablet, and allow it to soak in for 5 to 10 seconds. Add a second drop, letting it run from the tablet onto the specimen and filter paper.
- After 2 minutes, the filter paper will turn blue if the test result is positive. Don't read the color that appears on

(continued)

Common sites and causes of GI blood loss

Illustrated here are potential areas that can cause blood loss, resulting in positive fecal occult blood testing. Further clinical assessment and testing is needed to determine the specific area involved.

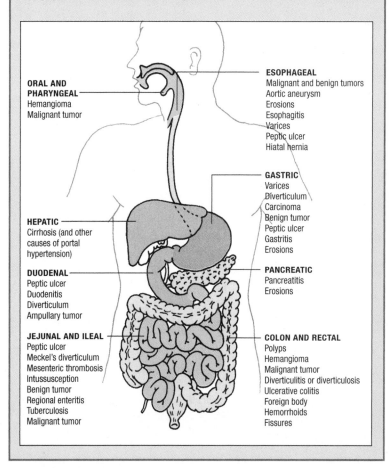

ORAL AND PHARYNGEAL
Hemangioma
Malignant tumor

HEPATIC
Cirrhosis (and other causes of portal hypertension)

DUODENAL
Peptic ulcer
Duodenitis
Diverticulum
Ampullary tumor

JEJUNAL AND ILEAL
Peptic ulcer
Meckel's diverticulum
Mesenteric thrombosis
Intussusception
Benign tumor
Regional enteritis
Tuberculosis
Malignant tumor

ESOPHAGEAL
Malignant and benign tumors
Aortic aneurysm
Erosions
Esophagitis
Varices
Peptic ulcer
Hiatal hernia

GASTRIC
Varices
Diverticulum
Carcinoma
Benign tumor
Peptic ulcer
Gastritis
Erosions

PANCREATIC
Pancreatitis
Erosions

COLON AND RECTAL
Polyps
Hemangioma
Malignant tumor
Diverticulitis or diverticulosis
Ulcerative colitis
Foreign body
Hemorrhoids
Fissures

the tablet itself or develops on the filter paper after the 2-minute period. Note the results and discard the filter paper. Remove and discard your gloves and wash your hands thoroughly.

Hemoccult test
- Open the flap on the slide pack and use a wooden applicator to apply a thin smear of the fecal specimen to the guaiac-impregnated filter paper exposed in box A. Apply a second smear from another part of the specimen to the filter paper exposed in box B.
- Let the specimen dry for 3 to 5 minutes. Open the flap at the rear of the slide package and place 2 drops of Hemoccult developing solution on the paper over each smear. A positive result yields a blue reaction in 30 to 60 seconds. Record the results and discard the slide package. Remove and discard your gloves and wash your hands thoroughly.

Instant-View fecal occult blood test
- Add a fecal sample to the collection tube. Shake it to mix the sample with the extraction buffer, and then dispense 4 drops into the sample well of the cassette.
- Results will appear on the test region and the control region of the cassette in 5 to 10 minutes, indicating whether the hemoglobin level is less than 0.05 mcg/ml of feces.

POSTPROCEDURE CARE
- Answer the patient's questions about the test.
- Tell the patient to resume his usual diet and medications, as ordered.

PRECAUTIONS
- Send the specimen to laboratory immediately or perform the test immediately.

COMPLICATIONS
- None

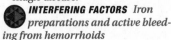

NORMAL RESULTS
- Green reactions indicate less than 2.5 ml of blood in feces.

ABNORMAL RESULTS
- A positive reaction indicates GI bleeding, which may result from varices, a peptic ulcer, carcinoma, ulcerative colitis, dysentery, or hemorrhagic disease.

INTERFERING FACTORS *Iron preparations and active bleeding from hemorrhoids*

Fecal urobilinogen test

DESCRIPTION

- Measures fecal urobilinogen (end product of bilirubin metabolism), brown pigment formed by bacterial enzymes in small intestine; excreted in feces or reabsorbed into portal blood, where it's returned to the liver and excreted in bile or in urine
- May be useful indicator of hepatobiliary and hemolytic disorders
- Rarely performed because serum bilirubin and urine urobilinogen are easily measured
- Proper bilirubin metabolism dependent on normal hepatobiliary system functioning and a normal erythrocyte life span

PURPOSE

- To help diagnose hepatobiliary and hemolytic disorders

PREPARATION

- Notify the laboratory and practitioner of drugs the patient is taking that may affect test results; they may be restricted.
- No dietary restrictions are required.

Teaching points

- Explain to the patient that the fecal urobilinogen test evaluates liver and bile duct function or detects red blood cell disorders.
- Tell the patient who will perform the test and where it will be done.
- Inform the patient that he need not restrict food and fluids.
- Tell the patient that the test requires collection of a random feces specimen.
- Tell the patient not to contaminate the feces specimen with toilet tissue or urine.

KEY STEPS

- Confirm the patient's identity using two patient identifiers according to facility policy.
- Collect a random feces specimen.
- Send the specimen to the laboratory immediately after collection.

POSTPROCEDURE CARE

- Tell the patient to resume his usual medications.

PRECAUTIONS

- Refrigerate the specimen if transport or testing is delayed more than 30 minutes; freeze the specimen if the test is to be performed by an outside laboratory.
- Use a light-resistant collection container because urobilinogen breaks down to urobilin when exposed to light.

COMPLICATIONS

- None

NORMAL RESULTS

- The level is 50 to 300 mg/24 hours (SI, 100 to 400 EU/100 g).

ABNORMAL RESULTS

- Absent or low levels of urobilinogen in the feces indicate obstructed bile flow, the result of intrahepatic disorders (hepatocellular jaundice caused by cirrhosis or hepatitis), extrahepatic disorders (choledocholithiasis, tumor of the head of the pancreas, ampulla of Vater, or bile duct), or depressed erythropoiesis (aplastic anemia).

Ferritin level test

DESCRIPTION

- Protein that stores iron in the body
- Provides information about the body's ability to store iron for later use
- Usually performed with iron testing and total iron-binding capacity

PURPOSE

- To measure a patient's iron level to determine whether blood has too much or too little iron

PREPARATION

- No dietary restrictions are needed.
- The test requires a blood sample.

Teaching points

- Explain the purpose of the test and how it's done.
- Tell the patient who will perform the test and where it will be done.
- Tell him that he doesn't need to restrict his diet.
- Inform him that he may experience discomfort from the tourniquet and needle puncture.
- Inform the patient that the test should take less than 5 minutes.

DIAGNOSTIC PROCEDURE

KEY STEPS

- Confirm the patient's identity using two patient identifiers according to facility policy.
- Perform a venipuncture and collect a blood sample.

POSTPROCEDURE CARE

- Apply direct pressure to the venipuncture site until bleeding stops.

PRECAUTIONS

- Maintain standard precautions while collecting the sample.
- Handle the sample gently to prevent hemolysis.

COMPLICATIONS

- Hematoma at the venipuncture site

INTERPRETATION

NORMAL RESULTS

- In men, the level is 20 to 300 ng/ml (SI, 20 to 300 µg/L).
- In women, the level is 20 to 120 ng/ml (SI, 20 to 120 µg/L).

ABNORMAL RESULTS

- Low levels may indicate iron deficiency, chronic GI bleeding, or heavy menstrual bleeding.
- High levels may indicate alcoholic liver disease, hemochromatosis, hemolytic anemia, Hodgkin's lymphoma, and megaloblastic anemia.

Fetal hemoglobin test

DESCRIPTION

- Normal hemoglobin produced in the red blood cells of a fetus and in smaller amounts in infants
- Constitutes 50% to 90% of hemoglobin level in a neonate; remaining hemoglobin level is Hb A_1 and Hb A_2 (hemoglobin level in adults); body stops making fetal hemoglobin (Hb F) during first years of life and then makes Hb A
- Hb F over 5% of hemoglobin level after age 6 months: indicates abnormality, particularly thalassemia

PURPOSE

- To diagnose thalassemia

PREPARATION

- The test requires a blood sample.
- Drawing the sample takes less than 5 minutes.
- No dietary restrictions are needed.

Teaching points

- Explain that the test detects thalassemia.
- Tell the patient who will perform the test and where it will be done.
- Explain that he may experience slight discomfort from the tourniquet and needle puncture.
- If the patient is a child, explain to his parents that a small amount of blood will be taken from his finger or earlobe.
- Tell the patient that he doesn't have to restrict his diet.
- Inform him that the test should take less than 5 minutes.

KEY STEPS

- Confirm the patient's identity using two patient identifiers according to facility policy.
- Perform a venipuncture and collect the blood sample in a 4.5-ml EDTA tube.
- For a young child, collect capillary blood in a microcollection device.
- Completely fill the collection tube and invert it gently several times to mix the sample and anticoagulant thoroughly.

POSTPROCEDURE CARE

- Apply direct pressure to the venipuncture site until bleeding stops.
- If a large hematoma develops at the venipuncture site, monitor pulses distal to the site.

PRECAUTIONS

- Make sure that subdermal bleeding has stopped before removing pressure.
- Handle the sample gently to prevent hemolysis.

COMPLICATIONS

- Hematoma at the venipuncture site

NORMAL RESULTS

- In neonates up to age 1 month, value is 60% to 90% (SI, 0.60 to 0.90).
- In children ages 1 to 23 months, value is 2% (SI, 0.02).
- From age 24 months to adult, value is 0% to 2% (SI, 0 to 0.02).

ABNORMAL RESULTS

- The Hb F value may be 30% or more of the total hemoglobin level in patients with beta-thalassemia major.
- The Hb F value may be slightly increased in unrelated hematologic disorders, such as aplastic anemia, homozygous sickle cell disease, and myeloproliferative disorders.
- The Hb F value commonly increases to as much as 5% during normal pregnancy.

Fetal-maternal erythrocyte distribution test

OVERVIEW

DESCRIPTION

- Measures number of fetal red blood cells (RBCs) in maternal circulation
- Some RBCs transferred from fetal to maternal circulation during most spontaneous or elective abortions and normal deliveries
- Minimal amount of blood transferred: no clinical significance
- Significant transfer of blood from Rh-positive fetus to Rh-negative mother: results in maternal immunization to D antigen and development of anti-D antibodies in maternal circulation
- In subsequent pregnancy: maternal immunization subjects an Rh-positive fetus to potentially fatal hemolysis and erythroblastosis

PURPOSE

- To detect and measure fetal-maternal blood transfer
- To determine the amount of $Rh_o(D)$ immune globulin needed to prevent maternal immunization to the D antigen

PREPARATION

- No food and fluid restrictions are needed.
- The test requires a blood sample.

Teaching points

- Explain that this test determines the amount of fetal blood transferred to the maternal circulation and helps determine the appropriate treatment, if necessary.
- Tell the patient who will perform the test and where it will be done.
- Tell her that no dietary restrictions are required.
- Explain to the patient that she may experience slight discomfort from the tourniquet and needle puncture.
- Inform her that the test should take less than 5 minutes.

DIAGNOSTIC PROCEDURE

KEY STEPS

- Confirm the patient's identity using two patient identifiers according to facility policy.
- Perform a venipuncture and collect the sample in a 7-ml EDTA tube.
- Label the sample with the patient's name, the hospital or blood bank number, the date, and the phlebotomist's initials.
- Send the sample to the laboratory immediately with a properly completed laboratory request.

POSTPROCEDURE CARE

- Apply direct pressure to the venipuncture site until bleeding stops.

PRECAUTIONS

- Maintain standard precautions while collecting the sample.
- Check the patient's history for recent administration of dextran, I.V. contrast media, or drugs that may alter results.

COMPLICATIONS

- Hematoma at the venipuncture site

INTERPRETATION

NORMAL RESULTS

- Maternal whole blood contains no fetal RBCs.

ABNORMAL RESULTS

- Increased fetal RBC volume in the maternal circulation requires more than one dose of $Rh_o(D)$ immune globulin.
- To determine the number of vials needed, divide the calculated milliliters of fetal-maternal hemorrhage by 30. (One vial of $Rh_o[D]$ immune globulin protects against a 30-ml fetal-maternal hemorrhage.)
- To prevent complications in later pregnancies in an unsensitized Rh-negative mother, give her $Rh_o(D)$ immune globulin as soon as possible (no later than 72 hours) after the birth of an Rh-positive infant or after a spontaneous or elective abortion. Most practitioners are now giving $Rh_o(D)$ immune globulin prophylactically at 28 weeks' gestation to women who are Rh-negative but have no detectable Rh antibodies.
- The following patients should be screened for Rh isoimmunization or irregular antibodies: all Rh-negative mothers during their first prenatal visit and at 28 weeks' gestation and all Rh-positive mothers with histories of transfusion, a jaundiced infant, stillbirth, cesarean delivery, or induced or spontaneous abortion.

Fibrin split products test

DESCRIPTION
- Fibrin clot formed in response to vascular injury; degraded by plasmin, a fibrin-dissolving enzyme
- Resulting fragments known as *fibrin split products* (FSP) or *fibrinogen degradation products*
- FSP detected in diluted serum that's left in blood sample after clotting

PURPOSE
- To detect FSP in the circulation
- To help determine the presence and severity of a hyperfibrinolytic state (such as disseminated intravascular coagulation [DIC]) that may result in primary fibrinogenolysis or hypercoagulability (see *Causes of disseminated intravascular coagulation*)

PREPARATION
- The test requires a blood sample.
- Notify the laboratory and practitioner of drugs the patient is taking that may affect test results; it may be necessary to restrict them.
- No dietary restrictions are needed.

Teaching points
- Explain that the FSP test determines whether blood clots normally.
- Tell the patient who will perform the test and where it will be done.
- Tell him that he doesn't have to restrict his diet.
- Explain that he may experience slight discomfort from the tourniquet and needle puncture.
- Inform him that the test should take less than 5 minutes.

DIAGNOSTIC PROCEDURE

KEY STEPS
- Confirm the patient's identity using two patient identifiers according to facility policy.
- Perform a venipuncture and draw 2 ml of blood into a plastic syringe.
- Draw the sample before giving heparin to avoid false-positive test results.

- Transfer the sample to the tube provided by the laboratory, which contains a soybean trypsin inhibitor and bovine thrombin.
- Gently invert the collection tube several times to mix the contents thoroughly.
- The blood clots within 2 seconds; after clotting, the sample must be sent immediately to the laboratory for incubation at 98.6° F (37° C) for 30 minutes before testing proceeds.

POSTPROCEDURE CARE
- Apply direct pressure to the venipuncture site until bleeding stops.
- If a large hematoma develops at the venipuncture site, monitor pulses distal to the site.
- After the test, tell the patient to resume his medications.

PRECAUTIONS
- Make sure that subdermal bleeding has stopped before removing pressure.
- Maintain standard precautions while collecting the sample.

COMPLICATIONS
- Hematoma at the venipuncture site

NORMAL RESULTS
- Serum contains less than 10 mcg/ml (SI, < 10 mg/L) of FSP. A quantitative assay shows levels of less than 3 mcg/ml (SI, < 3 mg/L).

ABNORMAL RESULTS
- FSP levels increase in primary fibrinolytic states because of increased levels of circulating profibrinolysin; in secondary states because of DIC and subsequent fibrinolysis; and in alcoholic cirrhosis, preeclampsia, abruptio placentae, congenital heart disease, sunstroke, burns, intrauterine death, pulmonary embolus, deep vein thrombosis (transient increase), and myocardial infarction (after 1 or 2 days).
- FSP levels are usually greater than 100 mcg/ml (SI, > 100 mg/L) in active renal disease or renal transplant rejection.

Causes of disseminated intravascular coagulation

Obstetric	Amniotic fluid embolism, eclampsia, retained dead fetus, retained placenta, abruptio placentae, and gestational hypertension
Neoplastic	Sarcoma, metastatic carcinoma, acute leukemia, prostate cancer, and giant hemangioma
Infectious	Acute bacteremia, septicemia, and rickettsemia; viral, fungal, or protozoal infection
Necrotic	Trauma, destruction of brain tissue, extensive burns, heatstroke, rejection of transplant, and hepatic necrosis
Cardiovascular	Fat embolism, acute venous thrombosis, cardiopulmonary bypass surgery, hypovolemic shock, cardiac arrest, and hypotension
Other	Snakebite, cirrhosis, transfusion of incompatible blood, purpura, and glomerulonephritis

Fluorescein angiography

DESCRIPTION

- Rapid-sequence blue-colored flash photographs of fundus taken with a special camera after I.V. injection of a vegetable-based dye, sodium fluorescein
- Enhances visibility of microvascular structures of the retina and choroids from fluorescein dye and sophisticated photographic equipment
- Permits evaluation of the entire retinal vascular bed, including retinal circulation
- May be used with a photographic technique called indocyanine green angiography in certain diseases to obtain further information

PURPOSE

- To document retinal circulation and the layers beneath the retina
- To help evaluate intraocular abnormalities

PREPARATION

- Make sure that the patient has signed an appropriate consent form.
- Note and report all allergies.
- Check the patient's history for glaucoma.

Teaching points

- Explain the purpose of the test and how it's done.
- Tell the patient who will perform the test and where it will be done.
- Tell him that no dietary restrictions are required.
- Warn him that he may experience a strobe-light effect during the test.
- Explain that the study is fairly painless and adverse effects are uncommon but may include nausea and mild urticaria.
- Inform the patient that skin and urine may appear yellow for 24 to 48 hours.
- Inform him that the test takes about 30 minutes.
- Caution him that his near vision will be blurred for up to 12 hours after the test.

- Instruct the patient not to drive and to avoid direct sunlight during the period of blurred vision.

DIAGNOSTIC PROCEDURE

KEY STEPS

- Confirm the patient's identity using two patient identifiers according to facility policy.
- The patient is given mydriatic eyedrops.
- The patient is positioned in an examination chair facing the camera with his chin on the chin rest and his forehead against the bar.
- He's asked to open his eyes as widely as possible and stare straight ahead.
- The contrast medium is injected rapidly into the antecubital vein. Photographs — 25 to 30 — are taken in rapid sequence (1 second apart). Photographs may be taken up to 1 hour after the injection.

POSTPROCEDURE CARE

- Encourage oral fluid intake to help excrete the dye.

PRECAUTIONS

- Don't give miotic eyedrops on the day of the test.
- Serious adverse effects (laryngeal edema, bronchospasm, and respiratory arrest) are possible. Have emergency equipment available.

COMPLICATIONS

- Extravasation of the dye (painful and toxic to the tissues)

NORMAL RESULTS

- After rapid injection, sodium fluorescein reaches the retina in 12 to 15 seconds (filling phase).
- The retinal background appears evenly mottled (choroidal flush) during choroidal vessel and choriocapillary filling.
- The contrast fills the arteries (arterial phase).
- No leakage of contrast from retinal vessels is visible.

ABNORMAL RESULTS

- Abnormalities in the early filling phase suggest possible microaneurysms, arteriovenous shunts, and neovascularization.
- Delayed or absent flow of the dye through the arteries may indicate arterial stenosis or occlusion.
- Dilation of the vessels and fluorescein leakage may suggest venous occlusion.
- Recanalization and collateral circulation suggest chronic obstruction.
- Increased vascular tortuosity suggests hypertensive retinopathy.
- Leaking of fluorescence, surrounded by hard, yellow exudate, suggests possible aneurysms and capillary hemangiomas.
- Vascular leakage in the disk area suggests papilledema.

Fluorescent treponemal antibody absorption test

DESCRIPTION

- Uses indirect immunofluorescence to detect serum antibodies to *Treponema pallidum*, the organism that causes syphilis
- Prepared *T. pallidum* fixed on a slide; absorbed preparation of *Reiter treponema* added, then the patient's serum
- Test specific for *T. pallidum* because *Reiter treponema* combines with most nonsyphilitic antibodies
- Treponemal organisms coated by syphilitic antibodies in test serum
- Slide then stained with fluorescein-labeled antiglobulin; attaches to coated spirochetes that fluoresce when viewed under an ultraviolet microscope
- Usually performed on serum sample to detect primary or secondary syphilis; cerebrospinal fluid (CSF) specimen required to detect tertiary syphilis
- Also known as *FTA-ABS* or *FTA*
- Because antibody levels are constant for long periods, FTA-ABS test not recommended for monitoring the patient's response to therapy (see *Two tests for* Treponema pallidum)

Two tests for *Treponema pallidum*

The microhemagglutination assay for the *Treponema pallidum* antibody increases the specificity of syphilis testing by eliminating methodologic interference. In this assay, tanned sheep red blood cells are coated with *T. pallidum* antigen and combined with absorbed test serum. Hemagglutination occurs in the presence of specific *anti-T. pallidum* antibodies in the serum.

In the enzyme-linked immunosorbent assay, tubes coated with *T. pallidum* are washed and then treated with enzyme-labeled antihuman globulin. After the substrate for the enzymes is added to the tubes, the enzymatic activity is measured by quantitating the reaction product formed.

PURPOSE

- To confirm primary and secondary syphilis
- To screen for suspected false-positive results of the Venereal Disease Research Laboratory tests

PREPARATION

- No food and fluid restrictions are required.
- The test requires a blood sample.

Teaching points

- Explain that this test can confirm or rule out syphilis.
- Tell the patient who will perform the test and where it will be done.
- Tell him that no dietary restrictions are required.
- Explain to the patient that he may experience discomfort from the tourniquet and needle puncture.
- Inform him that the test should take less than 5 minutes.

KEY STEPS

- Confirm the patient's identity using two identifiers according to policy.
- Perform a venipuncture and collect the sample in a 7-ml clot-activator tube.

POSTPROCEDURE CARE

- Apply direct pressure to the venipuncture site until bleeding stops.
- If the test is reactive, explain the nature of syphilis and stress the importance of proper treatment and the need to find and treat the patient's sexual contacts.
- Provide the patient with additional information about syphilis and how it's spread; emphasize the need for antibiotic therapy, if appropriate. Report positive results to state public health authorities and prepare the patient for mandatory inquiries.
- If the test is nonreactive or findings are borderline but syphilis hasn't been ruled out, instruct the patient to return for follow-up testing; explain that inconclusive results don't

necessarily indicate that he's free from the disease.

PRECAUTIONS

- Handle the sample gently to prevent hemolysis.
- Maintain standard precautions while collecting the sample.

COMPLICATIONS

- Hematoma at the venipuncture site

NORMAL RESULTS

- The result is nonreactive.

ABNORMAL RESULTS

- The presence of treponemal antibodies in the serum — a reactive test result — doesn't indicate the stage or severity of infection. (The presence of these antibodies in CSF is strong evidence of tertiary neurosyphilis.)
- Increased antibody levels appear in most patients with primary syphilis and in almost all patients with secondary syphilis.
- Antibody levels are elevated for several years, with or without treatment.
- The absence of treponemal antibodies, a nonreactive test result, doesn't rule out syphilis. *T. pallidum* causes no detectable immunologic changes in the blood for 14 to 21 days after the initial infection.
- Organisms may be detected earlier by examining suspicious lesions with a darkfield microscope.
- Low antibody levels and other nonspecific factors produce borderline findings. In such cases, repeated testing and a thorough review of the patient's history may be productive.
- Although the FTA-ABS test is specific, some patients with nonsyphilitic conditions, such as systemic lupus erythematosus, genital herpes, and increased or abnormal globulins, or those who are pregnant may show minimally reactive levels.
- The FTA-ABS test doesn't always distinguish *T. pallidum* from certain other treponemas such as those that cause pinta, yaws, and bejel.

Folic acid level test

DESCRIPTION

- Quantitative analysis of serum folic acid (also called pteroylglutamic acid, folacin, or folate) levels by radioisotope assay of competitive binding; usually combined with measurement of serum vitamin B_{12} levels
- Water-soluble vitamin that affects hematopoiesis, deoxyribonucleic acid synthesis, and overall body growth
- Occurs in organ meats, such as liver or kidneys, yeast, fruits, leafy vegetables, fortified breads and cereals, eggs, and milk
- Deficiency from inadequate dietary intake, especially during pregnancy
- Suspected hematologic abnormality usual indication for test because of folic acid's role in hematopoiesis

PURPOSE

- To aid in the differential diagnosis of megaloblastic anemia, which may result from folic acid or vitamin B_{12} deficiency
- To assess folate stores in pregnancy

PREPARATION

- Fasting overnight before the test is required.
- The test requires a blood sample.
- Check the patient's history for drugs that may affect test results, such as phenytoin or pyrimethamine.

Teaching points

- Explain that this test determines the folic acid level in the blood.
- Tell the patient who will perform the test and where it will be done.
- Instruct him to avoid food for at least 8 hours before the test.
- Explain to the patient that he may experience slight discomfort from the tourniquet and needle puncture.
- Inform the patient that the test should take less than 5 minutes.

KEY STEPS

- Confirm the patient's identity using two patient identifiers according to facility policy.
- Perform a venipuncture and collect the sample in a 4.5-ml tube without additives.
- Send the sample to the laboratory immediately.

POSTPROCEDURE CARE

- Apply direct pressure to the venipuncture site until bleeding stops.
- Tell the patient to resume his usual diet.

PRECAUTIONS

- Handle the sample gently to prevent hemolysis.
- Protect the sample from light.
- Maintain standard precautions while collecting the sample.

COMPLICATIONS

- Hematoma at the venipuncture site

NORMAL RESULTS

- Values are 1.8 to 20 ng/ml (SI, 4 to 45.3 nmol/L).

ABNORMAL RESULTS

- Low serum levels may indicate hematologic abnormalities, such as anemia (especially megaloblastic anemia), leukopenia, and thrombocytopenia.
- The Schilling test is usually performed to rule out vitamin B_{12} deficiency, which also causes megaloblastic anemia.
- Decreased folic acid levels can also result from hypermetabolic states (such as hyperthyroidism), inadequate dietary intake, small-bowel malabsorption syndrome, hepatic or renal diseases, chronic alcoholism, or pregnancy.
- Serum levels higher than normal may indicate excessive dietary intake of folic acid or folic acid supplements. Even when taken in large doses, the vitamin is nontoxic.

Follicle-stimulating hormone, serum

OVERVIEW

DESCRIPTION
◆ Test of gonadal function; measures levels of follicle-stimulating hormone (FSH), glycoprotein secreted by anterior pituitary gland
◆ Vital in infertility evaluation
◆ Performed more commonly on women than on men
◆ In women: spurs development of primary ovarian follicles into graafian follicles for ovulation (secretion varies diurnally and fluctuates during menstrual cycle, peaking at ovulation)
◆ In men: continuous secretion of FSH (and testosterone) stimulate and maintain spermatogenesis
◆ Widely fluctuating levels in women; for true baseline level, daily tests needed (for 3 to 5 days), or multiple samples may be drawn on the same day

PURPOSE
◆ To help diagnose and treat infertility and disorders of menstruation such as amenorrhea
◆ To help diagnose precocious puberty in girls (before age 9) and in boys (before age 10)
◆ To aid in the differential diagnosis of hypogonadism

PREPARATION
◆ The test requires a blood sample.
◆ Withhold drugs that may interfere with accurate determination of test results for 48 hours before the test. If the patient must continue them (for example, for infertility treatment), note this on the laboratory request.
◆ Make sure that the patient is relaxed and recumbent for 30 minutes before the test.

Teaching points
◆ Explain to the patient, or her parents if she's a minor, that this test helps determine if her hormonal secretion is normal.
◆ Tell the patient who will perform the test and where it will be done.
◆ Explain that the patient may experience slight discomfort from the tourniquet and needle puncture.
◆ Advise the patient of any medication restrictions.
◆ Tell her that the test should take about 45 minutes.

DIAGNOSTIC PROCEDURE

KEY STEPS
◆ Confirm the patient's identity using two patient identifiers according to facility policy.
◆ Perform a venipuncture, preferably between 6 a.m. and 8 a.m., and collect the sample in a 7-ml clot-activator tube. Send the sample to the laboratory immediately.
◆ If the patient is a woman, indicate the phase of her menstrual cycle on the laboratory request. If she's menopausal, note this on the laboratory request.

POSTPROCEDURE CARE
◆ Apply direct pressure to the venipuncture site until bleeding stops.
◆ Tell the patient to resume her medications.

PRECAUTIONS
◆ Handle the sample gently to prevent hemolysis.
◆ Maintain standard precautions while collecting the sample.

COMPLICATIONS
◆ Hematoma at the venipuncture site

INTERPRETATION

NORMAL RESULTS
◆ Reference values vary greatly, depending on the patient's age, stage of sexual development, and — for a woman — phase of her menstrual cycle.
◆ For the menstruating woman, FSH values are follicular phase, 5 to 20 mIU/ml (SI, 5 to 20 International Units/L); ovulatory phase, 15 to 30 mIU/ml (SI, 15 to 30 International Units/L); and luteal phase, 5 to 15 mIU/ml (SI, 5 to 15 International Units/L).
◆ FSH values for menopausal women range from 50 to 100 mIU/ml (SI, 50 to 100 International Units/L).
◆ FSH values for men range from 5 to 20 mIU/ml (SI, 5 to 20 International Units/L).

ABNORMAL RESULTS
◆ Low FSH levels may cause aspermatogenesis in men and anovulation in women.
◆ Low FSH levels may indicate secondary hypogonadotropic states, which can result from anorexia nervosa, panhypopituitarism, or hypothalamic lesions.
◆ High FSH levels in women may indicate ovarian failure from Turner's syndrome (primary hypogonadism) or Stein-Leventhal syndrome (polycystic ovary syndrome).
◆ High FSH levels may occur in patients with precocious puberty (idiopathic or with central nervous system lesions) and in postmenopausal women.
◆ High FSH levels in men may indicate destruction of the testes (from mumps orchitis or X-ray exposure), testicular failure, seminoma, or male climacteric.
◆ Congenital absence of the gonads and early-stage acromegaly may cause FSH levels to rise in both sexes.

Free erythrocyte porphyrins test

OVERVIEW

DESCRIPTION
- Porphyrins chelated with iron to form heme; incorporated into proteins to become functioning hemoproteins
- Small amount of porphyrin at end of heme synthesis known as *cell-free erythrocyte protoporphyrin*
- Levels elevated in conditions that decrease the iron supply

PURPOSE
- To screen disorders of red blood cells (RBCs) in children ages 6 months to 5 years
- To diagnose erythropoietic protoporphyria
- To evaluate lead poisoning

PREPARATION
- The test requires a blood sample.
- No dietary restrictions are needed.
- Review any medications that may be ordered to hold.

Teaching points
- Inform the patient or the parents of the child that this test helps determine the cause of anemia.
- Tell the patient who will perform the test and where it will be done.
- Tell the patient that no dietary restrictions are required.
- Tell the patient that he may experience slight discomfort from the tourniquet and needle puncture.
- Inform the patient that the test should take less than 5 minutes.

DIAGNOSTIC PROCEDURE

KEY STEPS
- Confirm the patient's identity using two patient identifiers according to facility policy.
- Perform a venipuncture and collect 5 ml of blood.
- Record the patient's hematocrit on the laboratory slip.
- Protect the specimen from light to prevent RBC breakdown and transport it directly to the laboratory.

POSTPROCEDURE CARE
- Apply pressure to the venipuncture site until bleeding stops.

PRECAUTIONS
- Maintain standard precautions while collecting the sample.
- The results are unreliable in infants younger than age 6 months.

COMPLICATIONS
- Hematoma at the venipuncture site

INTERPRETATION

NORMAL RESULTS
- The value is below 100 mcg/dl.
- The value may differ depending on the method used — check with the laboratory for their values.

ABNORMAL RESULTS
- An increased level indicates a decrease in the binding with iron and is usually indicative of an iron deficiency. This is seen in iron deficiency anemias, chronic lead poisoning, anemias associated with chronic diseases, and erythropoietic protoporphyria.

Free thyroxine and free triiodothyronine level tests

OVERVIEW

DESCRIPTION

◆ Measures serum levels of free thyroxine (FT_4) and free triiodothyronine (FT_3), the minute portions of T_4 and T_3 not bound to thyroxine-binding globulin (TBG) and other serum proteins
◆ Both measured because it's unclear if FT_4 or FT_3 is the better indicator of thyroid function
◆ Unbound hormones responsible for thyroid's effects on cellular metabolism
◆ Disadvantages: cumbersome and difficult laboratory method, inaccessibility, and cost
◆ May be useful in the 5% of patients in whom the standard T_3 or T_4 test don't produce diagnostic results

PURPOSE

◆ To measure the metabolically active form of the thyroid hormones
◆ To aid in the diagnosis of hyperthyroidism and hypothyroidism when TBG levels are abnormal

PREPARATION

◆ The test requires a blood sample.

Teaching points

◆ Explain that this test helps evaluate thyroid function.
◆ Tell the patient who will perform the test and where it will be done.
◆ Tell him that no dietary restrictions are required.
◆ Explain that he may experience slight discomfort from the tourniquet and needle puncture.
◆ Inform him that the test should take less than 5 minutes.

DIAGNOSTIC PROCEDURE

KEY STEPS

◆ Confirm the patient's identity using two patient identifiers according to facility policy.
◆ Perform a venipuncture and collect the sample in a 7-ml clot-activator tube.

POSTPROCEDURE CARE

◆ Apply direct pressure to the venipuncture site until bleeding stops.

PRECAUTIONS

◆ Handle the sample gently to prevent hemolysis.

COMPLICATIONS

◆ Hematoma at the venipuncture site

INTERPRETATION

NORMAL RESULTS

◆ The normal range for FT_4 is 0.9 to 2.3 ng/dl (SI, 10 to 30 nmol/L); for FT_3, 0.2 to 0.6 ng/dl (SI, 0.003 to 0.009 nmol/L).
◆ Values vary, depending on the laboratory.

ABNORMAL RESULTS

◆ High FT_4 and FT_3 levels indicate hyperthyroidism unless the patient has peripheral resistance to thyroid hormone.
◆ High FT_3 levels with normal or low FT_4 levels indicate T_3 toxicosis, a distinct form of hyperthyroidism.
◆ Low FT_4 levels usually indicate hypothyroidism, except in patients receiving replacement therapy with T_3.
◆ FT_4 and FT_3 levels may vary in patients receiving thyroid therapy, depending on the preparation used and the time of sample collection.

Fungal serology

OVERVIEW

DESCRIPTION

- Tests that use immunodiffusion, complement fixation, precipitin, latex agglutination, or agglutination methods to demonstrate the presence of specific mycotic antibodies (see *Serum test methods for fungal infections*)
- Occasionally provide sole evidence of mycosis
- Usual organism entry: as spores inhaled into lungs or infiltrated through wounds in skin or mucosa
- Body's defenses unable to destroy organisms initially; multiply to form lesions and mycosis spread by blood and lymph vessels
- Most people able to overcome initial mycotic infection; elderly people and those with deficient immune system more susceptible to acute or chronic mycotic infection and to disorders secondary to such infection
- Deep-seated (usually in the lungs) or superficial (in the skin or mucosal linings) mycosis

PURPOSE

- To rapidly detect the presence of antifungal antibodies, aiding in the diagnosis of mycosis
- To monitor the effectiveness of therapy for mycosis

PREPARATION

- The patient must fast for 12 to 24 hours before the test.
- The test requires a blood sample.

Teaching points

- Explain that this test aids in the diagnosis of certain fungal infections. If appropriate, tell the patient that this test monitors his response to antimycotic therapy and that it may be necessary to repeat the test.
- Tell the patient who will perform the test and where it will be done.
- Instruct him to fast for 12 hours before the test.

- Explain that the patient may experience slight discomfort from the tourniquet and needle puncture.
- Inform him that the test should take less than 5 minutes.

DIAGNOSTIC PROCEDURE

KEY STEPS

- Confirm the patient's identity using two patient identifiers according to facility policy.
- Perform a venipuncture and collect the sample in a 10-ml sterile clot-activator tube.
- Send the sample to the laboratory immediately.

POSTPROCEDURE CARE

- Apply direct pressure to the venipuncture site until bleeding stops.

PRECAUTIONS

- If transport to the laboratory is delayed, store the sample at 39.2° F (4° C).
- Maintain standard precautions while collecting the sample.

COMPLICATIONS

- Hematoma at the venipuncture site

INTERPRETATION

NORMAL RESULTS

- Depending on the test method, a negative result or normal titer is obtained.

ABNORMAL RESULTS

- Test results indicate aspergillosis, blastomycosis, coccidioidomycosis, cryptococcosis, histoplasmosis, or sporotrichosis.

INTERFERING FACTORS *Recent skin testing with fungal antigens (high titers); mycosis-caused immunosuppression (low titers or false-negative results)*

Serum test methods for fungal infections

DISEASE AND NORMAL VALUES	CLINICAL SIGNIFICANCE OF ABNORMAL RESULTS
Blastomycosis	
Complement fixation: titers < 1:8	Titers ranging from 1:8 to 1:16 suggest infection; titers > 1:32 denote active disease. A rising titer in serial samples taken every 3 to 4 weeks indicates disease progression; a falling titer indicates regression. This test has limited diagnostic value because of a high percentage of false-negatives.
Immunodiffusion: negative	A more sensitive test for blastomycosis; detects 80% of infected people.
Coccidioidomycosis	
Complement fixation: titers < 1:2	Most sensitive test for this fungus. Titers ranging from 1:2 to 1:4 suggest active infection; titers > 1:16 usually denote active disease. Test may remain active in mild infections.
Immunodiffusion: negative	Most useful for screening, followed by complement fixation test for confirmation.
Precipitin: titers < 1:16	Good screening test; titers > 1:16 usually indicate infection. About 80% of infected people show positive titers by 2 weeks; most revert to negative by 6 months. Early primary disease is shown by positive precipitin and negative complement fixation test. A positive complement fixation and negative precipitin test indicate chronic disease.
Histoplasmosis	
Complement fixation (histoplasmin): titers < 1:8	Titers ranging from 1:8 to 1:16 suggest infection; titers > 1:32 indicate active disease. Antibodies generally appear 10 to 21 days after initial infection. Test is positive in 10% to 15% of cases.
Complement fixation: titers < 1:18	Titers ranging from 1:8 to 1:16 suggest infection; titers > 1:32 indicate active disease. More sensitive than histoplasmin complement fixation test; gives positive results in 75% to 80% of cases. (Histoplasmin and yeast antigens are positive in 10% of cases.) A rising titer in serial samples taken every 2 to 3 weeks indicates progressive infection; a decreasing titer indicates regression.
Immunodiffusion (histoplasmin): negative	Appearance of H and M bands indicates active infection. If the M band appears first and lasts longer than the H band, the infection may be regressing. The M band alone may indicate early infection, chronic disease, or a recent skin test.
Aspergillosis	
Complement fixation: titers < 1:8	Titers > 1:8 suggest infection; 70% to 90% of patients with known pulmonary aspergillosis or aspergillus allergy present antibodies. This test can't detect invasive aspergillosis because patients with this disease don't have antibodies; biopsy is required.
Immunodiffusion: negative	One or more precipitin bands suggests infection. The number of bands is related to complement fixation titers; the more precipitin bands, the higher the titer.
Sporotrichosis	
Agglutination: titers < 1:40	Titers > 1:80 usually indicate active infection. The test usually is negative in cutaneous infections and positive in extracutaneous infections.
Cryptococcosis	
Latex agglutination for cryptococcal antigen: negative	About 90% of patients with cryptococcal meningitis exhibit positive latex agglutination in cerebrospinal fluid. Culturing is definitive because false-positives do occur. (Presence of rheumatoid factor may cause a positive reaction.) Serum antigen tests are positive in 33% of patients with pulmonary cryptococcosis; biopsy is usually required.

Galactose-1-phosphate uridyltransferase test

DESCRIPTION

- Measures enzyme that helps convert galactose to glucose during lactose metabolism
- Deficiency possible cause of galactosemia (hereditary disorder impairing eye, brain, and liver development and causing irreversible cataracts, mental retardation, and cirrhosis unless treated immediately)
- Qualitative test: screens for deficiency; required in some facilities for all neonates
- Quantitative test: done after positive qualitative test result; measures amount of fluorescent substance generated during a coupled enzyme reaction, and identifies adult galactosemia carriers
- Deficiency also detected by prenatal testing of amniotic fluid (rarely performed because neonatal screening detects deficiency in sufficient time to prevent irreversible damage)

PURPOSE

- To screen the infant for galactosemia
- To detect a heterozygous carrier of galactosemia

PATIENT PREPARATION

- The test requires a blood sample.
- No dietary restrictions are needed.

Teaching points

- Explain the purpose of the test and how it's done.
- When testing an adult, explain that this test identifies carriers of galactosemia, a genetic disorder that may be transmitted to offspring.
- If a blood sample wasn't taken from the umbilical cord at birth, tell the parents that a small amount of blood will be drawn from the infant's heel. Explain that the procedure is safe and quick.
- When testing a neonate, explain to the parents that the test screens for galactosemia, a potentially dangerous enzyme deficiency.
- Tell the patient who will perform the test and where it will be done.
- Tell him that no dietary restrictions are required.
- Explain that the patient may experience slight discomfort from the tourniquet and needle puncture.
- Inform him that the test should take less than 5 minutes.

DIAGNOSTIC PROCEDURE

KEY STEPS

- Confirm the patient's identity using two patient identifiers according to facility policy.
- For a qualitative (screening) test, collect cord blood or blood from a heel-stick on special filter paper, saturating all three circles.
- Perform a follow-up quantitative test soon after a positive qualitative test result.
- For a quantitative test, perform a venipuncture and collect a 4-ml sample in a heparinized or EDTA tube, depending on the laboratory method used.
- Indicate the patient's age on the laboratory request.
- Check the patient's history for a recent exchange transfusion.
- Note this on the laboratory request or postpone the test.
- Send the sample to the laboratory on wet ice.

POSTPROCEDURE CARE

- Apply direct pressure to the venipuncture site until bleeding stops.
- If test results indicate galactosemia, refer the parents for nutrition counseling and provide a galactose- and lactose-free diet for their infant.

PRECAUTIONS

- Maintain standard precautions while collecting the sample.
- Handle the sample gently to prevent hemolysis.

COMPLICATIONS

- Hematoma at the venipuncture site

INTERPRETATION

NORMAL RESULTS

- A negative qualitative test result is obtained.
- A quantitative test result is 18.5 to 28.5 units/g of hemoglobin (Hb). Confirm the normal range with the particular laboratory in case a different method is used.

ABNORMAL RESULTS

- A positive qualitative test result may indicate a transferase deficiency.
- A quantitative test result of below 5 units/g of Hb indicates galactosemia.
- A quantitative test result of 5 to 18.5 units/g of Hb may indicate that the patient is a carrier.

Gallium scanning

DESCRIPTION
◆ Total body scan performed 24 to 72 hours after I.V. injection of radioactive gallium citrate

PURPOSE
◆ To detect primary or metastatic neoplasms
◆ To detect inflammatory lesions
◆ To evaluate malignant lymphoma
◆ To identify recurrent tumors
◆ To clarify focal defects in the liver when scanning and ultrasonography are inconclusive
◆ To evaluate bronchogenic carcinoma
◆ To screen for the cause of a fever of unknown origin

PREPARATION
◆ Make sure that the patient has signed an appropriate consent form.
◆ Note and report all allergies.
◆ Inform the patient that he need not restrict food or fluids.
◆ Give the patient a laxative or cleansing enema (or both).
◆ Reassure the patient that radiation exposure is minimal.

Teaching points
◆ Explain the purpose of the test and how it's done.
◆ Tell the patient who will perform the test and where it will be done.
◆ Tell the patient that no dietary restrictions are needed.
◆ Inform the patient that the test takes about 30 to 60 minutes.

KEY STEPS
◆ Confirm the patient's identity using two patient identifiers according to facility policy.
◆ Various patient positions may be needed, depending on the condition.
◆ Scans or scintigrams are taken from various views 24, 48, and 72 hours after the injection of gallium.
◆ If bowel disease is suggested and additional scans are needed, give the patient a cleansing enema.

POSTPROCEDURE CARE
◆ Tell the patient to resume his previous activity.

PRECAUTIONS
◆ The test is contraindicated in children and in pregnant or breast-feeding women unless the benefit outweighs the risks.

COMPLICATIONS
◆ Infection at the injection site

NORMAL RESULTS
◆ Gallium activity is demonstrated in the liver, spleen, bones, and large bowel.

ABNORMAL RESULTS
◆ Abnormally high activity suggests inflammatory bowel disease and colon cancer.
◆ Abnormal activity in one or more lymph nodes or in extranodal locations suggests possible Hodgkin's disease and non-Hodgkin's lymphoma.
◆ Localization of gallium suggests possible hepatoma, abscess, or tumor.

Gamma globulin test

DESCRIPTION
◆ Form of protein electrophoresis that examines globulin proteins

PURPOSE
◆ To examine the amount of globulin proteins in the blood

PREPARATION
◆ The test requires a blood sample.
◆ Fasting is required for 4 hours before the test.
◆ Ask the patient what drugs he's taking; they may be restricted.

Teaching points
◆ Explain the purpose of the test and how it's done.
◆ Tell the patient who will perform the test and where it will be done.
◆ Instruct the patient to fast for at least 4 hours before the test.
◆ Inform the patient that the test should take less than 5 minutes.

KEY STEPS
◆ Confirm the patient's identity using two patient identifiers according to facility policy.
◆ Perform a venipuncture and collect the sample in a 7-ml clot-activator tube.

POSTPROCEDURE CARE
◆ Apply direct pressure to the venipuncture site.

PRECAUTIONS
◆ Maintain standard precautions while collecting the sample.

COMPLICATIONS
◆ Hematoma at the venipuncture site

NORMAL RESULTS
◆ Serum globulin count is 2 to 3.5 g/dl.
◆ Immunoglobulin (Ig) M component is 75 to 300 mg/dl.
◆ IgG component is 650 to 1,850 mg/dl.
◆ IgA component is 90 to 350 mg/dl.

ABNORMAL RESULTS
◆ Increased gamma globulin proteins may indicate multiple myeloma, chronic inflammatory disease (for example, rheumatoid arthritis and systemic lupus erythematosus), hyperimmunization, acute infection, or Waldenström's macroglobulinemia.

Gamma-glutamyltransferase level test

DESCRIPTION

- Measures level of serum gamma-glutamyltransferase (GGT), which helps transfer amino acids across cellular membranes and may aid in glutathione metabolism
- More sensitive indicator of hepatic necrosis than aspartate aminotransferase assay and at least as sensitive as alkaline phosphatase (ALP) assay because GGT isn't elevated in bone growth or pregnancy
- Sensitive to effects of alcohol on the liver (levels may be elevated after moderate alcohol intake and in chronic alcoholism, even without clinical evidence of hepatic injury)
- Nonspecific test; provides few data about the type of hepatic disease because increased levels also occur in renal, cardiac, and prostate disease and with some drugs
- Highest GGT levels found in the kidneys; also present in the liver, biliary tract, epithelium, pancreas, lymphocytes, brain, and testes

PURPOSE

- To provide information about hepatobiliary diseases, to assess liver function, and to detect alcohol ingestion
- To distinguish between skeletal and hepatic disease when the serum ALP level is elevated (a normal GGT level suggests that such elevation stems from skeletal disease)

PREPARATION

- This test requires a blood sample.
- No dietary restrictions are needed.

Teaching points

- Explain that this test evaluates liver function.
- Tell the patient who will perform the test and where it will be done.
- Tell him that no dietary restrictions are needed.
- Explain that the patient may experience slight discomfort from the tourniquet and needle puncture.

- Inform him that the test should take less than 5 minutes.

DIAGNOSTIC PROCEDURE

KEY STEPS

- Confirm the patient's identity using two patient identifiers according to facility policy.
- Perform a venipuncture and collect the sample in a 4-ml tube without additives.
- GGT activity is stable in serum at room temperature for 2 days.

POSTPROCEDURE CARE

- Apply direct pressure to the venipuncture site until bleeding stops.

PRECAUTIONS

- Maintain standard precautions while collecting the sample.
- Handle the sample gently to prevent hemolysis.

COMPLICATIONS

- Hematoma at the venipuncture site

NORMAL RESULTS

- In children, level is 3 to 30 units/L (SI, 0.05 to 0.51 µkat/L).
- In men age 16 and older, level is 6 to 38 units/L (SI, 0.10 to 0.63 µkat/L).
- In women ages 16 to 45, level is 4 to 27 units/L (SI, 0.08 to 0.46 µKat/L); age 45 and older, 6 to 37 units/L (SI, 0.10 to 0.63 µkat/L).

ABNORMAL RESULTS

- Serum GGT levels rise in acute hepatic disease.
- Moderate increases occur in acute pancreatitis, renal disease, and prostatic metastases; postoperatively; and in some patients with epilepsy or brain tumors.
- Levels also increase after alcohol ingestion because of enzyme induction. The sharpest elevations occur in patients with obstructive jaundice and hepatic metastatic infiltrations.
- Levels may also increase 5 to 10 days after acute myocardial infarction because of tissue granulation and healing or as an indication of the effects of cardiac insufficiency on the liver.

Gastric acid stimulation test

DESCRIPTION

- Measures secretion of gastric acid for 1 hour after subcutaneous injection of pentagastrin or a similar drug that stimulates gastric acid output
- Usually done after a basal secretion test suggests abnormal gastric acid secretion

PURPOSE

- To help diagnose duodenal ulcer, Zollinger-Ellison syndrome, pernicious anemia, and gastric carcinoma

PREPARATION

- Make sure that the patient has signed an appropriate consent form.
- Note and report all allergies.
- Check the patient's history for hypersensitivity to pentagastrin.
- The patient must fast from midnight before the test until the test takes place.
- Withhold antacids, anticholinergics, adrenergic-receptor blockers, histamine-2 receptor antagonists, corticosteroids, proton pump inhibitors, and reserpine before the test.

Teaching points

- Explain the purpose of the test and how it's done.
- Tell the patient who will perform the test and where it will be done.
- Tell him to refrain from eating, drinking, and smoking from midnight before the test until the test takes place.
- Inform the patient of any medications to withhold.
- Have the patient notify the practitioner immediately if adverse effects occur (such as abdominal pain, nausea, vomiting, flushing, transitory dizziness, faintness, and numbness of the extremities).
- Inform him that the test takes about 1 hour.

KEY STEPS

- Confirm the patient's identity using two patient identifiers according to facility policy.
- A nasogastric (NG) tube is inserted.
- Basal gastric secretions are collected using the NG tube.
- Pentagastrin is injected.
- Prevent contamination of specimens with saliva.
- After 15 minutes, a specimen is collected every 15 minutes for 1 hour.
- The color, odor, and presence of food, mucus, bile, or blood in specimens are noted and recorded.
- All specimens are labeled "stimulated contents," and numbered 1 through 4.
- Specimens are sent to the laboratory immediately.

POSTPROCEDURE CARE

- If the NG tube is to remain in place, clamp it or attach it to low intermittent suction.
- Watch for and report nausea, vomiting, abdominal distention, or pain after removal of the NG tube.
- Provide soothing lozenges for a sore throat.
- Tell the patient to resume his diet and medications, as ordered.

PRECAUTIONS

WARNING *Watch for adverse effects of pentagastrin, such as rash, hives, nausea, vomiting, abdominal pain, blurred vision, diaphoresis, and shortness of breath.*

COMPLICATIONS

- Adverse effects of pentagastrin

NORMAL RESULTS

- For men, levels are 8 to 28 mEq/hour.
- For women, levels are 11 to 21 mEq/hour.

ABNORMAL RESULTS

- Elevated gastric secretion may indicate duodenal ulcer.
- Markedly elevated secretion suggests Zollinger-Ellison syndrome.
- Depressed secretion may indicate gastric carcinoma.
- Achlorhydria may indicate pernicious anemia.

Gastric culture

DESCRIPTION

- Test for tuberculosis infection, useful when a sputum specimen can't be obtained by expectoration or nebulization
- Requires aspiration of gastric contents and cultivation of any microbes present
- Provides a specimen for rapid presumptive identification of bacteria (by Gram stain) in neonatal septicemia
- Accompanies a chest radiograph and a purified protein derivative skin test

PURPOSE

- To help diagnose mycobacterial infections
- To identify the infectious bacteria in neonatal septicemia

PREPARATION

- Fasting is required for 8 hours before the test.
- Just before the procedure, obtain baseline oxygen saturation and heart rate and rhythm. Assist the patient into high Fowler's position.
- Check the patient's history for recent antimicrobial therapy and inform the practitioner of your findings; it may be necessary to stop drugs before the test.

Teaching points

- Instruct the patient to remain in bed each morning until the specimen collection is complete to prevent premature emptying of stomach contents.
- Explain to the patient (or parents, if the patient is a child) that gastric culture helps diagnose tuberculosis.
- Tell the patient who will perform the test. Explain that it may be necessary to repeat the procedure on three consecutive mornings.
- Inform him that the nasogastric (NG) tube may make him gag but that it passes more easily if he relaxes and follows instructions about breathing and swallowing.
- Instruct the patient to fast for at least 8 hours before the test.
- Inform him (or his parents) that it may take a while to get test results because acid-fast bacteria grow slowly.

DIAGNOSTIC PROCEDURE

KEY STEPS

- Confirm the patient's identity using two patient identifiers according to facility policy.
- As soon as the patient awakens in the morning, put on gloves, perform the NG tube insertion, confirming the position, and obtain gastric washings.
- Clamp the tube before quickly removing it from the patient.
- Note recent antimicrobial therapy on the laboratory request, along with the site and time of collection.
- Label the specimen container with the patient's name, the practitioner's name, and the facility number.
- If possible, obtain the specimens before the start of antimicrobial therapy.
- Never inject water into an NG tube unless you're sure the tube is correctly placed in the patient's stomach. During lavage, use sterile distilled water to decrease the risk of contamination with saprophytic mycobacteria.
- Put the specimen in a tightly capped container, wipe the outside of the container with disinfectant, and place it upright in a plastic bag.

POSTPROCEDURE CARE

- Tell the patient to resume his usual diet and medications.
- Tell him not to blow his nose for 4 hours to prevent bleeding.

PRECAUTIONS

- Wear gloves when performing the procedure and when handling specimens and the NG tube.
- Check the patient's pulse rate for irregularities during this procedure to detect arrhythmias and monitor him for signs of hypoxia.

COMPLICATIONS

- Tube enters the trachea: coughing, cyanosis, decreasing oxygen saturation readings, and gasping result

INTERPRETATION

NORMAL RESULTS

- The culture specimen tests negative for pathogenic mycobacteria.

ABNORMAL RESULTS

- Isolation and identification of the organism *Mycobacterium tuberculosis* indicates the presence of active tuberculosis; other species, such as *M. bovis*, *M. kansasii*, and *M. avium-intracellulare*, may cause pulmonary disease that's clinically indistinguishable from tuberculosis.
- These mycobacterial infections may be difficult to treat and usually require susceptibility studies to determine the most effective antimicrobial therapy.
- Pathogenic bacteria causing neonatal septicemia may also be identified through culture.

Gastrin level test

DESCRIPTION

◆ Measures level of polypeptide hormone that facilitates digestion by triggering gastric acid secretion, stimulates release of enzymes, increases gastric and intestinal motility, and stimulates bile flow
◆ Useful in patients suspected of having gastrinoma (Zollinger-Ellison syndrome)

PURPOSE

◆ To confirm a diagnosis of gastrinoma, the gastrin-secreting tumor in Zollinger-Ellison syndrome
◆ To aid in the differential diagnosis of gastric and duodenal ulcers and pernicious anemia

PREPARATION

◆ Diet and medications are restricted.
◆ The test requires a blood sample.
◆ Withhold all drugs that may interfere with test results, especially insulin and anticholinergics, such as atropine and belladonna, as ordered. If the patient must continue them, note this on the laboratory request.

Teaching points

◆ Explain to the patient that this test helps determine the cause of GI symptoms.
◆ Tell the patient who will perform the test and where it will be done.
◆ Explain to the patient that he may experience slight discomfort from the tourniquet and needle puncture.
◆ Instruct the patient to abstain from alcohol for at least 24 hours before the test and to fast and avoid caffeinated drinks for 12 hours before the test, although he may drink water.
◆ Tell the patient to lie down and relax for at least 30 minutes before the test.
◆ Inform the patient that the test takes about 1 hour.

KEY STEPS

◆ Confirm the patient's identity using two patient identifiers according to facility policy.
◆ Perform a venipuncture and collect the sample in a 10- to 15-ml clot-activator tube.

POSTPROCEDURE CARE

◆ Apply direct pressure to the venipuncture site until bleeding stops.
◆ Tell the patient that he may resume his usual diet and medications, as ordered.

PRECAUTIONS

◆ Handle the sample gently to prevent hemolysis.
◆ To prevent destruction of serum gastrin by proteolytic enzymes, immediately send the sample to the laboratory to have the serum separated and frozen.

COMPLICATIONS

◆ Hematoma at the venipuncture site

NORMAL RESULTS

◆ Gastrin level is 50 to 150 pg/ml (SI, 50 to 150 ng/L).

ABNORMAL RESULTS

◆ Strikingly high serum gastrin levels (> 1,000 pg/ml [SI, > 1,000 ng/L]) confirm Zollinger-Ellison syndrome.
◆ Levels as high as 450,000 pg/ml (SI, 450,000 ng/L) have been reported.
◆ Increased serum levels of gastrin may occur in some patients with duodenal ulcers (< 1 %) and in patients with achlorhydria (with or without pernicious anemia) or extensive stomach carcinoma (because of hyposecretion of gastric juices and hydrochloric acid).

Gastroesophageal reflux scanning

OVERVIEW

DESCRIPTION
◆ Performed when results of a barium swallow X-ray are inconclusive

PURPOSE
◆ To identify reflux
◆ To evaluate for esophageal disorders such as regurgitation
◆ To help identify the cause of nausea and vomiting

PREPARATION
◆ Fasting is required from midnight before the test.

Teaching points
◆ Explain to the patient that the test will evaluate his reflux and identify possible causes for his complaints.
◆ Tell the patient that the test is performed in the nuclear medicine department and is painless and safe.
◆ Inform the patient that a binder with a balloonlike compression device will be applied to his abdomen. The binder will fit snugly and the balloon may be inflated to apply pressure.
◆ Instruct the patient not to have any food or fluids after midnight before the test.
◆ Tell the patient that he will be required to drink a solution, such as orange juice, or eat a small portion of scrambled eggs that contains a radioisotope.
◆ Tell the patient that after ingesting the solution or eggs, a machine is passed over his chest to monitor the radioisotope's passage.
◆ Inform the parents of an infant that the isotope will be given with milk.
◆ Inform the patient that the test takes about 2 hours.

DIAGNOSTIC PROCEDURE

KEY STEPS
◆ Confirm the patient's identity using two patient identifiers according to facility policy.
◆ Place the patient in a supine or upright position and place the binder on the abdomen.
◆ Have the patient swallow the solution containing the radiopharmaceutical.
◆ If needed, the solution may be given via a nasogastric (NG) tube. Remove the NG tube before images are taken to prevent false-positive results.
◆ The binder may be inflated to exert abdominal pressure at specific intervals while a gamma counter is passed over the patient's chest to record the passage of the radiopharmaceutical through the esophagus and into the stomach to determine transit time and evaluate esophageal function.
◆ Reposition the patient as his stomach distends with continuous recordings to visualize events.
◆ A computer analysis is done to calculate the percentage of reflux.

POSTPROCEDURE CARE
◆ Remove the binder from the abdomen.

PRECAUTIONS
◆ Endoscopic tube insertion is used with patients who have esophageal motor dysfunction, hiatal hernia, or difficulty swallowing.
◆ Apply the binder below the ribs to prevent fractures.

COMPLICATIONS
◆ None

INTERPRETATION

NORMAL RESULTS
◆ The radioisotope descends through the esophagus in about 6 seconds. Radioactivity is only seen in the stomach and small bowel.
◆ Gastric reflux is below 4%.

ABNORMAL RESULTS
◆ Diffuse spasm of the esophagus, achalasia, or other esophageal motility disorders prolong transit time.
◆ Radioactivity is detected in the esophagus with gastroesophageal reflux.

Gastrointestinal bleeding scanning

OVERVIEW

DESCRIPTION
◆ Nuclear medicine scan that localizes active GI bleeding

PURPOSE
◆ To detect and localize active GI tract bleeding to help in endoscopic or angiographic studies
◆ To detect and localize non-GI intra-abdominal hemorrhage

PREPARATION
◆ Obtain the patient's vital signs.
◆ Have the patient void before beginning the procedure.
◆ Administer a sedative if needed.

Teaching points
◆ Explain to the patient that this test helps determine the location of his bleeding.
◆ Tell the patient that only a small amount of nuclear material is administered during the test.
◆ Tell the patient who will perform the test and where it will be done.
◆ Inform the patient that he may feel as if he's going to have a bowel movement during the test, and to inform the technologist if this occurs.
◆ Tell the patient that he doesn't have to restrict food or drink, unless ordered.
◆ Instruct the patient to lie still during the procedure for the best images.
◆ Inform the patient that the test takes 1 to 4 hours.
◆ For 24 to 48 hours after the test, tell the patient to drink increased fluids.
◆ For 24 hours after the test, instruct the patient to flush the toilet immediately after voiding and to carefully wash his hands with soap and water.
◆ Instruct all caregivers to wear gloves when handling the patient's urine for 24 hours after the test.

DIAGNOSTIC PROCEDURE

KEY STEPS
◆ Confirm the patient's identity using two patient identifiers according to facility policy.
◆ Place the patient in a supine position on the table.
◆ Position the patient with foam wedges to help maintain his position.
◆ Inject the radionuclide into the patient and begin scanning.
◆ The abdomen is scanned every 1 minute, and then progress to every 5 to 15 minutes.
◆ Closely monitor the patient's vital signs during the procedure.

POSTPROCEDURE CARE
◆ Monitor the patient's vital signs.

PRECAUTIONS
◆ Use gloves when handling the radionuclide.
◆ If the patient is unstable, be aware that he may not tolerate the test.

COMPLICATIONS
◆ Reactions to the radionuclide

INTERPRETATION

NORMAL FINDINGS
◆ The radionuclide has normal distribution in the large vessels with no signs of bleeding.

ABNORMAL RESULTS
◆ The radionuclide accumulates at the site of active bleeding in the GI tract.
◆ The test won't identify the exact cause of the bleeding.
◆ The test isn't useful in the patient with chronic anemia.

Given diagnostic imaging

DESCRIPTION

◆ Records video images of stomach and small intestine, using a tiny video camera with light source and transmitter inside a capsule propelled through digestive tract by peristalsis
◆ Used to record images where other diagnostic techniques may not reach or make visible (see *Detecting disorders in the stomach and small intestine*)
◆ Also called the *camera pill*

PURPOSE

◆ To detect polyps or cancer
◆ To detect the causes of bleeding and anemia

PREPARATION

◆ Usually no bowel preparation is involved, but some patients may benefit from it.

Teaching points

◆ Explain that this test shows the stomach and small intestine, helping to detect disorders.
◆ Tell the patient who will perform the test and where it will be done.
◆ Inform him that he may need to fast for 12 hours before the test but may have fluids for up to 2 hours before the test.
◆ Explain to the patient that he'll need to swallow the camera pill and that it will send information to a receiver he'll wear on his belt.
◆ Tell him that the procedure is painless and that after swallowing the pill he can go home or go to work.
◆ Explain that walking helps facilitate movement of the pill.
◆ Tell him that he'll need to return to the facility in 24 hours (or as directed) so the recorder can be removed from his belt.
◆ Tell the patient that he will excrete the pill normally in his feces within 8 to 72 hours.

DIAGNOSTIC PROCEDURE

KEY STEPS

◆ Confirm the patient's identity using two patient identifiers according to facility policy.
◆ The patient ingests the camera pill, and a receiver is attached to his belt.
◆ The pill records images for up to 6 hours along its path through the stomach, small intestine, and mouth of the large intestine, transmitting the information to a data recorder on a belt worn around the patient's waist.
◆ The patient returns to the facility, as instructed, so the images can be transmitted to the computer, where they're displayed on the screen.

POSTPROCEDURE CARE

◆ After the images are obtained, tell the patient to resume his usual diet.

PRECAUTIONS

◆ The procedure is contraindicated in patients with a suspected obstruction, fistula, or stricture and in infants, young children, and others who can't swallow capsules.
◆ Because the battery is short lived, images of the large intestine can't be obtained.
◆ The capsule can't stop bleeding, take tissue samples, remove growths, or repair other detected problems (other invasive studies may be needed).

COMPLICATIONS

◆ None

INTERPRETATION

NORMAL RESULTS

◆ Normal anatomy of the stomach and small intestine is noted.

ABNORMAL RESULTS

◆ Bleeding sites or abnormalities of the stomach and small bowel, such as erosions, Crohn's disease, celiac disease, benign and malignant tumors of the small intestine, vascular disorders, medication-related small-bowel injuries, and pediatric small-bowel disorders are noted.

Detecting disorders in the stomach and small intestine

In the Given diagnostic imaging system, the patient swallows the capsule, which then travels through the body by the natural movement of the digestive tract. A receiver worn outside the body records the images. The strength of the signal indicates the capsule's location.

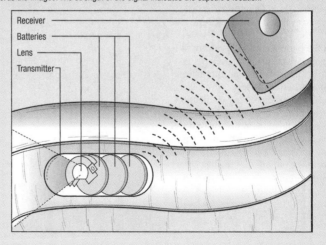

Receiver
Batteries
Lens
Transmitter

Glucagon level test

OVERVIEW

DESCRIPTION

- Radioimmunoassay for quantitative analysis of plasma glucagon, which promotes glucose production, controls its storage, and is secreted during hypoglycemia
- Evaluates patients suspected of having glucagonoma (alpha cell tumor) or hypoglycemia caused by idiopathic glucagon deficiency or pancreatic dysfunction
- Measured with glucose and insulin levels because these influence glucagon secretion

PURPOSE

- To help diagnose glucagonoma and hypoglycemia caused by chronic pancreatitis or idiopathic glucagon deficiency

PREPARATION

- Fasting is required for 10 to 12 hours before the test.
- Withhold insulin, catecholamines, and other drugs that may influence test results. If the patient must continue them, note this on the laboratory request.
- This test requires a blood sample.
- Have the patient lie down and relax for 30 minutes before the test.

Teaching points

- Explain to the patient that this test helps to evaluate pancreatic function.
- Tell the patient who will perform the test and where it will be done.
- Instruct the patient to fast for at least 10 hours before the test.
- Advise the patient of any medication restrictions.
- Explain to the patient that he may experience slight discomfort from the tourniquet and needle puncture.
- Inform the patient that the test takes about 45 minutes.

DIAGNOSTIC PROCEDURE

KEY STEPS

- Confirm the patient's identity using two patient identifiers according to facility policy.
- Perform a venipuncture and collect the sample in a chilled 10-ml EDTA tube.
- Place the sample on ice and send it to the laboratory immediately.

POSTPROCEDURE CARE

- Apply direct pressure to the venipuncture site until bleeding stops.
- Tell the patient to resume his usual diet and medications, as ordered.

PRECAUTIONS

- Maintain standard precautions while collecting the sample.
- Handle the sample gently to prevent hemolysis.

COMPLICATIONS

- Hematoma at the venipuncture site

INTERPRETATION

NORMAL RESULTS

- Level is below 60 pg/ml (SI, < 60 ng/L).

ABNORMAL RESULTS

- Elevated fasting levels (900 to 7,800 pg/ml [SI, 900 to 7,800 ng/L]) can occur in patients with glucagonoma, diabetes mellitus, acute pancreatitis, and pheochromocytoma.
- Abnormally low glucagon levels are linked to idiopathic glucagon deficiency and hypoglycemia caused by chronic pancreatitis.

INTERFERING FACTORS *Exercise, stress, prolonged fasting, insulin, or catecholamines (possible increase in glucagon level)*

Glucose oxidase test

DESCRIPTION

◆ Specific, qualitative test for glycosuria, to monitor urine glucose in patients with diabetes
◆ May be performed at home because of its simplicity and convenience (uses commercial, plastic-coated reagent strips [Clinistix, Diastix] or glucose enzymatic test strips)

PURPOSE

◆ To detect glycosuria and determine the renal threshold for glucose
◆ To monitor urine glucose levels during insulin therapy

PREPARATION

◆ Use Clinitest tablets if the patient is taking ascorbic acid, hypochlorites, levodopa, peroxides, phenazopyridine, or salicylates.
◆ No dietary restrictions are needed.

Teaching points

◆ Explain to the patient that the glucose oxidase test determines urine glucose level.
◆ Tell the patient who will perform the test and where it will be done.
◆ Tell him he doesn't have to restrict his diet.
◆ If the patient is newly diagnosed with diabetes, teach him how to perform a reagent strip test.
◆ Instruct him not to contaminate the urine specimen with toilet tissue or feces.
◆ Inform him that the test takes about 1 hour.

KEY STEPS

◆ Confirm the patient's identity using two patient identifiers according to facility policy.
◆ Have the patient void, and then give him a drink of water.
◆ Collect a second-voided specimen after 30 to 45 minutes.

Clinistix test

◆ Dip the test area of the reagent strip in the specimen for 2 seconds.
◆ Remove excess urine by tapping the strip against a clean surface or the side of the container and begin timing.
◆ Hold the Clinistix strip in the air and "read" the color exactly 10 seconds after taking the strip out of the urine by comparing it with the reference color blocks on the label of the container.
◆ Record the results; ignore color changes that develop after 10 seconds.

Diastix test

◆ Dip the reagent strip in the specimen for 2 seconds.
◆ Remove excess urine by tapping the strip against the container and begin timing.
◆ Hold the Diastix strip in the air and compare the color to the color chart exactly 30 seconds after taking the strip out of the urine.
◆ Record the results; ignore color changes that develop after 30 seconds.

Glucose enzymatic test strip

◆ Withdraw about 1″ (2.5 cm) of the reagent tape from the dispenser; dip ¼″ (0.6 cm) in the specimen for 2 seconds.
◆ Remove excess urine by tapping the strip against the side of the container and begin timing.
◆ Hold the glucose enzymatic test strip in the air and compare the color of the darkest part of the tape to the color chart exactly 60 seconds after taking the strip out of the urine.

◆ If the tape indicates 0.5% or higher, wait an additional 60 seconds to make the final color comparison.
◆ Record the results.

POSTPROCEDURE CARE

◆ Keep the test strip container tightly closed to prevent deterioration of the strips by exposure to light or moisture.

PRECAUTIONS

◆ Store the container under 86° F (30° C) to avoid heat degradation.
◆ Don't use discolored or darkened Clinistix or Diastix, or dark yellow or yellow-brown glucose enzymatic test strips.

COMPLICATIONS

◆ None

NORMAL RESULTS

◆ No glucose is detected in the urine.

ABNORMAL RESULTS

◆ Glycosuria occurs in diabetes mellitus, adrenal and thyroid disorders, hepatic and central nervous system diseases, conditions involving low renal threshold (such as Fanconi's syndrome), toxic renal tubular disease, heavy metal poisoning, glomerulonephritis, and nephrosis; in pregnant women; and in those receiving total parenteral nutrition.
◆ Glycosuria occurs with prolonged use of phenothiazines and with ingestion of large amounts of glucose and of certain drugs, such as ammonium chloride, asparaginase, carbamazepine, corticosteroids, dextrothyroxine, lithium carbonate, nicotinic acid, and thiazide diuretics.

Glucose-6-phosphate dehydrogenase test

DESCRIPTION

♦ Detects glucose-6-phosphate dehy-drogenase (G6PD) deficiency — hereditary, sex-linked condition impairing stability of red blood cell (RBC) membrane and allowing strong oxidizing agents to destroy RBCs
♦ Mild deficiency: young RBCs have enough G6PD to survive; inherited by 10% of black males in United States
♦ Severe deficiency: all RBCs destroyed; inherited by some people of Mediterranean descent
♦ Hemolytic episodes produced by fava bean consumption in some whites

PURPOSE

♦ To detect hemolytic anemia caused by G6PD deficiency
♦ To aid in the differential diagnosis of hemolytic anemia

PREPARATION

♦ The test requires a blood sample.
♦ No dietary restrictions are needed.
♦ Check the patient's history and report recent blood transfusion or ingestion of aspirin, sulfonamides, phenacetin, nitrofurantoin, vitamin K derivatives, antimalarials, or fava beans, which cause hemolysis in patients with G6PD deficiency.

Teaching points

♦ Explain that this test detects an inherited enzyme deficiency that may affect RBCs.
♦ Tell the patient who will perform the test and where it will be done.
♦ Explain that the patient may experience slight discomfort from the tourniquet and needle puncture.
♦ Tell him that no dietary restrictions are needed.
♦ Inform him that the test should take less than 5 minutes.

KEY STEPS

♦ Confirm the patient's identity using two patient identifiers according to facility policy.
♦ Perform a venipuncture and collect the sample in a 4-ml EDTA tube.
♦ Completely fill the collection tube and invert it gently several times to mix the sample and anticoagulant.

POSTPROCEDURE CARE

♦ Apply direct pressure to the venipuncture site until bleeding stops.

PRECAUTIONS

♦ Handle the sample gently to prevent hemolysis.
♦ Refrigerate the sample if you can't send it to the laboratory immediately.

COMPLICATIONS

♦ Hematoma at the venipuncture site

NORMAL RESULTS

♦ Values vary with the measurement method but range from 4.3 to 11.8 units/g (SI, 0.28 to 0.76 milliunits/mmol) of hemoglobin.

ABNORMAL RESULTS

♦ Fluorescent spot testing or staining for Heinz bodies or erythrocytes can test for G6PD deficiency.
♦ If results are positive, the kinetic quantitative assay for G6PD may be necessary.
♦ Electrophoretic techniques assess genetic variants of deficiencies (which may cause lifelong, mild, or asymptomatic anemia).
♦ Some variants produce symptoms only when the patient experiences stress or illness or has been exposed to drugs or agents that elicit hemolytic episodes.

Glycosylated hemoglobin test

OVERVIEW

DESCRIPTION
- Monitors diabetes therapy by measuring the glycosylated hemoglobin (HbA$_{1c}$) level; provides information about the average blood glucose level during the preceding 2 to 3 months
- Requires only one venipuncture every 6 to 8 weeks; evaluates long-term effectiveness of diabetes therapy
- Reports values as percentage of total Hb in an erythrocyte
- Also called *total fasting Hb*

PURPOSE
- To assess control of diabetes mellitus

PREPARATION
- The test requires a blood sample.

Teaching points
- Explain that the HbA$_{1c}$ test evaluates diabetes therapy.
- Tell the patient who will perform the test and where it will be done.
- Explain that the patient may experience slight discomfort from the tourniquet and needle puncture.
- Inform him that he need not restrict food and fluids, and instruct him to maintain his prescribed medication and diet regimens.
- Inform him that the test should take less than 5 minutes.

DIAGNOSTIC PROCEDURE

KEY STEPS
- Confirm the patient's identity using two patient identifiers according to facility policy.
- Perform a venipuncture and collect the sample in a 5-ml EDTA tube.
- Invert the sample gently several times to mix the sample and anticoagulant adequately.

POSTPROCEDURE CARE
- Apply direct pressure to the venipuncture site until bleeding stops.
- Schedule the patient for an appointment in 6 to 8 weeks for appropriate follow-up testing.

PRECAUTIONS
- Completely fill the collection tube.

COMPLICATIONS
- Hematoma at the venipuncture site

INTERPRETATION

NORMAL RESULTS
- HbA$_{1c}$ value is 4% to 7%.

ABNORMAL RESULTS
- In diabetes, the patient has good control of blood glucose levels when the HbA$_{1c}$ value is less than 8%.
- An HbA$_{1c}$ value greater than 10% indicates poor control.

Gonorrhea culture

OVERVIEW

- Stained smear of genital exudate to confirm gonorrhea in men with characteristic symptoms and in women (especially if asymptomatic)
- Culture sites: urethra (in men), endocervix (in women), rectum, and throat

PURPOSE
- To confirm gonorrhea

PREPARATION
- Female patients should avoid douching for 24 hours before the test.
- Male patients shouldn't void during the hour before the test.

Teaching points
- Explain the purpose of the test and how it's done.
- Tell the patient who will perform the test and where it will be done.
- Instruct the female patient to avoid douching for 24 hours before the test.
- Tell the male patient not to void during the hour before the test.
- Advise the patient of dietary restrictions, if ordered.
- Explain that the test take about 15 minutes.
- Advise the patient to avoid sexual contact until test results are available.
- Explain that treatment usually begins after confirming a positive culture, except in a person who has symptoms of gonorrhea or who has had intercourse with someone known to have gonorrhea.
- Advise the patient that a repeat culture is necessary 1 week after the end of treatment to evaluate the effectiveness of therapy.
- Inform the patient that positive culture findings must be reported to the local health department.

DIAGNOSTIC PROCEDURE

KEY STEPS
- Confirm the patient's identity using two patient identifiers according to facility policy.
- *Endocervical culture:* Place the patient in the lithotomy position and drape her appropriately.
- To obtain a culture, use gloved hands and insert a vaginal speculum that has been lubricated only with warm water. Clean mucus from the cervix, using cotton balls in a ring forceps.
- Insert a dry, sterile cotton swab into the endocervical canal and rotate it from side to side. Leave the swab in place for several seconds for optimum absorption of organisms.
- In cases of deep pelvic inflammatory disease, it may be necessary to take cultures of the endometrium or aspirations by laparoscopy or culdoscopy.
- *Urethral culture:* Place the patient in a supine position and drape him appropriately.
- Clean the urethral meatus with sterile gauze or a cotton swab and then insert a thin urogenital alginate swab or a wire bacteriologic loop ⅜″ to ¾″

Culturing for *Neisseria gonorrhoeae*

Culturing for *Neisseria gonorrhoeae* requires the use of a modified Thayer-Martin (MTM) medium. If a laboratory isn't readily available, you may use Transgrow medium.

MODIFIED THAYER-MARTIN MEDIUM

MTM medium is a combination of hemoglobin, gonococcal growth-enhancing chemicals, and antimicrobial agents for culturing endocervical, urethral, rectal, and throat specimens. To inoculate a culture plate treated with MTM medium and to spread organisms out of their associated mucus, take these steps:
- Roll the swab in a Z pattern (as shown).
- Using the swab or a sterile wire loop, immediately cross-streak the plate (as shown).
- Incubate within 15 minutes of streaking.

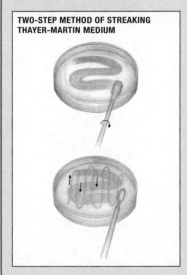

TWO-STEP METHOD OF STREAKING THAYER-MARTIN MEDIUM

TRANSGROW MEDIUM

A modification of MTM medium, Transgrow is available in a screw-cap bottle containing air and carbon dioxide. Transgrow bottles are used to transport suspect cultures when laboratory facilities aren't available at the site of specimen collection. Use this procedure:
- To prevent loss of carbon dioxide, inoculate the specimen bottle while it's upright.
- After uncapping the bottle, immediately insert the swab and soak up all excess moisture.
- Starting at the bottom of the bottle, roll the swab from side to side across the medium (as shown).
- Recap the bottle, and send it to the laboratory immediately. Subculturing should begin within 24 to 48 hours.

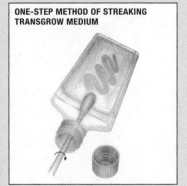

ONE-STEP METHOD OF STREAKING TRANSGROW MEDIUM

(1 to 2 cm) into the urethra, and rotate the swab or loop from side to side. Leave it in place for several seconds for optimum absorption of organisms.

◆ *Rectal culture:* After obtaining an endocervical or a urethral specimen, insert a sterile cotton swab into the anal canal about 1″ (2.5 cm), move the swab from side to side, and leave it in place for several seconds for optimum absorption.

– If the rectal swab is contaminated with stool, discard it and repeat the procedure with a clean swab.

◆ *Throat culture:* Position the patient with his head tilted back.

– Check his throat for inflamed areas using a tongue blade. Rub a sterile swab from side to side over the tonsillar areas, including inflamed or purulent sites.

◆ After specimen collection: Roll the swab in a Z pattern in a plate containing modified Thayer-Martin medium. Then cross-streak the medium with a sterile wire loop or the tip of the swab and cover the plate. (See *Culturing for* Neisseria gonorrhoeae.)

– Label the specimen with the appropriate information.

– Make direct smears of obtained material immediately to prepare the Gram stain. Quickly inoculate remaining material into selective culture media or into a transport system.

– Use a Culturette transport tube or a swab transport medium containing charcoal. Charcoal helps neutralize toxic materials in the specimen.

– If laboratory facilities aren't readily available, uncap the Transgrow medium specimen bottle just before inserting the swab of test material into the bottle. Keep the bottle upright to minimize loss of carbon dioxide. With the swab, absorb the excess moisture within the bottle and then roll the swab across the Transgrow medium. Discard the swab. Place the lid on the bottle and label it appropriately.

POSTPROCEDURE CARE

◆ The patient should avoid sexual relations until test results are available.

PRECAUTIONS

◆ Maintain standard precautions while collecting the specimen.

◆ Men sometimes experience nausea, sweating, weakness, and fainting from stress or discomfort when the cotton swab or wire loop enters the urethra.

COMPLICATIONS

◆ Vasovagal response in men

NORMAL RESULTS

◆ No *Neisseria gonorrhoeae* is detected in the culture.

ABNORMAL RESULTS

◆ A positive culture confirms gonorrhea.

Growth hormone suppression test

OVERVIEW

DESCRIPTION

- Evaluates excessive baseline levels of human growth hormone (hGH) from the anterior pituitary gland
- hGH: increases plasma glucose and fatty acid levels; insulin secretion increases to counteract these effects
- Also called *glucose loading*

PURPOSE

- To assess elevated baseline levels of hGH
- To confirm a diagnosis of gigantism in children and acromegaly in adults and adolescents

PREPARATION

- Withhold all steroids and other pituitary-based hormones. If the patient must continue these or other drugs, note this on the laboratory request.
- The test requires two blood samples.
- Withhold food and fluids and limit physical activity for at least 10 hours before the test.

Teaching points

- Explain to the patient, or his parents if the patient is a child, that this test helps determine the cause of his abnormal growth.
- Tell the patient who will perform the test and where it will be done.
- Tell the patient to lie down and relax for 30 minutes before the test.
- Instruct the patient to fast and limit physical activity for 10 to 12 hours before the test.
- Tell him that the test will require two blood samples. Warn him that he may experience nausea after drinking the glucose solution and some discomfort from the needle punctures and tourniquet.
- Inform the patient that the test takes about 1½ hours.

DIAGNOSTIC PROCEDURE

KEY STEPS

- Confirm the patient's identity using two patient identifiers according to facility policy.
- Perform a venipuncture and collect 6 ml of blood (basal sample) in a 7-ml clot-activator tube between 6 a.m. and 8 a.m.
- Give the patient 100 g of glucose solution by mouth. To prevent nausea, advise the patient to drink the glucose slowly.
- About 1 hour later, draw venous blood into a 7-ml clot-activator tube. Label the tubes appropriately and send them to the laboratory immediately.

POSTPROCEDURE CARE

- Apply direct pressure to the venipuncture site until bleeding stops.
- Tell the patient to resume his usual diet, activities, and medications, as ordered.

PRECAUTIONS

- Handle the samples gently to prevent hemolysis.
- Send each sample to the laboratory immediately because hGH has a half-life of only 20 to 25 minutes.

COMPLICATIONS

- Hematoma at the venipuncture site

INTERPRETATION

NORMAL RESULTS

- Glucose load suppresses hGH to levels ranging from undetectable to 3 ng/ml (SI, 3 µg/L) in 30 minutes to 2 hours.
- In children, rebound stimulation may occur after 2 to 5 hours.

ABNORMAL RESULTS

- In a patient with active acromegaly, elevated baseline hGH levels (5 ng/ml [SI, 5 µg/L]) aren't suppressed to less than 5 ng/ml during the test.
- Unchanged or rising hGH levels in response to glucose loading indicate hGH hypersecretion and may confirm suspected acromegaly and gigantism. This response may be verified by repeating the test after a 1-day rest.

Ham test

DESCRIPTION
- Determines the cause of hemolytic anemia, hemoglobinuria, and bone marrow aplasia and the stability of the red blood cell (RBC) membrane
- Helps diagnose paroxysmal nocturnal hemoglobinuria (PNH), a rare hematologic disease
- Washed RBCs mixed with ABO-compatible normal serum and acid; incubated at 98.6° F (37° C); examined for hemolysis
- Most PNH cells lysed in acidified human serum; normal RBCs not lysed
- Also known as *acidified serum lysis test*

PURPOSE
- To help diagnose PNH
- To determine cause of anemia

PREPARATION
- No dietary restrictions are needed.
- The test requires a blood sample.

Teaching points
- Explain to the patient that this test helps determine the cause of his anemia.
- Tell the patient who will perform the test and where it will be done.
- Explain that he may experience slight discomfort from the tourniquet and needle puncture.
- Tell him that he doesn't have to restrict his diet.
- Inform him that the test should take less than 5 minutes.

KEY STEPS
- Confirm the patient's identity using two patient identifiers according to facility policy.
- Because the blood sample must be defibrinated immediately, laboratory personnel perform the venipuncture and collect the sample.

POSTPROCEDURE CARE
- Apply direct pressure to the venipuncture site until bleeding stops.

PRECAUTIONS
- Only laboratory personnel should collect the sample.

COMPLICATIONS
- Hematoma at the venipuncture site

NORMAL RESULTS
- RBCs don't undergo hemolysis.
- Test results are negative.

ABNORMAL RESULTS
- Hemolysis of RBCs indicates PNH.

Haptoglobin level test

| |

OVERVIEW

DESCRIPTION

◆ Measures serum levels of haptoglobin (glycoprotein produced in the liver)
◆ Acute intravascular hemolysis: haptoglobin level decreases rapidly and may remain low for 5 to 7 days until the liver synthesizes more glycoprotein

PURPOSE

◆ To serve as an index of hemolysis
◆ To distinguish between hemoglobin and myoglobin in plasma; haptoglobin doesn't bind with myoglobin
◆ To investigate hemolytic transfusion reactions
◆ To establish proof of paternity using genetic (phenotypic) variations in haptoglobin structure

PREPARATION

◆ The test requires a blood sample.
◆ No dietary restrictions are needed.
◆ Notify the laboratory and practitioner of drugs the patient is taking that may affect test results; these medications may be restricted.

Teaching points

◆ Explain that this test determines the condition of red blood cells.
◆ Tell the patient who will perform the test and where it will be done.
◆ Tell him that no dietary restrictions are required.
◆ Explain that he may experience slight discomfort from the tourniquet and needle puncture.
◆ Inform the patient that the test should take less than 5 minutes.

DIAGNOSTIC PROCEDURE

KEY STEPS

◆ Confirm the patient's identity using two patient identifiers according to facility policy.
◆ Perform a venipuncture and collect the sample in a 7-ml clot-activator tube.

POSTPROCEDURE CARE

◆ Apply direct pressure to the venipuncture site until bleeding stops.
◆ Tell the patient to resume his usual medications.

PRECAUTIONS

⚡ **WARNING** *If serum haptoglobin values are very low, watch for symptoms of hemolysis, such as chills, fever, back pain, flushing, jugular vein distention, tachycardia, tachypnea, and hypotension.*
◆ Handle the sample gently to prevent hemolysis.

COMPLICATIONS

◆ Hematoma at the venipuncture site

INTERPRETATION

NORMAL RESULTS

◆ Serum haptoglobin levels, measured in terms of the protein's hemoglobin-binding capacity, range from 40 to 180 mg/dl (SI, 0.4 to 1.8 g/L).
◆ Nephelometric procedures yield lower results.
◆ Although haptoglobin is absent in 90% of neonates, levels gradually increase to normal by age 4 months.

ABNORMAL RESULTS

◆ Markedly decreased serum haptoglobin levels are characteristic in acute and chronic hemolysis, severe hepatocellular disease, infectious mononucleosis, and transfusion reactions.
◆ Hepatocellular disease inhibits haptoglobin synthesis.
◆ In hemolytic transfusion reactions, haptoglobin levels begin decreasing after 6 to 8 hours and fall to 40% of pretransfusion levels after 24 hours.
◆ In about 1% of the population, including 4% of blacks, haptoglobin is absent; this disorder is known as *congenital ahaptoglobinemia.*
◆ Elevated serum haptoglobin levels occur in diseases marked by chronic inflammatory reactions or tissue destruction, such as rheumatoid arthritis and malignant neoplasms.

Heinz bodies test

OVERVIEW

OVERVIEW

DESCRIPTION

- Detects Heinz bodies in a whole blood sample using phase microscopy or supravital stains
- If precipitation not spontaneous, various oxidant drugs added to the sample
- Heinz bodies: result of drug injury to red blood cells (RBCs), presence of unstable hemoglobin (Hb), unbalanced globin chain synthesis caused by thalassemia, or a red cell enzyme deficiency (such as glucose-6-phosphate dehydrogenase deficiency)
- Although removed from RBCs by the spleen, major cause of hemolytic anemias (see *Identifying Heinz bodies*)

PURPOSE

- To help detect causes of hemolytic anemia

PREPARATION

- The test requires a blood sample.
- No dietary restrictions are needed.
- Notify the laboratory and practitioner of drugs the patient is taking that may affect test results; they may be restricted.

Teaching points

- Explain that this test determines the cause of anemia.
- Tell the patient who will perform the test and where it will be done.
- Tell him that he doesn't have to restrict his diet.
- Explain that he may experience slight discomfort from the tourniquet and needle puncture.
- Inform the patient that the test should take less than 5 minutes.

DIAGNOSTIC PROCEDURE

KEY STEPS

- Confirm the patient's identity using two patient identifiers according to facility policy.
- Perform a venipuncture and collect the sample in a 3- or 4.5-ml EDTA tube.
- Invert the tube gently several times to mix the sample and anticoagulant.

POSTPROCEDURE CARE

- Apply direct pressure to the venipuncture site until bleeding stops.
- If a large hematoma develops at the venipuncture site, monitor pulses distal to the site.
- Tell the patient to resume his medications, as ordered.

PRECAUTIONS

- Maintain standard precautions while collecting the sample.
- Fill the sample collection tube completely.

COMPLICATIONS

- Hematoma at the venipuncture site

INTERPRETATION

NORMAL RESULTS

- A negative test result indicates an absence of Heinz bodies.

ABNORMAL RESULTS

- The presence of Heinz bodies may indicate an inherited RBC enzyme deficiency, the presence of unstable Hb, thalassemia, or drug-induced RBC injury.
- Heinz bodies may also be present after splenectomy.

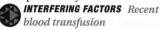 **INTERFERING FACTORS** *Recent blood transfusion*

Identifying Heinz bodies

After supravital staining, Heinz bodies (particles of denatured hemoglobin that are usually attached to the cell membrane) appear as small, purple inclusions at cell margins. Heinz bodies are present in certain hemolytic anemias.

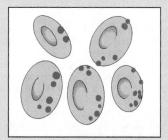

Helicobacter pylori antibody test

OVERVIEW

DESCRIPTION
- Noninvasive screening procedure for *Helicobacter pylori* that may be performed after gastric specimen obtained by endoscopy and cultured, using enzyme-linked immunosorbent assay (see *Other tests for* Helicobacter pylori)
- *H. pylori*: spiral, gram-negative bacterium linked to chronic gastritis and idiopathic chronic duodenal ulceration

PURPOSE
- To help diagnose *H. pylori* infection in patients with GI symptoms

PREPARATION
- No dietary restrictions are needed.
- The test requires a blood sample.

Teaching points
- Explain that this test diagnoses the infection that may cause ulcers.
- Tell him who will perform the test and where it will be done.
- Tell him that he doesn't have to restrict his diet.
- Explain that he may experience slight discomfort from the tourniquet and needle puncture.
- Tell the patient that the test should take less than 5 minutes.

DIAGNOSTIC PROCEDURE

KEY STEPS
- Confirm the patient's identity using two patient identifiers according to facility policy.
- Perform a venipuncture and collect the sample in a 7-ml clot-activator tube.
- Send the sample to the laboratory immediately.

POSTPROCEDURE CARE
- Apply direct pressure to the venipuncture site until bleeding stops.

PRECAUTIONS
- Maintain standard precautions while collecting the sample.
- This test should be performed only on patients with GI symptoms because many healthy people have *H. pylori* antibodies.

COMPLICATIONS
- Hematoma at the venipuncture site

INTERPRETATION

NORMAL RESULTS
- In a negative test result, no antibodies to *H. pylori* are found.

ABNORMAL RESULTS
- A positive *H. pylori* test result indicates that the patient has antibodies to the bacterium.
- Serologic results should be interpreted in light of clinical findings.

Other tests for *Helicobacter pylori*

H. pylori is detectable through blood, breath, feces, and tissue tests. Blood, breath, and feces tests are usually done before a tissue test because they are less invasive. Blood tests aren't used to detect *H. pylori* after treatment because a patient's blood can test positive even after *H. pylori* has been eliminated.

BLOOD TEST
The most common method, this test detects antibodies to *H. pylori* bacteria.

UREA BREATH TEST
Effective as a diagnostic tool for *H. pylori*, this test can also monitor whether treatment has been effective. In the practitioner's office, the patient drinks a urea solution that contains a special carbon atom. If *H. pylori* is present, it breaks down the urea, releasing the carbon. Blood carries the carbon to the lungs, and the patient exhales it. The breath test is 96% to 98% accurate.

FECES TEST
The *H. pylori* stool antigen test is another accurate way to detect *H. pylori* infection. It's a noninvasive test.

TISSUE TEST
Normally, this test uses a biopsy sample taken with an endoscope, using one of three types:
- The rapid urease test detects the enzyme disease caused by *H. pylori*.
- A histology test allows the physician to find and examine the actual bacteria.
- A culture test grows *H. pylori* in the tissue sample.

Hematocrit test

DESCRIPTION

- Performed separately or as part of a complete blood count
- Measures percentage by volume of packed red blood cells (RBCs) in a whole blood sample; for example, hematocrit (HCT) of 40% indicates that a 100-ml sample of blood contains 40 ml of packed RBCs
- Packing achieved by centrifuging anticoagulated whole blood in a capillary tube so that RBCs pack tightly without hemolysis
- Results used to calculate mean corpuscular volume and mean corpuscular hemoglobin concentration

PURPOSE

- To help diagnose polycythemia, anemia, or abnormal states of hydration
- To aid in the calculation of erythrocyte indices

PREPARATION

- The test requires a blood sample.
- No dietary restrictions are needed.

Teaching points

- Explain that the HCT test detects anemia and other abnormal blood conditions.
- Tell the patient who will perform the test and where it will be done.
- Tell him that there are no dietary restrictions.
- Explain to the patient that he may experience slight discomfort from the tourniquet and needle puncture.
- If the patient is a child, explain to him (if he's old enough) and his parents that a small amount of blood will be taken from his finger or earlobe.
- Tell him that the test should take less than 5 minutes. (See *How red blood cells work,* page 252.)

KEY STEPS

- Confirm the patient's identity using two patient identifiers according to facility policy.
- Perform a fingerstick using a heparinized capillary tube with a red band on the anticoagulant end. Fill the tube from the red-banded end to about two-thirds capacity; seal this end with clay.
- Or, perform a venipuncture and fill a 3- or 4.5-ml EDTA tube.
- Invert the tube gently several times to mix the sample.
- After testing, place the tube in the centrifuge with the red end pointing outward.

POSTPROCEDURE CARE

- Apply direct pressure to the venipuncture site until bleeding stops.
- Make sure that subdermal bleeding has stopped before removing pressure.
- If a large hematoma develops at the venipuncture site, monitor pulses distal to the site.

PRECAUTIONS

- Send the sample to the laboratory immediately.

COMPLICATIONS

- Hematoma at the venipuncture site

NORMAL RESULTS

- HCT is usually measured electronically; results are 3% lower than manual measurements, which trap plasma in the column of packed RBCs.
- In men, the value is 42% to 52% (SI, 0.42 to 0.52).
- In women, the value is 36% to 48% (SI, 0.36 to 0.48).
- In neonates younger than age 1 week, the value is 55% to 68% (SI, 0.55 to 0.68).
- In neonates age 1 week, the value is 47% to 65% (SI, 0.47 to 0.65).
- In infants age 1 month, the value is 37% to 49% (SI, 0.37 to 0.49).
- In infants age 3 months, the value is 30% to 36% (SI, 0.3 to 0.36).
- In infants age 1, the value is 29% to 41% (SI, 0.29 to 0.41).
- In children age 10, the value is 36% to 40% (SI, 0.36 to 0.4).

ABNORMAL RESULTS

- Low HCT suggests anemia, hemodilution, or massive blood loss.
- High HCT indicates polycythemia or hemoconcentration caused by blood loss and dehydration.

(continued)

How red blood cells work

If your patient thinks of iron deficiency anemia as just a minor malady, he may not comply with treatment. So encourage him to grasp the disorder's seriousness by explaining the oxygen-carrying role of red blood cells (RBCs) and describing how they develop. Highlight the crucial role played by iron.

WHERE DO RBCS COME FROM?

Explain that RBCs begin in stem cells in the bone marrow. During this process called *erythropoiesis,* a nucleated RBC precursor (hemocytoblast) matures into a nucleus-free RBC (reticulocyte). From the early basophil stage, during which hemoglobin synthesis begins, to the later normoblast stage, in which the cell nucleus wanes to allow greater mobility, the cell produces hemoglobin. This substance accounts for the blood cell's reddish color and allows it to carry oxygen. Hemoglobin also contains about two-thirds of the body's iron.

WHERE DO RBCS GO?

When the RBC's hemoglobin concentration reaches about 34%, the cell loses its nucleus and leaves the bone marrow to circulate in the bloodstream as a reticulocyte. Within about 24 hours, the young reticulocyte matures into an erythrocyte. The entire process (from hemocytoblast to erythrocyte) takes about 4 days and occurs continuously in the body.

WHAT HAPPENS TO OLD RBCS?

Explain that an RBC lives for about 120 days. When it completes its cycle, it attracts a macrophage. This scavenger cell — found in the spleen, liver, bone marrow, and other tissues — devours the worn-out RBC and breaks down the hemoglobin molecules into reusable elements. One of these elements — heme — gives the hemoglobin molecule its oxygen-carrying capacity. Iron released from the heme molecules mixes with a serum globulin called transferrin. This mixture then becomes new hemoglobin and also goes to the liver, spleen, and other cells for storage.

WHAT DIFFERENCE DOES IRON MAKE?

Tell the patient that with adequate intake, iron will circulate continuously through his body. On the other hand, inadequate intake will gradually deplete the body's iron reserves. As a result, erythrocytes, hemoglobin level, and RBC volume will diminish. This will impair the blood's oxygen-carrying capacity and lead to tissue hypoxia and, eventually, symptoms of iron deficiency anemia.

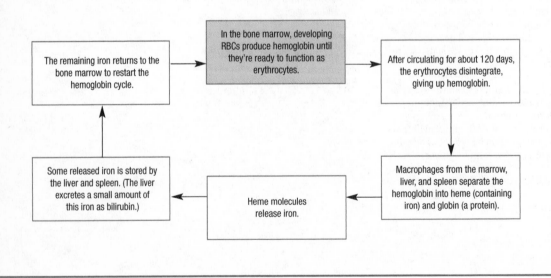

Hemoglobin electrophoresis

OVERVIEW

DESCRIPTION
◆ Most useful laboratory method for separating and measuring normal and abnormal hemoglobin (Hb)
◆ Separates different types of Hb to form series of distinctly pigmented bands in medium
◆ Results compared with a normal sample

PURPOSE
◆ To measure the amount of Hb A and to detect abnormal Hb
◆ To help diagnose thalassemia

PREPARATION
◆ The test requires a blood sample.
◆ No dietary restrictions are needed.

Teaching points
◆ Explain that Hb electrophoresis evaluates Hb.
◆ Tell the patient who will perform the test and where it will be done.
◆ Tell the patient that no dietary restrictions are required.
◆ If the patient is an infant or child, tell the parents that a small amount of blood will be taken from his finger.
◆ Inform the patient that the test should take less than 5 minutes.

DIAGNOSTIC PROCEDURE

KEY STEPS
◆ Confirm the patient's identity using two patient identifiers according to facility policy.
◆ Ask the patient if he has received a blood transfusion within the past 4 months.
◆ Perform a venipuncture and collect the sample in a 3- or 4.5-ml EDTA tube.
◆ For young children, collect capillary blood in a microcollection device.

POSTPROCEDURE CARE
◆ Apply pressure to the venipuncture site until bleeding stops.

PRECAUTIONS
◆ Completely fill the collection tube and invert it gently several times.
◆ Don't shake the tube vigorously.

COMPLICATIONS
◆ Hematoma at the venipuncture site

INTERPRETATION

NORMAL RESULTS
◆ In adults, Hb A accounts for 95% (SI, 0.95) of all Hb; Hb A_2, 1.5% to 3% (SI, 0.015 to 0.030); and Hb F, less than 2% (SI, < 0.02).
◆ In neonates, Hb F accounts for one-half the total. Hb S and Hb C are absent.

ABNORMAL RESULTS
◆ Hb electrophoresis allows the identification of various types of Hb; certain types may indicate hemolytic disease. (See *Variations of hemoglobin type and distribution*.)

Variations of hemoglobin type and distribution

Listed below are some of the variations of hemoglobin type and their clinical implications.

HEMOGLOBIN	PERCENTAGE OF TOTAL HEMOGLOBIN	CLINICAL IMPLICATIONS
Hb A	95% to 100% (SI, 0.95 to 1.0)	Normal
Hb A_2	4% to 5.8% (SI, 0.04 to 0.058)	ß-thalassemia minor
	1.5% to 3% (SI, 0.015 to 0.03)	Normal
	Under 1.5% (SI, < 0.015)	Hb H disease
Hb F	Under 1% (SI, < 0.01)	Normal
	2% to 5% (SI, 0.02 to 0.05)	ß-thalassemia minor
	10% to 90% (SI, 0.1 to 0.9)	ß-thalassemia major
	5% to 15% (SI, 0.05 to 0.15)	ß-thalassemia minor
	5% to 35% (SI, 0.05 to 0.35)	Heterozygous hereditary persistence of fetal Hb (HPFH)
	100% (SI, 1.0)	Homozygous HPFH
	15% (SI, 0.15)	Homozygous Hb S
Homozygous Hb S	70% to 98% (SI, 0.7 to 0.98)	Sickle cell disease
Homozygous Hb C	90% to 98% (SI, 0.9 to 0.98)	Hb C disease
Heterozygous Hb C	24% to 44% (SI, 0.24 to 0.44)	Hb C trait

Hemoglobin level test

OVERVIEW

DESCRIPTION
- Measures level of hemoglobin (Hb) in 100 ml (1 dl) of whole blood
- Correlates with red blood cell (RBC) count and affects the Hb-to-RBC ratio (mean corpuscular hemoglobin [MCH] and mean corpuscular hemoglobin concentration [MCHC])

PURPOSE
- To measure the severity of anemia or polycythemia and to monitor the patient's response to therapy
- To obtain data for calculating the MCH and MCHC

PREPARATION
- This test requires a blood sample.
- No dietary restrictions are needed.

Teaching points
- Explain that the Hb test detects anemia or polycythemia or assesses his response to treatment.
- Tell the patient who will perform the test and where it will be done.
- Tell him that there are no dietary restrictions.
- Explain that he may experience slight discomfort from the tourniquet and needle puncture.
- If the patient is an infant or a child, tell the parents that a small amount of blood will be taken from his finger or earlobe.
- Explain that the test should take less than 5 minutes.

DIAGNOSTIC PROCEDURE

KEY STEPS
- Confirm the patient's identity using two patient identifiers according to facility policy.
- For adults and older children, perform a venipuncture and collect the sample in a 3- or 4.5-ml EDTA tube.
- For younger children and infants, collect the sample by fingerstick or heelstick in a microcollection device with EDTA.
- Completely fill the collection tube and invert it gently several times to thoroughly mix the sample and anticoagulant.

POSTPROCEDURE CARE
- Apply direct pressure to the venipuncture site until bleeding stops.
- If a large hematoma develops at the venipuncture site, monitor pulses distal to the site.

PRECAUTIONS
- Handle the sample gently to prevent hemolysis.

COMPLICATIONS
- Hematoma at the venipuncture site

INTERPRETATION

NORMAL RESULTS
- In men, the level is 14 to 17.4 g/dl (SI, 140 to 174 g/L).
- In women, the level is 12 to 16 g/dl (SI, 120 to 160 g/L).
- In neonates younger than age 1 week, the level is 17 to 22 g/dl (SI, 170 to 220 g/L).
- In neonates age 1 week, the level is 15 to 20 g/dl (SI, 150 to 200 g/L).
- In infants age 1 month, the level is 11 to 15 g/dl (SI, 110 to 150 g/L).
- In children, the level is 11 to 13 g/dl (SI, 110 to 130 g/L).
- Persons who are more active or who live at high altitudes may have higher normal values.

ABNORMAL RESULTS
- A low Hb level may indicate anemia, recent hemorrhage, or fluid retention, causing hemodilution.
- A high Hb level suggests hemoconcentration from polycythemia or dehydration.

Hemoglobin level, urine

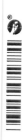

OVERVIEW

DESCRIPTION

- Detects hemoglobinuria, which occurs when plasma hemoglobin (Hb) level is higher than haptoglobin and excess free Hb is excreted in the urine
- Also identifies intact red blood cells (RBCs) in urine (hematuria), which can occur in the presence of free Hb
- Hb: contained in RBCs; consists of iron-protoporphyrin complex (heme) and polypeptide (globin)
- RBCs usually destroyed in reticuloendothelial system; if destroyed in circulation, free Hb enters the plasma and binds with haptoglobin

PURPOSE

- To help diagnose hemolytic anemias, infection, or severe intravascular hemolysis from a transfusion reaction

PREPARATION

- If a female patient is menstruating, reschedule the test; menstrual blood can interfere with test results.
- No dietary restrictions are needed.
- The test requires a random urine specimen.
- Notify the laboratory and practitioner of drugs the patient is taking that may affect test results.

Teaching points

- Explain that the urine hemoglobin test detects excessive RBC destruction.
- Tell the patient who will perform the test and where it will be done.
- Tell him he doesn't need to restrict his diet.
- Tell him that the test requires a random urine specimen, and teach him the proper collection technique.

DIAGNOSTIC PROCEDURE

KEY STEPS

- Confirm the patient's identity using two patient identifiers according to facility policy.
- Collect a random urine specimen. (See *Bedside testing for urine blood pigments*.)

Dipstik, Multistix, or Chemstrip method

- Dip the test stick into the specimen and withdraw it.
- After 30 seconds, read the results using the chart provided by the manufacturer.

Occult tablet test

- Put one drop of urine on filter paper, place the tablet on urine, and apply 2 drops of water to the tablet.
- After 2 minutes, inspect the filter paper.
- Blue indicates a positive test result.

Occult solution

- Place a drop of urine on filter paper, close the package, and turn it over.
- Apply 2 drops of solution to the site indicated. Inspect after 30 seconds.
- Blue indicates a positive test result.

POSTPROCEDURE CARE

- None

PRECAUTIONS

- Send the specimen to the laboratory immediately after collection.

COMPLICATIONS

- None

INTERPRETATION

NORMAL RESULTS

- The urine doesn't contain Hb.

ABNORMAL RESULTS

- Hemoglobinuria may result from severe intravascular hemolysis.
- Hemoglobinuria may result from acquired hemolytic anemias caused by chemical or drug intoxication or malaria; congenital hemolytic anemias; strenuous exercise; or paroxysmal nocturnal hemoglobinuria.
- Hemoglobinuria may signal cystitis, ureteral calculi, or urethritis.
- Hemoglobinuria and hematuria occur in renal epithelial damage, renal tumor, and tuberculosis.

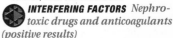 **INTERFERING FACTORS** *Nephrotoxic drugs and anticoagulants (positive results)*

Bedside testing for urine blood pigments

To test a patient's urine for blood pigments at the bedside, use one of these methods. Because these methods detect only blood pigments, immunochemical studies are necessary to differentiate hemoglobin from other blood pigments such as myoglobin.

REAGENT STRIP

- Collect a urine specimen.
- Dip the stick into the specimen and withdraw it.
- After 30 seconds, compare the stick to the color chart. Blue indicates a positive reaction; the intensity of color indicates pigment concentration.

OCCULT TABLET

- Collect a urine specimen.
- Put one drop of urine on the filter paper. Place the tablet on the urine, and then put two drops of water on the tablet.

- After 2 minutes, inspect the filter paper around the tablet. Blue indicates a positive reaction; the intensity of color indicates pigment concentration.

OCCULT SOLUTION

- Collect a urine specimen.
- After placing one drop of urine on the filter paper, close the package and turn it over. Open the opposite ends, and place two drops of solution on the filter paper.
- After 30 seconds, inspect the filter paper. Blue indicates a positive reaction; the intensity of color indicates pigment concentration.

Hemosiderin level, urine

DESCRIPTION
- Measures urine level of hemosiderin (collodial iron oxide and form of iron stored and deposited in body tissue)
- Hemochromatosis: occurs when storage mechanisms can't manage iron overload; excess iron damages cells unaccustomed to high iron levels
- May occur in rare hereditary form and in exogenous forms

PURPOSE
- To help diagnose hemochromatosis, hemolytic anemia associated with intravascular hemolysis

PREPARATION
- No dietary restrictions are needed.
- The test requires a urine sample.

Teaching points
- Explain that this test helps determine if his body is accumulating excess amounts of iron.
- Tell the patient who will perform the test and where it will be done.
- Tell him that he doesn't have to restrict his diet.
- Teach the patient how to collect a urine sample.

KEY STEPS
- Confirm the patient's identity using two patient identifiers according to facility policy.
- Collect a random urine specimen of about 30 ml, preferably the first void of the morning.

POSTPROCEDURE CARE
- Seal the container securely.

PRECAUTIONS
- Send the specimen to the laboratory immediately after collection.

COMPLICATIONS
- None

NORMAL RESULTS
- No hemosiderin is found in the urine.

ABNORMAL RESULTS
- The presence of hemosiderin indicates hemochromatosis.

Hepatitis A antibodies test

OVERVIEW

DESCRIPTION
- Identifies hepatitis A antibodies in serum or body fluid of patients with hepatitis A virus (HAV)
- Antibodies in blood and feces present only briefly before symptoms appear

PURPOSE
- To aid in the differential diagnosis of viral hepatitis

PREPARATION
- Check the patient's history for administration of hepatitis vaccine.
- No dietary restrictions are needed.
- The test requires a blood sample.

Teaching points
- Explain that this test helps identify a type of viral hepatitis.
- Tell the patient who will perform the test and where it will be done.
- Tell him that he doesn't have to restrict his diet.
- Explain that he may experience discomfort from the tourniquet and needle puncture.
- Inform the patient that the test should take less than 5 minutes.
- Tell him that confirmed viral hepatitis is reported to public health authorities in most states.

DIAGNOSTIC PROCEDURE

KEY STEPS
- Confirm the patient's identity using two patient identifiers according to facility policy.
- Perform a venipuncture and collect the sample in two 3- or 4.5-ml EDTA tubes.

POSTPROCEDURE CARE
- Apply direct pressure to the venipuncture site until bleeding stops.

PRECAUTIONS
- Maintain standard precautions while collecting the sample.

COMPLICATIONS
- Hematoma at the venipuncture site

INTERPRETATION

NORMAL RESULTS
- Serum is negative for hepatitis A antibodies.

ABNORMAL RESULTS
- A single positive test result may indicate previous exposure to the virus, but because these antibodies persist so long in the blood, only evidence of rising anti-HAV titers confirms HAV as the cause of current or very recent infection.

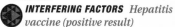 **INTERFERING FACTORS** *Hepatitis vaccine (positive result)*

Hepatitis B core antibodies test

DESCRIPTION
- Identifies past or present infection with hepatitis B virus (HBV)
- HBV core antibodies: protein molecules (immunoglobulins) in serum or body fluid that neutralize antigens or tag them for attack by other cells or chemicals, produced during or after acute HBV infection
- HBV core antigen antibodies: present in chronic carriers

PURPOSE
- To screen blood donors for hepatitis B
- To screen people at high risk for contracting hepatitis B, such as hemodialysis nurses
- To aid in the differential diagnosis of viral hepatitis

PREPARATION
- No dietary restrictions are needed.
- The test requires a blood sample.
- Check the patient's history for administration of hepatitis vaccine.

Teaching points
- Explain to the patient that this test helps identify a type of viral hepatitis.
- Tell the patient who will perform the test and where it will be done.
- Tell the patient that no dietary restrictions are required.
- Explain to the patient that he may experience discomfort from the tourniquet and needle puncture.
- Inform the patient that the test should take less than 5 minutes.
- Tell the patient that confirmed viral hepatitis is reported to public health authorities in most states.

KEY STEPS
- Confirm the patient's identity using two patient identifiers according to facility policy.
- Perform a venipuncture and collect the sample in two 3- or 4.5-ml EDTA tubes.

POSTPROCEDURE CARE
- Apply direct pressure to the venipuncture site until bleeding stops.

PRECAUTIONS
- Maintain standard precautions while collecting the sample.

COMPLICATIONS
- Hematoma at the venipuncture site

NORMAL RESULTS
- Serum is negative for hepatitis B core antibodies.

ABNORMAL RESULTS
- Positive findings may indicate that the patient is recovering from an acute HBV infection. (See *Typical sequence of hepatitis B and C markers after exposure*.)

  INTERFERING FACTORS *Hepatitis vaccine (positive result)*

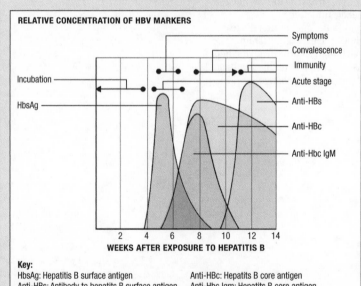

Typical sequence of hepatitis B and C markers after exposure

RELATIVE CONCENTRATION OF HBV MARKERS

Symptoms
Convalescence
Immunity
Acute stage
Anti-HBs
Anti-HBc
Anti-Hbc IgM

Incubation

HbsAg

WEEKS AFTER EXPOSURE TO HEPATITIS B
2   4   6   8   10   12   14

Key:
HbsAg: Hepatitis B surface antigen
Anti-HBs: Antibody to hepatits B surface antigen
Anti-HBc: Hepatits B core antigen
Anti-Hbc Igm: Hepatits B core antigen, immunoglobulin M antibody

Reprinted with permission from Serodiagnostic Assessment of Acute Viral Hepatitis. Abbott Park, Ill.: Abbott Laboratories, 1992.

Hepatitis B surface antibodies test

OVERVIEW

DESCRIPTION
◆ Identifies presence of hepatitis B antibodies, protein molecules (immunoglobulins) in serum or body fluid that neutralize antigens or tag them for attack by other cells or chemicals
◆ Indicates that patient who has been exposed to hepatitis B virus (HBV) isn't contagious
◆ Also indicates immunity to future HBV infection

PURPOSE
◆ To determine if immunity to HBV is present

PREPARATION
◆ No dietary restrictions are needed.
◆ This test requires a blood sample.
◆ Check the patient's history for administration of hepatitis vaccine.

Teaching points
◆ Explain to the patient that this test helps identify a type of viral hepatitis.
◆ Tell the patient who will perform the test and where it will be done.
◆ Tell the patient that no dietary restrictions are required.
◆ Explain to the patient that he may experience discomfort from the needle and tourniquet.
◆ Inform the patient that the test should take less than 5 minutes.

DIAGNOSTIC PROCEDURE

KEY STEPS
◆ Confirm the patient's identity using two patient identifiers according to facility policy.
◆ Perform a venipuncture and collect the sample in two 3- or 4.5-ml EDTA tubes.

POSTPROCEDURE CARE
◆ Apply direct pressure to the venipuncture site until bleeding stops.

PRECAUTIONS
◆ Maintain standard precautions while collecting the sample.

COMPLICATIONS
◆ Hematoma at the venipuncture site

INTERPRETATION

NORMAL RESULTS
◆ Serum is negative for hepatitis B surface antigens.

ABNORMAL RESULTS
◆ Positive findings indicate that the patient is immune to HBV infection.

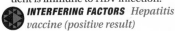 **INTERFERING FACTORS** *Hepatitis vaccine (positive result)*

Hepatitis B surface antigen test

OVERVIEW

DESCRIPTION
- Detects hepatitis B surface antigen, which appears in serum of patients with hepatitis B virus
- Uses radioimmunoassay or (less commonly) reverse passive hemagglutination during extended incubation period and usually during first 3 weeks of acute infection or when patient is a carrier
- Required by Food and Drug Administration's Bureau of Biologics to reduce incidence of hepatitis
- Donated blood screened for virus before it's stored
- Doesn't screen for hepatitis A virus (infectious hepatitis)
- Also called *hepatitis-associated antigen* or *Australia antigen*

PURPOSE
- To screen blood donors for hepatitis B
- To screen people at high risk for contracting hepatitis B such as hemodialysis nurses
- To aid in the differential diagnosis of viral hepatitis

PREPARATION
- No dietary restrictions are needed.
- This test requires a blood sample.
- Check the patient's history for administration of hepatitis B vaccine.

Teaching points
- Explain that this test helps identify a type of viral hepatitis.
- Tell the patient who will perform the test and where it will be done.
- Tell him he doesn't have to restrict his diet.
- Explain to the patient that he may experience slight discomfort from the tourniquet and needle puncture.
- Inform the patient that the test should take less than 5 minutes.
- If the patient is giving blood, explain the donation procedure to him.
- Tell the patient that confirmed viral hepatitis is reported to public health authorities in most states.

DIAGNOSTIC PROCEDURE

KEY STEPS
- Confirm the patient's identity using two patient identifiers according to facility policy.
- Perform a venipuncture and collect the sample in a 10-ml clot-activator tube.
- Wash your hands carefully after the procedure.

POSTPROCEDURE CARE
- Apply direct pressure to the venipuncture site until bleeding stops.

PRECAUTIONS
- Remember to wear gloves when drawing blood and dispose of the needle properly.

COMPLICATIONS
- Hematoma at the venipuncture site

INTERPRETATION

NORMAL RESULTS
- Normal serum is negative for hepatitis B surface antigen (HBsAg).

ABNORMAL RESULTS
- The presence of HBsAg in patients with hepatitis confirms hepatitis B.
- In chronic carriers and in patients with chronic active hepatitis, HBsAg may occur in the serum several months after the onset of acute infection.
- It may also occur in over 5% of patients with certain diseases other than hepatitis, such as hemophilia, Hodgkin's disease, and leukemia.
- If HBsAg is found in donor blood, that blood must be discarded because it carries a risk of transmitting hepatitis.
- Blood samples that test positive should be retested because inaccurate results occur.

Hepatitis C antibodies test

OVERVIEW

DESCRIPTION
- Detects hepatitis C virus (HCV) by checking for antibodies in the blood
- Performed in patients with risk factors for disease and in those who exhibit symptoms
- Indicates present or past infection

PURPOSE
- To test for the presence of HCV antibodies

PREPARATION
- The test doesn't indicate whether the HCV infection has been cured.
- The test requires a blood sample.

Teaching points
- Explain to the patient that the test can't distinguish between an acute or chronic infection.
- Tell the patient who will perform the test and where it will be done.
- Tell the patient that no dietary restrictions are required.
- Inform the patient that he may experience discomfort from the tourniquet and needle puncture.
- Inform the patient that the test should take less than 5 minutes.
- Tell the patient that confirmed viral hepatitis is reported to public health authorities in most states.

DIAGNOSTIC PROCEDURE

KEY STEPS
- Confirm the patient's identity using two patient identifiers according to facility policy.
- Perform the venipuncture and collect the sample in two 3- or 4.5-ml EDTA tubes.

POSTPROCEDURE CARE
- Apply direct pressure to the venipuncture site until bleeding stops.
- Offer appropriate referrals after testing.

PRECAUTIONS
- Maintain standard precautions while collecting the sample.

COMPLICATIONS
- Hematoma at the venipuncture site

INTERPRETATION

NORMAL RESULTS
- HCV antibodies are absent from the blood.

ABNORMAL RESULTS
- The absence of antibodies doesn't always mean the patient is free from hepatitis C; antibodies can take a few weeks to develop.
- Most people develop antibodies within 3 months of becoming infected.
- A positive sample for antibodies can't determine if the infection is current or from the past; further testing is required.
- False-positive results are possible; repeat the test to confirm.

Hepatitis D antibodies test

DESCRIPTION

◆ Detects hepatitis D virus (HDV), which occurs primarily in patients with acute or chronic episodes of hepatitis B virus
◆ HDV requires presence of hepatitis B surface antigen; needs double-shelled type B virus to replicate, thus can't outlast hepatitis B infection

PURPOSE

◆ To aid in the differential diagnosis of viral hepatitis

PREPARATION

◆ The test doesn't indicate whether the HDV infection is cured.
◆ The test requires a blood sample.

Teaching points

◆ Explain to the patient that the test can't distinguish between an acute and a chronic infection.
◆ Tell the patient who will perform the test and where it will be done.
◆ Tell the patient that no dietary restrictions are required.
◆ Inform the patient that he may experience discomfort from the tourniquet and needle puncture.
◆ Inform the patient that the test should take less than 5 minutes.
◆ Tell the patient that confirmed viral hepatitis is reported to public health authorities in most states.

KEY STEPS

◆ Confirm the patient's identity using two patient identifiers according to facility policy.
◆ Perform the venipuncture and collect the sample in two 3- or 4.5-ml EDTA tubes.

POSTPROCEDURE CARE

◆ Apply direct pressure to the venipuncture site until bleeding stops.

PRECAUTIONS

◆ Maintain standard precautions while collecting the sample.

COMPLICATIONS

◆ Hematoma at the venipuncture site

NORMAL RESULTS

◆ Serum is negative for HDV antibodies.

ABNORMAL RESULTS

◆ Detection of HDV antibodies indicates infection with HDV.

Herpes simplex virus antibodies test

DESCRIPTION

◆ Sensitive assays (indirect immuno-fluorescence and enzyme immuno-assay): detect immunoglobulin (Ig) M class antibodies to herpes simplex virus (HSV) or a fourfold or greater increase in IgG class antibodies between acute- and convalescent-phase sera
◆ HSV: member of herpesvirus group that causes genital lesions, keratitis or conjunctivitis, generalized dermal lesions, and pneumonia; associated with intrauterine or neonatal infections and encephalitis; most severe in immunosuppressed patients
◆ Type 1 HSV: causes infections above the waistline
◆ Type 2 HSV: involves external genitalia

PURPOSE

◆ To confirm infections caused by HSV
◆ To detect recent or past HSV infection

PREPARATION

◆ The test requires a blood sample.

Teaching points

◆ Explain the purpose of the test and how it's done.
◆ Tell the patient who will perform the test and where it will be done.
◆ Tell the patient that no dietary restrictions are required.
◆ Explain to the patient that he may experience slight discomfort from the tourniquet and needle puncture.
◆ Inform the patient that the test should take less than 5 minutes.

KEY STEPS

◆ Confirm the patient's identity using two patient identifiers according to facility policy.
◆ Perform a venipuncture and collect the sample in a 7-ml clot-activator tube.
◆ Allow the blood to clot for at least 1 hour at room temperature.
◆ Transfer the serum to a sterile tube or vial and send it to the laboratory promptly.

POSTPROCEDURE CARE

◆ Apply direct pressure to the venipuncture site until bleeding stops.
◆ If the patient's immune system is compromised, check the venipuncture site for changes and report them immediately.

PRECAUTIONS

◆ If transfer can't occur immediately, store the serum at 39.2° F (4° C) for 1 or 2 days or at –4° F (–20° C) for longer periods to avoid contamination.
◆ Handle the sample gently to prevent hemolysis.

COMPLICATIONS

◆ Hematoma at the venipuncture site

NORMAL RESULTS

◆ Sera from patients who have never been infected with HSV have no detectable antibodies (less than 1:5).
◆ HSV infection can be ruled out in a patient whose serum shows no detectable antibodies to the virus.

ABNORMAL RESULTS

◆ The presence of IgM or a fourfold or greater increase in IgG antibodies indicates active HSV infection.

Herpes simplex virus culture

DESCRIPTION

- Standard tube culture: about 50% of herpes simplex virus (HSV) strains detectable by characteristic cytopathic effects within 24 hours after receipt of specimen; 5 to 7 days required to detect remaining HSV strains
- Shell-vial culture: early HSV antigens detected within 16 hours after receipt of specimen with same sensitivity and specificity as standard tube cell cultures
- Herpesvirus group: Epstein-Barr virus, cytomegalovirus (CMV), varicella-zoster virus (VZV), human herpesvirus-6, herpesvirus-7, herpesvirus-8, and two closely related serotypes of HSV — types 1 and 2
- Only CMV, VZV, and HSV replicated in standard cell cultures of diagnostic laboratories

PURPOSE

- To confirm the diagnosis of HSV infection by culturing the virus from specimens

PREPARATION

- No dietary restrictions are needed.

Teaching points

- Explain to the patient that this test detects HSV infection.
- Tell the patient who will perform the test and where it will be done.
- Explain to the patient that specimens will be collected from suspected lesions during the prodromal and acute stages of clinical infection.
- Tell the patient that no dietary restrictions are required.
- Answer the patient's questions about testing procedures.

KEY STEPS

- Confirm the patient's identity using two patient identifiers according to facility policy.
- Collect a specimen for culture in the appropriate collection device.
- Obtain vesicle fluid with a 27G needle or a tuberculin syringe. If the fluid is scant, scrape the base of the ulcer with a swab to remove cells.
- For the throat, skin, eye, or genital area, use a microbiologic transport swab.
- For body fluids or other respiratory specimens (such as washings or lavage), use a sterile screw-capped jar.

POSTPROCEDURE CARE

- Answer any questions the patient may have about the virus.

PRECAUTIONS

- Wear gloves when obtaining and handling all specimens.
- Transport the specimen to the laboratory as soon as possible after collection. If the anticipated time between collection and inoculation of cell cultures is more than 3 hours, the specimen should be stored and transported at 39.2° F (4° C).
- Don't allow the specimen to dry.

COMPLICATIONS

- None

NORMAL RESULTS

- HSV is seldom recovered from an immunocompetent patient who shows no overt signs of the disease.

ABNORMAL RESULTS

- Detectable HSV in specimens taken from dermal lesions, the eye, or cerebrospinal fluid is highly significant.
- Specimens from the upper respiratory tract may be associated with intermittent shedding of the virus, particularly in an immunocompromised patient.
- Like other herpesviruses, HSV can be shed from the immunocompromised patient intermittently in the absence of apparent disease.
- For epidemiologic purposes, HSV detected by characteristic cytopathic effects in standard tube cell cultures is confirmed and identified as type 1 or 2.

Heterophil antibodies test

DESCRIPTION

◆ Detects and identifies two immunoglobulin (Ig) M antibodies in human serum that react against foreign red blood cells (RBCs): Epstein-Barr virus (EBV) antibodies and Forssman antibodies
◆ Paul-Bunnell test (also called presumptive test): EBV antibodies in sera of patients with infectious mononucleosis agglutinate with sheep RBCs
◆ Forssman antibodies, in sera of some healthy persons and in those with serum sickness, agglutinating with sheep RBCs; results inconclusive for infectious mononucleosis
◆ If Paul-Bunnell test establishes presumptive titer, Davidsohn differential absorption test used to distinguish EBV from Forssman antibodies

PURPOSE

◆ To aid in the differential diagnosis of infectious mononucleosis

PREPARATION

◆ The test requires a blood sample.

Teaching points

◆ Explain to the patient that this test helps detect infectious mononucleosis.
◆ Tell the patient who will perform the test and where it will be done.
◆ Tell the patient that no dietary restrictions are required.
◆ Explain to the patient that he may experience slight discomfort from the tourniquet and needle puncture.
◆ Inform the patient that the test should take less than 5 minutes.

KEY STEPS

◆ Confirm the patient's identity using two patient identifiers according to facility policy.
◆ Perform a venipuncture and collect the sample in a 7-ml clot-activator tube.

POSTPROCEDURE CARE

◆ Apply direct pressure to the venipuncture site until bleeding stops.
◆ If the titer is positive and infectious mononucleosis is confirmed, explain the treatment plan to the patient.
◆ If the titer is positive but infectious mononucleosis isn't confirmed, or if the titer is negative but symptoms persist, explain that additional testing is needed in a few days or weeks to confirm the diagnosis and plan ffective treatment.

PRECAUTIONS

◆ Maintain standard precautions while collecting the sample.

COMPLICATIONS

◆ Hematoma at the venipuncture site

NORMAL RESULTS

◆ The titer is less than 1:56; may be higher in elderly people.
◆ Some laboratories refer to a normal titer as "negative" or as having "no reaction."
◆ A negative titer doesn't always rule out this disorder; occasionally, the titer becomes reactive after 2 weeks. If symptoms persist, repeat the test in 2 weeks.

ABNORMAL RESULTS

◆ Although heterophil antibodies occur in the sera of about 80% of patients with infectious mononucleosis 1 month after its onset, a positive finding — a titer higher than 1:56 — doesn't confirm this disorder.
◆ A high titer can result from systemic lupus erythematosus, syphilis, cryoglobulinemia, or the presence of antibodies to nonsyphilitic treponemata, such as yaws, pinta, or bejel.
◆ A gradual increase in the titer during week 3 or 4 followed by a gradual decrease during weeks 4 to 8 is conclusive for infectious mononucleosis.
◆ Confirming infectious mononucleosis depends on heterophil agglutination and hematologic tests that show absolute lymphocytosis with 10% or more atypical lymphocytes.

Hexosaminidase A and B levels, serum

OVERVIEW

DESCRIPTION
- Fluorometric test that measures hexosaminidase A and B content of serum samples drawn by venipuncture or collected from neonate's umbilical cord or from amniotic fluid obtained by amniocentesis
- Alternative: test cultured skin fibroblasts, but procedure costly and complex
- Preferred screening method and specimen: may be recommended by reference center for congenital disease
- Hexosaminidase: group of enzymes needed for metabolism of gangliosides (water-soluble glycolipids found mainly in brain tissue)
- Hexosaminidase A deficiency: indicates Tay-Sachs disease (affects people of eastern European Jewish ancestry about 100 times more than general population); transmitted if both parents have defective gene
- Hexosaminidase A and B deficiency: indicates Sandhoff disease; not common or prevalent in any ethnic group

PURPOSE
- To confirm or rule out Tay-Sachs disease in the neonate
- To screen for a Tay-Sachs carrier
- To establish prenatal diagnosis of hexosaminidase A deficiency

PREPARATION
- The test requires a blood sample.
- No dietary restrictions are needed.

Teaching points
- Explain to the patient that this test identifies carriers of Tay-Sachs disease.
- When testing a neonate, explain to the parents that this test detects Tay-Sachs disease.
- Tell the patient who will perform the test and where it will be done.
- Tell the parents that blood will be drawn from the neonate's arm, neck, or umbilical cord; that the procedure is safe and quickly performed; and that the neonate will have a small bandage on the venipuncture site.
- If the test is prenatal, advise the patient of preparations for amniocentesis.
- Tell the patient that no dietary restrictions are required.
- Explain to the patient that he may experience slight discomfort from the tourniquet and needle puncture.

DIAGNOSTIC PROCEDURE

KEY STEPS
- Confirm the patient's identity using two patient identifiers according to facility policy.
- Perform a venipuncture, collect cord blood, or assist with amniocentesis, as appropriate.
- Collect the sample in a 7-ml clot-activator tube.
- If the test can't occur immediately, freeze the sample.

POSTPROCEDURE CARE
- Apply direct pressure to the venipuncture site until bleeding stops.

PRECAUTIONS
- Handle the sample gently to prevent hemolysis.
- Although the serum of a pregnant woman can't be tested, her leukocytes or amniotic fluid can be used if needed; if the father's blood test result is negative, the child won't inherit Tay-Sachs disease.

COMPLICATIONS
- Hematoma at the venipuncture site

INTERPRETATION

NORMAL RESULTS
- Total serum levels range from 5 to 12.9 units/L; hexosaminidase A accounts for 55% to 76% of the total.

ABNORMAL RESULTS
- Absence of hexosaminidase A indicates Tay-Sachs disease (total hexosaminidase levels may be normal).
- Absence of hexosaminidase A and B indicates Sandhoff disease, an uncommon, virulent variant of Tay-Sachs disease in which deterioration occurs more rapidly.

HIDA scan

DESCRIPTION
◆ Technetium-99m scan to measure the gamma rays emitted from bile

PURPOSE
◆ To diagnose suspected gallbladder disorders
◆ To help in the differential diagnosis of acute and chronic cholecystitis
◆ To evaluate the patency of the biliary enteric bypass
◆ To assess obstructive jaundice when done in conjunction with ultrasound or radiography
◆ To assess enterogastric reflux

PREPARATION
◆ Fasting is required for at least 2 hours before the test.
◆ Have the patient void before the procedure.
◆ Make sure the patient has a patent I.V. line.
◆ Make sure he has signed an appropriate consent form.

Teaching points
◆ Explain to the patient that this test helps evaluate his gallbladder function.
◆ Reassure the patient that the test uses only small amounts of radioactive material.
◆ Tell the patient who will perform the test and where it will be done.
◆ Advise the patient of any dietary and medication restrictions.
◆ Instruct the patient to lie still during the test for the best images.
◆ Inform the patient that the test takes about 1½ hours.

KEY STEPS
◆ Confirm the patient's identity using two patient identifiers according to facility policy.
◆ Place the patient on the table in a supine position.
◆ Administer the radionuclide into the I.V. access device.
◆ The right upper quadrant of the abdomen will be scanned at various intervals for 1 hour.
◆ During the test, morphine may be administered to initiate spasms of the sphincter of Oddi.
◆ If the test is assessing gallbladder function or bile reflux, the patient will be given a fatty meal 60 minutes after the radionuclide injection.

POSTPROCEDURE CARE
◆ Instruct the patient to drink increased fluids for 24 to 48 hours, unless contraindicated.

PRECAUTIONS
◆ Wear gloves while handling the radionuclide.

COMPLICATIONS
◆ None

NORMAL RESULTS
◆ The gallbladder is normal shape and size with normal function. A patent cystic and common bile duct is present.

ABNORMAL RESULTS
◆ The inability to see the gallbladder 1 or 2 hours after injection indicates an obstruction of the cystic duct.
◆ Delayed filling of the gallbladder indicates cholecystitis.
◆ Radionuclide seen in the biliary tree but not in the bowel indicates obstruction of the common bile duct.
◆ If morphine is used and there's no visualization of the radionuclide within 15 to 30 minutes, acute cholecystitis is indicated.

Holter monitoring

DESCRIPTION

- Continuous recording of heart activity as the patient follows his normal routine, usually for 24 hours
- Patient-activated monitor worn for 5 to 7 days; allows patient to manually initiate recording of heart activity when symptoms occur
- Also known as *ambulatory electrocardiography* or *dynamic monitoring*

PURPOSE

- To detect cardiac arrhythmias
- To evaluate chest pain
- To evaluate the effectiveness of antiarrhythmic drug therapy
- To monitor pacemaker function
- To correlate symptoms and palpitations with actual cardiac events and patient activities
- To detect sporadic arrhythmias missed by an exercise or resting electrocardiogram (ECG)

PREPARATION

- Make sure that the patient has signed an appropriate consent form.
- Note and report all allergies.
- Provide bathing instructions because some equipment must not get wet.
- Review all instructions and restrictions with the patient.

Teaching points

- Explain the purpose of the test and how it's done.
- Tell the patient who will perform the test and where it will be done.
- Instruct the patient to avoid magnets, metal detectors, high-voltage areas, and electric blankets.
- Explain the importance of logging activities as well as emotional upsets, physical symptoms, and ingestion of medication in a diary.
- Explain how to mark the tape at the onset of symptoms, if applicable.
- Explain how to check the recorder to make sure that it's working properly.

KEY STEPS

- Confirm the patient's identity using two patient identifiers according to facility policy.
- Electrodes are applied to the chest wall and securely attached to the lead wires and monitor.
- A new or fully charged battery is inserted in the recorder.
- A tape is inserted and the recorder is turned on.
- The electrode attachment circuit is tested by connecting the recorder to a standard ECG machine, noting artifact during normal patient movement.

POSTPROCEDURE CARE

- Remove all chest electrodes.
- Clean the electrode sites.

PRECAUTIONS

- Placing electrodes over large muscles masses, such as the pectorals, is avoided to limit artifact.

COMPLICATIONS

- Skin sensitivity to the electrodes

NORMAL RESULTS

- The ECG shows no significant arrhythmias or ST-segment changes.
- Changes in heart rate occur during various activities.

ABNORMAL RESULTS

- Abnormalities in cardiac rate or rhythm suggest possible serious arrhythmias, which may not always be causing symptoms.
- ST-T wave changes may coincide with patient symptoms or increased activity and may suggest possible myocardial ischemia.

Homocysteine level test

DESCRIPTION

- Measures homocysteine (tHcy), a sulfur-containing amino acid
- Transmethylation product of methionine
- Intermediate in cysteine synthesis; produced by enzymatic or acid hydrolysis of proteins

PURPOSE

- To make a biochemical diagnosis of inborn errors of methionine, folate, and vitamins B_6 and B_{12} metabolism
- To indicate acquired folate or cobalamin deficiency
- To evaluate the risk factors for atherosclerotic vascular disease
- To evaluate as a contributing factor in the pathogenesis of neural tube defects
- To evaluate the cause of recurrent spontaneous abortions
- To evaluate delayed child development or failure to thrive in infants

PREPARATION

- Fasting is required for 12 to 14 hours before the test.
- This test requires a blood sample.

Teaching points

- Inform the patient that this test detects tHcy levels in plasma.
- Tell the patient who will perform the test and where it will be done.
- Instruct the patient to fast for at least 12 hours before the test.
- Inform him that he may experience slight discomfort from the tourniquet and needle puncture.
- Inform the patient that the test should take less than 5 minutes.

KEY STEPS

- Confirm the patient's identity using two patient identifiers according to facility policy.
- Perform a venipuncture and collect the sample in a 5-ml tube with EDTA added.

POSTPROCEDURE CARE

- Apply direct pressure to the venipuncture site until bleeding stops.

PRECAUTIONS

- Handle the sample gently to prevent hemolysis.
- Immediately put the sample on ice and send it to the laboratory.

COMPLICATIONS

- Hematoma at the venipuncture site

NORMAL RESULTS

- Level of tHcy is 4 to 17 µmol/L.

ABNORMAL RESULTS

- Low levels indicate inborn or acquired folate or cobalamin deficiency and inborn B_6 or B_{12} deficiency.
- Elevated tHcy levels indicate a higher incidence of atherosclerotic vascular disease.
- In patients with type 2 diabetes mellitus, studies show that tHcy levels increase even with a modest deterioration in renal function.

Homovanillic acid level, urine

DESCRIPTION

- Quantitative analysis of urine levels of homovanillic acid (HVA), a metabolite of dopamine synthesized in the brain and precursor to epinephrine and norepinephrine
- Dopamine broken down by liver into HVA for excretion
- HVA levels measured with dopamine, epinephrine, and norepinephrine levels

PURPOSE

- To help diagnose neuroblastoma and ganglioneuroma
- To rule out pheochromocytoma

PREPARATION

- No dietary restrictions are needed.
- Have the patient avoid stressful situations and strenuous exercise for 24 hours before the test.
- Notify the laboratory and practitioner of medication the patient is taking that may affect test results; they may need to be discontinued.

Teaching points

- Explain that this test assesses hormone secretion.
- Tell the patient who will perform the test and where it will be done.
- Tell him that the test requires collection of urine over a 24-hour period.
- Teach the patient how to collect a 24-hour urine sample.

KEY STEPS

- Confirm the patient's identity using two patient identifiers according to facility policy.
- Collect the patient's urine over a 24-hour period, discarding the first specimen and retaining the last.
- Use a bottle containing a preservative to keep the specimen at a pH of 2.0 to 4.0.

POSTPROCEDURE CARE

- Tell the patient to resume his usual activities and medications.

PRECAUTIONS

- Keep the sample refrigerated or on ice during the collection period.
- Send the specimen to the laboratory immediately after collection is completed.

COMPLICATIONS

- None

NORMAL RESULTS

- The normal urine HVA value for adults is less than 10 mg/24 hours (SI, < 55 µmol/day).

ABNORMAL RESULTS

- Elevated HVA levels suggest neuroblastoma, a malignant soft-tissue tumor that develops in infants and young children.
- It may also suggest a ganglioneuroma, a tumor of the sympathetic nervous system that develops in older children and adults.
- An abnormally high HVA level rules out pheochromocytoma.

INTERFERING FACTORS *Monoamine oxidase inhibitors, aspirin, and levodopa*

Human chorionic gonadotropin level, serum

OVERVIEW

DESCRIPTION
- Confirms conception by detecting human chorionic gonadotropin (hCG), which occurs in blood 9 days after ovulation when fertilized ovum is implanted into uterine wall
- hCG and progesterone thought to maintain corpus luteum during early pregnancy; production peaking around 10 weeks' gestation, then falling to below 10% of first trimester peak levels for rest of pregnancy
- May not be detectable about 2 weeks after delivery (see *Production of hCG during pregnancy*)
- Serum immunoassay more sensitive (and costlier) than pregnancy test using urine sample
- Also known as *beta-subunit assay*

PURPOSE
- To detect early pregnancy
- To determine adequacy of hormone production in high-risk pregnancies (for example, habitual abortion)
- To help diagnose trophoblastic tumors, such as hydatidiform mole and choriocarcinoma, and tumors that ectopically secrete hCG
- To monitor treatment for induction of ovulation and conception

PREPARATION
- No dietary restrictions are needed.
- The test requires a blood sample.

Teaching points
- Explain to the patient that this test determines if she's pregnant.
- Tell the patient who will perform the test and where it will be done.
- If detection of pregnancy isn't the diagnostic objective, offer the appropriate explanation.
- Tell the patient that no dietary restrictions are needed.
- Explain to the patient that she may experience slight discomfort from the tourniquet and needle puncture.
- Inform the patient that the test should take less than 5 minutes.

DIAGNOSTIC PROCEDURE

KEY STEPS
- Confirm the patient's identity using two patient identifiers according to facility policy.
- Perform a venipuncture and collect the sample in a 7-ml clot-activator tube.

POSTPROCEDURE CARE
- Apply direct pressure to the venipuncture site until bleeding stops.

PRECAUTIONS
- Handle the sample gently to prevent hemolysis.
- Send the sample to the laboratory immediately.

COMPLICATIONS
- Hematoma at the venipuncture site

INTERPRETATION

NORMAL RESULTS
- Level is below 4 International Units/L.
- During pregnancy, hCG levels vary and depend on number of days after the last normal menstrual period.

ABNORMAL RESULTS
- Elevated hCG beta-subunit levels indicate pregnancy; significantly higher levels suggest a multiple pregnancy.
- Increased levels may also suggest hydatidiform mole, trophoblastic neoplasms of the placenta, and nontrophoblastic carcinomas that secrete hCG (including gastric, pancreatic, and ovarian adenocarcinomas).
- Low hCG beta-subunit levels can occur in an ectopic pregnancy or a pregnancy of less than 9 days.
- Beta-subunit levels can't differentiate pregnancy from tumor recurrence because they're high in both conditions.

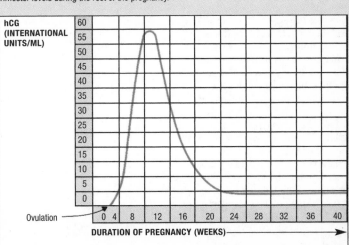

Production of hCG during pregnancy

Production of human chorionic gonadotropin (hCG) increases steadily during the first trimester, peaking around 10 weeks' gestation, as shown below. Levels then fall to less than 10% of first trimester levels during the rest of the pregnancy.

Human chorionic gonadotropin level, urine

OVERVIEW

DESCRIPTION
- Qualitative and quantitative analysis of urine levels of human chorionic gonadotropin (hCG)
- Detects pregnancy as early as 14 days after ovulation
- hCG and progesterone thought to maintain corpus luteum during early pregnancy; production peaking around 10 weeks' gestation, then falling to below 10% of first trimester peak levels for rest of pregnancy
- Easier and less expensive than serum hCG test (beta-subunit assay); a more common test for detecting pregnancy

PURPOSE
- To detect and confirm pregnancy
- To help diagnose hydatidiform mole or hCG-secreting tumors, threatened abortion, or a dead fetus

PREPARATION
- The test requires a first-voided morning specimen or urine collection over a 24-hour period, depending on whether the test is qualitative or quantitative.
- Notify the laboratory and practitioner of drugs the patient is taking that may affect test results; it may be necessary to restrict them.

Teaching points
- Explain the purpose of the test and how it's done.
- If appropriate, explain to the patient that the urine hCG test determines whether she's pregnant or determines the status of her pregnancy.
- Or, explain how the test functions as a screen for some types of cancer.
- Tell the patient who will perform the test and where it will be done.
- Tell the patient that she need not restrict food but should restrict fluids for 8 hours before the test.
- Teach the patient how to collect a 24-hour urine specimen.

DIAGNOSTIC PROCEDURE

KEY STEPS
- Confirm the patient's identity using two patient identifiers according to facility policy.
- For verification of pregnancy (qualitative analysis), collect a first-voided morning specimen. If this isn't possible, collect a random specimen.
- For quantitative analysis, collect the patient's urine over a 24-hour period in the appropriate container, discarding the first specimen and retaining the last.
- Specify the date of the patient's last menstrual period on the laboratory request.

POSTPROCEDURE CARE
- Tell the patient to resume her usual diet and medications.

PRECAUTIONS
- Refrigerate the 24-hour specimen or keep it on ice during the collection period.
- Make sure that the test occurs at least 5 days after a missed period to avoid a false-negative result.

COMPLICATIONS
- None

INTERPRETATION

NORMAL RESULTS
- In a qualitative immunoassay analysis, results are negative (nonpregnant) or positive (pregnant) for hCG.
- In a quantitative analysis, urine hCG levels in the first trimester of a normal pregnancy may be as high as 500,000 International Units/24 hours; in the second trimester, from 10,000 to 25,000 International Units/24 hours; and in the third trimester, from 5,000 to 15,000 International Units/24 hours.
- Measurable hCG levels don't normally appear in the urine of men or nonpregnant women.

ABNORMAL RESULTS
- During pregnancy, elevated urine hCG levels may indicate multiple pregnancy or erythroblastosis fetalis; depressed urine hCG levels may indicate threatened abortion or ectopic pregnancy.
- Measurable levels of hCG in men and nonpregnant women may indicate choriocarcinoma, ovarian or testicular tumors, melanoma, multiple myeloma, or gastric, hepatic, pancreatic, or breast cancer.

INTERFERING FACTORS *Early pregnancy, ectopic pregnancy, or threatened abortion (false-negative result)*

Human growth hormone level, serum

DESCRIPTION

- Quantitative analysis of levels of plasma human growth hormone (hGH), also called *somatotropin,* a protein secreted by pituitary gland and primary regulator of human growth
- Part of anterior pituitary stimulation or suppression test
- No defined feedback mechanism or single target gland; hGH affects many body tissues
- Like insulin, promotes protein synthesis and stimulates amino acid uptake by cells; raises plasma glucose levels by inhibiting glucose uptake and utilization by cells, and increases free fatty acid levels by enhancing lipolysis
- Regulates secretion by hypothalamus through a growth hormone–releasing factor and a growth hormone release-inhibiting factor (somatostatin)
- Secretion diurnal; varies with exercise, sleep, stress, and nutritional status
- Testing crucial because symptoms of hGH deficiency rarely reversible by therapy; dwarfism or gigantism induced by hyposecretion or hypersection, respectively

PURPOSE

- To differentiate between pituitary or thyroid hypofunction in the diagnosis of dwarfism
- To confirm the diagnosis of acromegaly and gigantism in the adult
- To help diagnose pituitary and hypothalamic tumors
- To help evaluate hGH therapy

PREPARATION

- The test requires a blood sample.
- Withhold all drugs that affect hGH levels such as pituitary-based steroids. If the patient must continue them, note this on the laboratory request.
- Make sure that the patient is relaxed and recumbent for 30 minutes before the test; stress and activity elevate hGH levels.

Teaching points

- Explain to the patient, or his parents if the patient is a child, that this test measures hormone levels and helps determine the cause of abnormal growth.
- Tell the patient who will perform the test and where it will be done.
- Inform the patient that another sample may be necessary the next day for comparison.
- Instruct the patient to fast and limit activity for 10 to 12 hours before the test.
- Tell the patient he may experience slight discomfort from the tourniquet and needle puncture.
- Inform the patient that the test takes about 1 hour.

KEY STEPS

- Confirm the patient's identity using two patient identifiers according to facility policy.
- Between 6 a.m. and 8 a.m. on 2 consecutive days, perform a venipuncture and collect at least 7 ml of blood in a clot-activator tube.

POSTPROCEDURE CARE

- Apply direct pressure to the venipuncture site until bleeding stops.
- Tell the patient to resume his usual diet, activities, and medications, as ordered.

PRECAUTIONS

- Handle the sample gently to prevent hemolysis.
- Send the sample to the laboratory immediately because hGH has a half-life of only 20 to 25 minutes.

COMPLICATIONS

- Hematoma at the venipuncture site

NORMAL RESULTS

- Normal hGH levels for men range from undetectable to 5 ng/ml (SI, 5 µg/L); for women, from undetectable to 10 ng/ml (SI, 10 µg/L).
- Children's values may range from undetectable to 16 ng/ml (SI, 16 µg/L) and are usually higher.

ABNORMAL RESULTS

- Increased hGH levels may indicate a pituitary or hypothalamic tumor, frequently an adenoma, which causes gigantism in children and acromegaly in adults and adolescents.
- Some patients with diabetes mellitus have elevated hGH levels without acromegaly.
- Suppression testing is required to confirm the diagnosis.
- Pituitary infarction, metastatic disease, and tumors may decrease hGH levels.
- Dwarfism may result from low hGH levels, although only 15% of all cases of growth failure relate to endocrine dysfunction.
- Confirming the diagnosis requires stimulation testing with arginine or insulin.

Human immunodeficiency virus antibodies test

DESCRIPTION

- Detects antibodies to human immunodeficiency virus (HIV), the cause of acquired immunodeficiency symdrome (AIDS), in serum
- HIV identified by enzyme-linked immunosorbent assay or other tests (see *Testing for HIV*); confirmed by Western blot test and immunofluorescence

PURPOSE

- To screen a high-risk patient for HIV
- To screen donated blood for HIV

PREPARATION

- Provide adequate counseling about the reasons for performing the test; usually, a patient's practitioner requests it.
- Have the patient sign a consent form.
- The test requires a blood sample.

Teaching points

- Explain that this test detects HIV infection.
- If the patient has questions about his condition, be sure to provide full and accurate information.
- Tell the patient who will perform the test and where it will be done.
- Tell him he doesn't need to restrict his diet.
- Explain that he may experience slight discomfort from the tourniquet and needle puncture.
- Inform him that the test should take less than 5 minutes.
- Tell the patient to report early signs of AIDS, such as fever, weight loss, axillary or inguinal lymphadenopathy, rash, and persistent cough or diarrhea. Women should also report gynecologic symptoms.
- Tell the patient to assume that he can transmit HIV to others until conclusively proved otherwise.
- To prevent virus transmission, advise the patient about safer sex practices.
- Instruct him not to share razors, toothbrushes, or utensils (which may be contaminated with blood) and to

clean such items with household bleach diluted 1:10 in water.
- Advise him against donating blood, tissues, or an organ.
- Warn the patient to inform his practitioner and dentist about his condition so that they can take proper precautions.

DIAGNOSTIC PROCEDURE

KEY STEPS

- Confirm the patient's identity using two patient identifiers according to facility policy.
- Perform a venipuncture and collect the sample in a 10-ml barrier tube.

POSTPROCEDURE CARE

- Apply direct pressure to the venipuncture site until bleeding stops.
- Keep the venipuncture site clean and dry because the patient may have a compromised immune system.
- Keep test results confidential.
- When the patient receives the results, let him ask questions.
- Encourage the patient with positive screening tests to seek medical follow-up care, even if he's asymptomatic.

PRECAUTIONS

- Barrier tubes help prevent contamination when pouring the serum.
- Observe standard precautions when drawing a blood sample.
- Use gloves, properly dispose of needles, and use blood-fluid precaution labels on tubes, as necessary.

COMPLICATIONS

- Hematoma at the venipuncture site
- Infection

INTERPRETATION

NORMAL RESULTS

- No HIV antibodies are present.

ABNORMAL RESULTS

- The test detects previous exposure to HIV — it doesn't identify patients

who have been exposed to the virus but haven't yet made antibodies.
- Most patients with AIDS have HIV antibodies.
- A positive result can't determine if a patient harbors active virus or when the patient will show signs and symptoms of AIDS.
- Many apparently healthy people have been exposed to HIV and have antibodies. Test results for such people aren't false-positives.
- Patients in the later stages of AIDS may show no detectable antibodies in their serum because they can no longer mount an antibody response.

Testing for HIV

Newer tests are available to help identify human immunodeficiency virus (HIV)-infected antibodies quicker and more conveniently, including a test to identify genetic changes that may alter the patient's course of treatment.

ORAQUICK RAPID HIV-1 ANTIBODY TEST

For the many people per year who don't check back for test results, rapid HIV testing may be done in any outpatient setting. The OraQuick rapid HIV-1 antibody test, approved by the U.S. Food and Drug Administration (FDA), allows results to be obtained in less than 20 minutes using 1 drop of blood. A color indicator similar to a home pregnancy test is used. If it's positive, another test must be done to confirm the results.

NUCLEIC ACID TEST

The FDA has also approved a nucleic acid test to screen plasma donation for HIV and hepatitis C. This test has been shown to dramatically reduce the waiting time involved until blood and blood products may be used.

GENE-BASED TEST

Spikes of HIV virus in the bloodstream commonly mean that the individual being treated for HIV is growing resistant to the drug treatment being used. The U.S. government has approved the first gene-based test to help determine if an HIV-infected person's virus is mutating, making therapy fail. This test can help the practitioner to select more appropriate treatment.

Human leukocyte antigen test

DESCRIPTION

- Identifies four types of human leukocyte antigen (HLA) — HLA-A, HLA-B, HLA-C, and HLA-D — present on surface of all nucleated cells; most easily detected on lymphocytes
- Essential to immunity and determine degree of histocompatibility between transplant recipients and donors
- Numerous antigenic determinants (over 60, for instance, at HLA-B locus) present for each site; one set of each antigen inherited from each parent
- High incidence of specific HLA types linked to specific diseases, such as rheumatoid arthritis and multiple sclerosis; findings have little diagnostic significance

PURPOSE

- To provide histocompatibility typing of transplant recipients and donors
- To aid in genetic counseling
- To aid in paternity testing

PREPARATION

- No dietary restrictions are needed.
- The test requires a blood sample.
- Check the patient's history for recent blood transfusions. It may be necessary to postpone HLA testing if he has recently undergone a transfusion.

Teaching points

- Explain that this test detects antigens on white blood cells.
- Tell the patient who will perform the test and where it will be done.
- Tell the patient that no dietary restrictions are needed.
- Explain to the patient that he may experience slight discomfort from the tourniquet and needle puncture.
- Inform the patient that the test should take less than 5 minutes.

KEY STEPS

- Confirm the patient's identity using two patient identifiers according to facility policy.
- Perform a venipuncture and collect the sample in a tube containing anticoagulant acid citrate dextrose solution.

POSTPROCEDURE CARE

- Apply direct pressure to the venipuncture site until bleeding stops.
- Refer the patient and his family to appropriate counseling services.

PRECAUTIONS

- Handle the sample gently to prevent hemolysis.

COMPLICATIONS

- Hematoma at the venipuncture site

NORMAL RESULTS

- There's no reaction of lymphocytes in HLA-A, HLA-B, and HLA-C testing.
- There's no reaction of leukocytes in HLA-D testing.

ABNORMAL RESULTS

- In HLA-A, HLA-B, and HLA-C testing, lymphocytes that react with the test antiserum undergo lysis; they're detectable by phase microscopy.
- In HLA-D testing, leukocyte incompatibility is marked by blast formation, deoxyribonucleic acid synthesis, and proliferation.
- Incompatible HLA-A, HLA-B, HLA-C, and HLA-D groups may cause unsuccessful tissue transplantation.
- Many diseases have a strong association with certain types of HLAs. For example, HLA-DR5 is associated with Hashimoto's thyroiditis.
- B8 and Dw3 are associated with Graves' disease, whereas B8 alone is associated with chronic autoimmune hepatitis, celiac disease, and myasthenia gravis.
- Dw3 alone is associated with Addison's disease, Sjögren's syndrome, dermatitis herpetiformis, and systemic lupus erythematosus.
- In paternity testing, a putative father who presents a phenotype (two haplotypes: one from the father and one from the mother) with no haplotype or antigen pair identical to one of the child's is excluded as the father.
- A putative father with one haplotype identical to one of the child's may be the father; the probability varies with the incidence of the haplotype in the population.

Human placental lactogen test

DESCRIPTION

- Radioimmunoassay measuring plasma levels of human placental lactogen (hPL), also known as *human chorionic somatomammotropin*
- With measurement of estriol levels, reliable indicator of placental function and fetal well-being
- Useful as a tumor marker in certain malignant states such as ectopic tumors that secrete hPL
- Used in high-risk pregnancies and suspected placental tissue dysfunction
- hPL: lactogenic and somatotropic (growth hormone) that, with prolactin, prepares breasts for lactation; indirectly provides energy for maternal metabolism and fetal nutrition; and facilitates protein synthesis and mobilization essential to fetal growth
- Autonomous secretion that begins at about 5 weeks' gestation and declines rapidly after delivery
- Values widely variable during latter half of pregnancy; serial determinations over several days most reliable

PURPOSE

- To assess placental function and fetal well-being
- To help diagnose hydatidiform mole and choriocarcinoma
- To help diagnose and monitor treatment of nontrophoblastic tumors that ectopically secrete hPL

PREPARATION

- No dietary restrictions are needed.
- This test requires collection of a blood sample.

Teaching points

- Explain that this test helps assess placental function and fetal well-being.
- If assessing fetal well-being isn't the diagnostic objective, offer an appropriate explanation.
- Tell the patient who will perform the test and where it will be done.
- Tell her that no dietary restrictions are needed.
- Explain that she may experience slight discomfort from the tourniquet and needle puncture.
- Inform the pregnant patient that it may be necessary to repeat this test during her pregnancy.
- Tell her that the test should take less than 5 minutes.

DIAGNOSTIC PROCEDURE

KEY STEPS

- Confirm the patient's identity using two patient identifiers according to facility policy.
- Perform a venipuncture and collect the sample in a 7-ml clot-activator tube.

POSTPROCEDURE CARE

- Apply direct pressure to the venipuncture site until bleeding stops.

PRECAUTIONS

- Maintain standard precautions while collecting the sample.
- Handle the sample gently to prevent hemolysis.

COMPLICATIONS

- Hematoma at the venipuncture site

INTERPRETATION

NORMAL RESULTS

- For pregnant women, normal hPL levels vary with the gestational phase and slowly increase throughout pregnancy, reaching 8.6 mcg/ml at term.
- At 5 to 27 weeks' gestation, the level is less than 4.6 mcg/ml.
- At 28 to 31 weeks' gestation, the level is 2.4 to 6.1 mcg/ml.
- At 32 to 35 weeks' gestation, the level is 3.7 to 7.7 mcg/ml.
- At 36 weeks' gestation to term, the level is 5 to 8.6 mcg/ml.
- At term in patients with diabetes, the mean level is 9 to 11 mcg/ml.
- For men and nonpregnant women, the level is below 0.5 mcg/ml.

ABNORMAL RESULTS

- For reliable interpretation, correlate hPL levels with gestational age; for example, after 30 weeks' gestation, levels below 4 mcg/ml may indicate placental dysfunction.
- Low hPL levels are characteristically associated with postmaturity syndrome, intrauterine growth retardation, preeclampsia, and eclampsia.
- Declining levels may help differentiate incomplete abortion from threatened abortion.
- Know that low hPL levels don't confirm fetal distress.
- Levels over 4 mcg/ml after 30 weeks' gestation don't guarantee fetal well-being because elevated levels have been reported after fetal death.
- An hPL value above 6 mcg/ml after 30 weeks' gestation may suggest an unusually large placenta, commonly occurring in a patient with diabetes mellitus, multiple pregnancy, or Rh isoimmunization.
- The test's usefulness in predicting fetal death in a patient with diabetes mellitus and in managing Rh isoimmunization during pregnancy is limited.
- Below-normal levels of hPL may indicate trophoblastic neoplastic disease, such as hydatidiform mole and choriocarcinoma.
- Abnormal levels of hPL have occurred in the sera of patients with other neoplastic disorders, including bronchogenic carcinoma, hepatoma, lymphoma, and pheochromocytoma. In these patients, hPL levels are used as tumor markers for evaluating chemotherapy, monitoring tumor growth and recurrence, and detecting residual tissue after excision.

17-hydroxycorticosteroid level, urine

DESCRIPTION

- Measures urine levels of 17-hydroxy-corticosteroid, metabolites of hormones that regulate glyconeogenesis (more than 80% are metabolites of cortisol, the primary adrenocortical steroid)
- Measures plasma cortisol, urine-free cortisol, and urine 17-ketosteroid levels; tests corticotropin stimulation and suppression to confirm results
- Reflects cortisol secretion and, indirectly, adrenocortical function
- Most accurately determined from a 24-hour specimen because cortisol secretion varies diurnally and in response to stress and other factors
- Uses column chromatography and spectrophotofluorimetry with the Porter-Silber reagent

PURPOSE

- To assess adrenocortical function

PREPARATION

- The test requires collection of urine over a 24-hour period.
- Notify the laboratory and practitioner of drugs the patient is taking that may affect test results; they may be restricted.

Teaching points

- Explain to the patient that this test evaluates how his adrenal glands are functioning.
- Teach him how to collect a 24-hour urine specimen.
- Tell the patient to restrict food and fluids that will alter test results (such as coffee or tea) and to avoid excessive physical exercise and stressful situations during the collection period.
- Tell the patient who will perform the test and where it will be done.

DIAGNOSTIC PROCEDURE

KEY STEPS

- Confirm the patient's identity using two patient identifiers according to facility policy.
- Collect the patient's urine over a 24-hour period, discarding the first specimen and retaining the last.
- Label the specimen appropriately, including the patient's gender, on the request forms.

POSTPROCEDURE CARE

- Tell the patient to resume his usual activities, diet, and medications.

PRECAUTIONS

- Use a bottle containing a preservative to prevent deterioration of the specimen.
- Refrigerate the specimen or place it on ice during the collection period.

COMPLICATIONS

- None

INTERPRETATION

NORMAL RESULTS

- In men, the level is 4.5 to 12 mg/24 hours (SI, 12.4 to 33.1 μmol/day).
- In women, the level is 2.5 to 10 mg/24 hours (SI, 6.9 to 27.6 μmol/day).
- In children ages 8 to 12, the level is less than 4.5 mg/24 hours (SI, < 12.4 μmol/day).
- In children younger than age 8, the level is less than 1.5 mg/24 hours (SI, < 4.14 μmol/day).

ABNORMAL RESULTS

- Increased levels may occur in Cushing's syndrome, adrenal carcinoma or adenoma, pituitary tumor, virilism, hyperthyroidism, severe hypertension, and extreme stress induced by such conditions as acute pancreatitis and eclampsia.
- Decreased levels may indicate Addison's disease, hypopituitarism, or myxedema.

Hypotonic duodenography

DESCRIPTION

◆ Fluoroscopic examination of duodenum after instillation of barium sulfate and air through an intestinal catheter to detect duodenal or pancreatic disease

◆ Involves passing a catheter through the patient's nose into the duodenum, I.V. infusion of glucagon or I.M. injection of propantheline bromide (or another anticholinergic) to induce duodenal atony

◆ Barium and air instilled to distend the relaxed duodenum, flatten its deep circular folds, and record the precise delineation of the duodenal anatomy

◆ Further studies needed despite films demonstrating small duodenal lesions and tumors of the head of the pancreas that impinge on the duodenal wall

PURPOSE

◆ To detect small, postbulbar duodenal lesions, tumors of the head of the pancreas, and tumors of the ampulla of Vater

◆ To help diagnose chronic pancreatitis

PREPARATION

◆ Fasting is required after midnight the night before the test.

◆ Just before the test, have the patient remove dentures, glasses, necklaces, hairpins, combs, and constricting undergarments; also ask him to void.

Teaching points

◆ Explain that hypotonic duodenography permits examination of the duodenum and pancreas after the instillation of barium and air.

◆ Tell the patient who will perform the test and where it will be done.

◆ Instruct him to fast from midnight the night before the test.

◆ Inform him that a tube will be passed through his nose into the duodenum to serve as a channel for the barium and air.

◆ Tell the patient that he may experience a cramping pain as air is introduced into the duodenum. Instruct him to breathe deeply and slowly through his mouth if he experiences this pain to help relax the abdominal muscles.

◆ If the patient is to receive glucagon or an anticholinergic during the procedure, describe the possible adverse effects of glucagon (nausea, vomiting, hives, flushing) or anticholinergics (dry mouth, thirst, tachycardia, urine retention, blurred vision). If an anticholinergic is given to an outpatient, advise him to have someone accompany him home.

◆ Inform the patient that the test takes about 1 hour.

◆ After the procedure, encourage the patient to drink extra fluids, unless contraindicated, to help eliminate the barium.

◆ Tell the patient that he may burp instilled air or pass flatus and that the barium colors the feces chalky white for 24 to 72 hours after the test.

KEY STEPS

◆ Confirm the patient's identity using two patient identifiers according to facility policy.

◆ While the patient is sitting, a catheter is passed through his nose and into the stomach.

◆ The patient is then placed into a supine position on an X-ray table; the catheter is advanced into the duodenum under fluoroscopic guidance.

◆ The patient is given I.V. glucagon, which quickly induces duodenal atony for about 20 minutes; or an I.M. anticholinergic is injected.

◆ Barium is instilled through the catheter; spot films are taken of the duodenum.

◆ Some of the barium is then withdrawn, air is instilled, and additional spot films are taken.

◆ When the required films have been obtained, the catheter is removed.

POSTPROCEDURE CARE

◆ If the patient received an anticholinergic, make sure that he voids within a few hours after the test.

◆ Advise the outpatient to rest in a waiting area until his vision clears (about 2 hours) unless someone can take him home.

◆ Give a cathartic.

◆ Record a description of feces the patient passed in the hospital and notify the practitioner if the patient hasn't expelled the barium after 2 to 3 days.

PRECAUTIONS

◆ The test is contraindicated in patients with upper GI tract strictures, particularly with ulcerations or large masses.

◆ Monitor the elderly or extremely ill patient for gastric reflux.

◆ Observe the patient for adverse reactions during the procedure. Know that such reactions may follow administration of glucagon or an anticholinergic.

COMPLICATIONS

◆ Adverse reaction to drugs

NORMAL RESULTS

◆ When barium and air distend the atonic duodenum, the mucosa normally appears smooth and even.

◆ The regular contour of the pancreas head also appears on the duodenal wall.

ABNORMAL RESULTS

◆ Irregular nodules or masses on the duodenal wall could mean duodenal lesions, tumors of the ampulla of Vater, tumors of the pancreas head, or chronic pancreatitis.

◆ A differential diagnosis requires further tests, such as endoscopic retrograde cholangiopancreatography, serum and urine amylase tests, ultrasonography of the pancreas, and computed tomography of the pancreas.

Hysterosalpingography

DESCRIPTION

+ Radiologic examination showing uterine cavity, fallopian tubes, and peritubal area
+ Fluoroscopic X-rays obtained as contrast medium flows through the uterus and fallopian tubes
+ Performed as part of an infertility evaluation

PURPOSE

+ To confirm tubal abnormalities such as adhesions
+ To confirm uterine abnormalities such as congenital malformations
+ To confirm the presence of fistulas or peritubal adhesions
+ To evaluate the cause of repeated miscarriage

PREPARATION

+ Make sure that the patient has signed an appropriate consent form.
+ Note and report all allergies, including iodinated contrast media.
+ Check the patient's history for recent pelvic infection.
+ A test for pelvic infections may be needed before the study.
+ Antibiotics may be prescribed before the test.

Teaching points

+ Explain the purpose of the test and how it's done.
+ Tell the patient who will perform the test and where it will be done.
+ Explain that the procedure should take place 2 to 5 days after menstruation ends.
+ Inform the patient that the test takes about 15 minutes.
+ Explain that she may receive a mild sedative or a nonprescription prostaglandin inhibitor 30 minutes before the procedure.
+ Tell the patient that a small amount of vaginal bleeding and pelvic cramping may occur for a few days after the study.
+ Tell the patient that additional tests and studies may be required to establish a precise diagnosis.

KEY STEPS

+ Confirm the patient's identity using two patient identifiers according to facility policy.
+ The patient is assisted into the lithotomy position; a scout film is taken.
+ A bimanual examination determines uterine size and position.
+ A speculum is inserted in the vagina, and the vagina and cervix are cleaned.
+ A cannula is inserted into the cervix and anchored to a tenaculum.
+ Contrast medium is injected through the cannula.
+ The uterus and fallopian tubes are viewed fluoroscopically and X-rays are taken.
+ For oblique views, the table is tilted or the patient is asked to change position.
+ Films may be taken later to evaluate the spillage of contrast medium into the peritoneal cavity.

POSTPROCEDURE CARE

+ Monitor the patient's vital signs.
+ Monitor the patient for signs and symptoms of infection and uterine perforation.
+ Monitor for bleeding.
+ Watch for an adverse reaction to the contrast medium.
+ Tell the patient to gradually return to normal activities.

PRECAUTIONS

+ The procedure is contraindicated during menstruation and in patients with undiagnosed vaginal bleeding and pelvic inflammatory disease.

COMPLICATIONS

+ Uterine perforation
+ Infection
+ Bleeding
+ Adverse reaction to the contrast medium

NORMAL RESULTS

+ The uterine cavity is symmetrical.
+ The fallopian tubes are a normal caliber.
+ Contrast medium spills freely into the peritoneal cavity.
+ Contrast medium doesn't leak from the uterus.

ABNORMAL RESULTS

+ The uterus is asymmetrical, suggesting intrauterine adhesions or masses.
+ Contrast medium flow through the fallopian tubes is impaired, suggesting partial or complete blockage.
+ Contrast medium leaks through the uterine wall, suggesting fistulas.

Hysteroscopy

DESCRIPTION
- Examination with a small-diameter endoscope, showing interior of uterus
- Usually performed in the practitioner's office after the patient is given a local anesthetic or mild sedative
- Performed during the first week after the end of a patient's menstrual cycle

PURPOSE
- To investigate abnormal uterine bleeding
- To remove polyps
- To evaluate infertile patients
- To direct the removal of intrauterine devices
- To help diagnose and treat intrauterine adhesions
- To diagnose uterine fibroids

PREPARATION
- Make sure that the patient has signed an appropriate consent form.
- Note and report all allergies.
- Check the patient's history for hypersensitivity to the anesthetic.
- Obtain the results of the patient's last Papanicolaou test.
- Fasting may be required before the test.
- Have the patient empty her bladder before the test.
- Recommend that the patient have a friend or relative drive her home after the procedure.

Teaching points
- Explain the purpose of the test and how it's done.
- Teach the patient how to collect a 24-hour urine specimen.
- Advise the patient of any dietary restrictions ordered.
- Warn the patient that the practitioner may inflate her uterus with carbon dioxide (CO_2); tell her that her body will absorb it but that it may cause upper abdominal or shoulder pain for 24 to 36 hours after the test.
- Inform the patient that some vaginal bleeding and mild abdominal cramping may occur after the test.

DIAGNOSTIC PROCEDURE

KEY STEPS
- Confirm the patient's identity using two patient identifiers according to facility policy.
- The patient is assisted into a modified dorsal lithotomy position with her legs in stirrups.
- A local anesthetic is given.
- The vagina is cleaned and the hysteroscope inserted.
- Visualization begins at the level of the internal os.
- In contact hysteroscopy, the uterus isn't distended; only the area in direct contact with the hysteroscope is visible.
- In panoramic hysteroscopy, an external illumination source and media (such as CO_2) for distention are used; this makes the tissue visible from a distance.
- Cultures of the vagina and cervix may be taken.

POSTPROCEDURE CARE
- Provide the patient with a sanitary pad if needed.
- Provide analgesics as needed.
- Monitor the patient's vital signs.
- Watch the patient for bleeding.

PRECAUTIONS
- Watch for adverse reaction to analgesics.
- Watch for signs and symptoms of infection, such as fever and pain.

COMPLICATIONS
- Severe cramps, dyspnea, upper abdominal and right shoulder pain (can develop if CO_2 passes into the peritoneal cavity)
- Adverse reaction to drugs
- Infection

INTERPRETATION

NORMAL RESULTS
- The interior of the uterus is normal in size and shape and free from adhesions and lesions.

ABNORMAL RESULTS
- The interior of the uterus is abnormally shaped, suggesting polyps, uterine wall tumors, or adhesions.

🔵 **INTERFERING FACTORS** *Heavy bleeding or a distended bladder (interferes with visualization)*

Immune complex assays

DESCRIPTION

◆ Detect immune complex diseases (postinfectious syndromes, serum sickness, drug sensitivity, rheumatoid arthritis, and systemic lupus erythematosus [SLE]), which may occur when immune complexes develop faster than the lymphoreticular system can clear them (See *Serum immunoglobulin levels in various disorders*)

◆ Detect complexes indirectly; more than one test needed to achieve accurate results

◆ Immune complexes: develop when antigen reacts with antibody of isotopes immunoglobulin (Ig) G 1, 2, 3, or IgM in tissues

◆ Complexes detected by histologic examination of biopsy tissue and fluorescence or peroxidase staining with antibodies specific for immunologic types

◆ Appropriate serum test methods: use of C1, rheumatoid factor, or cellular substrates, such as Raji cells, as reagents

PURPOSE

◆ To demonstrate circulating immune complexes in serum
◆ To monitor the patient's response to therapy
◆ To estimate disease severity

PREPARATION

◆ No dietary restrictions are required.
◆ This test requires a blood sample.
◆ If the patient is scheduled for C1q assay (a component of C1), check his history for recent heparin therapy and report such therapy to the laboratory.

Teaching points

◆ Explain that these tests help evaluate the immune system.
◆ Explain who will perform the test and where it'll be done.
◆ Inform the patient that the test may be repeated to monitor his response to therapy, if appropriate.

◆ Inform the patient that fasting isn't required before the test.
◆ Tell the patient that the test requires a blood sample and that he may experience slight discomfort from the tourniquet and needle puncture.
◆ Tell the patient that the test takes less than 5 minutes.

KEY STEPS

◆ Confirm the patient's identity using two patient identifiers according to facility policy.
◆ Perform a venipuncture and collect the sample in a 7-ml clot-activator tube.

Serum immunoglobulin levels in various disorders

This table lists various disorders and the associated changes in serum immunoglobulin levels.

DISORDER	IgG	IgA	IgM
Immunoglobulin disorders			
Lymphoid aplasia	D	D	D
Agammaglobulinemia	D	D	D
Type I dysgammaglobulinemia (selective immunoglobulin [Ig] G and IgA deficiency)	D	D	N or I
Type II dysgammaglobulinemia (absent IgA and IgM)	N	D	D
IgA globulinemia	N	D	N
Ataxia-telangiectasia	N	D	N
Multiple myeloma, macroglobulinemia, lymphomas			
Heavy chain disease (Franklin's disease)	D	D	D
IgG myeloma	I	D	D
IgA myeloma	D	I	D
Macroglobulinemia	D	D	I
Acute lymphocytic leukemia	N	D	N
Chronic lymphocytic leukemia	D	D	D
Acute myelocytic leukemia	N	N	N
Chronic myelocytic leukemia	N	D	N
Hodgkin's disease	N	N	N
Hepatic disorders			
Hepatitis	I	I	I
Laënnec's cirrhosis	I	I	N
Biliary cirrhosis	N	N	I
Hepatoma	N	N	D
Rheumatoid arthritis	I	I	I
Other disorders			
Systemic lupus erythematosus	I	I	I
Nephrotic syndrome	D	D	N
Trypanosomiasis	N	N	I
Pulmonary tuberculosis	I	N	N

Key: N=Normal; I=Increased; D=Decreased.

(continued)

POSTPROCEDURE CARE

◆ Apply direct pressure to the venipuncture site until the bleeding stops.
◆ Inform the practitioner of abnormal results.

PRECAUTIONS

◆ Because many patients with immune complexes have a compromised immune system, keep the venipuncture site clean and dry.
◆ Send the sample to the laboratory immediately to prevent deterioration of immune complexes.

COMPLICATIONS

◆ Hematoma at the venipuncture site

INTERPRETATION

NORMAL RESULTS

◆ Immune complexes aren't detected in serum.

ABNORMAL RESULTS

◆ The presence of detectable immune complexes in serum has etiologic importance in many autoimmune diseases, such as SLE and rheumatoid arthritis.
◆ For definitive diagnosis, the presence of these complexes must be considered with the results of other studies. For example, in SLE, immune complexes are associated with high titers of antinuclear antibodies and circulating antinative deoxyribonucleic acid antibodies.
◆ Because of their filtering function, renal glomeruli appear vulnerable to immune complex deposition, although blood vessel walls and choroid plexuses (vascular folds in the ventricles of the brain) can be affected.

Insulin, serum

DESCRIPTION

- Quantitative analysis of serum insulin levels
- Insulin usually measured with glucose levels; glucose is primary stimulus for insulin release from pancreatic islet cells
- Regulates metabolism and transport or mobilization of carbohydrates, amino acids, proteins, and lipids
- Stimulated by increased plasma glucose levels; secretion peaks after meals, when metabolism and food storage are highest

PURPOSE

- To help diagnose hyperinsulinemia as well as hypoglycemia resulting from a tumor or hyperplasia of pancreatic islet cells, glucocorticoid deficiency, or severe hepatic disease
- To help diagnose diabetes mellitus and insulin-resistant states

PREPARATION

- The patient must fast for at least 10 hours before the test.
- Withhold corticotropin, corticosteroids (including hormonal contraceptives), thyroid supplements, epinephrine, and other drugs that may interfere with test results. If the patient must continue them, note this on the laboratory request.
- Make sure the patient is relaxed and recumbent for 30 minutes before the test.
- This test requires a blood sample.

Teaching points

- Explain that this test helps determine if the pancreas is functioning normally.
- Tell the patient who will perform the test and where it'll be done.
- Instruct the patient to fast for at least 10 hours before the test.
- Tell the patient that the test requires a blood sample and that he may experience slight discomfort from the tourniquet and needle puncture.
- Explain that questionable results may require a repeat test or a simultaneous glucose tolerance test, which requires that he drink a glucose solution.
- Tell the patient the test takes about 45 minutes.

DIAGNOSTIC PROCEDURE

KEY STEPS

- Confirm the patient's identity using two patient identifiers according to facility policy.
- Perform a venipuncture and collect one sample for insulin level in a 7-ml EDTA tube.
- Collect a sample for glucose level in a tube with sodium fluoride and potassium oxalate.

POSTPROCEDURE CARE

- Apply pressure to the venipuncture site until bleeding stops.
- Inform the practitioner of abnormal results.
- After the test, tell the patient to resume his usual activities, diet, and medications.

PRECAUTIONS

WARNING *Fasting for this test may precipitate dangerously severe hypoglycemia in patients with insulinoma. Keep an ampule of dextrose 50% available to counteract possible hypoglycemia.*

- Pack the insulin sample in ice and send it with the glucose sample to the laboratory immediately.
- Handle the samples gently to prevent hemolysis.

COMPLICATIONS

- Hematoma at the venipuncture site

INTERPRETATION

NORMAL RESULTS

- Insulin level is 0 to 35 µU/ml (SI, 144 to 243 pmol/L).

ABNORMAL RESULTS

- Insulin levels are interpreted in light of the prevailing glucose level.
- A normal insulin level may be inappropriate for the glucose results.
- High insulin and low glucose levels after a significant fast suggest the presence of an insulinoma.
- Prolonged fasting or stimulation testing may be needed to confirm the diagnosis.
- In insulin-resistant diabetes mellitus, insulin levels are elevated; in noninsulin-resistant diabetes, they're low.

Insulin tolerance test

DESCRIPTION

- Measures serum levels of human growth hormone (hGH) and corticotropin after patient receives loading dose of insulin
- More reliable than direct measurement of hGH and corticotropin because many healthy people have undetectable fasting levels of these hormones
- Insulin-induced hypoglycemia: stimulates hGH and corticotropin secretion in people with an intact hypothalamic-pituitary-adrenal axis
- Not recommended for patients with cardiovascular or cerebrovascular disorders, epilepsy, or low basal plasma cortisol levels

PURPOSE

- To help diagnose hGH and corticotropin deficiency
- To identify pituitary dysfunction
- To aid differential diagnosis of primary and secondary adrenal hypofunction

PREPARATION

- Fasting and activity restriction are required for 10 to 12 hours before the test.
- The test requires several blood samples and I.V. insulin.

Teaching points

- Explain that this test evaluates hormonal secretion.
- Instruct the patient to fast and restrict physical activity for 10 to 12 hours before the test.
- Explain that the test involves I.V. infusion of insulin and the collection of multiple blood samples.
- Warn the patient that he may experience an increased heart rate, diaphoresis, hunger, and anxiety after administration of insulin. Reassure the patient that these symptoms are transient, and that if they become severe, the test will be stopped.
- Tell the patient to lie down and relax for 90 minutes before the test.

KEY STEPS

- Confirm the patient's identity using two patient identifiers according to facility policy.
- Between 6 a.m. and 8 a.m., perform a venipuncture and collect three 5-ml samples of blood for basal levels: one in a gray-top tube (for blood glucose) and two in green-top tubes (for hGH and corticotropin).
- Give an I.V. bolus of U-100 regular insulin (0.15 units/kg) over 1 or 2 minutes.
- Use an indwelling venous catheter to avoid repeated venipunctures.
- Collect additional blood samples 15, 30, 45, 60, 90, and 120 minutes after giving the insulin.
- At each interval, collect three samples: one in a tube with sodium fluoride and potassium oxidate and two in heparinized tubes.
- Label the tubes appropriately and send them to the laboratory immediately.

POSTPROCEDURE CARE

- Apply pressure to the venipuncture site until bleeding stops.
- Inform the practitioner of abnormal results.
- Instruct the patient that he may resume his usual diet, activities, and medications.

PRECAUTIONS

WARNING *Be sure to have concentrated glucose solution readily available in case the patient has severe hypoglycemic reaction to insulin.*

- Handle the samples gently to prevent hemolysis.

COMPLICATIONS

- Hematoma at the I.V. or venipuncture site
- Hypoglycemic reaction

NORMAL RESULTS

- Blood glucose falls to 50% of the fasting level 20 to 30 minutes after the patient receives insulin.
- This stimulates a 10- to 20-ng/dl (SI, 10 to 20 mcg/L) increase in baseline values for hGH and corticotropin, with peak levels occurring 60 to 90 minutes after the patient receives insulin.

ABNORMAL RESULTS

- Failure of stimulation indicates anterior pituitary or adrenal hypofunction and helps confirm hGH or a corticotropin deficiency.
- An hGH increase of less than 10 ng/dl (SI, < 10 mcg/L) above baseline suggests hGH deficiency.
- A definitive diagnosis of hGH deficiency requires a supplementary stimulation test such as the arginine test.
- Additional testing is needed to determine the site of the abnormality.
- An increase in corticotropin levels of less than 10 ng/dl above baseline suggests adrenal insufficiency.
- The metyrapone or corticotropin stimulation test then confirms the diagnosis and determines whether the insufficiency is primary or secondary.

Internal fetal monitoring

DESCRIPTION

- Invasive procedure involving attachment of electrode to fetal scalp to monitor fetal heart rate (FHR)
- Catheter introduced into uterine cavity; measures frequency and pressure of uterine contractions
- Performed only during labor, after membranes have ruptured and cervix has dilated 3 cm, with the fetal head lower than the –2 station and only if external monitoring provides inadequate data
- Provides more accurate information about fetal health than external monitoring; useful in determining if cesarean delivery is needed
- Minimal risks to patient (perforated uterus and intrauterine infection) and fetus (scalp abscess and hematoma)

PURPOSE

- To monitor FHR, especially beat-to-beat variability (short-term variability)
- To measure the frequency and pressure of uterine contractions to assess the progress of labor
- To evaluate intrapartum fetal health
- To supplement or replace external fetal monitoring

PREPARATION

- Make sure the patient has signed an informed consent form.
- No dietary restrictions are required.

Teaching points

- Explain that internal fetal monitoring accurately assesses fetal health and uterine activity and that it doesn't necessarily suggest a problem.
- Tell the patient who will perform the test and where it'll be done.
- Tell the patient that she doesn't need to restrict food or fluids.
- Warn the patient that she may feel mild discomfort when the uterine catheter and scalp electrode are inserted.

KEY STEPS

- Confirm the patient's identity using two patient identifiers according to facility policy.
- The steps vary depending on whether the procedure is being used to measure FHR or uterine contractions.

To measure fetal heart rate

- Assist the patient into the dorsal lithotomy position and prepare her perineal area for a vaginal examination, explaining each step of the procedure as it's performed by a physician or certified nurse-midwife.
- As the procedure begins, instruct the patient to breathe through her mouth and relax her abdominal muscles.
- After the vaginal examination, the fetal scalp is palpated and an appropriate site is identified.
- A plastic tube carrying the small electrode is introduced into the cervix, pressed firmly against the fetal scalp, and rotated clockwise to attach the electrode to the scalp.
- The electrode wire is tugged gently to ensure proper attachment and the tube is withdrawn, leaving the electrode in place.
- Apply a conduction medium to a leg plate and strap it to the patient's thigh. Attach electrode wires to the leg plate and plug a cable from the leg plate into the fetal monitor.
- To check proper placement of the scalp electrode, turn on the monitor and press the electrocardiogram button; an FHR signal indicates proper electrode attachment.

To measure uterine contractions

- Before the uterine catheter is inserted, fill it with sterile normal saline solution to prevent air emboli. Explain each step of the procedure to the patient.
- Ask the patient to breathe deeply through her mouth and to relax her abdominal muscles.
- After the vagina has been examined and the presenting part of the fetus palpated, the catheter and guide are inserted 3/8" to 3/4" (1 to 2 cm) into the cervix, usually between the fetal head and the posterior cervix.
- The catheter is then gently advanced into the uterus until the black mark on the catheter is flush with the vulva. (The catheter guide should never be passed deeply into the uterus.)
- The guide is removed and the catheter is connected to a transducer that converts the intrauterine pressure, as measured by the fluid in the catheter, to an electrical signal. (See *Understanding internal fetal monitoring,* page 286.)

POSTPROCEDURE CARE

- After removing the fetal scalp electrode, apply antiseptic or antibiotic solution to the attachment site.
- Be sure to remove the fetal scalp electrode and the uterine catheter before cesarean delivery.

PRECAUTIONS

- If FHR patterns indicate distress, fetal oxygenation can usually be improved by loading maternal fluids to increase placental perfusion, turning the mother on her side (preferably left) to alleviate supine hypotension, and giving oxygen to the mother. If these measures return FHR patterns to normal, labor may continue. If abnormal patterns persist, cesarean delivery may be required.

COMPLICATIONS

- Fetal scalp abscess or maternal intrauterine infection

(continued)

NORMAL RESULTS

◆ Heart rate is 120 to 160 beats/minute, with a variability of 5 to 25 beats/minute.

ABNORMAL RESULTS

◆ Bradycardia (FHR < 120 beats/minute) may indicate fetal heart block, malposition, or hypoxia.
◆ Fetal bradycardia may also result from maternal ingestion of certain drugs, such as propranolol (Inderal) and opioid analgesics.
◆ Tachycardia (FHR > 160 beats/minute) may result from early fetal hypoxia, fetal infection or arrhythmia, prematurity, or maternal fever, tachycardia, hyperthyroidism, or use of vagolytics.

◆ Decreased variability (fluctuation of < 5 beats/minute from baseline) may result from fetal arrhythmia or heart block, hypoxia, central nervous system malformation, or infections, or from maternal use of opioids or vagolytics.
◆ Early decelerations (slowing of FHR at the onset of a contraction with recovery to baseline within no more than 15 seconds after the contraction ends) are related to fetal head compression and usually ensure fetal health.
◆ Late decelerations (slowing of FHR after a contraction begins, a lag time of > 20 seconds, and a recovery time of > 15 seconds) may be related to uteroplacental insufficiency, fetal hypoxia, or acidosis.

◆ Recurrent and persistently late decelerations with decreased variability usually indicate serious fetal distress, possibly resulting from conduction (spinal, caudal, or epidural) anesthesia or fetal hypoxia.
◆ Variable decelerations (sudden precipitous drops in FHR unrelated to uterine contractions) are commonly related to cord compression.
◆ A severe drop in FHR (to < 70 beats/minute for more than 60 seconds) with a decrease in variability indicates fetal distress and may result in a compromised neonate.
◆ Poor beat-to-beat variability without periodic patterns may indicate fetal distress, requiring further evaluation such as analysis of fetal blood gas levels.
◆ Low intrauterine pressure during labor that isn't progressing normally may indicate a need for oxytocin (Pitocin) stimulation.
◆ High intrauterine pressure may indicate abruptio placentae or overstimulation from oxytocin, possibly resulting in fetal distress caused by decreased placental perfusion.

⬢ INTERFERING FACTORS *Drugs that affect the parasympathetic and sympathetic nervous systems*

Understanding internal fetal monitoring

Internal fetal monitoring uses an electrode attached to the fetal scalp. The resultant fetal electrocardiograms (FECGs) are transmitted to an amplifier. A cardiotachometer measures the interval between FECGs and plots a continuous fetal heart rate (FHR) graph, which is displayed on a two-channel oscilloscope screen. Intrauterine catheters attached to a transducer in a leg plate measure the frequency and pressure of uterine contractions, which are plotted below the FHR graph.

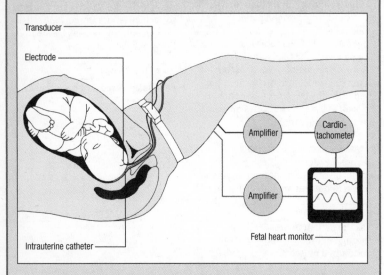

International normalized ratio

DESCRIPTION

- Also known as *INR system*
- Measures prothrombin time, to monitor oral anticoagulant therapy
- Not used to screen for coagulopathies

PURPOSE

- To evaluate the effectiveness of oral anticoagulant therapy

PREPARATION

- No dietary restrictions are required.
- This test requires a blood sample.

Teaching points

- Explain that the INR test determines the effectiveness of his oral anticoagulant therapy.
- Tell the patient who will perform the test and where it'll be done.
- Inform him that fasting isn't required.
- Tell the patient that the test requires a blood sample and that he may experience slight discomfort from the tourniquet and needle puncture.
- Tell the patient the test takes less than 5 minutes.

KEY STEPS

- Confirm the patient's identity using two patient identifiers according to facility policy.
- Perform a venipuncture and collect the sample in a 4.5-ml tube with sodium citrate added.
- Completely fill the collection tube; otherwise, an excess of citrate appears in the sample.
- Gently invert the tube several times to thoroughly mix the sample and the anticoagulant.

POSTPROCEDURE CARE

- Apply direct pressure to the venipuncture site until bleedings stops.
- Inform the practitioner of abnormal results.

PRECAUTIONS

- To prevent hemolysis, avoid excessive probing during venipuncture and handle the sample gently.
- Put the sample on ice and send it to the laboratory immediately.

COMPLICATIONS

- Hematoma at the venipuncture site; if large, monitor pulses distal to the venipuncture site

NORMAL RESULTS

- For patients receiving warfarin (Coumadin) therapy, INR is 2.0 to 3.0 (SI, 2.0 to 3.0).
- For those with mechanical prosthetic heart valves, INR is 2.5 to 3.5 (SI, 2.5 to 3.5).

ABNORMAL RESULTS

- Increased INR values may indicate disseminated intravascular coagulation, cirrhosis, hepatitis, vitamin K deficiency, salicylate intoxication, uncontrolled oral anticoagulation, or massive blood transfusion.

  INTERFERING FACTORS *Failure to fill the collection tube completely, to adequately mix the sample and the anticoagulant, or to send the sample to the laboratory immediately*

  Hemolysis from excessive probing at the venipuncture site or from rough handling of the sample

Iron and total iron-binding capacity

DESCRIPTION

- Measures amount of iron that would appear in plasma if all transferrin were saturated with iron (iron essential to formation and function of hemoglobin and other heme and nonheme compounds)
- About 70% of total body iron in blood
- Carried in hemoglobin of red blood cells
- Absorbed by intestines; then distributed to various body compartments for synthesis, storage and transport

PURPOSE

- To determine the serum iron level in the blood
- To estimate total iron storage
- To help diagnose hemochromatosis
- To help distinguish iron deficiency anemia from anemia of chronic disease (for information on another test used to differentiate anemias, see *Siderocyte stain*)
- To help evaluate nutritional status

PREPARATION

- No dietary restrictions are required.
- The test requires a blood test.

Teaching points

- Explain that this test evaluates the body's capacity to store iron.
- Tell the patient who will perform the test and where it'll be done.
- Tell him that the test requires a blood sample and that he may experience slight discomfort from the tourniquet and needle puncture.
- Explain to the patient that no dietary restrictions are required.
- Tell the patient the test takes less than 5 minutes.

KEY STEPS

- Confirm the patient's identity using two patient identifiers according to facility policy.
- Perform a venipuncture to collect the blood sample.

POSTPROCEDURE CARE

- Apply direct pressure to the venipuncture site until the bleeding stops.
- Inform the practitioner of abnormal results.

PRECAUTIONS

- Handle the sample gently to prevent hemolysis.
- Send the sample to the laboratory immediately.

COMPLICATIONS

- Hematoma at the venipuncture site

NORMAL RESULTS

- Serum iron level in males is 60 to 170 mcg/dl (SI, 10.7 to 30.4 µmol/L); in females, 50 to 130 mcg/dl (SI, 9 to 23.3 µmol/L).
- Total iron-binding capacity (TIBC) is 300 to 360 mcg/dl (SI, 54 to 64 µmol/L).
- Saturation is 20% to 50% (SI, 0.2 to 0.5).

ABNORMAL RESULTS

- In iron deficiency, serum iron levels decrease and TIBC increases, decreasing saturation.
- In chronic inflammation, serum iron may be low despite adequate body stores, but TIBC may be unchanged or decreased to preserve normal saturation.
- Iron overload may not alter serum levels until later, but serum iron increases and TIBC remains the same, increasing saturation.

Siderocyte stain

Siderocytes are red blood cells (RBCs) containing particles of nonhemoglobin iron known as *siderocytic granules*. In neonates, siderocytic granules occur in normoblasts and reticulocytes during hemoglobin synthesis. However, the spleen removes most of these granules from normal RBCs, and they disappear rapidly with age.

In adults, an elevated siderocyte level usually indicates abnormal erythropoiesis, which may occur in congenital spherocytic anemia, chronic hemolytic anemias (such as the thalassemias), pernicious anemia, hemochromatosis, toxicities (such as lead poisoning), infection, or severe burns. Elevated levels may also follow splenectomy because the spleen normally removes siderocytic granules.

PERFORMING THE TEST

The siderocyte stain test measures the number of circulating siderocytes. Venous blood is drawn into a 3- or 4.5-ml EDTA tube or, for infants and children, collected in a Microtainer or pipette and smeared directly on a 3″ × 5″ glass slide. When the blood smear is stained, siderocytic granules appear as purple-blue specks clustered around the periphery of mature erythrocytes. Cells containing these granules are counted as a percentage of total RBCs. The results aid differential diagnosis of the anemias and hemochromatosis and help detect toxicities.

INTERPRETING RESULTS

Normally, neonates have a slightly elevated siderocyte level that reaches the normal adult value of 0.5% (SI, 0.05) of total RBCs in 7 to 10 days. In patients with pernicious anemia, the siderocyte level is 8% to 14% (SI, 0.08 to 0.14); in chronic hemolytic anemia, 20% to 100% (SI, 0.2 to 1.0); in lead poisoning, 10% to 30% (SI, 0.1 to 0.3); and in hemochromatosis, 3% to 7% (SI, 0.03 to 0.07). A high siderocyte level calls for additional testing (including bone marrow examination) to determine the cause of abnormal erythropoiesis.

Ischemia-modified albumin test

DESCRIPTION

◆ Measures changes in human serum albumin when it comes in contact with ischemic tissue
◆ Ischemia-modified albumin (IMA): detectable in blood within minutes of ischemia
◆ Rises rapidly when oxygen supply to heart is compromised and oxygen supply doesn't meet oxygen demand; occurs sooner than other cardiac markers, such as troponin, and creatine kinase (see *IMA and necrosis markers*)
◆ Rises quickly in ischemia but not in necrosis of tissue
◆ Elevated in over 80% of patients with acute coronary syndrome
◆ Returns to normal within several hours of resolution of ischemia

PURPOSE

◆ Used with electrocardiogram (ECG) and troponin to rule out acute coronary syndrome
◆ For early identification of cardiac ischemia

PREPARATION

◆ No dietary restrictions are required.
◆ The test requires a blood test.

Teaching points

◆ Explain that this test helps determine if his heart is getting enough oxygen.
◆ Tell the patient who will perform the test and where it'll be done.
◆ Tell him that the test requires a blood sample and that he may experience slight discomfort from the tourniquet and needle puncture.
◆ Explain to the patient that no dietary restrictions are required.
◆ Tell the patient the test takes less than 5 minutes.

DIAGNOSTIC PROCEDURE

KEY STEPS

◆ Confirm the patient's identity using two patient identifiers according to facility policy.

◆ Perform a venipuncture to collect the blood sample.

POSTPROCEDURE CARE

◆ Apply direct pressure to the venipuncture site until the bleeding stops.
◆ Inform the practitioner of abnormal results.

PRECAUTIONS

◆ Handle the sample gently to prevent hemolysis.
◆ Send the sample to the laboratory immediately.

COMPLICATIONS

◆ Hematoma at the venipuncture site

INTERPRETATION

NORMAL RESULTS

◆ IMA isn't found in the blood.
◆ A normal ECG and negative troponin result rules out cardiac involvement.
◆ Negative results for IMA, ECG, and troponin have greater predictive value than other tests or combinations of tests.

ABNORMAL RESULTS

◆ IMA found in the blood indicates cardiac ischemia.

IMA and necrosis markers

Ischemia-modified albumin (IMA) rises much faster than other necrosis markers, allowing for earlier diagnosis of cardiac ischemia.

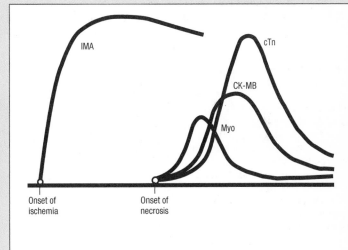

KEY:

IMA = Ischemia-modified albumin
cTn = Troponin
CK-MB = Creatine kinase MB
Myo = Myoglobin

Adapted with permission from *www.ischemia.com*

17-ketogenic steroids, urine

DESCRIPTION

- Determines urine levels of the 17-ketogenic steroids (17-KGS), using spectrophotofluorimetry
- 17-KGS: 17-hydroxycorticosteroids (for example, cortisol and its metabolites) and other adrenocortical steroids (such as pregnanetriol) that can be oxidized in laboratory to 17-ketosteroids
- Provides excellent overall assessment of adrenocortical function
- Results compared with those of other tests (such as plasma corticotropin, plasma cortisol, corticotropin stimulation, single-dose metyrapone, and dexamethasone suppression) for accurate diagnosis of specific disease

PURPOSE

- To evaluate adrenocortical and testicular function
- To help diagnose Cushing's syndrome and Addison's disease

PREPARATION

- Notify the laboratory and practitioner of drugs the patient is taking that may affect test results; they may be restricted.
- No fasting is required, but the patient should avoid strenuous exercise or stressful situations during the test.

Teaching points

- Explain that the urine 17-KGS test evaluates adrenal function.
- Inform the patient that fasting isn't required before the test but that he should avoid excessive physical exercise and stressful situations during the collection period.
- Tell him that the test requires urine collection over a 24-hour period; teach him how to collect the specimen correctly.

KEY STEPS

- Confirm the patient's identity using two patient identifiers according to facility policy.
- Collect the patient's urine over a 24-hour period, discarding the first specimen and retaining the last.
- Appropriately label the specimen and laboratory requests with the patient's name and gender.

POSTPROCEDURE CARE

- Inform the practitioner of abnormal results.
- After the test, tell the patient to resume his usual activities and medications.

PRECAUTIONS

- Use a bottle containing a preservative to keep the specimen at a pH of 4.0 to 4.5.
- Refrigerate the specimen or keep it on ice during the collection period.
- Send the specimen to the laboratory as soon as the collection is complete.

COMPLICATIONS

- None

NORMAL RESULTS

- In men, 4 to 14 mg/24 hours (SI, 13 to 49 µmol/day).
- In women, 2 to 12 mg/24 hours (SI, 7 to 42 µmol/day).
- In children ages 11 to 14, 2 to 9 mg/24 hours (SI, 7 to 31 µmol/day).
- In children younger than 11 and infants, 0.1 to 4 mg/24 hours (SI, 0.3 to 14 µmol/day).

ABNORMAL RESULTS

- Increased levels may be caused by hyperadrenalism, from Cushing's syndrome, adrenogenital syndrome (congenital adrenal hyperplasia), or adrenal carcinoma or adenoma; or by severe physical stress (such as that caused by burns, infections, or surgery) or emotional stress.
- Decreased levels may reflect hypoadrenalism, caused by Addison's disease, panhypopituitarism, cretinism, or cachexia.

Ketones, urine

DESCRIPTION

- Routine, semiquantitative screening test; commercially prepared product measures the urine level of ketone bodies
- Ketones: by-products of fat metabolism; include acetoacetic acid, acetone, and beta-hydroxybutyric acid
- Commercially available tests include Acetest tablet, Ketostix, or Keto-Diastix; each measures specific ketone body

PURPOSE

- To screen for ketonuria
- To identify diabetic ketoacidosis (DKA) and carbohydrate deprivation
- To distinguish between diabetic and nondiabetic coma
- To check for a metabolic complication of total parenteral nutrition (TPN)
- To monitor control of diabetes mellitus, ketogenic weight reduction, and treatment of DKA

PREPARATION

- No dietary restrictions are required.

Teaching points

- Explain that the ketone test evaluates fat metabolism.
- If the patient is newly diagnosed with diabetes, tell him how to perform the test.
- Tell the patient that no dietary restrictions are required.

DIAGNOSTIC PROCEDURE

KEY STEPS

- Confirm the patient's identity using two patient identifiers according to facility policy.
- Instruct the patient to void; then give him a drink of water.
- Collect a second-voided midstream specimen after 30 minutes.

Acetest

- Lay the tablet on a piece of white paper, and place 1 drop of urine on the tablet.
- Compare the tablet color (white, lavender, or purple) with the color chart after 30 seconds.

Ketostix

- Dip the reagent stick into the specimen and remove it immediately.
- Compare the stick color (buff or purple) with the color chart after 15 seconds. Record the results as negative, small, moderate, or large amounts of ketones.

Keto-Diastix

- Dip the reagent strip into the specimen and remove it immediately. Tap the edge of the strip against the container or a clean, dry surface to remove excess urine.
- Hold the Keto-Diastix strip horizontally to prevent mixing the chemicals from the two areas. Interpret each area of the strip separately. Compare the color of the ketone section (buff or purple) with the appropriate color chart after exactly 15 seconds; compare the color of the glucose section after 30 seconds.

All tests

- Ignore color changes that occur after the specified waiting periods. Record the results as negative or positive for small, moderate, or large amounts of ketones.
- Test the specimen within 1 hour after it's obtained, or refrigerate it until ready to test.
- Let refrigerated specimens return to room temperature before testing.
- Don't use tablets or strips that have become discolored or darkened.

POSTPROCEDURE CARE

- Answer the patient's questions.
- Inform the practitioner of abnormal results.

PRECAUTIONS

WARNING *If the patient is taking levodopa (Larodopa) or phenazopyridine (Pyridium) or has recently received sulfobromophthalein, use Acetest tablets because reagent strips may produce inaccurate results.*

COMPLICATIONS

- None

INTERPRETATION

NORMAL RESULTS

- No ketones are present.

ABNORMAL RESULTS

- Ketones are present in urine, indicating carbohydrate dehydration, which may suggest DKA, starvation, or a metabolic complication of TPN.

Kidney-ureter-bladder radiography

OVERVIEW

DESCRIPTION
- Surveys the abdomen even if renal function isn't intact
- Also known as a *flat plate of the abdomen*

PURPOSE
- To evaluate the size, structure, and position of the kidneys and bladder
- To screen for abnormalities, such as calcifications, in the area of the kidneys, ureters, and bladder

PREPARATION
- Make sure the patient has signed an appropriate consent form.
- Note and report allergies.

Teaching points
- Explain the purpose of the study and how it's done.
- Explain who will perform the test and where it'll be done.
- Tell the patient that fasting isn't required.
- Tell him the test takes only a few minutes.

DIAGNOSTIC PROCEDURE

KEY STEPS
- Confirm the patient's identity using two patient identifiers according to facility policy.
- The patient is assisted into a supine position with his arms extended over his head on an X-ray table. (See *Positioning the patient for KUB radiography.*)
- Symmetrical positioning of the iliac crests is noted.
- A single X-ray is taken.

POSTPROCEDURE CARE
- Answer the patient's questions.
- Inform the practitioner of abnormal results.

PRECAUTIONS
WARNING *During the X-ray, a man's gonads should be shielded; however, a woman's ovaries can't be shielded because they're too close to the kidneys, ureters, and bladder.*

COMPLICATIONS
- None

INTERPRETATION

NORMAL RESULTS
- Kidney shadows appear bilaterally, the right slightly lower than the left.
- Both kidneys are about the same size, with the superior poles tilted slightly toward the vertebral column, paralleling the shadows of the psoas muscles.
- The bladder shadow isn't as clearly visible as the kidney shadows.

ABNORMAL RESULTS
- Bilateral renal enlargement suggests possible polycystic kidney disease, multiple myeloma, lymphoma, amyloidosis, hydronephrosis, or compensatory renal hypertrophy.
- Unilateral renal enlargement suggests a possible tumor, cyst, or hydronephrosis.
- Abnormally small kidneys suggest possible end-stage glomerulonephritis or bilateral atrophic pyelonephritis.
- An apparent decrease in the size of one kidney suggests possible congenital hypoplasia, atrophic pyelonephritis, or ischemia.
- Renal displacement may be the result of a retroperitoneal tumor.
- Obliteration or bulging of a portion of the psoas muscle stripe suggests possible tumor, abscess, or hematoma.
- Abnormal location or absence of a kidney suggests possible congenital anomalies.
- A lobulated edge or border suggests possible polycystic kidney disease or patchy atrophic pyelonephritis.
- Opaque bodies suggest possible calculi, vascular calcification, cystic tumors, fecaliths, foreign bodies, soft tissue mass or abnormal fluid or gas collection.

Positioning the patient for KUB radiography

For kidney-ureter-bladder (KUB) radiography, the patient is instructed to lie in a supine position with his arms extended over his head. To prevent motion and ensure films of good quality, he's asked to lie still for the few seconds it takes to make the exposure. An obese patient may be asked to exhale and then hold his breath during the brief procedure. As an added precaution, the gonads of male patients should be shielded.

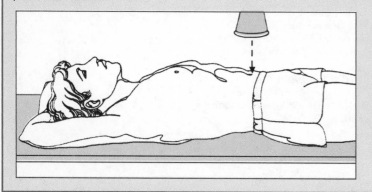

Lactate dehydrogenase test

OVERVIEW

DESCRIPTION

- Uses immunochemical separation and quantification or electrophoresis to identify and measure five tissue-specific isoenzymes: LD_1 and LD_2, which appear in the heart, red blood cells (RBCs), and kidneys; LD_3, primarily in the lungs; and LD_4 and LD_5, in the liver and skeletal muscles
- Lactate dehydrogenase (LD) in almost all body tissues; cellular damage increases total serum LD, limiting its diagnostic usefulness
- Catalyzes reversible conversion of muscle lactic acid into pyruvic acid; ultimately produces cellular energy
- Specificity of LD isoenzymes and distribution pattern useful in diagnosing hepatic, pulmonary, and erythrocyte damage (see *LD isoenzyme variations in disease*)

PURPOSE

- To aid in the differential diagnosis of a pulmonary infarction, anemias, hepatic disease, granulocytic leukemia, lymphomas, and platelet disorders
- To monitor patient's response to chemotherapy

PREPARATION

- No dietary restrictions are required.
- The test requires a blood sample.

Teaching points

- Explain that this test primarily detects tissue alterations.
- Explain who will perform the test and where it'll be done.
- Tell the patient that the test requires a blood sample and that he may experience slight discomfort from the tourniquet and needle puncture.
- Inform him that fasting isn't required before the test.
- Tell the patient the test takes less than 5 minutes.

DIAGNOSTIC PROCEDURE

KEY STEPS

- Confirm the patient's identity using two patient identifiers according to facility policy.
- Perform a venipuncture and collect the sample in a 4-ml clot-activator tube.
- Draw the samples on schedule to avoid missing peak levels, and mark the collection time on the laboratory request.

POSTPROCEDURE CARE

- Apply direct pressure to the venipuncture site until the bleeding stops.
- Inform the practitioner of abnormal results.

LD isoenzyme variations in disease

DISEASE	LD_1	LD_2	LD_3	LD_4	LD_5
Cardiovascular					
Rheumatic carditis	▓				
Myocarditis	▓				
Heart failure (decompensated)					▓
Shock	▓	▓			
Angina pectoris	▓				
Pulmonary					
Pulmonary embolism	▓				
Pulmonary infarction			▓		
Hematologic					
Pernicious anemia	▓	▓			
Hemolytic anemia	▓	▓			
Sickle cell anemia	▓	▓			
Hepatobiliary					
Hepatitis					▓
Active cirrhosis					▓
Hepatic congestion					▓

Key

▓ Normal   ▓ Diagnostic   ☐ Not diagnostic

(continued)

PRECAUTIONS

♦ Maintain standard precautions while collecting the sample.
♦ Handle the sample gently to prevent artifact blood sample hemolysis because RBCs contain LD_1.
♦ Send the sample to the laboratory immediately or, if transport is delayed, keep the sample at room temperature. Changes in temperature inactivate LD_5, thus altering isoenzyme patterns.

COMPLICATIONS

♦ Hematoma at the venipuncture site

INTERPRETATION

NORMAL RESULTS

♦ Total LD levels are 71 to 207 units/L (SI, 1.2 to 3.52 µkat/L).
♦ LD_1 level is 14% to 26% (SI, 0.14 to 0.26) of total.
♦ LD_2 level is 29% to 39% (SI, 0.29 to 0.39) of total.
♦ LD_3 level is 20% to 26% (SI, 0.20 to 0.26) of total.
♦ LD_4 level is 8% to 16% (SI, 0.08 to 0.16) of total.
♦ LD_5 level is 6% to 16% (SI, 0.06 to 0.16) of total.

ABNORMAL RESULTS

♦ Because many diseases increase total LD levels, isoenzyme electrophoresis is needed for diagnosis.
♦ Although in some disorders, total LD may be within normal limits, abnormal proportions of each enzyme indicate specific organ tissue damage.
♦ Increased midzone fractions (LD_2, LD_3, and LD_4) can indicate granulocytic leukemia, lymphomas, and platelet disorders.

Lactic acid and pyruvic acid test

OVERVIEW

DESCRIPTION

◆ Lactic acid: present in blood as lactate ions; derived from muscle cells and erythrocytes
◆ Intermediate product of carbohydrate metabolism; usually metabolized by liver
◆ Serum lactate level dependent on rates of production and metabolism; may increase significantly during exercise
◆ Lactate and pyruvate form reversible reaction; regulated by oxygen supply
◆ If oxygen levels deficient, pyruvate converts to lactate; if oxygen levels adequate, lactate converts to pyruvate
◆ Results in lactic acidosis when hepatic system fails to metabolize lactose sufficiently or if excess pyruvate converts to lactate
◆ Measurement of serum lactate levels recommended for patients with symptoms of lactic acidosis such as Kussmaul's respiration
◆ Comparison of pyruvate and lactate levels yields reliable information about tissue oxidation; measurement of pyruvate is difficult and occurs infrequently

PURPOSE

◆ To assess tissue oxidation
◆ To help determine the cause of lactic acidosis

PREPARATION

◆ Withhold food overnight and make sure the patient rests for at least 1 hour before the test.
◆ The test requires a blood sample.

Teaching points

◆ Explain that this blood test evaluates the oxygen level in tissues.
◆ Explain who will perform the test and where it'll be done.
◆ Explain to the patient to fast overnight and to rest for at least 1 hour before the test.
◆ Tell him that the test requires a blood sample and that he may experience slight discomfort from the tourniquet and needle puncture (if needed).
◆ Tell the patient the test should take less than 5 minutes.

DIAGNOSTIC PROCEDURE

KEY STEPS

◆ Confirm the patient's identity using two patient identifiers according to facility policy.
◆ Perform a venipuncture and collect the sample in a 5-ml tube with sodium fluoride and potassium oxalate added.
◆ Because lactate and pyruvate are extremely unstable, place the sample container in an ice-filled cup and send it to the laboratory immediately.

POSTPROCEDURE CARE

◆ Apply direct pressure to the venipuncture site until the bleeding stops.
◆ Inform the practitioner of abnormal results.
◆ Tell the patient to resume his usual diet and activity.

PRECAUTIONS

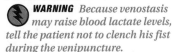 **WARNING** *Because venostasis may raise blood lactate levels, tell the patient not to clench his fist during the venipuncture.*
◆ Avoid using a tourniquet; however, if it's needed, release it at least 2 minutes before collecting the sample so blood can circulate.

COMPLICATIONS

◆ Hematoma at the venipuncture site

INTERPRETATION

NORMAL RESULTS

◆ Blood lactate values range from 0.93 to 1.65 mEq/L (SI, 0.93 to 1.65 mmol/L); pyruvate levels, from 0.08 to 0.16 mEq/L (SI, 0.08 to 0.16 mmol/L).
◆ The lactate-pyruvate ratio is less than 10:1.

ABNORMAL RESULTS

◆ Elevated blood lactate levels associated with hypoxia may result from strenuous muscle exercise, shock, hemorrhage, septicemia, myocardial infarction, pulmonary embolism, and cardiac arrest.
◆ When no reason for diminished tissue perfusion is apparent, increased lactate levels may result from systemic disorders, such as diabetes mellitus, leukemias and lymphomas, hepatic disease, and renal failure, or from enzymatic defects, such as von Gierke's disease (glycogen storage disease) and fructose 1,6-diphosphatase deficiency.
◆ Lactic acidosis can follow ingestion of large doses of acetaminophen (Tylenol) and ethanol as well as I.V. infusion of epinephrine, glucagon, fructose, or sorbitol.

Laparoscopy

DESCRIPTION
- Allows visualization of peritoneal cavity through a small fiber-optic telescope (laparoscope) inserted through the anterior abdominal wall
- Requires small incision, resulting in lower cost and faster recovery
- Allows many types of abdominal surgery, such as tubal ligation and cholecystectomy, to be done simultaneously

PURPOSE
- To identify the cause of pelvic pain
- To detect endometriosis, ectopic pregnancy, or pelvic inflammatory disease (PID)
- To evaluate pelvic masses
- To evaluate infertility
- To stage a carcinoma

PREPARATION
- Make sure the patient has signed an appropriate consent form.
- Note and report allergies.
- Check the patient's history for hypersensitivity to the anesthetic.
- Fasting is required for at least 8 hours before the test.
- Tell the practitioner if the patient takes aspirin, nonsteroidal anti-inflammatory drugs, or other drugs that affect clotting.

Teaching points
- Explain who will perform the test and where it'll be done.
- Tell the patient to fast after midnight before the test or for at least 8 hours before surgery.
- Warn the patient that she may experience pain at the puncture site and in the shoulder.
- Instruct the patient to void just before the test.
- Tell the patient the test takes about 15 to 30 minutes.
- Explain the use of a local or general anesthetic. (See *Learning about laparoscopy.*)
- Instruct the patient to restrict activity for 2 to 7 days after the procedure.
- Explain that abdominal and shoulder pain should disappear within 24 to 36 hours after the procedure.

DIAGNOSTIC PROCEDURE

KEY STEPS
- Confirm the patient's identity using two patient identifiers according to facility policy.
- The patient is anesthetized and helped into the lithotomy position.
- The bladder is catheterized.
- A bimanual examination of the pelvic area may be performed to detect abnormalities.
- An incision is made at the inferior rim of the umbilicus.
- The peritoneal cavity is insufflated with carbon dioxide or nitrous oxide.
- A laparoscope is inserted to examine the pelvis and abdomen.
- A second incision may be made just above the pubic hair line for some procedures.
- After the examination, minor surgical procedures, such as ovarian biopsy, may be performed.

POSTPROCEDURE CARE
- Provide analgesics.
- Monitor vital signs.
- Monitor the patient for adverse reactions to anesthetic.
- Monitor intake and output.
- Tell the patient to resume her usual diet.

PRECAUTIONS
- Watch for bleeding and signs and symptoms of infection.

COMPLICATIONS
- Bleeding
- Punctured visceral organ
- Peritonitis

INTERPRETATION

NORMAL RESULTS
- The uterus and fallopian tubes are a normal size and shape, free from adhesions, and mobile.
- The ovaries are a normal size and shape.
- No cysts and no endometriosis are found.

ABNORMAL RESULTS
- A bubble on the surface of the ovary suggests a possible ovarian cyst.
- Sheets or strands of tissue suggest possible adhesions.
- Small, blue powder burns on the peritoneum or serosa suggest endometriosis.
- Growths on the uterus suggests fibroids.
- An enlarged fallopian tube suggests possible hydrosalpinx.
- An enlarged or ruptured fallopian tube suggests a possible ectopic pregnancy.
- Infection or abscess suggests possible PID.

Learning about laparoscopy

Dear Patient,

Your health care provider has scheduled you for a laparoscopy. This procedure lets him see your reproductive and upper abdominal organs through a slender, telescope-like instrument. Laparoscopy allows for diagnosis and, sometimes, treatment of your disorder during the same procedure.

Laparoscopy takes about 1 hour. It's performed in the operating room, and you'll probably receive a general anesthetic. Usually, you can go home the same day.

GETTING READY

A few routine laboratory tests will be done to assess your general health, including a complete blood count, blood chemistry studies, and urinalysis.

Because you'll be receiving an anesthetic, don't eat or drink anything after midnight on the night before the procedure. If you're a smoker, don't smoke for about 12 hours before surgery. Remove eye makeup and nail polish beforehand.

DURING THE PROCEDURE

When the anesthetic takes effect, the health care provider will make a small incision in the lower part of your navel. Then he'll insert a needle through the incision and inject carbon dioxide or nitrous oxide to inflate your pelvic area. This creates a viewing space by lifting the abdominal wall away from the organs.

Next, the health care provider will insert a thin, flexible, optical instrument called a *laparoscope* through the incision. This instrument magnifies the view of your organs.

REMOVING IMPLANTS

If the findings confirm endometriosis, the health care provider may decide to remove the implants and adhesions by making a smaller incision just above your pubic hairline. He'll insert a special instrument for moving your internal organs aside. He may also insert a blunt instrument called a *cannula* through your vagina and into your uterus to move your uterus. The implants and adhesions will be removed by inserting instruments through the laparoscope.

Next, the health care provider will release the gas through the incision and remove the laparoscope. Then he'll close the incision and apply an adhesive bandage.

AFTER THE PROCEDURE

After laparoscopy, you'll go to the postanesthesia care unit, where nurses will monitor you until you're fully alert. If necessary, you'll receive an analgesic for minor discomfort in the incisional area when the anesthetic wears off. Expect vaginal bleeding similar to a menstrual period for a few days.

TIPS FOR RECOVERY

When you get home:
- Wait until the day after surgery to remove your bandage and bathe.
- Eat lightly because some gas will remain in your abdomen; you'll probably belch or feel bloated for 1 or 2 days.
- Take acetaminophen (Tylenol) or ibuprofen to relieve shoulder pain from the remaining gas in your abdomen.
- Resume your normal activities after 1 or 2 days, but avoid strenuous work or sports for about 1 week.
- Resume sexual activity when the bleeding stops or when your health care provider gives approval.

WHEN TO CALL THE HEALTH CARE PROVIDER

In rare instances, a laparoscopy may be complicated by infection, hemorrhage, or a burn or a small cut on an organ. Call your health care provider if you experience these signs or symptoms:
- a fever of 100.4° F (38° C) or higher
- persistent or excessive vaginal bleeding
- severe abdominal pain
- redness, puffiness, or drainage from your incision
- nausea, vomiting, or diarrhea.

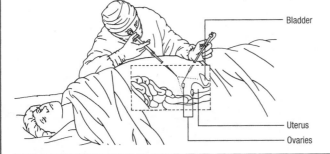

Bladder
Uterus
Ovaries

Laryngoscopy, direct

OVERVIEW

DESCRIPTION
- Allows visualization of the larynx; a fiber-optic endoscope, or laryngoscope, passed through the mouth or nose and pharynx to the larynx
- Usually follows indirect laryngoscopy

PURPOSE
- To detect lesions, strictures, or foreign bodies in the larynx
- To help diagnose laryngeal cancer or vocal cord impairment
- To remove benign lesions or foreign bodies from the larynx
- To examine the larynx when the view provided by indirect laryngoscopy is inadequate
- To evaluate signs and symptoms of pharyngeal or laryngeal disease (stridor or hemoptysis)

PREPARATION
- Make sure the patient has signed an appropriate consent form.
- Note and report allergies.
- Check the patient's history for hypersensitivity to the anesthetic.
- Fasting is required for at least 6 hours before the test.
- Give the patient a sedative to help him relax and a drug to reduce secretions.
- Give a general or local anesthetic to numb the gag reflex.

Teaching points
- Instruct the patient to fast for 6 to 8 hours before the test.
- Explain who will perform the test and where it'll be done.
- Tell the patient the test takes at least 30 minutes, and may take longer.

DIAGNOSTIC PROCEDURE

KEY STEPS
- Confirm the patient's identity using two patient identifiers according to facility policy.
- The patient is assisted into a supine position.
- A general anesthetic is given, or the mouth or nose and throat are sprayed with local anesthetic.
- The laryngoscope is inserted through the mouth.
- The larynx is examined for abnormalities.
- Specimens may be collected for further study.
- Minor surgery (polyp removal) may occur at this time.

POSTPROCEDURE CARE
- Assist the patient onto his side with his head slightly elevated to prevent aspiration.
- Restrict food and fluids until the gag reflex returns (usually 2 hours).
- Reassure the patient that voice loss, hoarseness, and sore throat are most likely temporary.
- Provide throat lozenges or a soothing liquid gargle after the gag reflex returns.
- Monitor the patient and immediately notify the practitioner if any adverse reactions to the anesthetic or sedative occur.
- Apply an ice collar to prevent or minimize laryngeal edema.
- Observe sputum for blood and notify the practitioner immediately if excessive bleeding or respiratory compromise occurs.
- Monitor vital signs, respiratory status, sputum, and voice quality.
- After a biopsy, instruct the patient to refrain from clearing his throat and coughing, and to avoid smoking.

PRECAUTIONS
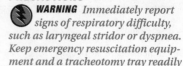 **WARNING** *Immediately report signs of respiratory difficulty, such as laryngeal stridor or dyspnea. Keep emergency resuscitation equipment and a tracheotomy tray readily available for 24 hours.*
- Watch for edema, bleeding, and subcutaneous emphysema.

COMPLICATIONS
- Subcutaneous crepitus around the patient's face and neck (sign of tracheal perforation)
- Airway obstruction (in patients with epiglottiditis)
- Adverse reaction to anesthetic
- Bleeding

INTERPRETATION

NORMAL RESULTS
- No inflammation, lesions, strictures, or foreign bodies are found.

ABNORMAL RESULTS
- Combined with the results of a biopsy, abnormal lesions suggest possible laryngeal cancer or benign lesions.
- Narrowing suggests stricture.
- Inflammation suggests possible laryngeal edema secondary to radiation or tumor.
- Asynchronous vocal cords suggest possible vocal cord dysfunction.

Leucine aminopeptidase level test

DESCRIPTION

- Measures serum levels of leucine aminopeptidase (LAP)
- LAP: isoenzyme of alkaline phosphatase (ALP); occurs widely in body tissues
- Highest levels in hepatobiliary tissues, pancreas, and small intestine
- Serum levels parallel serum ALP levels in hepatic disease

PURPOSE

- To provide information about suspected liver, pancreatic, and biliary diseases
- To differentiate skeletal disease from hepatobiliary or pancreatic disease
- To evaluate neonatal jaundice

PREPARATION

- Fasting is required for 8 hours before the test.
- The test requires a blood sample.
- Notify the laboratory and practitioner of drugs the patient is taking that may affect test results; they may need to be restricted.

Teaching points

- Explain that this test evaluates liver and pancreatic function.
- Explain who will perform the test and where it'll be done.
- Tell the patient to fast for at least 8 hours before the test.
- Tell him that the test requires a blood sample and that he may experience slight discomfort from the tourniquet and needle puncture.
- Inform the patient the test should take less than 5 minutes.

KEY STEPS

- Confirm the patient's identity using two patient identifiers according to facility policy.
- Perform a venipuncture and collect the sample in a 4-ml clot-activator tube.

POSTPROCEDURE CARE

- Apply direct pressure to the venipuncture site until the bleeding stops.
- Inform the practitioner of abnormal results.
- After the test, instruct the patient to resume his usual diet and medications.

PRECAUTIONS

- Handle the sample gently to prevent hemolysis.
- Transport the sample to the laboratory immediately.

COMPLICATIONS

- Hematoma at the venipuncture site

NORMAL RESULTS

- In men, the serum level is 80 to 200 units/ml (SI, 80 to 200 kU/L).
- In women, the serum level is 75 to 185 units/ml (SI, 75 to 185 kU/L).

ABNORMAL RESULTS

- Elevated levels can occur in biliary obstruction, tumors, strictures, and atresia; advanced pregnancy; and therapy with drugs containing estrogen or progesterone.

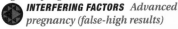 **INTERFERING FACTORS** *Advanced pregnancy (false-high results)*

Leukoagglutinins test

DESCRIPTION

- Detects leukoagglutinins (also known as *white blood cell [WBC] antibodies* or *human leukocyte antigen [HLA] antibodies*)
- Antibodies: react with WBCs and may cause a transfusion reaction; develop after exposure to foreign WBCs through transfusions, pregnancies, and allografts
- If blood recipient has antibodies, may result in febrile nonhemolytic reaction 1 to 4 hours after start of whole blood, red blood cell, platelet, or granulocyte transfusion (reaction must be distinguished from true hemolytic reaction before transfusion can proceed)
- Microlymphocytotoxicity test used for detecting leukoagglutinins: recipient serum tested against donor lymphocytes or against panel of lymphocytes of known HLA phenotype
- Antibodies in recipient serum bind to corresponding antigen in lymphocytes; cause cell membrane injury when complement added to test system
- Cell injury detected by examining lymphocytes under microscope

PURPOSE

- To detect leukoagglutinins in blood recipients who develop transfusion reactions, thus differentiating between hemolytic and febrile nonhemolytic transfusion reactions
- To detect leukoagglutinins in blood donors after transfusion of donor blood causes a reaction

PREPARATION

- The test requires a blood sample.
- No dietary restrictions are required.
- Check the patient's history for recent administration of blood, dextran, or I.V. contrast media and note this on the laboratory request.

Teaching points

- Explain that this test helps determine the cause of his transfusion reaction.

- Explain who will perform the test and where it'll be done.
- Tell the patient that the test requires a blood sample and that he may experience slight discomfort from the tourniquet and needle puncture.
- Tell him the test takes less than 5 minutes.

KEY STEPS

- Confirm the patient's identity using two patient identifiers according to facility policy.
- Perform a venipuncture and collect a sample in a 10-ml clot-activator tube. The laboratory requires 3 to 4 ml of serum for testing.
- Label the sample with the patient's name, the hospital or blood bank number, the date, and the phlebotomist's initials.
- Be sure to include on the laboratory request the patient's suspected diagnosis and history of blood transfusions, pregnancies, and drug therapy.

POSTPROCEDURE CARE

- Apply direct pressure to the venipuncture site until the bleeding stops.
- Inform the practitioner of abnormal results.

PRECAUTIONS

- If a transfusion recipient has a positive leukoagglutinin test, know that continued transfusions require premedication with acetaminophen (Tylenol) 1 or 2 hours before the transfusion, specially prepared leukocyte-poor blood, or use of leukocyte-removal blood filters to prevent further reactions.
- Note that tests for these antibodies aren't useful in deciding which patient should receive leukocyte-poor blood components; the decision must be based on clinical experience.

COMPLICATIONS

- Hematoma at the venipuncture site

NORMAL RESULTS

- If the lymphocytes don't absorb the added dye, the test result is negative.
- Agglutination doesn't occur because the serum contains no antibodies.

ABNORMAL RESULTS

- If the lymphocytes show dye uptake, the test result is positive.
- A positive result in a transfusion recipient indicates the presence of leukoagglutinins in his blood, identifying his transfusion reaction as a febrile nonhemolytic reaction to these antibodies.
- Recipients who test positive for HLA antibodies may need HLA-matched platelets to control bleeding episodes caused by thrombocytopenia.

Lipase test

OVERVIEW

DESCRIPTION

- Originates in pancreas and secreted into duodenum; converts triglycerides and other fats into fatty acids and glycerol
- Destruction of pancreatic cells (as in acute pancreatitis): causes large amounts of lipase to release into the blood (see *Blocked enzyme pathway*)
- Measures serum lipase levels; most useful when done with serum or urine amylase test

PURPOSE

- To help diagnose acute pancreatitis

PREPARATION

- The test requires a blood sample.
- Fasting is required from midnight before the test.
- Notify the laboratory of drugs the patient is taking that may affect test results; they may need to be restricted.

Teaching points

- Explain that this test evaluates pancreatic function.
- Explain who will perform the test and where it'll be done.
- Instruct the patient to fast overnight before the test.
- Tell the patient that the test requires a blood sample and that he may experience slight discomfort from the tourniquet and needle puncture.
- Tell him the test takes less than 5 minutes.

DIAGNOSTIC PROCEDURE

KEY STEPS

- Confirm the patient's identity using two patient identifiers according to facility policy.
- Perform a venipuncture and collect the sample in a 4-ml clot-activator tube.

POSTPROCEDURE CARE

- Apply direct pressure to the venipuncture site until the bleeding stops.
- Inform the practitioner of abnormal results.
- After the test, instruct the patient to resume his usual diet and medications.

PRECAUTIONS

- Maintain standard precautions while collecting the sample.
- Handle the sample gently to prevent hemolysis.

COMPLICATIONS

- Hematoma at the venipuncture site

INTERPRETATION

NORMAL RESULTS

- Level is less than 160 units/L (SI, < 2.72 µkat/L).

ABNORMAL RESULTS

- Increased levels suggest acute pancreatitis or pancreatic duct obstruction. After an acute attack, levels remain elevated for up to 14 days.
- Increased levels may occur in other pancreatic injuries, such as perforated peptic ulcer with chemical pancreatitis caused by gastric juices, and in a patient with high intestinal obstruction, pancreatic cancer, or renal disease with impaired excretion.

Blocked enzyme pathway

The pancreas secretes lipase, amylase, and other enzymes that pass through the pancreatic duct into the duodenum. In pancreatitis and obstruction of the pancreatic duct by a tumor or calculus (shown below), these enzymes can't reach their intended destination. Instead, they're diverted into the bloodstream by a mechanism that isn't fully understood.

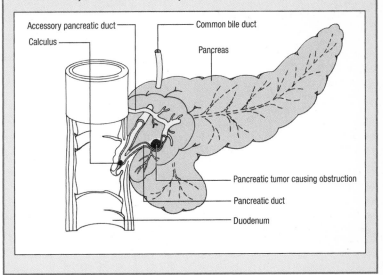

Lipoprotein electrophoresis

DESCRIPTION

- Isolates and measures types of cholesterol in serum: low-density lipoproteins (LDLs) and high-density lipoproteins (HDLs)
- HDL level inversely related to risk of coronary artery disease (CAD); higher the HDL level, lower the incidence of CAD (conversely, higher the LDL level, higher the incidence of CAD)

PURPOSE

- To assess the risk of CAD
- To assess the efficacy of lipid-lowering drug therapy

PREPARATION

- The test requires a blood sample.
- The patient should abstain from alcohol for 24 hours before the test and avoid food and exercise for 12 to 14 hours before the test.
- Notify the laboratory and practitioner of drugs the patient is taking that may affect test results; they may need to be restricted.

Teaching points

- Explain that this test determines the patient's risk of CAD.
- Explain who will perform the venipuncture and when it'll be done.
- Instruct the patient to maintain his normal diet for 2 weeks before the test, to abstain from alcohol for 24 hours before the test, and to fast and avoid exercise for 12 to 14 hours before the test.
- Tell the patient that the test requires a blood sample and that he may experience slight discomfort from the tourniquet and needle puncture.
- Tell him the test takes less than 5 minutes.

KEY STEPS

- Confirm the patient's identity using two patient identifiers according to facility policy.
- Perform a venipuncture and collect the sample in a 7-ml EDTA tube.

POSTPROCEDURE CARE

- Apply direct pressure to the venipuncture site until the bleeding stops.
- Inform the practitioner of abnormal results.
- After the test, instruct the patient to resume his usual diet and medications.

PRECAUTIONS

- Send the sample to the laboratory immediately to avoid spontaneous redistribution among the lipoproteins.
- If the sample can't be transported immediately, refrigerate it but don't freeze it.

COMPLICATIONS

- Hematoma at the venipuncture site

NORMAL RESULTS

- Normal lipoprotein values vary by age, sex, geographic area, and ethnic group; check the laboratory for reference values.
- Desirable HDL levels are greater than 60 mg/dl (SI, > 1.55 mmol/L).
- Optimal LDL levels are less than 100 mg/dl (SI, < 2.59 mmol/L); above optimal levels range from 100 to 129 mg/dl (SI, 2.59 to 3.34 mmol/L).

ABNORMAL RESULTS

- Undesirable HDL levels are below 40 mg/dl (SI, < 1.03 mmol/L).
- Borderline high LDL levels range from 130 to 159 mg/dl (SI, 3.36 to 4.12 mmol/L); high levels range from 160 to 189 mg/dl (SI, 4.14 to 4.90 mmol/L). LDL levels above 190 mg/dl (SI, > 4.92 mmol/L) are considered very high.

Lipoprotein phenotyping

DESCRIPTION

- Determines levels of the four major lipoproteins: chylomicrons, very-low-density (prebeta) lipoproteins, low-density (beta) lipoproteins, and high-density (alpha) lipoproteins
- Familial lipoprotein disorders are hyperlipoproteinemias or hypolipoproteinemias; detecting altered lipoprotein patterns is essential in identifying these disorders (see *Familial hyperlipoproteinemias*)
- Types of hyperlipoproteinemias and hypolipoproteinemias are characterized by electrophoretic patterns
- Six types of hyperlipoproteinemias: I, IIa, IIb, III, IV, and V (types IIa, IIb, and IV are relatively common)
- Hypolipoproteinemias are rare, including hypobetalipoproteinemia, betalipoproteinemia, and alpha-lipoprotein deficiency

PURPOSE

- To determine the classification of hyperlipoproteinemia and hypolipoproteinemia

PREPARATION

- Check the patient's drug history for heparin use. Withhold antilipemics, such as cholestyramine (Questran), about 2 weeks before the test.
- Notify the laboratory if the patient is receiving treatment for another condition that might significantly alter lipoprotein metabolism, such as diabetes mellitus, nephrosis, or hypothyroidism.
- Provide a low-fat meal the night before the test and withhold food and fluid after midnight before the test.
- The test requires a blood sample.

Teaching points

- Explain that lipoprotein typing determines how the body metabolizes fats.
- Explain who will perform the test and where it'll be done.

Familial hyperlipoproteinemias

TYPE	CAUSES AND INCIDENCE	CLINICAL SIGNS	LABORATORY FINDINGS
I	• Deficient lipoprotein lipase, resulting in increased chylomicrons • May be induced by alcoholism • Incidence: rare	• Eruptive xanthomas • Lipemia retinalis • Abdominal pain	• Increased chylomicron, total cholesterol, and triglyceride levels • Normal or slightly increased VLDLs • Normal or decreased LDLs and high-density lipoproteins • Cholesterol-triglyceride ratio < 0.2
IIa	• Deficient cell receptor, resulting in increased low-density lipoproteins (LDL) and excessive cholesterol synthesis • May be induced by hypothyroidism • Incidence: common	• Premature coronary artery disease (CAD) • Arcus cornea • Xanthelasma • Tendinous and tuberous xanthomas	• Increased LDL • Normal VLDL • Cholesterol-triglyceride ratio > 2.0
IIb	• Deficient cell receptor, resulting in increased LDL and excessive cholesterol synthesis • May be induced by dysgammaglobulinemia, hypothyroidism, uncontrolled diabetes mellitus, and nephrotic syndrome • Incidence: common	• Premature CAD • Obesity • Possible xanthelasma	• Increased LDL, VLDL, total cholesterol, and triglycerides
III	• Unknown cause, resulting in deficient very-low-density lipoproteins (VLDL)-to-LDL conversion • May be induced by hypothyroidism, uncontrolled diabetes mellitus, and paraproteinemia • Incidence: rare	• Premature CAD • Arcus cornea • Eruptive tuberous xanthomas	• Increased total cholesterol, VLDL, and triglycerides • Normal or decreased LDL • Cholesterol-triglyceride ratio > 0.4 • Broad beta band observed on electrophoresis
IV	• Unknown cause, resulting in decreased levels of lipase • May be induced by uncontrolled diabetes mellitus, alcoholism, pregnancy, steroid or estrogen therapy, dysgammaglobulinemia, and hyperthyroidism • Incidence: common	• Possible premature CAD • Obesity • Hypertension • Peripheral neuropathy	• Increased VLDL and triglycerides • Normal LDL • Cholesterol-triglyceride ratio < 0.25
V	• Unknown cause, resulting in defective triglyceride clearance • May be induced by alcoholism, dysgammaglobulinemia, uncontrolled diabetes mellitus, nephrotic syndrome, pancreatitis, and steroid therapy • Incidence: rare	• Premature CAD • Abdominal pain • Lipemia retinalis • Eruptive xanthomas • Hepatosplenomegaly	• Increased VLDL, total cholesterol, and triglyceride levels • Chylomicrons present • Cholesterol-triglyceride ratio < 0.6

(continued)

- Instruct the patient to abstain from alcohol for 24 hours before the test and to fast after midnight before the test.
- Tell the patient that the test requires a blood sample and that he may experience slight discomfort from the tourniquet and needle puncture.
- Tell the patient the test takes less than 5 minutes.

KEY STEPS
- Confirm the patient's identity using two patient identifiers according to facility policy.
- Perform a venipuncture and collect the sample in a 4-ml EDTA tube.
- Fill the collection tube completely and invert it gently several times to mix the sample and the anticoagulant thoroughly.

POSTPROCEDURE CARE
- Apply direct pressure to venipuncture site until bleeding stops.
- Inform the practitioner of abnormal results.

PRECAUTIONS
- When you draw multiple samples, collect the sample for lipoprotein phenotyping first because venous obstruction for 2 minutes can affect test results.
- Handle the sample gently to prevent hemolysis.

COMPLICATIONS
- Hematoma at the venipuncture site

INTERPRETATION

NORMAL RESULTS
- No altered lipoprotein patterns are detected.

ABNORMAL RESULTS
- Altered lipoprotein patterns are noted. (See *PLAC test*.)

PLAC test

The PLAC test is a blood test that can help determine who might be at risk for coronary artery disease (CAD).

The PLAC test works by measuring lipoprotein-associated phospholipase A_2, an enzyme produced by macrophages, a type of white blood cell. When heart disease is present, macrophages increase production of the enzyme. According to the FDA, studies have shown an elevated PLAC test result, in conjunction with a low-density-lipoprotein (LDL) cholesterol level of less than 130 mg/dl, generally indicates that a patient has two to three times the risk of CAD compared with similar patients with lower PLAC test results. Studies also found that those people with the highest PLAC test results and LDL cholesterol levels lower than 130 mg/dl had the greatest risk of heart disease.

Liver-spleen scanning

DESCRIPTION

◆ Involves distribution of radioactivity within the liver and spleen; recorded by gamma camera after I.V. injection of radioactive colloid, technetium 99m (^{99m}Tc)
◆ Demonstrates focal disease non-specifically as a cold spot (defect that fails to take up the colloid)
◆ With flow studies, may help distinguish metastasis, tumors, cysts, and abscesses
◆ May not show focal lesions smaller than ¾" (2 cm) in diameter or early hepatocellular disease

PURPOSE

◆ To screen for hepatic metastasis and hepatocellular disease
◆ To detect focal disease (such as tumors, cysts, or abscesses)
◆ To demonstrate hepatomegaly, splenomegaly, and splenic infarcts
◆ To assess the condition of the liver and spleen after abdominal trauma

PREPARATION

◆ Make sure the patient has signed an appropriate consent form.
◆ Note and report allergies.

◆ Stress the importance of lying still during the study.
◆ No dietary restrictions are required.

Teaching points

◆ Explain the purpose of the test and how it's done.
◆ Explain who will perform the test and where it'll be done.
◆ Tell the patient that he need not fast before the test.
◆ Tell him the test takes about 1 hour.

DIAGNOSTIC PROCEDURE

KEY STEPS

◆ Confirm the patient's identity using two patient identifiers according to facility policy.
◆ ^{99m}Tc is injected I.V.
◆ After 10 to 15 minutes the abdomen is scanned using various views.
◆ Scintigraphs are reviewed for clarity.
◆ Additional views are obtained as needed.

POSTPROCEDURE CARE

◆ Encourage oral fluid intake (unless contraindicated) to assist elimination of the radioactive material.
◆ Monitor vital signs and respiratory status.

◆ Monitor intake and output.
◆ Inform the practitioner of abnormal results.
◆ After the test, instruct the patient to flush the toilet immediately after urinating to reduce exposure to radiation in the urine.

PRECAUTIONS

◆ More than one radionuclide scan shouldn't occur in the same day.

COMPLICATIONS

WARNING *Watch for anaphylactoid reactions (such as shortness of breath, chest tightness, itching, and headache) or pyrogenic reactions that may result from a stabilizer, such as dextran or gelatin, added to ^{99m}Tc.*

INTERPRETATION

NORMAL RESULTS

◆ The liver and spleen appear equally bright on images.
◆ The distribution of radioactive colloid is usually more homogeneous in the spleen than in the liver.
◆ The liver has various normal indentations and impressions that may mimic focal disease. (See *Identifying liver indentations in nuclear imaging*.)

ABNORMAL RESULTS

◆ A uniformly decreased or patchy appearance suggests hepatocellular disease.
◆ Uniformly decreased distribution of the colloid suggests hepatitis.
◆ Failure to take up the radioactive colloid and the appearance of solitary or multiple focal defects suggest cysts, abscesses, hematomas, and tumors.
◆ Lentiform defects on the periphery of the liver suggest subcapsular hematoma.
◆ Linear defects suggest hepatic laceration.
◆ Focal defects in or next to the spleen, which may transect it, suggest splenic hematoma.

Identifying liver indentations in nuclear imaging

In nuclear imaging, normal indentations and impressions may be mistaken for focal lesions. These drawings of the liver — anterior and posterior view — identify the contours and impressions that may be misread.

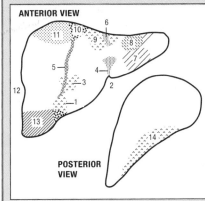

ANTERIOR VIEW

POSTERIOR VIEW

KEY
1. Gallbladder fossa
2. Ligamentum teres and falciform ligament
3. Hilum, main branching of the portal vein
4. Pars umbilicalis portion, left portal vein
5. Variable stripe of lobar fissure between right and left lobes
6. Variable stripe of semental fissure, left lobe
7. Thinning of left lobe
8. Impression of pectus excavatum
9. Cardiac impression
10. Hepatic veins and inferior vena cava
11. Shielding from right female breast
12. Harrison's groove or costal impression
13. Impression of hepatic flexure of colon
14. Right renal impression

Loop electrosurgical excision procedure

DESCRIPTION

- Used to obtain tissue specimens of the cervix for biopsy and to remove abnormal tissue from the cervix and high in the endocervical canal
- Usually performed after a Papanicolaou (Pap) test and colposcopy as follow-up to ensure accuracy of results
- Also known as *LEEP*

PURPOSE

- To confirm results of colposcopy and Pap test
- To identify lesions as benign or cancerous, invasive or noninvasive
- To remove cervical dysplasia and noninvasive cervical cancers

PREPARATION

- Help allay the patient's anxiety about a possible diagnosis of cervical cancer.
- No dietary restrictions are required.
- Make sure the patient or responsible family member has signed an informed consent.

Teaching points

- Describe the procedure to the patient and tell her that it provides a cervical tissue specimen for microscopic study and treats abnormal tissue growth.
- Explain who will perform the test and where it'll be done.
- Advise the outpatient to have someone accompany her home after the procedure.
- Tell the patient that she may experience mild discomfort during and after the procedure and that she may have some vaginal drainage afterward.
- Tell the patient that fasting isn't needed before the test.
- Tell the patient the test takes about 30 minutes.
- Advise the patient not to douche, use tampons or bubble bath, or engage in sexual intercourse for about 3 or 4 weeks after the test.

DIAGNOSTIC PROCEDURE

KEY STEPS

- Confirm the patient's identity using two patient identifiers according to facility policy.
- Place the patient into the lithotomy position and encourage her to relax.
- The examiner inserts a vaginal speculum and applies a local anesthetic to the area.
- The cervix is cleaned with a mild vinegar solution (3% acetic acid solution) or iodine to remove any debris or mucus. The solution also helps identify normal and abnormal tissues.
- The examiner inserts a thin wire loop attached to a high-frequency current, uses the loop to remove the suspected tissue, and sends the tissue to the laboratory.
- The examiner applies a cervical paste to the area where the tissue was removed to reduce bleeding.

POSTPROCEDURE CARE

- Inform the patient that she may experience some vaginal bleeding and mild cramping after the procedure.
- Inform the patient that she may experience black-brown vaginal discharge or a white watery discharge for about 1 week after the procedure with possible spotting for up to 4 weeks.
- Instruct the patient to notify the practitioner if she experiences fever, bleeding greater than a normal menstrual flow, increasing pelvic pain or severe abdominal pain, or a foul-smelling or malodorous vaginal discharge.
- Urge the patient to follow up with her practitioner as indicated for information about results.

PRECAUTIONS

- The test is contraindicated in patients with active menstrual bleeding and during pregnancy.

COMPLICATIONS

- Heavy bleeding
- Severe cramping
- Infection
- Cervical stenosis
- Accidental cutting or burning of normal tissue

NORMAL RESULTS

- Normal squamous cells of the cervix that flatten as they grow are noted.

ABNORMAL RESULTS

- Abnormal results include evidence of dysplastic cervical cells or more extensive invasion of the cancerous cells deeper into the cervix.

Lower leg venography

DESCRIPTION

- Radiographically examines veins in the leg to assess the condition of the deep leg veins after injection of a contrast medium
- Used in patients whose duplex ultrasound findings are equivocal
- Not used for routine screening due to high doses of radiation, which can cause phlebitis, local tissue damage and, occasionally, deep vein thrombosis (DVT)
- Also known as *ascending contrast phlebography*

PURPOSE

- To confirm a diagnosis of DVT
- To distinguish clot formation from venous obstruction (such as a large tumor of the pelvis impinging on the venous system)
- To evaluate congenital venous abnormalities
- To assess deep vein valvular competence
- To locate a suitable vein for arterial bypass grafting
- To evaluate chronic venous disease

PREPARATION

- Make sure the patient has signed a consent form.
- Note and report allergies.
- Report hypersensitivity to iodine, iodine-containing foods, or contrast media.
- Give the patient only liquids for 4 hours before the test.
- Stop anticoagulant therapy.
- Reassure the patient that contrast media complications are rare.
- Give the patient a sedative.

Teaching points

- Explain that this test evaluates deep leg veins.
- Explain who will perform the test and where it'll be done.
- Instruct the patient to restrict food and to drink only clear liquids for 4 hours before the test.
- Warn the patient that he might experience a burning sensation in the leg when the contrast medium is injected and some discomfort during the procedure.
- Inform him that contrast media complications are rare, but tell him to report nausea, severe burning or itching, constriction in the throat or chest, or dyspnea at once.
- Tell the patient the test takes 30 to 45 minutes.

DIAGNOSTIC PROCEDURE

KEY STEPS

- Confirm the patient's identity using two patient identifiers according to facility policy.
- Position the patient on a tilting X-ray table so that the leg being tested doesn't bear any weight.
- Tie a tourniquet around the ankle to expedite venous filling.
- Normal saline solution is injected into a superficial vein in the dorsum of the patient's foot, and a contrast medium is injected after placement has been confirmed.
- Using a fluoroscope, the distribution of the contrast medium is monitored, and spot films of the thigh and femoroiliac regions are taken from the anteroposterior and oblique views.
- Overhead films are taken of the calf, knee, thigh, and femoral area.
- After filming, reposition the patient horizontally, quickly elevate the leg being tested, and infuse normal saline solution to flush the contrast medium from the veins.
- The fluoroscope is checked to confirm complete emptying.
- After the needle is removed, apply a dressing to the injection site.

POSTPROCEDURE CARE

- Give the patient analgesics.
- Encourage the patient's oral fluid intake.
- If DVT is documented, initiate therapy (such as heparin infusion, bed rest, and leg elevation or support).
- Monitor vital signs and fluid intake and output.
- Monitor the injection site for bleeding, infection, hematoma, and erythema.
- Inform the practitioner of abnormal results.
- After the test, tell the patient to resume usual diet and medications.

PRECAUTIONS

- Because of the high volume of contrast used, especially if bilateral venography is necessary, monitor renal function and hydration status carefully.
- Because most allergic reactions to the contrast medium occur within 30 minutes of injection, observe the patient for signs and symptoms of anaphylaxis, such as flushing, urticaria, and laryngeal stridor.

COMPLICATIONS

- Adverse reactions to contrast media or drugs
- Thrombophlebitis
- Local tissue damage
- Renal insufficiency or failure
- Tissue necrosis and ulceration may occur with large extravasations and in patients with arterial insufficiency

INTERPRETATION

NORMAL RESULTS

- Steady opacification of the superficial and deep vasculature with no filling defects is noted.

ABNORMAL RESULTS

- Consistent filling defects, abrupt termination of a column of contrast material, unfilled major deep veins, or diversion of flow (through collaterals, for example) suggest DVT.
- Improper needle placement in a superficial vein, weight bearing or muscle contraction, or use of tourniquets can produce artifacts of poor filling.
- Diagnosis errors commonly result from incomplete filling.
- Fluoroscopy is essential for establishing that the contrast medium has reached the vessels being filmed and that opacification is adequate.

Lumbar puncture

DESCRIPTION

◆ Permits sampling of cerebral spinal fluid (CSF) for qualitative analysis
◆ Also known as a *spinal tap*

PURPOSE

◆ To measure CSF pressure
◆ To help diagnose viral or bacterial meningitis; subarachnoid or intracranial hemorrhage; tumors and brain abscesses; neurosyphilis and chronic central nervous system infections

PREPARATION

◆ Make sure the patient has signed a consent form.
◆ No dietary restrictions are required.
◆ Note and report allergies.

Teaching points

◆ Explain the purpose of the test and how it's done.
◆ Explain who will perform the test and where it'll be done.
◆ Tell the patient that fasting isn't required.
◆ Inform the patient that headache is the most common adverse effect.
◆ Tell the patient that the test takes at least 15 minutes.

DIAGNOSTIC PROCEDURE

KEY STEPS

◆ Confirm the patient's identity using two patient identifiers according to facility policy.
◆ Position the patient on his side at the edge of the bed with his knees drawn up to his abdomen and his chin tucked against his chest (the fetal position); or position the patient sitting while leaning over a bedside table.
◆ If the patient is in a supine position, provide pillows to support the spine on a horizontal plane.
◆ The skin site is prepared and draped.
◆ A local anesthetic is injected.

◆ The spinal needle is inserted in the midline between the spinous processes of the vertebrae (usually between the third and fourth lumbar vertebrae or between the fourth and fifth).
◆ The stylet is removed from the needle; CSF will drip out of the needle if properly positioned.
◆ A stopcock and manometer are attached to the needle to measure the initial (opening) CSF pressure.
◆ Specimens are collected and placed in the appropriate containers.
◆ The needle is removed and a small sterile dressing applied.

⚡ **WARNING** *During the procedure, observe the patient closely for signs of an adverse reaction (such as an elevated pulse rate, pallor, or clammy skin).*

POSTPROCEDURE CARE

◆ Keep the patient lying flat for 4 to 6 hours but tell him that he can turn from side to side.
◆ Encourage the patient to drink fluids and assist him as needed.
◆ Provide analgesics as needed.
◆ Monitor the patient's vital signs, neurologic status, and intake and output.
◆ Monitor the puncture site for redness, swelling, and drainage.
◆ Inform the practitioner of abnormal results.

PRECAUTIONS

◆ The test is contraindicated in patients with skin infection at the puncture site.

⚡ **WARNING** *In patients with increased intracranial pressure (ICP), CSF should be removed with extreme caution because cerebellar herniation and medullary compression can result.*

COMPLICATIONS

◆ Adverse reaction to the anesthetic
◆ Infection
◆ Meningitis
◆ Bleeding into the spinal canal
◆ Leakage of CSF
◆ Cerebellar herniation
◆ Medullary compression

NORMAL RESULTS

◆ Pressure is 50 to 180 mm H_2O.
◆ CSF appears clear and colorless.
◆ Protein level is 15 to 45 mg/dl (SI, 150 to 450 mg/L).
◆ Gamma globulin level is 3% to 12% of total protein.
◆ Glucose level is 40 to 70 mg/dl (2.2 to 3.9 mmol/L).
◆ Cell count is 0 to 5 white blood cells; no red blood cells (RBCs).
◆ Venereal Disease Research Laboratories (VDRL) test is nonreactive.
◆ Chloride level is 118 to 130 mEq/L (118 to 130 mmol/L).
◆ Gram stain shows no organisms.

ABNORMAL RESULTS

◆ Increased ICP indicates tumor, hemorrhage, or edema caused by trauma.
◆ Decreased ICP indicates spinal subarachnoid obstruction.
◆ Cloudy appearance of CSF suggests infection.
◆ Yellow or bloody appearance suggests intracranial hemorrhage or spinal cord obstruction.
◆ Brown or orange appearance indicates increased protein levels or RBC breakdown.
◆ Increased protein suggests tumor, trauma, diabetes mellitus, or blood in CSF.
◆ Decreased protein indicates rapid CSF production.
◆ Increased gamma globulin is associated with demyelinating disease or Guillain-Barré syndrome.
◆ Increased glucose level suggests hyperglycemia.
◆ Decreased glucose level could result from hypoglycemia, infection, or meningitis.
◆ Increased cell count indicates meningitis, tumor, abscess, or demyelinating disease.
◆ RBCs present due to hemorrhage.
◆ A positive VDRL test result indicates neurosyphilis.
◆ Decreased chloride level suggests infected meninges.
◆ Gram-positive or gram-negative organisms indicate bacterial meningitis.

Lung biopsy

DESCRIPTION

- Obtains a pulmonary tissue specimen for histologic examination (three types)
- Needle biopsy: performed when lesion is readily accessible, originates in lung parenchyma, or affixed to chest wall
- Transbronchial biopsy: removal of multiple tissue specimens through a fiber-optic bronchoscope; used for diffuse infiltrative pulmonary disease, tumors, or severe debilitation that contraindicates open biopsy
- Open biopsy: appropriate for well-circumscribed lesion requiring resection

PURPOSE

- To confirm the diagnosis of diffuse parenchymal pulmonary disease
- To confirm the diagnosis of pulmonary lesions

PREPARATION

- Make sure the patient has signed an appropriate consent form.
- Note and report allergies.
- Fasting is required after midnight before the procedure.
- Obtain results of prestudy tests; report abnormal results to the practitioner.
- Check the patient's history for hypersensitivity to local anesthetic.
- The patient will receive chest X-ray and blood studies before the biopsy.
- Give him a mild sedative 30 minutes before the biopsy.

Teaching points

- Explain the purpose of the test and how it's done.
- Explain who will perform the biopsy and where it'll be done.
- Instruct the patient to fast after midnight before the procedure.
- Tell the patient the test takes 30 to 60 minutes.

KEY STEPS

- Confirm the patient's identity using two patient identifiers according to facility policy.
- The procedure depends on the type of approach: needle, transbronchial, or open biopsy.
- Tissue specimens are obtained for histologic examination.
- Specimens are placed in appropriate and properly labeled containers.
- Repeat the chest X-ray immediately after the biopsy is complete.

POSTPROCEDURE CARE

- Monitor vital signs, intake and output, respiratory status, pulse oximetry, and breath sounds.
- Watch for bleeding and infection.
- Inform the practitioner of abnormal results.
- After the test, instruct the patient to resume his normal diet.

PRECAUTIONS

- The procedure is contraindicated in patients with severe uncorrected coagulopathy and severe pulmonary or cardiac disease.
- Coughing or movement during the biopsy can cause pneumothorax.

COMPLICATIONS

- Bleeding
- Infection
- Pneumothorax

NORMAL RESULTS

- Pulmonary tissue exhibits uniform texture of the alveolar ducts, alveolar walls, bronchioles, and small vessels.

ABNORMAL RESULTS

- Histologic examination of a pulmonary tissue specimen reveals possible squamous cell or oat-cell carcinoma and adenocarcinoma.

Lung perfusion and ventilation scanning

OVERVIEW

DESCRIPTION
- Produces a visual image of pulmonary blood flow after I.V. injection of a radiopharmaceutical
- Nuclear scan after inhalation of air mixed with radioactive gas
- Differentiates areas of ventilated lung from areas of underventilated lung

PURPOSE
- To assess arterial perfusion of the lungs
- To detect pulmonary emboli
- To evaluate pulmonary function
- To identify areas of the lung capable of ventilation, evaluate regional respiratory function and locate regional hypoventilation

PREPARATION
- Make sure the patient has signed an appropriate consent form.
- Note and report allergies.
- Stress the importance of lying still during imaging.
- No dietary restrictions are required.
- Make sure the patient has I.V. access.

Teaching points
- Explain the purpose of the test and how it's done.
- Explain who will perform the test and where it'll be done.
- Inform the patient that the amount of radioactivity is minimal.
- Tell him that fasting isn't required before the test.
- Tell the patient the test takes about 30 minutes.

DIAGNOSTIC PROCEDURE

KEY STEPS
- Confirm the patient's identity using two patient identifiers according to facility policy.

Lung perfusion scan
- With the patient in a supine position and taking moderately deep breaths, the radiopharmaceutical is injected I.V. slowly over 5 to 10 seconds to allow more even distribution of pulmonary blood flow.
- After the injection the gamma camera takes a series of single, stationary images in the anterior, posterior, oblique, and both lateral chest views.
- The images are projected onto an oscilloscope screen and show the distribution of radioactive particles.

Lung ventilation scan
- After the patient inhales air mixed with a small amount of radioactive gas through a mask, its distribution in the lungs is monitored on a nuclear scanner.
- The patient's chest is scanned as he exhales.

POSTPROCEDURE CARE
- Monitor the injection site for hematoma and apply warm soaks if one develops.
- Inform the practitioner of abnormal results.

PRECAUTIONS
- This scan is contraindicated in patients hypersensitive to the radiopharmaceutical.

COMPLICATIONS
- Hematoma at the injection site
- Sensitivity to the radiopharmaceutical

INTERPRETATION

NORMAL RESULTS
- Hot spots (areas of high uptake) indicate normal blood perfusion.
- The uptake pattern is uniform.
- In the ventilation scan, both lungs have an equal distribution and normal wash-in and wash-out phases.

ABNORMAL RESULTS
- Cold spots (areas of low uptake) indicate poor perfusion, suggesting an embolism.
- Decreased regional blood flow, without vessel obstruction, suggests possible pneumonitis.
- Unequal gas distribution in both lungs indicates poor ventilation or airway obstruction.

INTERFERING FACTORS *Chronic obstructive pulmonary disease, vasculitis, pulmonary edema, tumor, or sickle cell disease (poor imaging results)*

Lupus erythematosus cell preparation

DESCRIPTION

◆ In vitro procedure used to diagnose systemic lupus erythematosus (SLE)
◆ Less sensitive and reliable than antinuclear antibody (ANA) or antideoxyribonucleic acid (DNA) antibody test; used because it requires minimal equipment and reagents
◆ Blood sample mixed with laboratory-treated nucleoprotein (antigen)
◆ ANAs in sample react with nucleoprotein; cause swelling and rupture
◆ Phagocytes in serum engulf extruded nuclei, forming lupus erythematosus (LE) cells; detected by microscopic examination of sample

PURPOSE

◆ To help diagnose SLE
◆ To monitor treatment of SLE (about 60% of successfully treated patients fail to show LE cells after 4 to 6 weeks of therapy)

PREPARATION

◆ No dietary restrictions are required.
◆ The test requires a blood sample.
◆ Check the patient's medication history for drugs that may affect test results, such as isoniazid (Laniazid), hydralazine (Apresoline), and procainamide (Procanbid). If the patient must continue such drugs, be sure to note this on the laboratory request.

Teaching points

◆ Explain that this test helps detect antibodies to the patient's own tissue.
◆ Explain who will perform the test and where it'll be done.
◆ If appropriate, inform the patient that the test will be repeated to monitor his response to therapy.
◆ Inform the patient that fasting isn't required before the test.
◆ Tell him that the test requires a blood sample and that he may experience slight discomfort from the tourniquet and needle puncture.
◆ Tell the patient the test takes less than 5 minutes.

KEY STEPS

◆ Confirm the patient's identity using two patient identifiers according to facility policy.
◆ Perform a venipuncture and collect the sample in a 7-ml red-top tube.
◆ Handle the sample gently to prevent hemolysis.

POSTPROCEDURE CARE

◆ Apply direct pressure to the venipuncture site until the bleeding stops.
◆ If test results indicate SLE, tell the patient further tests may be required to monitor treatment.
◆ Inform the practitioner of abnormal results.

PRECAUTIONS

◆ Because the patient with SLE may have a compromised immune system, keep a clean, dry bandage over the venipuncture site for at least 24 hours and check for infection.

COMPLICATIONS

◆ Hematoma at the venipuncture site

NORMAL RESULTS

◆ No LE cells are present in the serum.

ABNORMAL RESULTS

◆ The presence of at least two LE cells may indicate SLE. Although these cells occur primarily in SLE, they may also appear in chronic active hepatitis, rheumatoid arthritis, scleroderma, and certain drug reactions.
◆ Up to 25% of patients with SLE demonstrate no LE cells.
◆ Apart from supportive clinical signs, a definitive diagnosis of SLE may require a confirming ANA or anti-DNA test.
◆ The ANA test detects autoantibodies in the serum of many patients with SLE who have negative LE cell tests.
◆ Anti-DNA antibodies appear in two-thirds of all patients with SLE but are rare in other conditions; thus, the presence of these antibodies is strong evidence of SLE.

INTERFERING FACTORS Isoniazid, hydralazine, and procainamide (syndrome resembling SLE)

Chlorpromazine (Thorazine), ethosuximide (Zarontin), gold salts, griseofulvin (Grifulvin), hormonal contraceptives, methyldopa (Aldomet), methysergide, para-aminosalicylic acid, penicillin, phenytoin (Dilantin), primidone (Mysoline), propylthiouracil (PTU), quinidine (Quinidex), reserpine, streptomycin, sulfonamides, and tetracyclines (false-positive or lupus-like syndrome)

Luteinizing hormone, plasma

DESCRIPTION

- Quantitative analysis of plasma luteinizing hormone (LH) or interstitial cell-stimulating hormone levels to test for anovulation and infertility in women
- For accurate diagnosis, results evaluated with findings from related hormone tests (such as follicle-stimulating hormone [FSH], estrogen, and testosterone)
- LH: glycoprotein secreted by basophilic cells of anterior pituitary gland
- In women: cyclic LH secretion (with FSH) causes ovulation and transforms ovarian follicle into corpus luteum, which secretes progesterone
- In men: continuous LH secretion stimulates interstitial (Leydig) cells of testes to release testosterone, which stimulates and maintains spermatogenesis (with FSH)

PURPOSE

- To detect ovulation
- To assess male or female infertility
- To evaluate amenorrhea
- To monitor therapy designed to induce ovulation

PREPARATION

- The test requires a blood sample.
- Because there's no evidence that plasma LH levels are affected by fasting, eating, or exercise, such pretest restrictions may not be needed.
- Withhold drugs that may interfere with plasma LH levels, such as corticosteroids (including estrogens and progesterone), for 48 hours before the test as ordered. If the patient must continue them, note this on the laboratory request.

Teaching points

- Explain to the female patient that this test helps determine if her secretion of female hormones is normal.
- Explain who will perform the test and where it'll be done.

- Tell the patient that the test requires a blood sample and that she may experience slight discomfort from the tourniquet and needle puncture.
- Review medication restrictions with the patient.
- Tell the patient the test takes less than 5 minutes.

DIAGNOSTIC PROCEDURE

KEY STEPS

- Confirm the patient's identity using two patient identifiers according to facility policy.
- Perform a venipuncture, and collect the sample in a 7-ml clot-activator tube.
- If the patient is a woman, indicate the phase of her menstrual cycle on the laboratory request. Make a note if the patient is menopausal.

POSTPROCEDURE CARE

- Apply direct pressure to the venipuncture site until the bleeding stops.
- Inform the practitioner of abnormal results.
- After the test, instruct the patient that she may resume medications.

PRECAUTIONS

- Maintain standard precautions while collecting the sample.
- Handle the sample gently to prevent hemolysis.

COMPLICATIONS

- Hematoma at the venipuncture site

INTERPRETATION

NORMAL RESULTS

- In women in the follicular phase, 5 to 15 mIU/ml (SI, 5 to 15 International Units/L); ovulatory phase, 30 to 60 mIU/ml (SI, 30 to 60 International Units/L); luteal phase, 5 to 15 mIU/ml (SI, 5 to 15 International Units/L).
- In postmenopausal women, 50 to 100 mIU/ml (SI, 50 to 100 International Units/L).
- In men, 5 to 20 mIU/ml (SI, 5 to 20 International Units/L).
- In children, 4 to 20 mIU/ml (SI, 4 to 20 International Units/L).

ABNORMAL RESULTS

- In women, absence of a midcycle peak in plasma LH levels may indicate anovulation.
- Decreased or low-normal plasma LH levels may indicate hypogonadism; these findings are commonly linked to amenorrhea.
- High plasma LH levels may indicate congenital absence of ovaries or ovarian failure from Stein-Leventhal syndrome (polycystic ovary syndrome), Turner's syndrome (ovarian dysgenesis), menopause, or early-stage acromegaly.
- Infertility can result from primary or secondary gonadal dysfunction.
- In men, low plasma LH values may indicate secondary gonadal dysfunction (of hypothalamic or pituitary origin); high values may indicate testicular failure (primary hypogonadism) or destruction, or congenital absence of testes.

  INTERFERING FACTORS *Steroids, including estrogens, progesterone, and testosterone (decreased levels)*

Lyme disease serology

DESCRIPTION

- Multisystem disorder characterized by dermatologic, neurologic, cardiac, and rheumatic manifestations in various stages
- Epidemiologic and serologic studies suggest tick-borne spirochete, *Borrelia burgdorferi,* is causative agent
- Tests for Lyme disease: indirect immunofluorescent and enzyme-linked immunosorbent assays measure antibody response to spirochete and indicate current infection or past exposure
- Tests identify 50% of patients with early-stage Lyme disease and all patients with later complications of carditis, neuritis, and arthritis, or patients in remission
- Indirect immunofluorescent assay: *B. burgdorferi* grown in culture, fixed to microscope slide, and incubated with human serum sample
- Fluorescein-labeled antiglobulin introduced into antigen-antibody complex
- Human antibody that binds to spirochete detected by viewing (under ultraviolet microscope) the fluorescent antiglobulin that attaches to it

PURPOSE

- To confirm a diagnosis of Lyme disease

PREPARATION

- The test requires a blood sample.
- Fasting is required for at least 12 hours before the test.

Teaching points

- Explain that this test helps determine whether the patient's symptoms are caused by Lyme disease.
- Explain who will perform the test and where it'll be done.
- Instruct the patient to fast for 12 hours before the sample is drawn, but not to restrict fluids.
- Tell the patient that the test requires a blood sample and that he may experience slight discomfort from the tourniquet and needle puncture.
- Tell the patient the test should take less than 5 minutes.

KEY STEPS

- Confirm the patient's identity using two patient identifiers according to facility policy.
- Perform a venipuncture and collect the sample in a 7-ml clot-activator tube.

POSTPROCEDURE CARE

- Apply direct pressure to the venipuncture site until the bleeding stops.
- Inform the practitioner of abnormal results.

PRECAUTIONS

- Handle the sample gently to prevent hemolysis.
- Send the sample to the laboratory immediately.

COMPLICATIONS

- Hematoma at the venipuncture site

NORMAL RESULTS

- Normal serum values are nonreactive.

ABNORMAL RESULTS

- A positive result can help confirm the diagnosis, but it isn't definitive.
- Other treponemal diseases and high rheumatoid factor titers can cause false-positive results.
- More than 15% of patients with Lyme disease fail to develop antibodies.

Lymphangiography

DESCRIPTION

- Radiographic examination of lymphatic system after injection of an oil-based contrast medium
- X-rays taken immediately after injection show lymphatic system; after 24 hours, show lymph nodes
- Contrast medium remains in nodes for 2 years
- Subsequent X-rays assess disease progression and monitor treatment effectiveness
- Staging of lymphoma determined by number of nodes affected, unilateral or bilateral node involvement, or extent of extranodal involvement
- Also known as *lymphography*

PURPOSE

- To detect and stage lymphomas
- To identify metastatic involvement of the lymph nodes
- To distinguish primary from secondary lymphedema
- To evaluate effectiveness of chemotherapy or radiation therapy
- To investigate enlarged lymph nodes

PREPARATION

- Make sure the patient has signed an appropriate consent form.
- Note and report allergies.
- Check the patient's history for hypersensitivity to iodine, seafood, or iodinated contrast media.
- No dietary restrictions are required.

Teaching points

- Explain the purpose of the test and how it's done.
- Explain who will perform the test and where it'll be done.
- Tell the patient that fasting isn't required before the test.
- Advise the patient that he'll receive a local anesthetic.
- Explain that the incision site may be sore for several days.
- Tell the patient the test takes about 3 hours.
- Explain that additional X-rays will be taken the next day (taking less than 30 minutes).
- Explain that the contrast medium discolors urine, feces, and skin, and that vision will have a bluish tinge for 48 hours.

DIAGNOSTIC PROCEDURE

KEY STEPS

- Confirm the patient's identity using two patient identifiers according to facility policy.
- A preliminary chest X-ray is taken.
- The skin is cleaned over the dorsum of each foot.
- Blue contrast medium is injected intradermally into the area between the toes of each foot (usually into the first and fourth toe webs) and makes the lymphatic vessels appear as small blue lines on the upper surface of each instep.
- A local anesthetic is injected into the dorsum of each foot.
- A 1" (2.5-cm) transverse incision is made to expose the lymphatic vessels.
- Each vessel is catheterized, and contrast injected.
- Fluoroscopy may be used to monitor filling of the lymphatic system.
- Needles are removed, incisions sutured, and sterile dressings applied.
- X-rays of the legs, pelvis, abdomen, and chest are taken.
- Injection into the foot allows visualization of the lymphatics of the leg, inguinal and iliac regions, and the retroperitoneum up to the thoracic duct.
- Injection into the hand allows visualization of the axillary and supraclavicular nodes.

POSTPROCEDURE CARE

- Apply ice packs to the incision sites.
- Give the patient analgesics.
- Prepare the patient for follow-up X-rays as needed.
- Monitor vital signs and respiratory status.
- Inform the practitioner of abnormal results.
- After the test, instruct the patient to maintain bed rest for 24 hours and keep his feet elevated.

PRECAUTIONS

 WARNING *Watch for signs and symptoms of pulmonary complications caused by embolization of contrast medium, such as shortness of breath, pleuritic pain, hypotension, low-grade fever, and cyanosis.*

- Watch for bleeding and infection.
- Observe incision sites.

COMPLICATIONS

- Bleeding
- Infection

INTERPRETATION

NORMAL RESULTS

- Homogeneous and complete filling with contrast medium is evident on the initial X-rays.
- On 24-hour X-rays, the lymph nodes are fully opacified and well circumscribed; lymph nodes should be of normal size and architecture.
- Lymphatic channels empty a few hours after injection.

ABNORMAL RESULTS

- Enlarged, foamy-looking nodes suggest lymphoma.
- Filling defects or lack of opacification suggests metastatic involvement.
- Shortened or decreased lymphatic vessels suggest primary lymphedema.
- Abruptly terminating lymphatic vessels suggest secondary lymphedema.

Lymph node biopsy

OVERVIEW

DESCRIPTION
- Surgical excision of an active lymph node or the needle aspiration of a nodal specimen for histologic examination

PURPOSE
- To determine the cause of lymph node enlargement
- To distinguish between benign and malignant lymph node tumors
- To stage metastatic cancer

PREPARATION
- Make sure the patient has signed an appropriate consent form.
- Note and report allergies.
- Check the patient's history for hypersensitivity to anesthetic.
- For a needle biopsy, fasting isn't necessary.

Teaching points
- Explain the purpose of the test and how it's done.
- Explain who will perform the test and where it'll be done.
- For excisional biopsy, instruct the patient to restrict food from midnight and to drink clear liquids only.
- If the patient will receive a general anesthetic, instruct him to restrict fluids.
- Tell the patient the test takes 15 to 30 minutes.

DIAGNOSTIC PROCEDURE

KEY STEPS
- Confirm the patient's identity using two patient identifiers according to facility policy.

Excisional biopsy
- The skin over the biopsy site is prepared and draped.
- An anesthetic is given; an incision is made and an entire node removed.
- The specimen is placed in an appropriate, properly labeled container.
- After the wound is sutured, a sterile dressing is applied.

Needle biopsy
- The biopsy site is prepared and draped.
- A local anesthetic is given.
- The biopsy needle is directed into the node and a small core specimen obtained.
- The specimen is placed in a properly labeled container.
- Pressure is applied to the biopsy site to control bleeding.
- A dressing is applied after bleeding stops.

POSTPROCEDURE CARE
- Monitor vital signs.
- Observe the biopsy site.
- Inform the practitioner of abnormal results.
- After the test, tell the patient to resume his usual diet and activity.

PRECAUTIONS
- Watch for bleeding and infection.

COMPLICATIONS
- Bleeding
- Infection

INTERPRETATION

NORMAL RESULTS
- The lymph node is encapsulated by collagenous connective tissue.
- The lymph node is divided into smaller lobes by tissue strands called *trabeculae.*
- The outer cortex is composed of lymphoid cells and nodules or follicles containing lymphocytes.
- The inner medulla is composed of reticular phagocytic cells.

ABNORMAL RESULTS
- Histologic examination may be necessary to distinguish between malignant and nonmalignant causes of lymph node enlargement.
- A lymphoma affecting the entire lymph system suggests possible Hodgkin's disease.
- Lymph node malignancy suggests possible metastatic cancer. (See *Staging non-Hodgkin's lymphoma.*)

Staging non-Hodgkin's lymphoma

Stage I: Involvement of a single lymph node region or of a single extralymphatic organ or site

Stage II: Involvement of two or more lymph node regions on the same side of the diaphragm, or localized involvement of an extralymphatic organ or the site of one or more lymph node regions on the same side of the diaphragm

Stage III: Involvement of lymph node regions on both sides of the diaphragm, which may also be accompanied by localized involvement of an extralymphatic organ or site or of the spleen (or both)

Stage IV: Diffuse or disseminated involvement of one or more extralymphatic organs or tissue with or without associated lymph node enlargement

---

Lymphocytes test

DESCRIPTION

- Class of leukocytes
- Two types: T lymphocytes and B lymphocytes

PURPOSE

- To determine lymphocyte blood count

PREPARATION

- The test requires a blood sample.
- No dietary restrictions are required.

Teaching points

- Explain who will perform the test and where it'll be done.
- No dietary restrictions are required.
- Inform the patient that he may feel slight discomfort from the tourniquet and needle puncture.
- Tell the patient the test takes less than 5 minutes.

KEY STEPS

- Confirm the patient's identity using two patient identifiers according to facility policy.
- Perform the venipuncture and collect the sample in a 5-ml EDTA tube.

PREPARATION

- Apply direct pressure to venipuncture site until bleeding stops.
- Inform the practitioner of abnormal results.

PRECAUTIONS

- Maintain standard precautions while collecting the sample.

COMPLICATIONS

- Hematoma at the venipuncture site

NORMAL RESULTS

- Total lymphocyte count is 800 to 2,600/µl (SI, 0.8×10^9/L to 2.6×10^9/L).

ABNORMAL RESULTS

- Increased absolute lymphocyte count is greater than 4,500/µl (SI, 4.5×10^9/L).
- Increased counts can occur in such conditions as influenza and mononucleosis.
- Decreased counts occur in such conditions as acquired immunodeficiency syndrome, aplastic anemia, and bone marrow suppression.

Lymphocyte transformation test

DESCRIPTION

- Evaluates lymphocyte competency without injection of antigens into patient's skin
- In vitro tests: eliminate risk of adverse effects but can still accurately assess ability of lymphocytes to proliferate, recognize, and respond to antigens
- Mitogen assay: evaluates mitotic response of T and B lymphocytes to foreign antigen
- Antigen assay: uses specific substances (such as purified protein derivative, *Candida*, mumps, tetanus toxoid, and streptokinase) to stimulate lymphocyte transformation
- Mixed lymphocyte culture (MLC) assay: used to match transplant recipients and donors and to test for immunocompetence
- Can determine ability of neutrophils to engulf and destroy bacteria and foreign particles (see *Neutrophil function tests*)

PURPOSE

- To assess and monitor genetic and acquired immunodeficiency states
- To provide histocompatibility typing of tissue transplant recipients and donors
- To detect whether a patient has been exposed to various pathogens, such as those that cause malaria, hepatitis, and mycoplasmal pneumonia

PREPARATION

- If the patient will receive a radioisotope scan, be sure to draw the serum sample for this test first.
- The test requires a blood sample.
- No dietary restrictions are required.

Teaching points

- Explain that this test evaluates lymphocyte function, which is crucial to the immune system.
- Inform the patient that the test monitors his response to therapy, if appropriate.
- Explain who will perform the test and where it'll be done.

- For histocompatibility typing, explain that this test helps determine the best match for a transplant.
- Inform the patient that fasting isn't required.
- Tell the patient that the test requires a blood sample and that he may experience slight discomfort from the tourniquet and needle puncture.
- Tell the patient the test takes less than 5 minutes.

KEY STEPS

- Confirm the patient's identity using two patient identifiers according to facility policy.
- Perform a venipuncture.
- If the patient is an adult, collect the sample in a 7-ml heparinized tube; for a child, use a 5-ml heparinized tube.
- Completely fill the collection tube and invert it gently several times to mix the sample and the anticoagulant.

POSTPROCEDURE CARE

- Because the patient may have a compromised immune system, take care to keep the venipuncture site clean and dry.
- Apply direct pressure to the venipuncture site until the bleeding stops.

- Inform the practitioner of abnormal results.

PRECAUTIONS

- Send the sample to the laboratory immediately.

COMPLICATIONS

- Hematoma at the venipuncture site

NORMAL RESULTS

- Results depend on the mitogens used. Reference ranges accompany test results.
- A positive test is normal; a negative test indicates a deficiency.

ABNORMAL RESULTS

- In the mitogen and antigen assays, a low stimulation index or unresponsiveness indicates a depressed or defective immune system.
- In the MLC test, the stimulation index is a measure of compatibility. A high index indicates poor compatibility.
- A low stimulation index indicates good compatibility.
- A high stimulation index, in response to the relevant pathogen, can also demonstrate exposure to malaria, hepatitis, mycoplasmal pneumonia, periodontal disease, and certain viral infections in a patient who no longer has detectable serum antibodies.

Neutrophil function tests

Neutrophil function tests may reveal the inability of neutrophils to kill a target bacteria or to migrate to the bacterial site (chemotaxis). The killing ability can be evaluated by the nitro-blue tetrazolium (NBT) test, which relies on neutrophil generation of bactericidal enzymes and toxins during killing. This action results in increased oxygen consumption and glucose metabolism, which reduces colorless NBT to blue formazan. The reduced dye is then extracted with pyridine and measured photometrically; the level of reduction indicates phagocytic activity.

Neutrophil killing activity can also be evaluated by noting the neutrophil's chemi-luminescence, its ability to emit light. After a neutrophil phagocytizes a microorganism, oxygen-containing substances form within phagocytic vacuoles. As the cell is stimulated, it emits light in proportion to the amount of oxygen-containing substances that are formed, providing an indirect measurement of phagocytosis.

Chemotaxis can be assessed in vitro by placing bacteria in the lower half of a two-part chamber and phagocytic neutrophils in the upper half. After incubation, migrating cells are counted microscopically and compared with standard values.

Lysozyme test

DESCRIPTION

- Also known as *muramidase:* low-molecular-weight enzyme present in mucus, saliva, tears, skin secretions, and various internal body cells and fluids
- Splits, or lyses, cell walls of gram-positive bacteria and, with complement and other blood factors, destroys them
- Synthesized in granulocytes and monocytes; first appears in serum after destruction of these cells
- Appears in urine when serum level exceeds three times normal level (renal tissue also contains lysozyme, and renal injury alone can cause measurable excretion of enzyme)
- Measures urine levels with a turbidimeter; measures serum levels to confirm the results of urine testing

PURPOSE

- To help diagnose acute monocytic or granulocytic leukemia and to monitor the progression of these diseases
- To evaluate proximal tubular function and to diagnose renal impairment
- To detect rejection or infarction of kidney transplantation

PREPARATION

- The test requires collection of urine over 24 hours.
- No dietary restrictions are required.

Teaching points

- Explain that this test evaluates renal function and the immune system.
- Tell the patient that fasting isn't required.
- Tell the patient that the test requires collection of urine over a 24-hour period, and teach him how to collect the specimen correctly.

KEY STEPS

- Confirm the patient's identity using two patient identifiers according to facility policy.
- Collect the patient's urine over a 24-hour period, discarding the first specimen and retaining the last specimen in the appropriate container.
- Keep the collection bag on ice if the patient has an indwelling urinary catheter in place.

POSTPROCEDURE CARE

- Inform the practitioner of abnormal results.

PRECAUTIONS

- If a woman is menstruating, anticipate possible test rescheduling.
- Tell the patient to avoid contaminating the urine specimen with toilet tissue or feces.
- Cover and refrigerate the specimen throughout the collection period.
- Send the specimen to the laboratory as soon as the test is complete.

COMPLICATIONS

- None

NORMAL RESULTS

- Urine lysozyme values are 0 to 3 mg/24 hours.

ABNORMAL RESULTS

- Elevated urine lysozyme levels are characteristic of impaired renal proximal tubular reabsorption, acute pyelonephritis, nephrotic syndrome, tuberculosis of the kidney, severe extrarenal infection, rejection or infarction of kidney transplantation (levels normally increase during the first few days after transplantation), and polycythemia vera.
- Urine levels rise markedly after the acute onset or relapse of monocytic or myelomonocytic leukemia and rise moderately after acute onset or relapse of granulocytic (myeloid) leukemia.
- Urine lysozyme levels remain normal or decrease in lymphocytic leukemia and remain normal in myeloblastic and myelocytic leukemias.

Magnesium level test

DESCRIPTION

- Measures serum levels of magnesium
- Electrolyte vital for neuromuscular function: aids intracellular metabolism, activates many essential enzymes, affects the metabolism of nucleic acids and proteins, helps transport sodium and potassium across cell membranes, and influences intracellular calcium levels
- Occurs mostly in bone and intracellular fluid; small amount in extracellular fluid
- Absorbed by small intestine and excreted in urine and stools

PURPOSE

- To evaluate electrolyte status
- To assess neuromuscular and renal function

PREPARATION

- The test requires a blood sample.
- Magnesium salts should be avoided for 3 days before the test.

Teaching points

- Explain that the serum magnesium test determines the magnesium content of the blood.
- Explain who will perform the test and where it'll be done.
- Instruct the patient to avoid magnesium salts (such as milk of magnesia or Epsom salts) for at least 3 days before the test, but tell him that he doesn't need to restrict food and fluids.
- Tell the patient that the test requires a blood sample and that he may experience slight discomfort from the tourniquet and needle puncture.
- Tell the patient the test takes less than 5 minutes.

KEY STEPS

- Confirm the patient's identity using two patient identifiers according to facility policy.
- Perform a venipuncture without a tourniquet, if possible, and collect the sample in a 3- or 4-ml clot-activator tube.

POSTPROCEDURE CARE

- Apply direct pressure to the venipuncture site until the bleeding stops.
- Inform the practitioner of abnormal results.

PRECAUTIONS

- Handle the sample gently to prevent hemolysis.
- In hypermagnesemia, watch for lethargy; flushing; diaphoresis; decreased blood pressure; slow, weak pulse; muscle weakness; diminished deep tendon reflexes; slow, shallow respiration; and electrocardiogram changes (such as prolonged PR interval, wide QRS complex, elevated T waves, atrioventricular block, and premature ventricular contractions [PVCs]).
- In hypomagnesemia, watch for leg and foot cramps, hyperactive deep tendon reflexes, arrhythmias, muscle weakness, seizures, twitching, tetany, tremors, PVCs, and ventricular fibrillation.

COMPLICATIONS

- Hematoma at the venipuncture site

NORMAL RESULTS

- Level ranges from 1.3 to 2.1 mg/dl (SI, 0.65 to 1.05 mmol/L).

ABNORMAL RESULTS

- Hypermagnesemia most commonly occurs in renal failure, when the kidneys excrete inadequate amounts of magnesium, in magnesium administration or ingestion, and in adrenal insufficiency (Addison's disease).
- Hypomagnesemia is most common in chronic alcoholism; also in malabsorption syndrome, diarrhea, faulty absorption after bowel resection, prolonged bowel or gastric aspiration, acute pancreatitis, primary aldosteronism, severe burns, hypercalcemic conditions (including hyperparathyroidism), malnutrition, and certain diuretic therapy.

Magnetic resonance imaging

DESCRIPTION

◆ Uses a powerful magnetic field and radiofrequency waves to produce computerized images of internal organs and tissues
◆ Eliminates risks associated with exposure to X-ray beams and isn't harmful to cells
◆ Also known as *MRI*

PURPOSE

◆ To obtain images of internal organs and tissues not readily visible on standard X-rays

PREPARATION

◆ Because patients requiring life support equipment, including ventilators, require special preparation, contact MRI staff in advance of the test.
◆ Make sure the patient has signed an appropriate consent form.
◆ Note and report allergies.
◆ No dietary restrictions are required.
◆ A claustrophobic patient may require sedation or an open MRI to reduce anxiety. (See *Open MRI*.)

Teaching points

◆ Explain who will perform the test and where it'll be done.
◆ Tell the patient that fasting isn't required.
◆ Instruct the patient to remove any metal objects he's wearing or carrying.
◆ Advise the patient that he'll be asked to remain still during the procedure.
◆ Warn the patient that the machine makes loud clacking sounds.
◆ Tell the patient the test takes 30 to 60 minutes.

DIAGNOSTIC PROCEDURE

KEY STEPS

◆ Confirm the patient's identity using two patient identifiers according to facility policy.
◆ If the patient will receive a contrast medium, an I.V. line is started and the medium is administered before the procedure.
◆ Check the patient for metal objects at the scanner room door.
◆ Place the patient in the supine position on a padded scanning table.
◆ The table is positioned in the opening of the scanning gantry.
◆ Use a call bell or intercom to maintain verbal contact.
◆ The patient may wear earplugs if needed.
◆ Varying radiofrequency waves are directed at the area being scanned.
◆ A computer reconstructs information as images on a television screen.

POSTPROCEDURE CARE

◆ Monitor the patient's vital signs.
◆ Watch for orthostatic hypotension.
◆ Inform the practitioner of abnormal results.

PRECAUTIONS

◆ Because MRI works through a powerful magnetic field, it can't be performed on patients with a pacemaker, an aneurysm clip, or other ferrous metal implants.
◆ Because of the strong magnetic field, metallic or computer-based equipment (such as ventilators and I.V. pumps) can't enter the MRI area.

COMPLICATIONS

◆ Orthostatic hypotension
◆ Anxiety
◆ Claustrophobia

INTERPRETATION

NORMAL RESULTS

◆ Refer to the specific type of MRI.

ABNORMAL RESULTS

◆ Refer to the specific type of MRI.

Open MRI

With an open magnetic resonance imaging (MRI) unit, the patient isn't completely enclosed in a tunnel. This is ideal for patients with claustrophobia. Open MRI units are low-field units (0.2 to 0.5 Tesla) as opposed to closed MRI units, which are typically high-field units (1.0 to 1.5 or greater Tesla). The image quality is almost always better in a high-field unit, not only because of the field strength, but also because of the gradient speed and strength, surface coils, and software.

Accurate diagnosis may be difficult unless the interpreting radiologist has experience reading low-field units. If results with an open MRI are equivocal, a repeat closed MRI should be done. For small body parts (such as the hand, wrist, foot, ankle, or elbow), a high-resolution closed MRI is recommended. Some practitioners prefer a high-resolution MRI for the cervical spine as well, because small extradural defects in the neural foramina are difficult to see even when using a high-field unit.

Magnetic resonance imaging of bone and soft tissue

DESCRIPTION

◆ Noninvasive technique that produces clear and sensitive tomographic images of bone and soft tissue
◆ Provides superior contrast of body tissues and allows imaging of multiple planes, including direct sagittal and coronal views
◆ Eliminates risks associated with exposure to radiation from X-rays and isn't harmful to cells

PURPOSE

◆ To evaluate bony and soft-tissue tumors
◆ To identify changes in the bone marrow cavity
◆ To identify spinal disorders

PREPARATION

◆ Make sure the patient has signed an appropriate consent form.
◆ Note and report allergies.
◆ Make sure the scanner can accommodate the patient's weight and abdominal girth.
◆ Screen for surgically implanted joints, pins, clips, valves, pumps, or pacemakers containing metal.
◆ Stop I.V. infusion pumps, feeding tubes with metal tips, pulmonary artery catheters, and similar devices before the test.
◆ For certain types of magnetic resonance imaging (MRI), start an I.V. for injection of a contrast medium.
◆ A claustrophobic patient may require sedation or an open MRI to reduce anxiety.
◆ An anesthesiologist may need to be present to monitor a heavily sedated patient.
◆ No dietary restrictions are required.

Teaching points

◆ Explain that MRI is painless and doesn't involve exposure to radiation.
◆ Explain who will perform the test and where it'll be done.
◆ Reassure the patient that he'll be able to communicate with the technician at all times.

◆ Tell the patient that he need not restrict food or fluids.
◆ Explain to the patient that he'll hear the scanner clicking, whirring, and thumping, and that he may use earplugs.
◆ Instruct the patient to remove all metallic objects, such as jewelry, hairpins, and wristwatch, before the test.
◆ Tell the patient the test takes 30 to 90 minutes.

KEY STEPS

◆ Confirm the patient's identity using two patient identifiers according to facility policy.
◆ Check the patient for metal objects at the scanner room door.
◆ Place the patient on a narrow, padded, nonmetallic table that moves into the scanner tunnel.
◆ Use a call bell or intercom to maintain verbal contact.
◆ Instruct the patient to remain still during the procedure.
◆ Monitor the patient for claustrophobia and anxiety.
◆ The area to be studied is stimulated with radiofrequency waves.
◆ A computer measures resulting energy changes at these body sections and uses them to generate images.

POSTPROCEDURE CARE

◆ Provide the patient with comfort measures as needed.
◆ Monitor the patient's vital signs.
◆ Monitor the patient for orthostatic hypotension.
◆ Inform the practitioner of abnormal results.
◆ After the test, tell the patient that he may resume his normal activities.

PRECAUTIONS

◆ If the patient is unstable, make sure an I.V. line without metal components is in place and that all equipment is compatible with MRI imaging; monitor oxygen saturation, cardiac rhythm, and respiratory status during the test.

COMPLICATIONS

◆ Orthostatic hypotension
◆ Anxiety
◆ Claustrophobia

NORMAL RESULTS

◆ No evidence of disease is found in bone, muscles, and joints.

ABNORMAL RESULTS

◆ Structural abnormalities may suggest primary and metastatic tumors and various disorders of the bone, muscles, and joints.

Magnetic resonance imaging of the ear

OVERVIEW

DESCRIPTION
- Noninvasive technique to assesses cranial nerves and bone
- Provides high-quality, cross-sectional images of the body without X-rays or other radiation
- Fast spin echo (FSE) magnetic resonance imaging (MRI): for otologic assessment, especially with suspected retrocochlear lesion

PURPOSE
- To assess the cause of sudden unilateral sensorineural hearing loss
- To show early nonossified soft-tissue scarring in the membranous labyrinth
- To investigate lesions of the petrous apex
- To diagnose vestibular schwannomas as small as 2 mm
- To make visible cranial nerves VII and VIII, especially when anticipating excision of an auditory neuroma

PREPARATION
- Make sure the patient has signed an appropriate consent form.
- Note and report allergies.
- No dietary restrictions are required.
- Inform the practitioner of a patient's pacemaker or other implants.
- Have the patient remove all jewelry and metal objects.

Teaching points
- Explain the purpose of the test and how it's done
- Explain who will perform the test and where it'll be done.
- Tell the patient that he'll hear loud noises from the machine during the test but may receive earplugs or a music headset to decrease this noise.
- Explain the need to remain still during the procedure.
- Tell the patient that fasting isn't needed before the test.
- Tell the patient without I.V. contrast, the test takes about 15 minutes; FSE MRI is faster.

DIAGNOSTIC PROCEDURE

KEY STEPS
- Confirm the patient's identity using two patient identifiers according to facility policy.
- Each MRI protocol depends on the purpose of the test.
- The patient is prepared and placed on the MRI table.
- The patient's head is moved into a large, hollow, cylindrical magnet.
- The scan is performed and images obtained.

POSTPROCEDURE CARE
- Monitor the patient's vital signs.
- Monitor the patient for orthostatic hypotension.
- Inform the practitioner of abnormal results.

PRECAUTIONS
- A claustrophobic patient may require sedation or an open MRI to reduce anxiety.

COMPLICATIONS
- Orthostatic hypotension
- Anxiety
- Claustrophobia

INTERPRETATION

NORMAL RESULTS
- Cranial nerves and auditory bones appear normal.

ABNORMAL RESULTS
- Structural abnormalities suggest possible disorders, such as viral labyrinthitis, increased intracranial pressure, or paragangliomas.

Magnetic resonance imaging of the neurologic system

OVERVIEW

DESCRIPTION

- Produces cross-sectional images of the brain and spine in multiple planes
- Enables ability to "see through" bone and to delineate fluid-filled soft tissue
- Research continues on optimal magnetic fields and radiofrequency waves for each type of tissue (see *New methods of monitoring cerebral function;* also see *MRI techniques,* page 324)

PURPOSE

- To help diagnose intracranial and spinal lesions
- To help diagnose soft-tissue abnormalities
- To detect small tumors and hemorrhages and cerebral infarction earlier than possible with computed tomography scanning

PREPARATION

- Make sure the patient has signed an appropriate consent form.
- Note and report allergies.
- Screen for surgically implanted joints, pins, clips, valves, pumps, or pacemakers containing metal.
- Remove all metallic objects from the patient.
- A claustrophobic patient may require sedation or an open magnetic resonance imaging (MRI) to reduce anxiety.
- Reassure the patient that he'll be able to communicate with the technician at all times.
- No dietary restrictions are required.

Teaching points

- Explain the purpose of the test and how it's done.
- Explain who will perform the test and where it'll be done.
- Inform the patient that MRI is painless and doesn't involve exposure to radiation.
- Stress the need for the patient to remain still for the entire procedure.
- Warn the patient that he'll hear clicking, whirring, and thumping sounds during the procedure, and that he may wear earplugs.
- Tell the patient he doesn't need to fast before the test.
- Tell the patient that the test may take up to 90 minutes.

DIAGNOSTIC PROCEDURE

KEY STEPS

- Confirm the patient's identity using two patient identifiers according to facility policy.
- The patient is placed in a supine position on a narrow table.
- The table is moved to the desired position inside the scanner.
- Radiofrequency energy is directed at the head or spine.
- Resulting images are displayed on a monitor.
- Images are recorded on film or magnetic tape.

New methods of monitoring cerebral function

OPTICAL IMAGING

Optical imaging uses fiber-optic light and a camera to produce visual images of the brain as it responds to stimulation. This technique produces higher-resolution pictures of the brain than magnetic resonance imaging (MRI) or positron emission tomography scans. Researchers believe it may be valuable during neurosurgery to minimize damage to crucial areas of the brain that control speech, movement, and other activities. Because the procedure scans only the brain's surface, it's meant to be used with other diagnostic techniques.

FAST MRI

Fast MRI produces pictures less than a second apart. These images display blood flow through the brain and the changes that occur in blood flow when the patient performs different tasks. Neuroscientists believe that active areas of the brain must consume more oxygen and that areas of the brain that are currently working become laden with oxygen. Fast MRI can distinguish between oxygen-laden and oxygen-depleted blood. Thus, this test may be used to help identify which areas of the normal brain are involved in certain activities and emotions. Possible applications for fast MRI include guiding neurosurgeons during surgery and helping researchers better understand epilepsy, brain tumors, and even psychiatric illnesses.

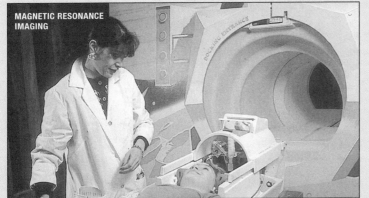

MAGNETIC RESONANCE IMAGING

Photo from Timby, B.K. *Fundamental Nursing Skills and Concepts,* 8th ed. Philadelphia: Lippincott Williams & Wilkins, 2005.

(continued)

POSTPROCEDURE CARE

◆ Monitor the patient's vital signs.
◆ Monitor the patient for orthostatic hypotension.
◆ Inform the practitioner of abnormal results.
◆ After the test, tell the patient to resume his normal activities.

PRECAUTIONS

◆ Because of powerful magnetic fields, MRI is contraindicated in patients with pacemakers, intracranial clips, ferrous metal implants, or gunshot wounds to the head.
◆ Metallic or computer-based equipment (such as ventilators and I.V. pumps) must not enter the MRI area.

COMPLICATIONS

◆ Orthostatic hypotension
◆ Anxiety
◆ Claustrophobia

INTERPRETATION

NORMAL RESULTS

◆ The appearance of brain and spinal cord structures is defined and distinct.

ABNORMAL RESULTS

◆ Structural changes that increase tissue water content suggest possible cerebral edema, demyelinating disease, and pontine and cerebellar tumors.
◆ Areas of demyelination (curdlike gray or gray-white areas) around the edges of ventricles suggest multiple sclerosis lesions.
◆ Changes in normal anatomy suggest possible tumors.

MRI techniques

Magnetic resonance imaging (MRI) is used to provide clear images of parts of the brain, such as the brain stem and cerebellum that are difficult to image by other methods. Four MRI techniques are available to examine other aspects of the brain.

MAGNETIC RESONANCE ANGIOGRAPHY

Magnetic resonance angiography allows the visualization of blood flowing through the cerebral vessels. Images of blood vessels done with magnetic resonance angiography aren't as clear as those obtained by angiography, but this technique is less invasive.

MAGNETIC RESONANCE SPECTROSCOPY

Magnetic resonance spectroscopy creates images over time that show the metabolism of certain chemical markers in a specific area of the brain. Some researchers have dubbed this test a "metabolic biopsy" because it reveals pathologic neurochemistry over time.

DIFFUSION-PERFUSION IMAGING

Diffusion-perfusion imaging uses a stronger-than-normal magnetic gradient to reveal areas of focal cerebral ischemia within minutes. Currently used in stroke research, this MRI technique may be used by diagnosticians to distinguish permanent from reversible ischemia.

NEUROGRAPHY

Neurograms provide a three-dimensional image of nerves. They may be used to find the exact location of nerves that are damaged, crimped, or in disarray.

Magnetic resonance imaging of the urinary tract

DESCRIPTION

- Uses radiofrequency waves and magnetic fields to show specific structures (kidney or prostate), which are then converted to computer-generated images
- May reveal blood vessel size and anatomy when imaging soft-tissue structures of kidneys; not useful for detecting calculi or calcified tumors

PURPOSE

- To diagnose urinary tract disorders
- To evaluate genitourinary tumors and abdominal or pelvic masses
- To detect prostate calculi and cysts
- To detect cancer invasion into seminal vesicles and pelvic lymph nodes

PREPARATION

- Make sure that the patient or family member has signed an appropriate consent form.
- If the patient will receive a contrast medium, obtain a history of allergies or hypersensitivity to these drugs. Mark sensitivities on the chart and notify the practitioner.
- Ask the patient if he has any implanted metal devices or prostheses, such as vascular clips, shrapnel, pacemakers, joint implants, filters, and intrauterine devices. If so, the patient may not be able to have the test.
- Just before the procedure, have the patient void.

Teaching points

- Explain that magnetic resonance imaging (MRI) of the urinary tract helps evaluate abnormalities in the urinary system.
- Explain who will perform the test and where it'll be done.
- Instruct the patient to avoid alcohol, caffeine-containing beverages, and smoking for at least 2 hours, and food for at least 1 hour, before the test.

- Tell the patient to continue taking medications, except for iron, which interferes with the imaging.
- Before the test, tell the patient that he'll need to remove all clothing, jewelry, and metallic objects and wear a special hospital gown without snaps or closures.
- Inform the patient that he won't feel pain but may feel claustrophobic while lying supine in the tubular MRI chamber. Tell him the practitioner may order an anxiolytic.
- Tell the patient that he'll hear loud noises from the machine during the test but may receive earplugs or a music headset to decrease this noise.
- Tell the patient the test takes between 30 and 90 minutes.
- After the procedure, instruct the patient that he may resume his usual diet, fluids, and medications.

KEY STEPS

- Confirm the patient's identity using two patient identifiers according to facility policy.
- The patient is placed in the supine position on a narrow, flat table.
- If the patient will receive a contrast medium, start an I.V. line so that the medium is infused before the procedure.
- The table is moved to the enclosed cylindrical scanner.
- Tell the patient to lie still in the scanner while the images are being produced.
- Varying radiofrequency waves are directed at the area being scanned.
- Although the patient's face remains uncovered to allow him to see out, advise him to keep his eyes closed to promote relaxation and prevent a closed-in feeling.
- If the patient feels nauseated because of claustrophobia, encourage him to take deep breaths.

POSTPROCEDURE CARE

- If the patient received sedatives, monitor his vital signs until he's awake and responsive.
- Monitor the patient for adverse reactions to the contrast medium (such as flushing, nausea, urticaria, and sneezing).
- Inform the practitioner of abnormal results.

PRECAUTIONS

- Because of powerful magnetic fields, MRI is contraindicated in patients with pacemakers, intracranial clips, ferrous metal implants, or gunshot wounds to the head.
- Metallic or computer-based equipment (such as ventilators and I.V. pumps) must not enter the MRI area.

COMPLICATIONS

- Anxiety
- Adverse reactions to contrast medium

NORMAL RESULTS

- The soft tissue structures of the kidneys are visible.
- Blood vessels can be seen.

ABNORMAL RESULTS

- Visual images suggest tumors, strictures, stenosis, thrombosis, malformations, abscess, inflammation, edema, fluid collection, bleeding, hemorrhage, or organ atrophy.

Mammography

DESCRIPTION

- Detects breast cysts or tumors, especially those not palpable on physical examination
- Questionable findings may require a follow-up ultrasound (see *Using ultrasonography to detect breast cancer*)
- Follows American Cancer Society guidelines
- May not reveal all cancers; never substitute for biopsy
- Yields many false-positive results
- New digital image approved by U.S. Food and Drug Administration is used similarly to mammography (see *Digital mammography*)

PURPOSE

- To screen for malignant breast tumors
- To investigate breast masses, breast pain, or nipple discharge
- To differentiate between benign breast disease and malignant tumors
- To monitor patients with breast cancer who are treated with breast-conserving surgery and radiation

PREPARATION

- When scheduling the test, inform the staff if the patient has breast implants.
- Make sure the patient has signed an appropriate consent form.
- No dietary restrictions are required.
- Note and report allergies.

Teaching points

- Explain the purpose of the test and how it's done.
- Explain who will perform the test and where it'll be done.
- Instruct the patient to avoid using underarm deodorant or powder the day of the examination.
- Tell the patient that she may be asked to wait while the films are checked.
- Tell her that fasting isn't required.
- Inform the patient the test takes about 15 minutes.

DIAGNOSTIC PROCEDURE

KEY STEPS

- Confirm the patient's identity using two patient identifiers according to facility policy.
- The patient rests one breast on a table above the X-ray cassette.
- The compressor is placed on the breast.
- The patient holds her breath until the X-ray is taken and she's told to breathe again.
- An X-ray of the craniocaudal view is taken.
- The machine is rotated, and the breast is compressed again.
- An X-ray of the lateral view is taken.
- The procedure is repeated for the other breast.
- The film is developed and checked for quality.

POSTPROCEDURE CARE

- Answer the patient's questions.
- Inform the practitioner of abnormal results.

PRECAUTIONS

- None

COMPLICATIONS

- Vasovagal reaction during compression

INTERPRETATION

NORMAL RESULTS

- The test reveals normal ducts, glandular tissue, and fat architecture.
- No abnormal masses or calcifications are present.

ABNORMAL RESULTS

- Irregular, poorly outlined, opaque areas suggest malignant tumor, especially if solitary and unilateral.
- Well-outlined, regular, clear spots may be benign, especially if bilateral.

Digital mammography

Digital mammography produces pictures of the breast using X-rays. Instead of film, this process uses detectors that change the X-rays into electrical signals, which are then converted to an image. Digital mammography is used for screening and diagnosis. For the patient, the procedure is the same as with ordinary mammography.

Digital mammography may offer advantages over conventional mammography:

- The images can be stored and retrieved electronically, which makes long-distance consultations with other mammography specialists easier.
- Because the images can be adjusted by the radiologist, subtle differences between tissues may be noted.
- The number of follow-up procedures required may be reduced.
- The need for fewer exposures with digital mammography can reduce the already low levels of radiation.

The U.S. Food and Drug Administration has recently approved the Lorad Digital Breast Imager to be used with the Lorad M-IV Mammography X-ray System for this digital procedure.

Digital mammography has been shown to be effective in the detection of breast cancer and other abnormalities.

Using ultrasonography to detect breast cancer

Ultrasonography is especially usedful for diagnosing tumors less than 0.6 cm in diameter and in distinguishing cysts from solid tumors in dense breast tissue. As with other ultrasound techniques, a transducer sends a beam of high-frequency sound waves through the patient's skin and into the breast. The sound waves are then processed and displayed for interpretation.

A benefit to ultrasonography is that it can show all areas of the breast, including the area close to the chest wall, which is difficult to study with X-rays. When used as an adjunct to mammography, ultrasound increases diagnostic accuracy; when used alone, it's more accurate than mammography in examining the denser breast tissue of a young patient.

Manganese level test

OVERVIEW

DESCRIPTION

◆ Analysis by atomic absorption spectroscopy, to measure serum levels of manganese
◆ Trace element that activates several enzymes (including cholinesterase and arginase) essential to metabolism
◆ Found in unrefined cereals, green leafy vegetables, and nuts
◆ Toxicity: from inhaling manganese dust or fumes (hazard in steel and dry-cell battery industries) or drinking contaminated water

PURPOSE

◆ To detect manganese toxicity

PREPARATION

◆ No dietary restrictions are required.
◆ The test requires a blood sample.
◆ Check the patient's history for drugs that may influence serum manganese levels, such as estrogens and glucocorticoids.

Teaching points

◆ Explain that this test determines the level of manganese in the blood.
◆ Explain who will perform the test and where it'll be done.
◆ Inform the patient that he need not restrict food or fluids.
◆ Tell him that the test requires a blood sample and that he may experience slight discomfort from the tourniquet and needle puncture.
◆ Tell the patient the test takes less than 5 minutes.

DIAGNOSTIC PROCEDURE

KEY STEPS

◆ Confirm the patient's identity using two patient identifiers according to facility policy.
◆ Perform a venipuncture and collect the sample in a metal-free collection tube. Laboratories supply a special kit for this test on request.

POSTPROCEDURE CARE

◆ Apply direct pressure to the venipuncture site until the bleeding stops.
◆ Inform the practitioner of abnormal results.

PRECAUTIONS

◆ Handle the sample gently to prevent hemolysis.
◆ Send the sample to the laboratory immediately.

COMPLICATIONS

◆ Hematoma at the venipuncture site

INTERPRETATION

NORMAL RESULTS

◆ Level is 0.4 to 1.4 mcg/ml (SI, 7.28 to 25.5 nmol/L).

ABNORMAL RESULTS

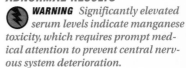 **WARNING** *Significantly elevated serum levels indicate manganese toxicity, which requires prompt medical attention to prevent central nervous system deterioration.*
◆ Low serum manganese levels may indicate deficient dietary intake, although not necessarily disease.

Mediastinoscopy

DESCRIPTION

◆ Operative procedure that shows mediastinal structures through a mediastinoscope with a built-in light source
◆ Used when sputum cytology, lung scans, radiography, and bronchoscopic biopsy fail to confirm a diagnosis

PURPOSE

◆ To detect bronchogenic carcinoma, lymphoma, and sarcoidosis
◆ To stage lung cancer
◆ To permit biopsy of paratracheal and carinal lymph nodes

PREPARATION

◆ Make sure the patient has signed an appropriate consent form.
◆ Note and report allergies.
◆ Check the patient's history for hypersensitivity to the anesthetic.
◆ The patient shouldn't have food or fluids after midnight before the test.

Teaching points

◆ Explain the purpose of the test and how it's done.
◆ Explain who will perform the test and where it'll be done.
◆ Instruct the patient to fast after midnight before the test.
◆ Inform the patient that he'll receive a general anesthetic.
◆ Warn the patient that he may have temporary chest pain, tenderness at the incision site, and a sore throat (from intubation).
◆ Explain to the patient that he'll have an incision above the suprasternal notch.
◆ Tell the patient the test takes about 1 hour.

KEY STEPS

◆ Confirm the patient's identity using two patient identifiers according to facility policy.
◆ The patient is intubated and anesthetized.
◆ A small transverse suprasternal incision is made.
◆ A channel is formed using finger dissection, and lymph nodes are palpated.
◆ The mediastinoscope is inserted.
◆ Tissue specimens are collected and sent to the laboratory for frozen section examination.
◆ If analysis confirms malignancy of a resectable tumor, thoracotomy and pneumonectomy may follow immediately.

POSTPROCEDURE CARE

◆ Give the prescribed analgesic.
◆ Monitor the patient's vital signs and intake and output.
◆ Watch the patient for bleeding and signs of infection.
◆ Observe the incision and dressings.
◆ Monitor the patient's respiratory and neurologic status.
◆ After the test, have the patient resume his normal diet and activities.

PRECAUTIONS

◆ Observe the patient for signs and symptoms of complications such as fever (mediastinitis); crepitus (subcutaneous emphysema); dyspnea, cyanosis, and diminished breath sounds (pneumothorax); tachycardia and hypotension (hemorrhage or cardiac tamponade); or loss of voice and obstruction of breathing (laryngeal nerve damage).

COMPLICATIONS

◆ Pneumothorax
◆ Perforated esophagus
◆ Mediastinitis
◆ Infection
◆ Hemorrhage
◆ Laryngeal nerve damage
◆ Cardiac tamponade

NORMAL RESULTS

◆ The lymph nodes appear as small, smooth, flat oval bodies of lymphoid tissue.

ABNORMAL RESULTS

◆ Anatomical abnormalities suggest various disorders including lung or esophageal cancer, and lymphomas such as Hodgkin's disease.

Melanin, urine

DESCRIPTION

- Measures urine levels of melanin: black-brown pigment produced by specialized cells and melanocytes that covers the skin, hair, and eyes
- Cutaneous malignant melanomas: produce excessive melanin, develop most commonly around head and neck but may originate in mucous membranes (such as rectum), retina, or central nervous system
- Melanin precursor, melanogen: may be excreted in urine; if urine left standing, exposure to air converts melanogen to melanin in 24 hours
- Thormählen's test: sodium nitroprusside (nitroferricyanide) detects melanin in urine, based on characteristic color changes
- Chromatography: isolates and measures pigment

PURPOSE

- To help diagnose malignant melanomas

PREPARATION

- No dietary restrictions are required.
- The test requires a random urine specimen.

Teaching points

- Explain what melanin is, and tell the patient the urine melanin test detects its presence in urine.
- Tell the patient that fasting isn't required.
- Inform the patient that the test requires a random urine specimen, and teach him how to collect the specimen.

KEY STEPS

- Confirm the patient's identity using two patient identifiers according to facility policy.
- Collect a random urine specimen.

POSTPROCEDURE CARE

- Answer the patient's questions.
- Inform the practitioner of abnormal results.

PRECAUTIONS

- Send the specimen to the laboratory immediately.

COMPLICATIONS

- None

NORMAL RESULTS

- No melanogen or melanin is found.

ABNORMAL RESULTS

- In a patient with a visible skin tumor, the presence of melanin or melanogen in urine indicates advanced internal metastasis.
- In a patient without a visible skin tumor, because malignant melanomas may also develop in internal organs, the presence of melanin or melanogen in urine indicates an internal melanoma.

Methemoglobin level test

DESCRIPTION

- Detects methemoglobin (MetHb): structural hemoglobin (Hb) variant formed when heme portion of de-oxygenated Hb is oxidized to ferric state
- Prevents heme from combining with oxygen and transporting it to the tissues; patient becomes cyanotic

PURPOSE

- To detect methemoglobinemia acquired from excessive radiation or the toxic effects of chemicals or drugs
- To detect congenital methemoglobinemia

PREPARATION

- If possible, obtain a history of the patient's hematologic status and Hb disorder, conditions that produce nitrite, and exposure to sources of nitrites in drugs.
- Notify the laboratory and practitioner of drugs the patient is taking that may affect test results; they may need to be restricted.
- No dietary restrictions are required.
- The test requires a blood sample.

Teaching points

- Explain that this test detects abnormal Hb in the blood.
- Explain who will perform the test and where it'll be done.
- Tell the patient that the test requires a blood sample and that he may experience slight discomfort from the tourniquet and needle puncture.
- Tell the patient that fasting isn't required before the test.
- Inform the patient the test takes less than 5 minutes.

KEY STEPS

- Confirm the patient's identity using two patient identifiers according to facility policy.
- Perform a venipuncture and collect the sample in a 4.5-ml heparinized tube.
- Fill the collection tube completely and invert it gently several times.

POSTPROCEDURE CARE

- Apply direct pressure until bleeding stops.
- If a large hematoma develops at the venipuncture site, monitor pulses distal to the site.
- Inform the practitioner of abnormal results.

PRECAUTIONS

- To prevent hemolysis, don't shake the tube vigorously.
- Place the collection tube on ice and send it to the laboratory immediately.

COMPLICATIONS

- Hematoma at the venipuncture site

NORMAL RESULTS

- Level is 0% to 1.5% (SI, 0 to 0.015) of total Hb.

ABNORMAL RESULTS

- Increased MetHb levels may indicate acquired or hereditary methemoglobinemia, carbon monoxide poisoning, ingestion of certain drugs, or being exposed to certain substances.
- Decreased MetHb levels may occur in pancreatitis.

Monocytes test

DESCRIPTION
- Mononuclear cells: type of white blood cell
- Phagocytic; develop into macrophages
- Help protect the body against infection

PURPOSE
- To help diagnose an illness, such as infection or inflammatory disease

PREPARATION
- No dietary restrictions are required.
- The test requires a blood sample.

Teaching points
- Explain who will perform the test and where it'll be done.
- Tell the patient that the test requires a blood sample and that he may experience slight discomfort from the tourniquet and needle puncture.
- Tell the patient he need not restrict food or fluids.
- Inform the patient the test takes less than 5 minutes.

KEY STEPS
- Confirm the patient's identity using two patient identifiers according to facility policy.
- Perform a venipuncture and collect the blood sample.

POSTPROCEDURE CARE
- Apply direct pressure to the venipuncture site until the bleeding stops.
- Inform the practitioner of abnormal results.

PRECAUTIONS
- Send the specimen to the laboratory promptly.

COMPLICATIONS
- Hematoma at the venipuncture site

NORMAL RESULTS
- Count is 0.21 to 0.92 $\times$ 10^9/L.

ABNORMAL RESULTS
- Increased counts may indicate carcinomas, monocytic leukemia, lymphomas, collagen vascular disease such as systemic lupus erythematosus and rheumatoid arthritis infections, subacute bacterial endocarditis, tuberculosis, hepatitis, or malaria.

Multiple-gated acquisition scanning

OVERVIEW

DESCRIPTION

◆ Shows moving image of the beating heart and important features that reveal health of cardiac ventricles
◆ Useful, noninvasive tool for assessing heart function
◆ Commonly given at rest and then repeated with exercise or after patient receives certain drugs

PURPOSE

◆ To assess the function of the heart
◆ To detect certain heart conditions

PREPARATION

◆ Make sure the patient or a responsible family member has signed an informed consent form.
◆ Reassure the patient that the tracer poses no radiation hazard and rarely produces adverse effects.
◆ No dietary restrictions are required.

Teaching points

◆ Tell the patient that he'll receive an I.V. injection of a radioactive tracer and that a detector positioned above his chest will record the circulation of this tracer through the heart.
◆ Explain who will perform the test and where it'll be done.
◆ Tell the patient that fasting isn't needed before the test.
◆ Inform the patient that he may experience slight discomfort from the needle puncture, but that the imaging itself is painless.
◆ Instruct the patient to remain silent and motionless during imaging, unless otherwise instructed.

DIAGNOSTIC PROCEDURE

KEY STEPS

◆ Confirm the patient's identity using two patient identifiers according to facility policy.
◆ A radioactive isotope is injected into the patient's vein.
◆ Radioactive isotopes attach to red blood cells and pass through the heart in the circulation.
◆ The isotopes are traced through the heart by a scintillation camera.
◆ For the next minute, the scintillation camera records the first pass of the isotope through the heart so that the aortic and mitral valves can be located.
◆ Using an electrocardiogram, the camera is gated for selected 60-msec intervals, representing end-systole and end-diastole, and 500 to 1,000 cardiac cycles are recorded on X-ray or Polaroid film.

POSTPROCEDURE CARE

◆ Answer the patient's questions.
◆ Inform the practitioner of abnormal results.

PRECAUTIONS

◆ Movement during the examination may interfere with the image. Have the patient remain as still as possible.

COMPLICATIONS

◆ None

INTERPRETATION

NORMAL RESULTS

◆ The left ventricle contracts symmetrically, and the isotope appears evenly distributed in the scans.

ABNORMAL RESULTS

◆ Patients with coronary artery disease usually have asymmetrical blood distribution to the myocardium, which produces segmental abnormalities of ventricular wall motion; such abnormalities may also result from preexisting conditions such as myocarditis.
◆ Patients with cardiomyopathy show globally reduced ejection fractions. In patients with left-to-right shunts, the recirculating radioisotope prolongs the downslope of the curve of scintigraphic data; early arrival of activity in the left ventricle or aorta signifies a right-to-left shunt.

Myelography

DESCRIPTION
- Combines fluoroscopy and radiography to evaluate the spinal subarachnoid space after injection of a contrast medium
- Fluoroscopy: shows flow of contrast medium and outlines subarachnoid space

PURPOSE
- To demonstrate lesions partially or totally blocking cerebrospinal fluid (CSF) flow in the subarachnoid space (such as tumors and herniated intervertebral disks)
- To detect arachnoiditis, spinal nerve root injury, or tumors in the posterior fossa of the skull

PREPARATION
- Make sure the patient has signed a consent form.
- Withhold food and fluid for 8 hours before the test.
- Check the patient's history for hypersensitivity to iodine and iodine-containing substances (such as shellfish) and contrast media.
- A patient undergoing lumbar puncture may need an enema.
- Give the patient a sedative and an anticholinergic.

Teaching points
- Explain the purpose of the test and how it's done.
- Explain who will perform the test and where it'll be done.
- Instruct the patient to fast for 8 hours before the test.
- Warn the patient that he may feel transient burning, flushing, warmth, headache, salty taste, or nausea and vomiting when the contrast medium is injected.
- Instruct the patient to resume his usual diet and activities 1 day after the test.

DIAGNOSTIC PROCEDURE

KEY STEPS
- Confirm the patient's identity using two patient identifiers according to facility policy.
- The patient is positioned on his side at the edge of the table with his knees drawn up to his abdomen and his chin on his chest.
- The patient may receive a cisternal puncture if lumbar deformity or infection at the puncture site exists.
- A lumbar puncture is performed.
- Fluoroscopy verifies proper needle position in the subarachnoid space.
- Some CSF may be removed for routine laboratory analysis.
- The patient is placed in the prone position.
- The contrast medium is injected.
- If a subarachnoid space obstruction blocks the upward flow of the contrast medium, a cisternal puncture may be performed.
- The flow of the contrast medium is studied with fluoroscopy; X-rays are taken.
- The contrast medium is withdrawn, if oil-based, and the needle is removed.
- The puncture site is cleaned and a small dressing applied.
- If a spinal tumor is confirmed, the patient may go directly to the operating room.

POSTPROCEDURE CARE
- If the patient received an oil-based contrast medium, keep him flat in bed for 8 to 12 hours.
- If he received a water-based contrast medium, elevate the head of the bed for 6 to 8 hours.
- If the test involved a water-based contrast, make sure that the large dye load doesn't reach the surface of the brain; to prevent this, keep the patient's head elevated 30 to 45 degrees after the procedure.
- Encourage the patient to drink fluids to assist the kidneys in eliminating the contrast medium.
- Notify the practitioner if the patient fails to void within 8 hours.

- Monitor the patient's vital signs and intake and output.
- Monitor the patient's neurologic status.
- Observe the puncture site.
- Watch for bleeding and infection.
- Monitor the patient for seizure activity.

PRECAUTIONS
WARNING *If radicular pain, fever, back pain, or signs and symptoms of meningeal irritation (such as headache, irritability, or neck stiffness) develop, inform the practitioner immediately. Keep the room quiet and dark, and provide an analgesic or an antipyretic.*
- Notify the radiologist if the patient has a history of epilepsy or of antidepressant or phenothiazine use; phenothiazines given with metrizamide during myelography increases the risk of toxicity.

COMPLICATIONS
- Bleeding
- Infection
- Meningeal irritation
- Seizures
- Dehydration

INTERPRETATION

NORMAL RESULTS
- The contrast medium flows freely through the subarachnoid space.
- No obstruction or structural abnormality is found.

ABNORMAL RESULTS
- Extradural lesions suggest herniated intervertebral disks, or metastatic tumors.
- Lesions within the subarachnoid space suggest neurofibromas or meningiomas.
- Lesions within the spinal cord suggest ependymomas or astrocytomas.
- Fluid-filled cavities in the spinal cord and widening of the cord itself suggest possible syringomyelia.

Myoglobin test

DESCRIPTION

- Oxygen-binding muscle protein found in skeletal and cardiac muscle
- Muscle ischemia, trauma, and inflammation: cause myoglobin's release into blood
- Release into blood important when determining damaged cardiac muscle
- Creatine kinase (CK) and its isoform CK-MB: released more slowly than myoglobin during myocardial infarction (MI)
- Myoglobin: detected as soon as 2 hours after onset of chest pain; peaks in 4 hours; can be early indicator of MI

PURPOSE

- To estimate damage to skeletal or cardiac muscle tissue (nonspecific test)
- To determine if an MI has occurred (specific test)
- To predict flare-ups of polymyositis

PREPARATION

- Obtain a patient history, including disorders that may be associated with increased myoglobin levels.
- The test requires a blood sample.
- No dietary restrictions are required.

Teaching points

- Explain the purpose of the test.
- Explain who will perform the test and where it'll be done.
- Tell the patient he need not restrict food or fluids.
- Tell him that the test requires a blood sample and that he may experience slight discomfort from the tourniquet and needle puncture.
- Inform the patient that the results need to be correlated with other tests for a definitive diagnosis.
- Tell him that the test takes less than 5 minutes.

KEY STEPS

- Confirm the patient's identity using two patient identifiers according to facility policy.
- Perform a venipuncture and collect the sample in a 4-ml tube with no additives.
- Expect to collect blood samples 4 to 8 hours after the onset of an acute MI.

POSTPROCEDURE CARE

- Apply direct pressure to the venipuncture site until the bleeding stops.
- Inform the practitioner of abnormal results.

PRECAUTIONS

- Handle the sample gently to prevent hemolysis.
- Send the sample to the laboratory immediately.

COMPLICATIONS

- Hematoma at the venipuncture site

NORMAL RESULTS

- Value is 0 to 0.09 mcg/ml (SI, 5 to 70 nmol/L).

ABNORMAL RESULTS

- Besides MI, increased myoglobin levels may occur in acute alcohol intoxication, dermatomyositis, hypothermia (with prolonged shivering), muscular dystrophy, polymyositis, rhabdomyolysis, severe burns, trauma, severe renal failure, and systemic lupus erythematosus.

  INTERFERING FACTORS *Recent angina or cardioversion (may increase levels)*

Myoglobin, urine

DESCRIPTION

- Detects presence of myoglobin (red pigment in cytoplasm of cardiac and skeletal muscle cells) in urine
- In extensively damaged muscle cells (such as disease or severe crushing trauma): myoglobin released into blood, quickly cleared by renal glomerular filtration, and eliminated in urine (myoglobinuria)
- Appears in urine within 24 hours after myocardial infarction (MI)
- Must be differentiated from urine hemoglobin because of marked structural similarities: Hemoglobin, bound to haptoglobin: precipitates in urine mixed with ammonium sulfate; myoglobin remains soluble and can be measured
- Differential precipitation test commonly used

PURPOSE

- To help diagnose muscular disease or rhabdomyolysis
- To detect extensive infarction of muscle tissue
- To assess the extent of muscular damage from crushing trauma

PREPARATION

- No dietary restrictions are required.
- The test requires a random urine specimen.

Teaching points

- Explain that the urine myoglobin test detects a red pigment found in muscle cells and helps evaluate muscle injury or disease.
- Inform the patient that he need not restrict food or fluids.
- Tell the patient that this test requires a random urine specimen, and teach him the proper collection technique.
- Tell the patient that the test should take less than 10 minutes.

KEY STEPS

- Confirm the patient's identity using two patient identifiers according to facility policy.
- Collect a random urine specimen.

POSTPROCEDURE CARE

- Answer the patient's questions.
- Inform the practitioner of abnormal results.

PRECAUTIONS

- Send the specimen to the laboratory immediately.

COMPLICATIONS

- None

NORMAL RESULTS

- Myoglobin doesn't appear in urine.

ABNORMAL RESULTS

- Myoglobinuria occurs in acute or chronic muscular disease, alcoholic polymyopathy, familial myoglobinuria, extensive MI, and in severe trauma to the skeletal muscles (resulting from a crush injury, extreme hyperthermia, or severe burns).
- It also occurs in strenuous or prolonged exercise but disappears after rest.

Nasopharyngeal culture

DESCRIPTION
◆ Makes preliminary identification of organisms to guide clinical management and determine the need for additional testing
◆ Requires subsequent susceptibility testing to determine appropriate antimicrobial therapy

PURPOSE
◆ To identify pathogens causing upper respiratory tract symptoms
◆ To identify *Bordetella pertussis* and *Neisseria meningitidis*, especially in very young, elderly, or debilitated patients and asymptomatic carriers
◆ To isolate viruses, especially in carriers of influenza viruses A and B

PREPARATION
◆ No dietary restrictions are required.

Teaching points
◆ Explain that this test isolates the cause of nasopharyngeal infection.
◆ Explain who will perform the test and where it'll be done.
◆ Tell the patient he need not restrict food or fluids.
◆ Tell the patient that secretions will be obtained from the back of his nose and throat, using a cotton-tipped swab.
◆ Warn the patient that he may experience slight discomfort and gagging.
◆ Reassure the patient that obtaining the specimen takes less than 15 seconds.

DIAGNOSTIC PROCEDURE

KEY STEPS
◆ Confirm the patient's identity using two patient identifiers according to facility policy.
◆ Moisten the swab with sterile water or saline solution.
◆ Have the patient cough before beginning to collect the specimen.
◆ Position the patient with his head tilted back.

◆ Using a penlight and a tongue blade, inspect the nasopharyngeal area.
◆ Gently pass the swab through the nostril and into the nasopharynx, keeping the swab near the septum and floor of the nose. Rotate the swab quickly and remove it.
◆ Or, place a glass tube in the patient's nostril and carefully pass the swab through the tube into the nasopharynx. Rotate the swab for 5 seconds and then place it in the culture tube with transport medium. Remove the glass tube. (See *Obtaining a nasopharyngeal specimen.*)
◆ Label the specimen with the patient's name, the practitioner's name, the date and time of collection, the origin of the material, and the suspected organism.
◆ Ideally, fresh culture medium should be inoculated with specimens for *B. pertussis* at the patient's bedside because of the organism's susceptibility to environmental changes.
◆ If specimen collection is to isolate a virus, follow the laboratory's recommended collection technique.
◆ To prevent specimen contamination, don't let the swab touch the sides of the patient's nostril or his tongue.
◆ Note antimicrobial therapy or chemotherapy on the laboratory request.
◆ Keep the container upright.

Obtaining a nasopharyngeal specimen

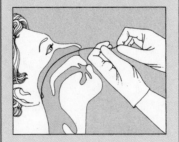

When the swab passes into the nasopharynx, gently but quickly rotate it to collect a specimen. Then remove the swab, taking care not to injure the nasal mucous membrane.

◆ Tell the laboratory if the suspected organism is *Corynebacterium diphtheriae* or *B. pertussis* because these need special growth media.
◆ If *B. pertussis* is suspected, use Dacron or calcium alginate mini-tipped swabs for collection.
◆ When specimens can't be directly placed onto growth media, the best media-based transport is one supplemented with antibiotics to reduce the growth of normal flora.

POSTPROCEDURE CARE
◆ Answer the patient's questions.
◆ Inform the practitioner of abnormal results.

PRECAUTIONS
◆ Refrigerate a viral specimen according to the laboratory's procedure.
◆ Wear gloves when performing the procedure and handling the specimen.

COMPLICATIONS
WARNING *Laryngospasm may occur after the culture is obtained if the patient has epiglottiditis or diphtheria. Have resuscitation equipment available.*

INTERPRETATION

NORMAL RESULTS
◆ Nonhemolytic streptococci, alpha-hemolytic streptococci, *Neisseria* species (except *N. meningitidis* and *N. gonorrhoeae*), coagulase-negative staphylococci such as *Staphylococcus epidermidis,* and occasionally coagulase-positive *S. aureus* are present.

ABNORMAL RESULTS
◆ Group A beta-hemolytic *streptococci;* occasionally groups B, C, and G beta-hemolytic *streptococci; B. pertussis, C. diphtheriae,* and *S. aureus;* large numbers of pneumococci; *Haemophilus influenzae;* myxovirus influenzae; paramyxoviruses; *Candida albicans; mycoplasma* species; and *Mycobacterium* tuberculosis are present.

Neonatal thyroid-stimulating hormone test

DESCRIPTION
- Immunoassay confirms congenital hypothyroidism after screening test detects low thyroxine (T_4) levels
- Thyroid-stimulating hormone (TSH): levels surge after birth, triggering a rise in thyroid hormone (essential for neurologic development)
- Congenital hypothyroidism: thyroid gland doesn't respond to TSH stimulation; results in diminished thyroid hormone levels and elevated TSH levels; early detection and treatment critical to prevent mental retardation and cretinism

PURPOSE
- To confirm diagnosis of congenital hypothyroidism

PREPARATION
- No dietary restrictions are required.

Teaching points
- Explain that this test helps confirm the diagnosis of congenital hypothyroidism.
- Stress the importance of detecting the disorder early so that prompt therapy can prevent irreversible brain damage.
- Explain who will perform the test and where it'll be done.
- Tell the parents that no dietary restrictions are required.
- Tell the parents that the test should take less than 5 minutes.

KEY STEPS
- Confirm the patient's identity using two patient identifiers according to facility policy.

Filter paper sample
- Assemble the necessary equipment, wash your hands thoroughly, and put on gloves.
- Wipe the infant's heel with an alcohol or povidone-iodine swab, and then dry it thoroughly with a gauze pad.
- Perform a heelstick. Squeezing the infant's heel gently, fill the circles on the filter paper with blood. Make sure the blood saturates the paper.
- Allow the filter paper to dry, label it appropriately, and send it to the laboratory.

Serum sample
- Perform a venipuncture and collect the sample in a 3-ml clot-activator tube.

POSTPROCEDURE CARE
- Apply direct pressure to the venipuncture or heelstick site until bleeding stops.
- Inform the practitioner of abnormal results.

PRECAUTIONS
- Maintain standard precautions while collecting the sample.
- Label the sample and send it to the laboratory immediately.

COMPLICATIONS
- Hematoma at the venipuncture site

NORMAL RESULTS
- TSH level at age 1 to 2 days, 25 to 30 µIU/ml (SI, 25 to 30 mU/L).
- TSH level after age 1 to 2 days, less than 25 µIU/ml (SI, < 25 mU/L).

ABNORMAL RESULTS
- Neonatal TSH levels must be interpreted in light of the T_4 level.
- Increased TSH levels with decreased T_4 levels indicate primary congenital hypothyroidism (thyroid gland dysfunction).
- Decreased TSH and T_4 levels may indicate secondary congenital hypothyroidism (pituitary or hypothalamic dysfunction).
- Normal TSH levels with decreased T_4 levels may indicate hypothyroidism caused by a congenital defect in T_4-binding globulin or transient congenital hypothyroidism caused by prematurity or prenatal hypoxia. A complete thyroid workup must be done to confirm the cause of hypothyroidism before starting treatment.

Nephrotomography

DESCRIPTION

◆ Presents images as "slices" or linear layers of the kidneys; structures in front of and behind the selected planes appear blurry
◆ Produces film images of the renal arterial network and parenchyma before and after opacification with contrast medium
◆ Separate procedure or adjunct to excretory urography

PURPOSE

◆ To differentiate between a simple renal cyst and a solid neoplasm
◆ To assess renal lacerations
◆ To assess posttraumatic nonperfused areas of the kidneys
◆ To localize adrenal tumors
◆ To show space-occupying lesions

PREPARATION

◆ Make sure the patient has signed an appropriate consent form.
◆ Note and report allergies.
◆ Check the patient's history for hypersensitivity to iodine or iodine-containing foods (such as shellfish) or to iodinated contrast media.
◆ If the patient has a history of I.V. contrast hypersensitivity, inform the practitioner so that a prophylaxis (such as diphenhydramine [Benadryl]) or a low osmolar contrast medium can be used.
◆ Check the serum creatinine level and inform the practitioner if it's greater than 1.5 mg/dl. (I.V. fluids may be ordered.)
◆ The diet must be restricted for 8 hours before the test.

Teaching points

◆ Explain the purpose of the test and how it's done.
◆ Explain who will perform the test and where it'll be done.
◆ Instruct the patient to fast for 8 hours before the test.

◆ Warn the patient that he may experience transient adverse effects from the contrast medium injection (such as burning, stinging at the injection site, flushing, and a metallic taste).
◆ Tell him that he may hear loud, clacking sounds as the films are exposed.
◆ Tell the patient the test takes less than 1 hour.

DIAGNOSTIC PROCEDURE

KEY STEPS

◆ Confirm the patient's identity using two patient identifiers according to facility policy.
◆ A plain film of the kidneys is obtained.
◆ Preliminary tomograms are obtained and reviewed.
◆ A contrast medium is administered I.V., using either a bolus or infusion method.
◆ Serial tomograms are obtained.

POSTPROCEDURE CARE

◆ Ensure adequate hydration.
◆ Monitor the patient's vital signs and intake and output.
◆ Monitor the patient's serum creatinine levels.
◆ Observe him for signs and symptoms of a posttest allergic reaction to the contrast medium (such as flushing, nausea, urticaria, and sneezing) or an anaphylactic reaction.

◆ Inform the practitioner of abnormal results.
◆ After the test, tell the patient to resume his normal diet and activity.

PRECAUTIONS

◆ The procedure is performed with extreme caution in patients with impaired renal function (serum creatinine levels above 1.5 mg/dl) and especially in elderly and dehydrated patients.

COMPLICATIONS

◆ Adverse reaction to the contrast medium
◆ Impaired renal function

INTERPRETATION

NORMAL RESULTS

◆ The size, shape, and position of the kidneys are normal.
◆ No space-occupying lesions or other abnormalities are noted.

ABNORMAL RESULTS

◆ Various structural abnormalities, such as simple cysts and solid tumors, are noted. (See *Simple cyst or solid tumor: Differential diagnosis in nephrotomography.*)

Simple cyst or solid tumor: Differential diagnosis in nephrotomography

FEATURE	CYST	TUMOR
Consistency	Homogeneous	Irregular
Contact with healthy renal tissue	Sharply distinct	Poorly resolved
Density	Radiolucent	Variable radiolucent patches (or same as normal renal parenchyma)
Shape	Spheric	Variable
Wall of lesion	Thin and well defined	Thick and irregular

Neutrophils test

DESCRIPTION

- One of five types of white blood cells (WBCs)
- Help protect the body against infection and aid immune system
- More than 50% of WBCs in peripheral circulation
- Quickly phagocytize significant quantities of microorganisms; body's first line of defense against infection
- Each mature neutrophil inactivates 5 to 20 bacteria

PURPOSE

- To reveal whether neutrophils are present in normal proportion to one another, if one cell type is increased or decreased, or if immature cells are present
- To help diagnose specific types of illnesses that affect the immune system

PREPARATION

- No dietary restrictions are required.
- The test requires a blood sample.

Teaching points

- Explain the purpose of the test and how it's done.
- Explain who will perform the test and where it'll be done.
- Tell the patient that fasting isn't required before the test.
- Inform the patient that the test requires a blood sample and that he may experience slight discomfort from the tourniquet and needle puncture.
- Tell him the test takes less than 5 minutes.

KEY STEPS

- Confirm the patient's identity using two patient identifiers according to facility policy.
- Perform the venipuncture.

POSTPROCEDURE CARE

- Apply direct pressure to the venipuncture site until the bleeding stops.
- Inform the practitioner of abnormal results.

PRECAUTIONS

- Maintain standard precautions while collecting the sample.

COMPLICATIONS

- Hematoma at the venipuncture site

NORMAL RESULTS

- A small number of slightly immature neutrophils, known as *band cells,* are present in peripheral blood.

ABNORMAL RESULTS

- The presence of many band cells and their precursors, known as a *shift to the left,* indicates infection.
- The presence of mature, hypersegmented neutrophils that have more nuclear segments than normal, known as a *shift to the right,* indicates pernicious anemia and hepatic disease.
- Increased band cells and a low total WBC count, known as a *degenerative shift,* indicate bone marrow depression (as in typhoid fever).
- Increased band cells, metamyelocytes, and myelocytes and a high WBC count, known as a *regenerative shift,* indicate stimulation of the bone marrow (as in pneumonia and appendicitis).

Nuclear medicine scanning

OVERVIEW

DESCRIPTION

◆ Imaging of specific body organs or systems by a scintillating scanning camera after I.V. injection, inhalation, or oral ingestion of a radioactive tracer compound

PURPOSE

◆ To produce tissue analysis and images not readily seen on standard X-rays
◆ To detect or rule out malignant lesions when X-ray findings are normal or questionable

PREPARATION

◆ Make sure the patient has signed an appropriate consent form.
◆ Note and report allergies.
◆ Note prior nuclear medicine procedures.
◆ Review dietary restrictions based on exact test.
◆ It's important that the patient remain still during the procedure.

Teaching points

◆ Explain the purpose of the test and how it's done.
◆ Explain who will perform the test and where it'll be done.
◆ Advise the patient to remain still during the procedure and that he'll be asked to take various positions on a scanner table.
◆ Tell him the test takes about 1½ hours, but the time may vary based on the exact test.
◆ Explain dietary restrictions based on exact test.

DIAGNOSTIC PROCEDURE

KEY STEPS

◆ Confirm the patient's identity using two patient identifiers according to facility policy.
◆ If the patient will receive an I.V. tracer isotope, an I.V. line is started.
◆ The detector of a scintillation camera is directed at the area being scanned and displays the image on a monitor.
◆ Scintigraphs are obtained and reviewed for clarity.
◆ If necessary, additional views are obtained.

POSTPROCEDURE CARE

◆ Monitor the patient's vital signs.
◆ Observe the injection site.
◆ Watch the patient for infection and orthostatic hypotension.
◆ Inform the practitioner of abnormal results.
◆ Tell the patient to resume his normal diet and activities.

PRECAUTIONS

◆ Make sure the patient isn't scheduled for more than one radionuclide scan on the same day.

COMPLICATIONS

◆ Infection
◆ Orthostatic hypotension

INTERPRETATION

NORMAL RESULTS

◆ See the specific nuclear medicine scan.

ABNORMAL RESULTS

◆ See the specific nuclear medicine scan.

5′-nucleotidase level test

DESCRIPTION

- More difficult than alkaline phosphatase (ALP) assay
- Measures level of serum 5′-nucleotidase (5′NT) — phosphatase formed almost entirely in hepatobiliary tract
- Unlike ALP, 5′NT hydrolyzes nucleoside 58-phosphate groups only
- Helps determine whether ALP elevation is caused by skeletal or hepatic disease
- 5′NT remains normal in skeletal disease and pregnancy; more specific for assessing hepatic dysfunction than ALP or leucine aminopeptidase
- Not widely used as liver function study but may be more sensitive than ALP to diagnose cholangitis, biliary cirrhosis, and malignant infiltrations of the liver
- Used to determine if ALP elevation is caused by skeletal or hepatic disease

PURPOSE

- To distinguish between hepatobiliary and skeletal disease when the source of increased ALP levels is uncertain
- To help differentiate biliary obstruction from acute hepatocellular damage
- To detect hepatic metastasis in the absence of jaundice

PREPARATION

- The test requires a blood sample.
- No dietary restrictions are required.

Teaching points

- Explain that this test evaluates liver function.
- Explain who will perform the test and where it'll be done.
- Tell the patient that the test requires a blood sample and that he may experience slight discomfort from the tourniquet and needle puncture.
- Inform the patient that he need not restrict food or fluids.
- Tell him the test takes less than 5 minutes.

KEY STEPS

- Confirm the patient's identity using two patient identifiers according to facility policy.
- Perform a venipuncture and collect the sample in a 4-ml tube without additives.

POSTPROCEDURE CARE

- Apply direct pressure to the venipuncture site until the bleeding stops.
- Inform the practitioner of abnormal results.

PRECAUTIONS

- Maintain standard precautions while collecting the sample.
- Handle the sample gently to prevent hemolysis.

COMPLICATIONS

- Hematoma at the venipuncture site

NORMAL RESULTS

- Levels in adults range from 2 to 17 units/L (SI, 0.03 to 0.29 µkat/L); values for children are lower.

ABNORMAL RESULTS

- Extremely high levels of 5′NT occur in common bile duct obstruction by calculi or tumors in diseases that cause severe intrahepatic cholestasis such as neoplastic infiltrations of the liver.
- Slight to moderate increases may reflect acute hepatocellular damage or active cirrhosis.

Ocular ultrasonography

DESCRIPTION

- Transmits high-frequency sound waves through the eye and measures their reflection from ocular structures
- Provides one-dimensional image; scan converts echoes into waveforms whose crests represent positions of different structures
- B-scan: converts echoes into patterns of dots that form a two-dimensional, cross-sectional image of ocular structure
- Scan measures eye's axial length and characterizes tissue texture of abnormal lesions
- B-scan easier to interpret than A-scan; used more often to evaluate ocular structures and to diagnose abnormalities
- A- and B-scan combination yields most useful results
- Helps evaluate fundus clouded by an opaque medium (such as a cataract)
- May be done before cataract removal to ensure integrity of retina or to measure length of eye and curvature of cornea if implanting an intraocular lens
- Readily available and provides immediate information
- Identifies intraocular foreign bodies and determines their position in relation to ocular structures; also assesses severity of resulting ocular damage

PURPOSE

- To aid in evaluating the fundus in an eye with opacity such as a cataract
- To help diagnose vitreous disorders and retinal detachment
- To diagnose and differentiate between intraocular and orbital lesions and to follow their progression through serial examinations
- To locate intraocular foreign bodies
- To measure the dimensions of other tumors detectable by ophthalmoscopy

PREPARATION

- No dietary restrictions are required.

Teaching points

- Describe the procedure and explain that ocular ultrasonography evaluates the eye's structures.
- Explain who will perform the test and where it'll be done.
- Tell the patient that a small transducer will be placed on his closed eyelid and that the transducer transmits high-frequency sound waves that are reflected by the structures in the eye.
- Inform the patient that he may be asked to move his eyes or change his gaze during the procedure and that his cooperation is required to ensure accurate test results.
- Tell him that fasting isn't required.

KEY STEPS

- Confirm the patient's identity using two patient identifiers according to facility policy.
- The patient is placed in a supine position on an X-ray table.
- For the B-scan, the patient is asked to close his eyes, and a water-soluble gel (such as Goniosol) is applied to his eyelid. The transducer is then placed on the eyelid.
- For the A-scan, anesthetizing drops are instilled in the patient's eye, and a clear plastic eye cup is placed directly on the eyeball.
- A water-soluble gel is then applied to the eye cup, and the transducer is positioned on the medium.
- The transducer then transmits high-frequency sound waves into the patient's eye, and the resulting echoes are transformed into images or waveforms on the oscilloscope screen.

POSTPROCEDURE CARE

- After the test, remove the water-soluble gel from the patient's eyelid.
- Inform the practitioner of abnormal results.

PRECAUTIONS

- None

COMPLICATIONS

- None

NORMAL RESULTS

- The optic nerve and the posterior lens capsule produce echoes that take on characteristic forms on A- and B-scan images.
- The posterior wall of the eye appears as a smooth, concave curve; retrobulbar fat is also visible.
- The lens and vitreous humor are also visible.
- Normal orbital echo patterns depend on the position of the transducer and the position of the patient's gaze during the procedure.

ABNORMAL RESULTS

- In eyes clouded by a vitreous hemorrhage, organization of the hemorrhage is identifiable by the degree of density that appears on the image. The cause, prognosis, and associated abnormalities may be determined.
- Massive vitreous organization and vitreous bands are noted.
- Retinal detachment characteristically produces a dense, sheetlike echo on a B-scan and is commonly found in patients with an opacity.
- Intraocular tumors may be diagnosed and differentiated according to size, shape, location, and texture.
- Melanomas, metastatic tumors, hemangiomas, retinoblastomas, and cystic lesions may be present.
- Evidence of meningiomas, neurofibromas, gliomas, neurilemomas, or the inflammatory changes associated with Graves' disease may be observed.

Oculoplethysmography

DESCRIPTION

◆ Noninvasive procedure that indirectly measures blood flow in the ophthalmic artery
◆ Reflects carotid blood flow and cerebral circulation; not a reliable screening or diagnostic test for carotid artery disease
◆ Also called *OPG*
◆ Ocular pneumoplethysmography (OPG-Gee): indirectly measures ophthalmic artery pressures
◆ Carotid phonoangiography commonly used as complement to OPG

PURPOSE

◆ To help detect and evaluate carotid artery disease
◆ To evaluate symptoms of transient ischemic attacks
◆ To evaluate asymptomatic carotid bruits
◆ To evaluate nonhemispheric neurologic symptoms (such as dizziness, ataxia, or syncope)

PREPARATION

◆ Make sure the patient has signed an appropriate consent form.
◆ Note and report allergies.
◆ Have the patient remove his contact lenses before the procedure.
◆ Administer glaucoma medications and eyedrops as usual.
◆ No dietary restrictions are required.

Teaching points

◆ Explain the purpose of the test and how it's done.
◆ Explain who will perform the test and where it'll be done.
◆ Tell the patient that he need not restrict food or fluids.
◆ Advise the patient to take his usual glaucoma medications and eyedrops.
◆ Tell the patient that his eyes may burn slightly after instillation of the anesthetic eyedrops.
◆ Warn the patient that, if OPG-Gee is scheduled, he may experience transient loss of vision when his eyes receive suction.
◆ Instruct the patient to avoid blinking or moving during the procedure.
◆ Tell the patient that the test takes only a few minutes.
◆ Instruct the patient not to rub his eyes for 2 hours after the test to prevent corneal abrasions.
◆ Instruct the patient not to reinsert contact lenses for about 2 hours after OPG.

KEY STEPS

◆ Confirm the patient's identity using two patient identifiers according to facility policy.

OPG

◆ Anesthetic eyedrops are instilled and small photoelectric cells are attached to the patient's earlobes.
◆ Tracings for both ears are taken and compared.
◆ Eyecups resembling contact lenses are applied to the corneas and held in place with light suction (40 to 50 mm Hg).
◆ Tracings of the pulsations within each eye are compared with each other and with right ear tracings.

OPG-Gee

◆ Anesthetic eyedrops are instilled.
◆ Eyecups are attached to the sclerae.
◆ A vacuum of 300 mm Hg is applied to each eye, corresponding to a mean pressure of 100 mm Hg in the ophthalmic artery.
◆ When suction is applied, the pulse in both eyes disappears.
◆ The pressure is gradually released.
◆ The eye pulses should return simultaneously.
◆ Pulse arrival times are converted to ophthalmic artery pressures and then compared.
◆ Both brachial pressures are taken.
◆ The higher systolic pressure is compared with the ophthalmic artery pressures. (See *OPG examination and tracings*, page 344.)
◆ Pulse arrival times in the eyes and ears are measured and compared.
◆ If indicated, cerebral angiography may follow.

POSTPROCEDURE CARE

◆ Tell the patient that mild burning is normal as the eyedrops wear off, but to report severe burning.

PRECAUTIONS

◆ Observe for and immediately report symptoms of corneal abrasion, such as pain and photophobia.

COMPLICATIONS

◆ Corneal abrasion
◆ Scleral hematoma

(continued)

OPG examination and tracings

The patient shown here is undergoing oculoplethysmography (OPG). The eyecups on the patient's corneas detect ocular pulsations, which are compared with each other and with the blood flow in the ear. Blood flow in the ear is detected by a small photoelectric cell (not shown).

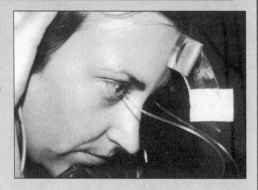

The OPG tracing at right is normal, showing simultaneous pulsations in the right and left eyes and in the right ear. The differential waveform of ocular pulses (horizontal waveform), which amplifies pulse differences, and the vertical lines drawn on valleys and peaks of pulses, to indicate pulse delays, confirm simultaneous pulsation.

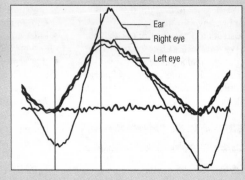

Ear
Right eye
Left eye

The OPG tracing at right is abnormal; the left-eye pulsation (vertical lines) arrives later than the other two pulsations, indicating left internal carotid artery stenosis. Note the elevation of the differential waveform.

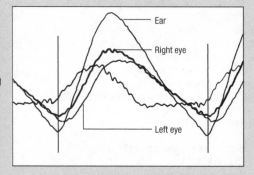

Ear
Right eye
Left eye

NORMAL RESULTS

- In OPG, all pulses occur simultaneously.
- In OPG-Gee, the difference between ophthalmic artery pressures should be less than 5 mm Hg.
- Ophthalmic artery pressure divided by the higher brachial systolic pressure should exceed 0.67.

ABNORMAL RESULTS
OPG

- Reduced rate of blood flow during systole and delayed arrival of a pulse in the ipsilateral eye suggest carotid occlusive disease.
- Reveals only severe narrowing or occlusion and can't be used as a reliable screening or diagnostic test for carotid artery disease.

OPG-Gee

- A difference between ophthalmic artery pressures of more than 5 mm Hg suggests the presence of carotid occlusive disease on the side with the lower pressure.
- A ratio between the ophthalmic artery pressure and the higher brachial systolic pressure of less than 0.67 reinforces the diagnosis of carotid occlusive disease.
- The lower the ratio, the more severe the stenosis.

Oral cholecystography

OVERVIEW

DESCRIPTION
- Radiographic examination of the gallbladder after administration of a contrast medium
- Indicated for patients with symptoms of biliary tract disease
- Usually done to confirm gallbladder disease

PURPOSE
- To detect gallstones
- To help diagnose inflammatory disease and tumors of the gallbladder

PREPARATION
- Make sure the patient has signed an appropriate consent form.
- Note and report allergies.
- Make sure that the patient has nothing to eat or drink, except water, after the evening meal.
- Give the patient an oral contrast agent (usually tablets), 2 to 3 hours after the evening meal.
- Examine vomitus or diarrhea for undigested tablets. If noted, notify the practitioner and the radiography department.
- Give an enema the morning of the test if ordered.

Teaching points
- Explain the purpose of the test and how it's done.
- Explain who will perform the test and where it'll be done.
- Instruct the patient to eat a meal containing fat at noon the day before the test to stimulate release of bile from the gallbladder.
- Instruct him to eat a fat-free meal in the evening to inhibit gallbladder contraction and to promote bile accumulation.
- Tell the patient the test usually takes 30 to 45 minutes.

DIAGNOSTIC PROCEDURE

KEY STEPS
- Confirm the patient's identity using two patient identifiers according to facility policy.
- A fluoroscopic examination is performed to evaluate gallbladder opacification.
- Various positions are used to detect filling defects.
- A fat stimulus, such as a high-fat meal or a synthetic fat-containing agent, may be given.
- The emptying of the gallbladder is observed in response to the fat stimulus and spot films are taken to show the common bile duct.
- If the gallbladder empties slowly or not at all, delayed films are taken.

POSTPROCEDURE CARE
- If the test results are normal, instruct the patient to resume his usual diet.
- Inform the practitioner of abnormal results.
- If gallstones are present, the patient needs an appropriate diet, usually fat-restricted, to help prevent acute attacks.

PRECAUTIONS
- Before repeating oral cholecystography, the patient must continue a low-fat diet until a definitive diagnosis can be made.

COMPLICATIONS
- Adverse reaction to contrast medium

INTERPRETATION

NORMAL RESULTS
- Opacification of the gallbladder is observed.
- The gallbladder appears pear-shaped with smooth, thin walls.

ABNORMAL RESULTS
- Filling defects may indicate gallstones.
- Fixed defects may indicate polyps or a benign tumor.
- Failed or faint opacification may indicate inflammatory disease, such as cholecystitis, with or without gallstones.
- Failure of the gallbladder to contract following stimulation by a fatty meal may indicate cholecystitis or common bile duct obstruction.

Oral glucose tolerance test

OVERVIEW

DESCRIPTION

- Most sensitive method of evaluating borderline cases of diabetes mellitus
- Involves monitoring of plasma and urine glucose levels for 3 hours after ingestion of a challenge dose of glucose to assess insulin secretion and the body's ability to metabolize glucose

PURPOSE

- To confirm diabetes mellitus in selected patients
- To help diagnose hypoglycemia and malabsorption syndrome

PREPARATION

- Notify the laboratory and practitioner of drugs the patient is taking that may affect test results; they may be restricted.
- The test requires five blood samples and usually five urine specimens.

Teaching points

- Explain that the oral glucose tolerance test evaluates glucose metabolism.
- Explain who will perform the test and where it'll be done.
- Instruct the patient to maintain a high-carbohydrate diet for 3 days and then to fast for 10 to 16 hours before the test.
- Tell him not to smoke, drink coffee or alcohol, or exercise strenuously for 8 hours before or during the test.
- Tell the patient that this test requires five blood samples and usually five urine specimens.
- Warn him about the symptoms of hypoglycemia (such as weakness, restlessness, nervousness, hunger, and sweating) and tell him to report them immediately.
- Tell the patient the procedure usually takes 3 hours but can last as long as 6 hours.

DIAGNOSTIC PROCEDURE

KEY STEPS

- Confirm the patient's identity using two patient identifiers according to facility policy.
- Between 7 a.m. and 9 a.m., perform a venipuncture to obtain a fasting blood sample in a 7-ml clot-activator tube.
- A saline lock may be inserted and used to collect the multiple blood samples per facility protocol.
- Collect a urine specimen at the same time if your facility includes this as part of the test.
- After collecting these samples and specimens, give the test load of oral glucose and record the time of ingestion. Encourage the patient to drink the entire glucose solution within 5 minutes.
- Encourage the patient to drink water during the test to promote adequate urine excretion.
- Draw blood samples 30 minutes, 1 hour, 2 hours, and 3 hours after giving the loading dose, using 7-ml clot-activator tubes.
- Collect urine specimens at the same intervals.
- Specify when the patient last ate and the blood and urine collection times.
- Record the time the patient received his last pretest dose of insulin or oral antidiabetic drug.
- Tell the patient to lie down if he feels faint.

POSTPROCEDURE CARE

- Apply direct pressure to the venipuncture site until the bleeding stops.
- Inform the practitioner of abnormal results.

PRECAUTIONS

- Maintain standard precautions while collecting the samples and specimens.
- Send the blood samples and urine specimens to the laboratory immediately or refrigerate them.

COMPLICATIONS

- Hematoma at the venipuncture site

  WARNING *For severe hypoglycemia, notify the practitioner; draw a blood sample, record the time on the laboratory request, and stop the test (have the patient drink a glass of orange juice with sugar added or give I.V. glucose to reverse the reaction).*

INTERPRETATION

NORMAL RESULTS

- Plasma glucose levels peak at 160 to 180 mg/dl (SI, 8.8 to 9.9 mmol/L) within 30 minutes to 1 hour after the patient receives an oral glucose test dose; they return to fasting levels or lower within 2 to 3 hours.
- Urine glucose tests remain negative.

ABNORMAL RESULTS

- Decreased glucose tolerance, in which levels peak sharply before falling slowly to fasting levels, may confirm diabetes mellitus or may result from Cushing's disease, hemochromatosis, pheochromocytoma, or central nervous system lesions.
- Increased glucose tolerance, in which levels may peak at less than normal levels, may indicate insulinoma, malabsorption syndrome, adrenocortical insufficiency (Addison's disease), hypothyroidism, or hypopituitarism.

Oral lactose tolerance test

DESCRIPTION

- Measures plasma glucose levels after ingestion of a challenge dose of lactose
- Screens for lactose intolerance caused by lactase deficiency
- Absence or deficiency of lactase causes undigested lactose to remain in intestinal lumen, producing symptoms such as abdominal cramps and watery diarrhea
- True congenital lactase deficiency: rare
- Intolerance: develops with age-related decreased lactase levels

PURPOSE

- To detect lactose intolerance

PREPARATION

- Notify the laboratory and practitioner of drugs the patient is taking that may affect test results; they may be restricted.
- The patient should avoid food and fluids and strenuous activity for 8 hours before the test.
- The test requires four blood samples.

Teaching points

- Explain that this test determines if the patient's symptoms are caused by an inability to digest lactose.
- Explain who will perform the test and where it'll be done.
- Instruct the patient to fast and to avoid strenuous activity for 8 hours before the test.
- Tell him that the test requires four blood samples and that he may experience slight discomfort from the tourniquet and needle puncture.
- Tell the patient that the test may take up to 2 hours.

KEY STEPS

- Confirm the patient's identity using two patient identifiers according to facility policy.
- After the patient has fasted for 8 hours, perform a venipuncture and collect a blood sample in a 4-ml tube with sodium fluoride and potassium oxalate added.
- Give the test load of lactose: for an adult, 50 g of lactose dissolved in 400 ml of water; for a child, 50 g/m^2 of body surface area. Record the time of ingestion.
- Draw a blood sample 30, 60, and 120 minutes after giving the loading dose. Use a 4-ml tube with sodium fluoride and potassium oxalate added.
- If ordered, collect a feces specimen 5 hours after giving the loading dose.
- Send blood samples and feces specimen to the laboratory immediately or refrigerate them if transport is delayed.

POSTPROCEDURE CARE

- Apply direct pressure to the venipuncture site until the bleeding stops.
- Instruct the patient to resume his usual diet, medications, and activity stopped before the test.
- Inform the practitioner of abnormal results.

PRECAUTIONS

- Maintain standard precautions while collecting the samples.
- Specify the collection time on the laboratory requests.
- Watch for symptoms of lactose intolerance (such as abdominal cramps, nausea, bloating, flatulence, and watery diarrhea) caused by the loading dose.

COMPLICATIONS

- Hematoma at the venipuncture site

NORMAL RESULTS

- Plasma glucose levels rise over 20 mg/dl (SI, > 1.1 mmol/L) over fasting levels within 15 to 60 minutes after ingestion of the lactose loading dose.

ABNORMAL RESULTS

- A rise in plasma glucose of less than 20 mg/dl (SI, < 1.1 mmol/L) indicates lactose intolerance, as does feces acidity (pH, 5.5 or less) and high glucose content (> 1+ on the dipstick).
- Accompanying signs and symptoms provoked by the test also suggest, but don't confirm, the diagnosis because such signs and symptoms may appear in patients with normal lactase activity after a loading dose of lactose.
- Small-bowel biopsy with lactase assay may be needed to confirm the diagnosis.

Orbital computed tomography

DESCRIPTION

◆ Orbital computed tomography (CT): shows abnormalities not readily seen on standard X-rays; delineates their size, position, and relationship to adjoining structures
◆ Series of tomograms reconstructed by a computer and displayed as anatomic slices on a monitor
◆ Identifies space-occupying lesions earlier and more accurately than other radiographic techniques; also provides three-dimensional images of orbital structures, especially ocular muscles and optic nerve

PURPOSE

◆ To evaluate pathologies of the orbit and eye — especially expanding lesions and bone destruction
◆ To evaluate fractures of the orbit and adjoining structures, showing a complete three-dimensional view
◆ To determine the cause of unilateral exophthalmos

PREPARATION

◆ Make sure the patient has signed an appropriate consent form, if required.
◆ Check the patient's history for hypersensitivity reactions to iodine, shellfish, or contrast media; notify the practitioner of any sensitivity present.
◆ Withhold food and fluid, as appropriate, depending on type of procedure chosen for the patient.

Teaching points

◆ Describe the procedure and explain that the orbital CT scan shows the anatomy of the eye and its surrounding structures.
◆ Explain who will perform the test and where it'll be done.
◆ Tell the patient to remove jewelry, hairpins, or other metal objects in the X-ray field to allow for precise imaging of the orbital structures.
◆ If the patient won't be receiving contrast enhancement, tell him that fasting isn't required; if contrast enhancement is to be used, tell him to fast for 4 hours before the test.
◆ If the patient will receive a contrast medium, tell him that he may feel flushed and warm and may experience a transient headache, a salty or metallic taste, and nausea or vomiting after the injection.
◆ Tell the patient that a series of X-rays will be taken.
◆ Tell the patient that he'll lie on an X-ray table and that the head of the table will be moved into the scanner, which will rotate around his head and make loud clacking sounds.

DIAGNOSTIC PROCEDURE

KEY STEPS

◆ Confirm the patient's identity using two patient identifiers according to facility policy.
◆ Assist the patient into a supine position on the X-ray table with his head immobilized by straps, if required. Ask him to lie still.
◆ The head of the table is moved into the scanner, which rotates around the patient's head, taking X-rays.
◆ Information from the scan is stored on magnetic tapes, and the images are displayed on a monitor. It's possible to make photographs if a permanent record is needed.
◆ When this series of X-rays is complete, contrast enhancement is performed.
◆ The contrast medium is injected I.V., and a second series of scans is recorded.

POSTPROCEDURE CARE

◆ Inform the practitioner of abnormal results.
◆ After the test, instruct the patient to resume his usual diet.

PRECAUTIONS

◆ If the patient received a contrast medium, watch for its residual adverse effects, including headache, nausea, or vomiting.

COMPLICATIONS

◆ Adverse reaction to the contrast medium

NORMAL RESULTS

◆ Dense orbital bone provides a marked contrast to less dense periocular fat.
◆ The optic nerve and the medial and lateral rectus muscles are clearly defined.
◆ The rectus muscles appear as thin, dense bands on each side, behind the eye.
◆ The optic canals appear equal in size.

ABNORMAL RESULTS

◆ Intraorbital and extraorbital space-occupying lesions obscure the normal structures or cause orbital enlargement, indentation of the orbital walls, or bone destruction.
◆ Infiltrative lesions, such as lymphomas and metastatic carcinomas, appear as irregular areas of density.
◆ Encapsulated tumors, such as benign hemangiomas and meningiomas, appear as clearly defined masses of consistent density.
◆ Intracranial tumors may invade the orbit; thickening of the optic nerve may occur with gliomas, meningiomas, and secondary tumors that may cause enlargement of the optic canal.
◆ Early erosion or expansion of the medial orbital wall may arise from lesions in the ethmoidal cells (determines the cause of unilateral exophthalmos).
◆ Space-occupying lesions appear in the orbit or paranasal sinuses (causes exophthalmos).
◆ The medial and lateral rectus muscles thicken in proptosis (resulting from Graves' disease).
◆ Contrast medium may provide information about the circulation through abnormal ocular tissues.

Orbital radiography

OVERVIEW

DESCRIPTION
- Involves X-rays of the orbital structures, eyebrow, bridge of the nose, and cheekbone
- Tomograms may be taken with standard X-rays

PURPOSE
- To identify orbital fractures and disease
- To locate intraorbital or intraocular foreign bodies and changes to the structure of the eye, which may indicate various diseases
- To detect problems resulting from injury and trauma to the eye

PREPARATION
- Make sure the patient has signed an appropriate consent form.
- Note and report allergies.
- Have the patient remove any jewelry or metal objects that may interfere with a clear image.
- No dietary restrictions are required.

Teaching points
- Explain the purpose of the test and how it's done.
- Explain who will perform the test and where it'll be done.
- Tell the patient he need not restrict food or fluids.
- Advise the patient that positioning may cause some discomfort
- Tell the patient the test takes about 15 minutes.

DIAGNOSTIC PROCEDURE

KEY STEPS
- Confirm the patient's identity using two patient identifiers according to facility policy.
- Assist the patient into a supine position on the radiographic table, or seat him in a chair.
- If the patient is in severe pain from injury or trauma, give him an analgesic.
- A series of orbital X-rays is taken, including projections of the optical canal.
- Images of the unaffected eye may also be taken to compare its shapes and structures to those of the affected eye.
- Films are developed and checked for quality.

POSTPROCEDURE CARE
- Monitor the patient's response to the test.
- Inform the practitioner of abnormal results.

PRECAUTIONS
- Screen women for pregnancy.

COMPLICATIONS
- None

INTERPRETATION

NORMAL RESULTS
- Each orbit is composed of a roof, floor, and medial and lateral walls.
- The medial walls of both orbits are parallel to each other.
- The lateral walls of both orbits project toward each other.
- The superior orbital fissure lies in the back of the orbit, between the lateral wall and the roof. (See *Radiographic view of orbital structures.*)

ABNORMAL RESULTS
- Enlargement of an orbit suggests the presence of a lesion.
- Superior orbital fissure enlargement suggests possible orbital meningioma, intracranial conditions (such as pituitary tumors), or vascular anomalies.
- Optic canal enlargement suggests possible extraocular extension of a retinoblastoma, or indicates irritation from an injury or foreign body.
- Destruction of the orbital walls suggests possible malignant neoplasm or infection.
- A child's orbit is more likely to be enlarged by a fast-growing lesion because the orbital bones aren't fully developed.
- Clear-cut local indentations of the orbital wall suggest a benign tumor or cyst.
- Increased bone density suggests possible conditions, such as osteoblastic metastasis, sphenoid ridge meningioma, or Paget's disease.

Radiographic view of orbital structures

Illustrated below are the structures demonstrated by orbital radiography.

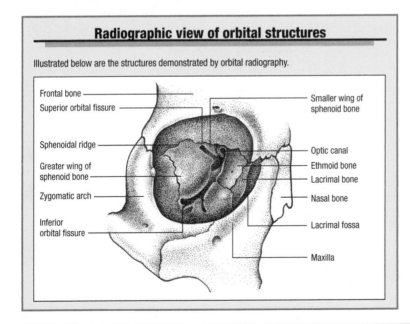

Frontal bone
Superior orbital fissure
Sphenoidal ridge
Greater wing of sphenoid bone
Zygomatic arch
Inferior orbital fissure

Smaller wing of sphenoid bone
Optic canal
Ethmoid bone
Lacrimal bone
Nasal bone
Lacrimal fossa
Maxilla

Osmolality, serum

DESCRIPTION

- Evaluates the concentration of dissolved particles in blood
- Osmolality: high in concentrated blood, low in dilute blood; increases with dehydration, decreases with fluid overload
- Helps in evaluating hydration status and suspected antidiuretic hormone (ADH) abnormalities

PURPOSE

- To help evaluate ADH function
- To evaluate acid-base balance
- To evaluate hydration status

PREPARATION

- The test requires a blood sample.
- No dietary restrictions are required.

Teaching points

- Explain that this test helps evaluate hydration status.
- Explain who will perform the test and where it'll be done.
- Inform the patient that fasting isn't required.
- Tell him that the test requires a blood sample and that he may experience slight discomfort from the tourniquet and needle puncture.
- Tell the patient the test should take less than 5 minutes.

KEY STEPS

- Confirm the patient's identity using two patient identifiers according to facility policy.
- Perform a venipuncture, collecting the sample in a 5-ml plain tube.

POSTPROCEDURE CARE

- Apply direct pressure to the venipuncture site until the bleeding stops.
- Inform the practitioner of abnormal results.

PRECAUTIONS

- Maintain standard precautions while collecting the sample.
- Handle the sample gently to prevent hemolysis.

COMPLICATIONS

- Hematoma at the venipuncture site

NORMAL RESULTS

- Serum osmolality is 275 to 295 mOsm/kg (SI, 275 to 295 mmol/kg).

ABNORMAL RESULTS

- Decreased serum osmolality indicates overhydration.
- Decreased levels may occur with hyponatremia, syndrome of inappropriate antidiuretic hormone secretion, adrenocorticoid insufficiency, and water intoxication.
- Increased serum osmolality levels are consistent with dehydration; increased levels may result from hypernatremia, overuse of diuretics, mannitol (Osmitrol) administration, diabetes insipidus, hyperglycemia, and renal tubular necrosis.
- A serum osmolality level greater than 360 mOsm/kg (SI, 360 mmol/kg) has been associated with respiratory arrest. Generalized tonic-clonic seizures or death may occur with levels exceeding 420 mOsm/kg (SI, 420 mmol/kg).

WARNING *Signs of critically high serum osmolality include decreased skin turgor, lethargy, coma, and shock.*

Osmolality, urine

DESCRIPTION

- Evaluates concentrating ability of the kidneys in acute and chronic renal failure by measuring number of osmotically active ions or particles present per kilogram of water
- Osmolality: high in concentrated urine, low in dilute urine; determined by effect of solute particles on freezing point of fluid
- Fluid intake determines if kidneys concentrate or dilute urine: excessive intake, more water excreted in urine, less in limited intake
- Distal segment of tubule varies permeability to water in response to antidiuretic hormone
- Osmolality is more sensitive indicator of renal function than dilution techniques that measure specific gravity

PURPOSE

- To evaluate renal tubular function
- To detect renal impairment

PREPARATION

- No dietary restrictions are required.
- Withhold diuretics.
- Emphasize to the patient that his cooperation is required to obtain accurate results.

Teaching points

- Explain that this test evaluates kidney function.
- Tell the patient that the test requires a urine specimen and collection of blood within 1 hour before or after the urine is collected.
- Tell him that fasting isn't required.
- Teach the patient how to collect a 24-hour urine specimen if required.

KEY STEPS

- Confirm the patient's identity using two patient identifiers according to facility policy.
- Collect a random urine specimen and draw a blood sample within 1 hour of urine collection.
- If a 24-hour urine collection is needed, record the total urine volume on the laboratory request. (Preservatives aren't required for a 24-hour container.)
- If the patient can't urinate into the specimen containers, give him a clean bedpan, urinal, or toilet specimen pan.
- Rinse the collection device after each use.
- If the patient is catheterized, empty the drainage bag before the test. Obtain the specimen from the catheter.

POSTPROCEDURE CARE

- After collecting the final specimen, provide the patient with a balanced meal or snack.
- Make sure the patient voids within 8 to 10 hours after the catheter has been removed.
- Inform the practitioner of abnormal results.

PRECAUTIONS

- Send each specimen to the laboratory immediately after collection.

COMPLICATIONS

- None

NORMAL RESULTS

- In a random specimen, 50 to 1,400 mOsm/kg.
- In a 24-hour urine specimen, 300 to 900 mOsm/kg.

ABNORMAL RESULTS

- Decreased renal capacity to concentrate urine in response to fluid deprivation, or to dilute urine in response to fluid overload, may indicate tubular epithelial damage, decreased renal blood flow, loss of functional nephrons, or pituitary or cardiac dysfunction.

Osmotic fragility test

DESCRIPTION

- Based on osmosis, test that measures resistance of red blood cells (RBCs) to hemolysis when exposed to increasingly dilute saline solutions: the sooner the hemolysis, the greater the osmotic fragility
- Offers quantitative confirmation of RBC morphology and supplements stained cell examination
- In isotonic saline solution, same salt concentration (osmotic pressure) as normal plasma (0.85 g/dl): RBCs keep their shape
- In hypotonic solution: RBCs take up water until they burst
- In hypertonic solution: RBCs shrink
- Degree of hypotonicity needed to produce hemolysis varies inversely with RBCs' osmotic fragility; closer the saline tonicity is to normal physiologic values when hemolysis occurs, more fragile the cells
- RBCs incubated in solution for 24 hours to improve test sensitivity if they don't hemolyze immediately
- Offers quantitative confirmation of RBC morphology and supplements stained cell examination.

PURPOSE

- To help diagnose hereditary spherocytosis
- To confirm morphologic RBC abnormalities

PREPARATION

- The test requires a blood sample.
- No dietary restrictions are required.

Teaching points

- Explain that the osmotic fragility test identifies the cause of anemia.
- Explain who will perform the test and where it'll be done.
- Inform the patient that food and fluids need not be restricted.
- Tell the patient that the test requires a blood sample and that he may experience slight discomfort from the tourniquet and needle puncture.
- Tell him the test should take less than 5 minutes.

KEY STEPS

- Confirm the patient's identity using two patient identifiers according to facility policy.
- Perform a venipuncture, collecting the sample in a 4.5-ml heparinized tube.
- Completely fill the collection tube and invert it gently several times to mix the sample and the anticoagulant thoroughly.

POSTPROCEDURE CARE

- Apply direct pressure to the venipuncture site until the bleeding stops.
- Inform the practitioner of abnormal results.

PRECAUTIONS

- Maintain standard precautions while collecting the sample.
- Handle the sample gently to prevent hemolysis.

COMPLICATIONS

- Hematoma at the venipuncture site

NORMAL RESULTS

- Osmotic fragility values (percentage of RBCs hemolyzed) that have been obtained photometrically are plotted against decreasing saline tonicity to produce an S-shaped curve with a slope characteristic of the disorder. Reference values differ with tonicities.

ABNORMAL RESULTS

- Low osmotic fragility (increased resistance to hemolysis) is characteristic of thalassemia, iron deficiency anemia, sickle cell anemia, and other RBC disorders in which target cells are found.
- Low osmotic fragility also occurs after splenectomy.
- High osmotic fragility (increased tendency to hemolyze) occurs in hereditary spherocytosis; and in spherocytosis associated with autoimmune hemolytic anemia, severe burns, or chemical poisoning.
- High osmotic fragility may also be found in hemolytic disease of the neonate (erythroblastosis fetalis).

Otoacoustic emissions test

DESCRIPTION

- Rapid screening method to assess the function of outer hair cells of the cochlea; shows abnormalities that may precede hearing loss
- Screens for cochlear hearing loss; outer hair cells are usually lost before inner cells are damaged
- Emissions absent when hearing loss is more than slight to mild
- Shows subtle changes in otoacoustic emissions in patients with normal hearing who are carriers of recessive hearing loss genes
- Provides a cost-effective method of neonatal screening; doesn't need patient participation
- Measures outer hair cell function, assists in patient triage during diagnostic testing, and provides a rapid indication of whether the outer hair cells are intact
- Helps detect nonorganic hearing loss (hearing loss that develops after birth may not be identified)
- May not detect slight (minimal) hearing loss

PURPOSE

- To screen and assess the health of the outer hair cells of the cochlea
- To screen the hearing of neonates

PREPARATION

- Remove significant cerumen accumulation from the patient's ear canals.
- No dietary restrictions are required.

Teaching points

- Explain the purpose of the test and how it's done.
- Explain who will perform the test and where it'll be done.
- Tell the patient fasting isn't required.
- Inform the patient that the test takes about 1 minute per ear, or slightly longer if findings aren't immediately found to be normal.

KEY STEPS

- Confirm the patient's identity using two patient identifiers according to facility policy.
- In screening, the technician places the probe in the patient's ear after having cleared it of debris, such as vernix, which is present in a neonate's ear.
- The audiologist adjusts signal levels and, in the case of distortion-product otoacoustic emissions, the frequency characteristics.
- The emission level is monitored and compared with the background noise level.

POSTPROCEDURE CARE

- Answer the patient's questions.
- Inform the practitioner of abnormal results.

PRECAUTIONS

- None

COMPLICATIONS

- None

NORMAL RESULTS

- Emission is 500 to 6,000 Hz, with signal-to-noise ratios of at least 5 dB.
- Emissions are sufficiently higher than the background physiologic and ambient noise levels.
- Results are frequency specific.

ABNORMAL RESULTS

- An absence of otoacoustic emissions at any test frequency suggests outer hair cell dysfunction and hearing loss of at least 25 dB.
- The presence of otoacoustic emissions at traditional screening levels indicates no more than a slight cochlear hearing disorder.
- A reduction in size or elimination of the otoacoustic emission can occur because of significant conductive hearing loss.

Otoscopy

DESCRIPTION

- Shows the external auditory canal and tympanic membrane by use of an otoscope
- Provides indirect information about the eustachian tube and middle ear cavity

PURPOSE

- To detect foreign bodies, cerumen, or stenosis in the external canal
- To detect external or middle ear disorders (infection or perforation)
- To evaluate integrity and appearance of the tympanic membrane

PREPARATION

- Make sure the patient has signed a consent form.

Teaching points

- Explain the purpose of the test and how it's done.
- Explain who will perform the test and where it'll be done.
- Warn the patient that with pneumatic otoscopy, he may experience dizziness with nystagmus.
- Tell the patient the procedure takes about 5 minutes.

DIAGNOSTIC PROCEDURE

KEY STEPS

- Confirm the patient's identity using two patient identifiers according to facility policy.
- The patient's head is tilted slightly away from the examiner with the ear to be examined pointed up.
- The auricle is pulled up, back, and away from the head to straighten an adult's ear canal; to straighten a child's canal, the auricle is pulled down.
- The largest speculum that will comfortably fit is selected.
- The otoscope is gently inserted into the ear canal with a downward and forward motion.
- The tympanic membrane is located and examined.

- The malleus is located; it should be partially visible through the translucent tympanic membrane.
- The tympanic membrane and surrounding fibrous rim (annulus) are examined.

POSTPROCEDURE CARE

- Answer the patient's questions.
- Inform the practitioner of abnormal results.

PRECAUTIONS

- If the patient has ear pain, the unaffected ear is assessed first; then the affected ear is assessed.

COMPLICATIONS

- Perforation of the tympanic membrane

INTERPRETATION

NORMAL RESULTS

- The tympanic membrane is thin, translucent, shiny, and slightly concave. It appears pearl gray or pale pink, and reflects light in its inferior portion (cone of light) with clearly defined landmarks.
- The short process of the malleus, manubrium, and umbo are visible but not prominent.
- Blood vessels should be visible only in the periphery.

ABNORMAL RESULTS

- Scarring, discoloration, retraction, or bulging of the tympanic membrane and the presence of drainage and scaly surface areas suggests presence of disease.
- Movement of the tympanic membrane in tandem with respiration suggests abnormal patency of the eustachian tube.
- A dry, flaky auditory canal lining may suggest eczema.
- An inflamed, swollen, and narrowed auditory canal, possibly with discharge, suggests otitis externa. (See *Common abnormalities of the tympanic membrane*.)

Common abnormalities of the tympanic membrane

Visual examination of the tympanic membrane may reveal abnormal findings. This table lists some of the more common findings and their typical causes.

ABNORMAL FINDINGS	USUAL CAUSE
Bright red color	Inflammation (otitis media)
Yellowish color	Pus or serum behind the tympanic membrane (acute or chronic otitis media)
Bubble behind the tympanic membrane	Serous fluid in the middle ear (serous otitis media)
Absent light reflection	Bulging tympanic membrane (acute otitis media)
Absent or diminishing landmarks	Thickened tympanic membrane (chronic otitis media, otitis externa, or tympanosclerosis)
Oval-dark areas	Perforated or scarred tympanic membrane (otitis media or trauma)
Prominent malleus	Retracted tympanic membrane (nonfunctional eustachian tube)
Reduced mobility	Stiffened middle-ear system (serous otitis media or, less commonly, middle-ear adhesions)

Oximetry

OVERVIEW

DESCRIPTION

- Used intermittently or continuously to monitor arterial oxygen saturation (Sao_2) noninvasively
- Photodetector slipped over finger measures transmitted light as it passes through vascular bed, detects relative amount of color absorbed by arterial blood, and calculates exact mixed venous oxygen saturation without interference from surrounding venous blood, skin, connective tissue, or bone
- With ear probe: oximetry monitors transmission of light waves through vascular bed of earlobe; results are inaccurate if earlobe is poorly perfuse, such as from low cardiac output (see *How oximetry works*)

PURPOSE

- To monitor the patient's oxygenation status

PREPARATION

- Remove false fingernails and nail polish from the test finger.
- Rub the location where the probe is to be applied to increase blood flow.
- No dietary restrictions are required.

Teaching points

- Explain that the test measures the amount of oxygen in his blood.
- Explain who will perform the test and where it'll be done.
- Tell the patient that the test is painless.
- Inform the patient that he need not restrict food or fluids.
- Tell the patient the test takes about 10 minutes, depending on how long he'll be monitored.

DIAGNOSTIC PROCEDURE

KEY STEPS

- Confirm the patient's identity using two patient identifiers according to facility policy.

- Place the transducer probe over the patient's finger so the light beams and sensors oppose each other.
- A beam of light passes through the tissue and the sensor measures the amount of light absorbed by the tissue.
- The pulse rate on the oximeter should correspond to the patient's actual pulse. If it doesn't, assess the patient, check the oximeter, and reposition the probe.
- If Sao_2 is used to guide weaning the patient from forced inspiratory oxygen, obtain arterial blood gas analysis occasionally to correlate pulse oximetry reading with Sao_2 levels in the blood.

POSTPROCEDURE CARE

- Inform the practitioner of abnormal results.

PRECAUTIONS

- If a finger is to be used, make sure the fingernail is free from nail polish. This will impair the results.
- If no reading is obtained, try warming the extremity or repositioning the probe.

COMPLICATIONS

- None

INTERPRETATION

NORMAL RESULTS

- Normal Sao_2 levels via oximetry for adults are 95% to 100%.
- For healthy, full-term neonates, by 1 hour after birth, Sao_2 should be 93% to 100%.

ABNORMAL RESULTS

- Levels below 95% indicate hypoxia that may warrant intervention.
- Patients with chronic lung disorders, such as chronic obstructive pulmonary disease, may have low Sao_2 levels that their body has compensated for, and they don't require extra oxygenation.
- Always evaluate the Sao_2 level with the patient's clinical status.
- Sao_2 levels below 75% require immediate medical attention.

  INTERFERING FACTORS *Elevated carboxyhemoglobin or methemoglobin (falsely elevated Sao_2 readings)*

How oximetry works

The pulse oximeter allows noninvasive monitoring of a patient's arterial oxygen saturation (Sao_2) levels by measuring absorption (amplitude) of light waves as they pass through areas of the body that are highly perfused by arterial blood. Oximetry also monitors pulse rate and amplitude.

Light-emitting diodes in a transducer (photodetector) attached to the patient's body (shown below on index finger) send red and infrared light beams through tissue. The photodetector records the relative amount of each color absorbed by arterial blood and transmits the data to a monitor, which displays the information with each heartbeat. If the Sao_2 level or pulse rate varies from preset limits, the monitor triggers visual and audible alarms.

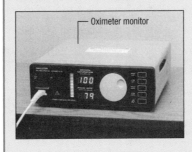

Oximeter monitor

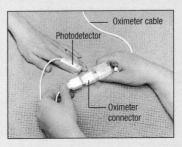

Oximeter cable

Photodetector

Oximeter connector

Papanicolaou test

DESCRIPTION
- Widely used for early detection of cervical cancer
- Permits cytologic evaluation of the vaginal pool, prostatic secretions, urine, gastric secretions, cavity fluids, bronchial aspirates, sputum, and solid tumor cells obtained by fine-needle aspiration
- Also known as a *Pap test* or *ThinPrep Pap test*

PURPOSE
- To detect malignant cells
- To detect inflammatory changes in tissue
- To assess response to chemotherapy and radiation therapy
- To detect viral, fungal, and, occasionally, parasitic invasion

PREPARATION
- Make sure the patient has signed an appropriate consent form.
- Note and report allergies.
- Schedule the study for the middle of the menstrual cycle.

Teaching points
- Explain the purpose of the test and how it's done.
- Explain who will perform the test and where it'll be done.
- Advise the patient that she may experience slight discomfort from the speculum.
- Stress the need to avoid activities that can wash away cellular deposits and change vaginal pH, including sexual intercourse for 24 hours, douching for 48 hours, and using vaginal creams or medications for 1 week.
- Tell the patient the test takes about 15 minutes.

DIAGNOSTIC PROCEDURE

KEY STEPS
- Confirm the patient's identity using two patient identifiers according to facility policy.

- The patient is assisted into the lithotomy position with her feet in stirrups.
- An unlubricated speculum is inserted into the vagina.
- The cervix is located.
- Secretions from the cervix and material from the endocervical canal are collected with an endocervical brush and a wooden spatula.
- Specimens are spread on slides and immediately immersed in or sprayed with a fixative.
- Specimens are appropriately labeled with date of last menses, collection site, and method.
- If vaginal or vulval lesions exist, scrapings taken directly from the lesion are preferred.

POSTPROCEDURE CARE
- If the patient bleeds, give her a sanitary napkin.
- Schedule a return appointment for the patient's next Pap test.

PRECAUTIONS
- The slides are preserved immediately.

COMPLICATIONS
- Bleeding

NORMAL RESULTS
- No malignant cells or abnormalities are present.

ABNORMAL RESULTS
- Cells with relatively large nuclei, only small amounts of cytoplasm, abnormal nuclear chromatin patterns, and marked variation in size, shape, and staining properties, with prominent nucleoli, suggest malignancy.
- Atypical but nonmalignant cells suggest a benign abnormality.
- Atypical cells may suggest dysplasia.
- Human papillomavirus (HPV) has been identified as a major risk factor for cervical cancer. A test is available that detects the types of HPV via their deoxyribonucleic acid. (See *Testing for cervical cancer.*)

Testing for cervical cancer

THINPREP TEST
Cervical cells for ThinPrep test analysis may be collected in the same manner as those of a Papanicolaou (Pap) test, using a cytobrush and plastic spatula. The specimens are deposited in a bottle provided with a fixative and sent to the laboratory. A filter is then inserted into the bottle, and excess mucus, blood, and inflammatory cells are filtered out by centrifuge. Remaining cells are then placed on a slide in a uniform, thin layer and read as a Pap test. This procedure causes fewer slides to be classified as unreadable, significantly reducing the incidence of false negatives and the need for repeat tests.

HPV DNA TEST
When using the ThinPrep test, screening can also be easily done for the human papillomavirus (HPV), of which certain strains have been identified as the primary cause of cervical cancer. The Digene hc2 HPV deoxyribonucleic acid (DNA) test has been approved by the U.S. Food and Drug Administration to determine if those identified at high risk for developing cervical cancer have been exposed to HPV. The specimen is collected as a Pap smear, but is dispersed with ThinPrep solution. Separate aliquots are used for each test, from brushings of the endocervix. The brush is then inserted into the specialized tube, snapped off at the shaft, and capped securely. The target solution in the tube disrupts the virus and releases target DNA, which combines with specific ribonucleic acid (RNA) probes creating RNA:DNA hybrids. The hybrids are captured, bound, and magnified and measured using a luminometer.

If the patient is found to be positive for HPV, she has been infected with the virus. Depending on the type of HPV found through DNA testing, the patient harboring high-risk HPV strains has a higher risk of developing cervical cancer. It's recommended that the patient undergo colposcopy, in which the cervix is viewed under a microscope and a biopsy is taken from the tissue sample.

Paracentesis

DESCRIPTION
- Obtains samples of ascitic fluid for diagnostic and therapeutic purposes by insertion of a trocar and cannula through the abdominal wall
- May be performed using image-guidance
- In four-quadrant tap, aspirates fluid from each quadrant of the abdomen to verify abdominal trauma and the need for surgery
- In peritoneal fluid analysis, assesses gross appearance, red blood cell (RBC) and white blood cell (WBC) counts, cytologic studies, microbiological studies for bacteria and fungi, and determinations of protein, glucose, amylase, ammonia, and alkaline phosphatase levels

PURPOSE
- To determine the cause of ascites
- To detect abdominal trauma
- To remove accumulated ascitic fluid

PREPARATION
- Make sure the patient has signed an appropriate consent form.
- Note and report allergies.
- No dietary restrictions are required.

Teaching points
- If the patient has severe ascites, inform him that the procedure will relieve his discomfort and allow him to breathe easier.
- Explain who will perform the test and where it'll be done.
- Inform the patient that he'll receive a local anesthetic.
- Explain that a blood sample may be taken for analysis.
- Tell the patient that he doesn't have to restrict his diet.
- Tell him the test takes 45 to 60 minutes.

DIAGNOSTIC PROCEDURE

KEY STEPS
- Confirm the patient's identity using two patient identifiers according to facility policy.
- Obtain baseline vital signs, weight, and abdominal girth measurement.
- Assist the patient onto a chair.
- If the patient can't tolerate being out of bed, assist him into high Fowler's position.
- Prepare and drape the puncture site.
- Local anesthetic is injected.
- The needle or trocar and cannula are inserted, usually 1″ or 2″ (2.5 to 5 cm) below the umbilicus, or in each quadrant of the abdomen.
- Fluid specimens are aspirated.
- Specimens are placed in appropriately labeled containers.
- The trocar or needle is removed, and a dressing is applied.

POSTPROCEDURE CARE
- Give I.V. infusions and albumin.
- Monitor vital signs and intake and output.
- Observe the puncture site and drainage for bleeding and infection.
- Obtain the patient's daily weight and daily abdominal girth measurement.
- Observe the patient for hematuria, which may indicate bladder trauma.
- Monitor serum electrolyte (especially sodium) and protein levels.

PRECAUTIONS
- If a large amount of fluid was removed, watch for signs of vascular collapse (such as tachycardia, tachypnea, hypotension, dizziness, and changes in mental status).
- Watch for signs and symptoms of hemorrhage and shock and for increasing pain and abdominal tenderness; these may indicate a perforated intestine, puncture of the inferior epigastric artery, hematoma of the anterior cecal wall, or rupture of the iliac vein or bladder.
- Observe the patient with severe hepatic disease for signs of hepatic coma, which may result from loss of sodium and potassium accompanying hypovolemia.

COMPLICATIONS
- Bleeding, hemorrhage
- Infection
- Bladder trauma
- Shock
- Perforated intestine
- Inferior epigastric artery puncture
- Anterior cecal wall hematoma
- Iliac vein rupture

INTERPRETATION

NORMAL RESULTS
- Fluid is odorless, clear to pale yellow.

ABNORMAL RESULTS
- Milk-colored fluid may indicate chylous ascites.
- Bloody fluid may indicate a tumor, hemorrhagic pancreatitis, or perforated intestine or duodenal ulcer.
- Cloudy or turbid fluid may indicate peritonitis or an infectious process.
- RBC count above 100/µl (SI, > 100/L) suggests neoplasm or tuberculosis.
- RBC count above 100,000/µl (SI, > 100,000/L) suggests intra-abdominal trauma.
- WBC count above 300/µl, with more than 25% neutrophils, suggests spontaneous bacterial peritonitis or cirrhosis.
- A high percentage of lymphocytes suggests tuberculous peritonitis or chylous ascites.
- A protein ascitic fluid-serum ratio of 0.5 or greater may suggest a malignancy or tuberculous or pancreatic ascites.
- Protein levels rise above 3 g/dl (SI, > 3 g/L) in malignancy and above 4 g/dl (SI, > 4 g/L) in tuberculosis.
- Albumin gradient between ascitic fluid and serum greater than 1 g/dl (SI, > 1 g/L) indicates chronic hepatic disease.
- Gram-positive cocci usually indicate primary peritonitis; gram-negative organisms indicate secondary peritonitis.
- Fungi may indicate histoplasmosis, candidiasis, or coccidioidomycosis.

Parathyroid hormone test

OVERVIEW

DESCRIPTION
- Evaluates parathyroid function
- Regulates calcium and phosphorus levels
- Also known as *PTH* or *parathormone*
- Measures serum calcium, phosphorus, and creatinine levels with serum PTH to understand the causes and effects of pathologic parathyroid function
- Release regulated by a negative feedback mechanism involving calcium level: normal or elevated circulating calcium (especially ionized) level inhibits PTH release, decreased level stimulates PTH release
- Circulating PTH occurs in three molecular forms: intact PTH molecule, which originates in the parathyroid glands, and two smaller circulating forms, N-terminal fragments and C-terminal fragments

PURPOSE
- To aid in the differential diagnosis of hyperparathyroidism and hypoparathyroidism
- *C-terminal PTH assay:* to diagnose chronic disturbances in PTH metabolism, such as secondary and tertiary hyperparathyroidism; to differentiate ectopic from primary hyperparathyroidism
- *Intact PTH and the N-terminal fragment assays:* to reflect acute changes in PTH metabolism and monitor patient's response to PTH therapy

PREPARATION
- Fasting overnight for at least 8 hours before the test is required.
- The test requires a blood sample.

Teaching points
- Explain that this test helps evaluate parathyroid function.
- Explain who will perform the test and where it'll be done.
- Instruct the patient to observe an overnight fast because food may affect PTH levels and interfere with results.

- Tell the patient that the test requires a blood sample and that he may experience slight discomfort from the tourniquet and needle puncture.
- Tell the patient the test takes less than 5 minutes.

DIAGNOSTIC PROCEDURE

KEY STEPS
- Confirm the patient's identity using two patient identifiers according to facility policy.
- Perform a venipuncture, and collect 3 ml of blood into two separate 7-ml clot-activator tubes.

POSTPROCEDURE CARE
- Apply direct pressure to the venipuncture site until bleeding stops.
- Inform the practitioner of abnormal results.
- Tell the patient to resume his usual diet.

PRECAUTIONS
- Maintain standard precautions while collecting the sample.
- Handle the sample gently to prevent hemolysis.

- Send the sample to the laboratory immediately so the serum can be separated and frozen for assay.

COMPLICATIONS
- Hematoma at the venipuncture site

INTERPRETATION

NORMAL RESULTS
- Levels vary, depending on the laboratory; they must be interpreted depending on calcium levels.
- Intact PTH level is 10 to 50 pg/ml (SI, 1.1 to 5.3 pmol/L).
- N-terminal fraction is 8 to 24 pg/ml (SI, 0.8 to 2.5 pmol/L).
- C-terminal fraction is 0 to 340 pg/ml (SI, 0 to 35.8 pmol/L).

ABNORMAL RESULTS
- Measured with serum calcium levels, abnormally elevated PTH values may indicate primary, secondary, or tertiary hyperparathyroidism.
- Abnormally low PTH levels may result from hypoparathyroidism or certain malignant diseases. (See *Clinical implications of abnormal parathyroid secretion.*)

Clinical implications of abnormal parathyroid secretion

CONDITIONS	CAUSES	PTH LEVELS	IONIZED CALCIUM LEVELS
Primary hyperparathyroidism	• Parathyroid adenoma or carcinoma	High	High to Normal
Secondary hyperparathyroidism	• Chronic renal disease • Severe vitamin D deficiency • Calcium malabsorption • Pregnancy and lactation	High	Low
Tertiary hyperparathyroidism	• Progressive secondary hyperparathyroidism	High	High to Low
Hypoparathyroidism	• Accidental removal of the parathyroid glands • Autoimmune disease	Low	Low
Malignant tumors	• Squamous-cell carcinoma of the lung • Renal, pancreatic, or ovarian carcinoma	High to Normal	High

Key: High ●   Normal ○   Low ○

Partial thromboplastin time

OVERVIEW

DESCRIPTION
- Used to evaluate all the clotting factors of the intrinsic pathway—except platelets—by measuring the time required for formation of a fibrin clot after the addition of calcium and phospholipid emulsion to a plasma sample
- Used with an activator, such as kaolin, to shorten clotting time

PURPOSE
- To screen for deficiencies of the clotting factors in the intrinsic pathways
- To monitor response to heparin therapy

PREPARATION
- No dietary restrictions are required.
- The test requires a blood sample.

Teaching points
- Explain that the partial thromboplastin time (PTT) test determines whether blood clots normally.
- Explain who will perform the test and where it'll be done.
- Inform the patient that no dietary restrictions are required.
- Tell the patient that the test requires a blood sample and that he may experience slight discomfort from the tourniquet and needle puncture.
- When appropriate, tell the patient receiving heparin therapy that this test may be repeated at regular intervals to assess his response to treatment.
- Tell the patient the test takes less than 5 minutes.

DIAGNOSTIC PROCEDURE

KEY STEPS
- Confirm the patient's identity using two patient identifiers according to facility policy.
- Perform a venipuncture, and collect the sample in a 7-ml tube with sodium citrate added.
- Completely fill the collection tube, invert it gently several times, and send it to the laboratory on ice.

POSTPROCEDURE CARE
- Apply direct pressure to the venipuncture site until bleeding stops.
- For a patient on anticoagulant therapy, additional pressure at the venipuncture site to control bleeding may be needed.
- If a large hematoma develops at the venipuncture site, monitor distal pulses.
- Inform the practitioner of abnormal results.

PRECAUTIONS
- Maintain standard precautions while collecting the sample.
- Avoid excessive probing at the venipuncture site, and handle the sample gently to prevent hemolysis.
- If the patient is receiving heparin therapy, perform the venipuncture on the arm opposite the heparin infusion.

COMPLICATIONS
- Hematoma at the venipuncture site

INTERPRETATION

NORMAL RESULTS
- A fibrin clot forms 21 to 35 seconds (SI, 21 to 35 s) after adding reagents.
- For a patient receiving an anticoagulant, ask the practitioner to specify the reference values for the therapy being delivered.

ABNORMAL RESULTS
- A prolonged PTT may indicate a deficiency of certain plasma clotting factors, the presence of heparin, or the presence of fibrin split products, fibrinolysins, or circulating anticoagulants that are antibodies to specific clotting factors.

Parvovirus B-19 antibodies test

OVERVIEW

DESCRIPTION
- An enzyme-linked immunosorbent assay and immunofluorescence test to detect immunoglobulin (Ig) G and IgM antibodies to parvovirus B-19 (small, single-stranded deoxyribonucleic acid virus belonging to *Parvoviridae;* destroys red blood cell [RBC] precursors and interferes with normal RBC production)
- Disease linked to erythema infectiosum (self-limiting, low-grade fever and rash in young children) and aplastic crisis (in patients with chronic hemolytic anemia and immunodeficient patients with bone marrow failure)

PURPOSE
- To detect parvovirus B-19 antibody, especially in prospective organ donors
- To diagnose erythema infectiosum, parvovirus B-19, aplastic crisis, and related parvovirus B-19 diseases

PREPARATION
- No dietary restrictions are required.
- The test requires a blood sample.

Teaching points
- To a potential organ donor, explain that the test is part of a panel of tests that occur before organ donation to protect the organ recipient from potential infection.
- Explain who will perform the test and where it'll be done.
- Inform the patient that no dietary restrictions are required.
- Tell the patient that the test requires a blood sample and that he may experience slight discomfort from the tourniquet and needle puncture.
- Tell the patient the test takes less than 5 minutes.

DIAGNOSTIC PROCEDURE

KEY STEPS
- Confirm the patient's identity using two patient identifiers according to facility policy.
- Perform a venipuncture, collect the sample in a 5-ml clot-activator tube, and store it on ice.

POSTPROCEDURE CARE
- Apply direct pressure to the venipuncture site until bleeding stops.
- Inform the practitioner of abnormal results.

PRECAUTIONS
- Handle the sample gently to prevent hemolysis.

COMPLICATIONS
- Hematoma at the venipuncture site

INTERPRETATION

NORMAL RESULTS
- Test is negative for IgG- and IgM-specific antibodies to parvovirus B-19.

ABNORMAL RESULTS
- About 50% of all adults lack immunity to parvovirus B-19; up to 20% of susceptible adults become infected after exposure.
- Positive results for IgG- and IgM-specific antibodies to parvovirus B-19 are linked to joint arthralgia, hydrops fetalis, fetal loss, transient aplastic anemia, chronic anemia in immunocompromised patients, and bone marrow failure.
- A positive result for parvovirus B-19 should be confirmed using the Western blot test.

Percutaneous liver biopsy

DESCRIPTION
- Needle aspiration of a core of liver tissue for histologic analysis
- Usually performed under local anesthesia with image-guidance

PURPOSE
- To diagnose hepatic parenchymal disease
- To diagnose malignant tumors and granulomatous infections

PREPARATION
- Make sure the patient has signed an appropriate consent form.
- Note and report allergies.
- Check the patient's history for hypersensitivity to the local anesthetic.
- Withhold food and fluid for 4 to 8 hours before the procedure.
- Report abnormal coagulation study results to the practitioner.
- Make sure that all aspirin products and nonsteroidal anti-inflammatory drugs are stopped at least 5 days before the procedure.

Teaching points
- Explain the purpose of the test and how it's done.
- Explain who will perform the test and where it'll be done.
- Instruct the patient to fast for 4 to 8 hours before the procedure.
- Warn the patient that he might experience right shoulder pain.
- Tell the patient that the procedure takes about 30 minutes.

DIAGNOSTIC PROCEDURE

KEY STEPS
- Confirm the patient's identity using two patient identifiers according to facility policy.
- The patient is placed in a supine position with his right hand under his head.
- After the biopsy site is selected, a local anesthetic is injected.

- The patient takes a deep breath, exhales, then holds his breath at the end of expiration.
- The biopsy needle is quickly inserted into the liver and withdrawn in 1 second while the patient is holding his breath. (See *Using a Menghini needle*.)
- After the needle is withdrawn, the patient resumes normal breathing.
- The tissue specimen is placed in a properly labeled specimen cup.

POSTPROCEDURE CARE
- Apply direct pressure to the biopsy site to stop bleeding.
- Position the patient on his right side for 2 to 4 hours, with a small pillow or sandbag under the costal margin to provide extra pressure. Advise bed rest for at least 24 hours.
- Give the patient an analgesic.
- Check the patient's vital signs every 15 minutes for 1 hour, every 30 minutes for 4 hours, and every 4 hours thereafter for 24 hours.
- Monitor the patient for bleeding and respiratory distress.
- Tell the patient to resume his normal diet, as ordered.

PRECAUTIONS
- Watch for and immediately notify the practitioner if bleeding or signs and symptoms of bile peritonitis (such as tenderness and rigidity around the biopsy site) occur.
- Watch for signs and symptoms of pneumothorax (such as tachypnea, decreased breath sounds, dyspnea, persistent shoulder pain, and pleuritic chest pain).

COMPLICATIONS
WARNING *Abdominal pain or dyspnea after the biopsy may indicate perforation of an abdominal organ or pneumothorax.*
- Peritonitis
- Bleeding
- Infection

NORMAL RESULTS
- The normal liver consists of sheets of hepatocytes supported by a reticulum framework.

ABNORMAL RESULTS
- Examination of hepatic tissue may indicate diffuse hepatic disease, such as cirrhosis and hepatitis, or granulomatous infections such as tuberculosis.
- Primary malignant tumors suggest possible hepatocellular carcinoma, cholangiocellular carcinoma, and angiosarcoma.

Using a Menghini needle

In percutaneous liver biopsy, a Menghini needle attached to a 5-ml syringe containing normal saline solution is introduced through the chest wall and intercostal space. First, negative pressure is created in the syringe. Then the needle is pushed rapidly into the liver and pulled out of the body entirely to obtain a tissue specimen.

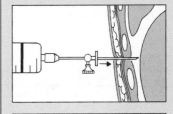

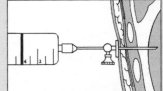

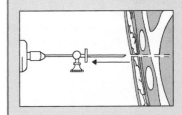

Percutaneous renal biopsy

OVERVIEW

DESCRIPTION
- Needle excision of a core of kidney tissue for histologic examination
- May help assess histologic changes caused by acute or chronic glomerulonephritis, pyelonephritis, renal vein thrombosis, amyloid infiltration, and systemic lupus erythematosus
- Can differentiate a primary renal cancer from a metastatic lesion in patients with a mass

PURPOSE
- To help diagnose renal parenchymal disease
- To monitor the progression of renal disease and assess the effectiveness of therapy

PREPARATION
- Make sure that blood samples and urine specimens are collected and tested before the biopsy and that results of other tests are available.
- The patient must fast for at least 8 hours before the test.
- Check the patient's history for hemorrhagic tendencies and hypersensitivity to the local anesthetic.
- Give a mild sedative 30 minutes to 1 hour before the biopsy to help the patient relax.
- Check the patient's vital signs, and tell him to void just before the test.
- Make sure that the patient has signed an appropriate consent form.

Teaching points
- Explain that this test diagnoses kidney disorders.
- Explain who will perform the test and where it'll be done.
- Instruct the patient to fast for 8 hours before the test.
- Inform the patient that he may experience a pinching sensation when the needle is inserted through his back into the kidney.
- Tell the patient that the test takes about 1 hour.

DIAGNOSTIC PROCEDURE

KEY STEPS
- Confirm the patient's identity using two patient identifiers according to facility policy.
- Assist the patient into a prone position on a firm surface with a sandbag beneath his abdomen.
- Tell the patient to take a deep breath while his kidney is being palpated.
- A 7″ 20G needle is used to inject the local anesthetic into the skin at the biopsy site.
- Instruct the patient to hold his breath and remain still as the needle is inserted.
- After the needle is inserted, tell the patient to take several deep breaths. If the needle swings smoothly during deep breathing, it has penetrated the kidney capsule.
- After the penetration depth is marked on the needle shaft, instruct the patient to hold his breath and remain as still as possible while the needle is withdrawn.
- After a small incision is made in the anesthetized skin, instruct the patient to hold his breath and remain still while the Vim-Silverman needle with stylet is inserted to the measured depth.
- Tell the patient to breathe deeply. Then tell him to remain still while the tissue specimen is obtained.
- The tissue is examined immediately under a hand lens to make sure that the specimen contains tissue from the cortex and medulla.
- Next, it's placed on a saline-soaked gauze pad and put in a properly labeled container.
- If an adequate tissue specimen hasn't been obtained, the procedure is repeated immediately.

POSTPROCEDURE CARE
- After an adequate specimen is secured, apply pressure to the biopsy site for 3 to 5 minutes to stop superficial bleeding, then apply a pressure dressing.
- Instruct the patient to lie flat on his back without moving for at least 12 hours to prevent bleeding. Check his vital signs every 15 minutes for 4 hours, every 30 minutes for the next 4 hours, every hour for the next 4 hours, and finally, every 4 hours. Report any changes.
- Examine the patient's urine for blood; small amounts may be present after the biopsy but should disappear within 8 hours.
- Hematocrit may be monitored after the procedure.
- Encourage the patient to drink fluids.
- Discourage the patient from engaging in strenuous activities for several days after the procedure.

PRECAUTIONS
- The test is contraindicated in patients with uncorrected bleeding disorders, severe hypertension, hydronephrosis, and only one kidney.

COMPLICATIONS
- Bleeding or infection

INTERPRETATION

NORMAL RESULTS
- Bowman's capsule in a section of kidney (the area between two layers of flat epithelial cells), the glomerular tuft, and the capillary lumen are noted.
- There is one layer of epithelial cells with microvilli (the proximal tubule) that form a brush border.
- Flat, squamous epithelial cells in the descending loop of Henle are seen.
- The ascending loop is distally convoluted, with collecting tubules lined with squamous epithelial cells.

ABNORMAL RESULTS
- Findings suggest cancer or renal disease.
- Malignant tumors (including Wilms' tumor and renal cell carcinoma) may be indicated.
- Disseminated lupus erythematosus, amyloid infiltration, acute or chronic glomerulonephritis, renal vein thrombosis, and pyelonephritis may be indicated.

Percutaneous transhepatic cholangiography

DESCRIPTION

- Fluoroscopic examination of the biliary ducts after injection of an iodinated contrast medium directly into a biliary radicle
- Used in patients with previous GI surgery and endoscopically inaccessible bilioenteric anastomosis to perform a contrast study of the biliary ducts
- May be performed for unsuccessful endoscopic cholangiopancreatography
- Also called *PTHC*

PURPOSE

- To evaluate upper abdominal pain after cholecystectomy
- To evaluate patients with severe jaundice
- To distinguish between obstructive and nonobstructive jaundice
- To determine location, extent, and, in many cases, cause of mechanical obstruction

PREPARATION

- Make sure the patient has signed a consent form.
- Note and report allergies.
- Check the patient's history for abnormal coagulation study results.
- Check the patient's history for hypersensitivity to iodine, seafood, the local anesthetic, and iodinated contrast media.
- Withhold food and fluids for 8 hours before the test.

Teaching points

- Explain the purpose of the test and how it's done.
- Explain who will perform the test and where it'll be done.
- Instruct the patient to fast for 8 hours before the test.
- Explain the possible need for a laxative the night before and a cleansing enema the morning of the test.
- Tell the patient that he'll receive a local anesthetic and I.V. sedation.

- Inform the patient that he may feel transient pain as the liver capsule is entered.
- Warn the patient that injection of the contrast medium may cause a sensation of pressure and epigastric fullness.
- Tell the patient the test takes about 1 or 2 hours.

DIAGNOSTIC PROCEDURE

KEY STEPS

- Confirm the patient's identity using two patient identifiers according to facility policy.
- The patient is given preprocedure antibiotics.
- The patient is given a sedative and analgesic.
- The patient is placed in a supine position on the table.
- The right upper quadrant of the abdomen is draped.
- The skin, subcutaneous tissue, and liver capsule are infiltrated with local anesthetic.
- A flexible needle is inserted under fluoroscopic guidance through the 10th or 11th intercostal space at the right midclavicular line.
- A contrast medium is injected.
- Spot films of significant findings are taken in various views.
- A drainage tube may be inserted to allow percutaneous drainage of bile, if dilated ducts are caused by obstruction.
- An internal stent may be inserted to allow bile drainage into the bowel, when the dilation and inflammation have diminished.

POSTPROCEDURE CARE

- Apply a sterile dressing to the puncture site.
- Enforce bed rest for at least 6 hours with the patient lying on his right side.
- Monitor the patient's vital signs and intake and output.
- Check the access site for bleeding, swelling, and tenderness.
- Instruct the patient to resume his usual diet.

PRECAUTIONS

- Watch for signs and symptoms of peritonitis: chills, temperature between 102° and 103° F (38.9° to 39.4° C), and abdominal pain, tenderness, and distention.

COMPLICATIONS

- Adverse effects of iodinated contrast media
- Adverse effects of sedation
- Pneumothorax
- Vasovagal reactions
- Peritonitis
- Bleeding
- Infection or sepsis
- Bile leakage

INTERPRETATION

NORMAL RESULTS

- Biliary ducts are of normal diameter and appear as regular channels homogeneously filled with the contrast medium.

ABNORMAL RESULTS

- Dilated biliary ducts may suggest cholelithiasis, biliary tract cancer, cancer of the pancreas, or cancer of the ampulla of Vater.
- Persistent filling defects may suggest calculi.
- A short and irregular stricture with a rat-tail appearance and gross dilation of the proximal ducts may suggest pancreatic or biliary carcinoma.
- Diffuse intrahepatic and extrahepatic stricture may suggest advanced sclerosing cholangitis or infiltrating cholangiocarcinoma.
- Ducts filled with debris, with possible abscesses of various sizes in communication with the ducts, may suggest acute supportive cholangitis.

Pericardial fluid analysis

DESCRIPTION

- Analyzes pericardial fluid in patients with pericardial effusion (accumulation of excess pericardial fluid), which may result from inflammation (as in pericarditis), rupture, or penetrating trauma
- To determine the effusion site, echocardiography performed before pericardiocentesis to minimize complications

PURPOSE

- To help identify the cause of pericardial effusion and to help determine appropriate therapy

PREPARATION

- Check the patient's history for current antimicrobial usage and record such usage on the test request form.
- No dietary restrictions are required.
- Make sure that the patient has signed an appropriate consent form.

Teaching points

- Explain to the patient that pericardial fluid analysis helps detect extra fluid around the heart.
- Explain who will perform the test and where it'll be done.
- Tell the patient that the diet doesn't need to be restricted.
- Tell the patient that an I.V. line will be started at a slow rate in case he needs medication.
- Inform the patient that he will receive a local anesthetic before aspiration needle insertion.
- Warn the patient that although fluid aspiration isn't painful, he may feel pressure when the needle is inserted into the pericardial sac.
- Tell the patient that he may be asked to hold his breath briefly to aid needle insertion and placement.
- Tell the patient that the procedure takes about 20 minutes.

DIAGNOSTIC PROCEDURE

KEY STEPS

- Confirm the patient's identity using two patient identifiers according to facility policy.
- Assist the patient into a supine position with the thorax elevated 60 degrees.
- When the patient is comfortable and well supported, instruct him to remain still during the procedure.
- A local anesthetic is given at the insertion site after the skin is prepared with alcohol or povidone-iodine solution from the left costal margin to the xiphoid process.
- With the three-way stopcock open, a 50-ml syringe is aseptically attached to one end and the cardiac needle to the other end.
- The electrocardiogram (ECG) leadwire is attached to the needle hub with an alligator clip. The ECG is set to lead V_1 and turned on (or the patient is connected to a bedside monitor).
- The needle is inserted through the chest wall into the pericardial sac, maintaining gentle aspiration until fluid appears in the syringe.
- The needle is angled 35 to 45 degrees toward the tip of the right scapula between the left costal margin and the xiphoid process. A Kelly clamp is attached at the skin surface after the needle is properly positioned so it won't advance further.
- While the fluid is being aspirated, label and number the specimen tubes.
- Watch for grossly bloody aspirate—a sign of inadvertent puncture of a cardiac chamber.
- Use specimen tubes with the proper additives.
- If the patient will receive bacterial culture and sensitivity tests, record antimicrobial therapy the patient is receiving on the laboratory request.
- If anaerobic organisms are suspected, consult the laboratory concerning the proper collection technique to avoid exposing the aspirate to air.

POSTPROCEDURE CARE

- When the needle is withdrawn, apply pressure immediately with sterile gauze pads for 3 to 5 minutes. Then apply a bandage.
- Check blood pressure readings, pulse, respiration, and heart sounds every 15 minutes until stable, every 30 minutes for 2 hours, every hour for 4 hours, and then every 4 hours thereafter.

PRECAUTIONS

- **WARNING** *Watch for signs of cardiac tamponade: muffled and distant heart sounds, distended jugular veins, paradoxical pulse, and shock.*
- Carefully observe the ECG tracing during insertion of the cardiac needle; an ST-segment elevation indicates that the needle has reached the epicardial surface and should be retracted slightly; an abnormally shaped QRS complex may indicate perforation of the myocardium. Premature ventricular contractions usually indicate that the needle has touched the ventricular wall.

COMPLICATIONS

- Puncture of a cardiac chamber

INTERPRETATION

NORMAL RESULTS

- There are between 10 ml and 50 ml of sterile fluid in the pericardium.
- Pericardial fluid is clear or straw-colored, without evidence of pathogens, blood, or malignant cells.
- Fewer than 1,000/µl (SI, < 1 × 10^9/L) white blood cells (WBCs) are found in pericardial fluid.
- Level of glucose in pericardial fluid equals level in whole blood.

ABNORMAL RESULTS

- Transudates are protein-poor effusions that arise from mechanical factors altering fluid formation or resorption, such as increased hydrostatic pressure, decreased plasma oncotic pressure, or obstruction of the pericardial lymphatic drainage system by a tumor.
- Exudate effusions may occur in pericarditis, neoplasms, acute myocardial infarction, tuberculosis (TB), rheumatoid disease, and systemic lupus erythematosus.
- An elevated WBC count or neutrophil fraction may accompany inflammatory conditions; a high lymphocyte fraction may indicate fungal or tuberculous pericarditis.
- Turbid or milky effusions may result from lymph or pus accumulation in the pericardial sac, TB, or rheumatoid disease.
- Bloody pericardial fluid may indicate hemopericardium, hemorrhagic pericarditis, or a traumatic tap.
- Hemorrhagic effusions may indicate a malignant tumor, closed chest trauma, Dressler's syndrome, or postcardiotomy syndrome.
- A glucose level below that of whole blood may reflect increased local metabolism because of malignancy, inflammation, or infection.

Pericardiocentesis

DESCRIPTION

- Needle aspiration and analysis of pericardial fluid
- Useful as an emergency measure to treat cardiac tamponade

PURPOSE

- To identify the cause of pericardial effusion
- To determine appropriate therapy
- To treat cardiac tamponade

PREPARATION

- Make sure the patient has signed an appropriate consent form if the clinical situation permits.
- Note and report allergies.
- Fasting before the test usually isn't needed.
- Administer I.V. sedation as ordered.

Teaching points

- Explain the purpose of the study and how it's done.
- Explain who will perform the test and where it'll be done.
- Explain the need to use a local anesthetic.
- Advise that the patient will feel pressure when the needle is inserted into the pericardial sac.
- Explain the need to insert an I.V. line before the procedure.
- Explain the need to monitor vital signs and heart rhythm during the procedure.
- Tell the patient the procedure takes 10 to 20 minutes.

KEY STEPS

- Confirm the patient's identity using two patient identifiers according to facility policy.
- The patient is placed in a supine position with the thorax elevated 20 degrees.
- The skin is prepared and draped from the left costal margin to the xiphoid process.
- A local anesthetic is injected.
- The needle is inserted through the chest wall into the pericardial sac. (See *Understanding pericardiocentesis.*)
- Needle insertion is usually guided by electrocardiogram (ECG) or echocardiogram.

  WARNING *Carefully observe the ECG tracing when the cardiac needle is being inserted; ST-segment elevation indicates that the needle has reached the epicardial surface and should be retracted slightly; an abnormally shaped QRS complex may indicate perforation of the myocardium. Premature ventricular contractions usually indicate that the needle has touched the ventricular wall.*

- After the needle is properly positioned, a Kelly clamp is attached to it at the skin surface so it won't advance further.
- Fluid is aspirated with a syringe of a pericardial catheter.
- A pericardial catheter may be connected to a drainage bag or to low-suction drainage.
- The insertion site is cleaned and dressed.
- Fluid samples are placed in appropriately labeled containers and sent to the laboratory for analysis as ordered.

Understanding pericardiocentesis

In pericardiocentesis, a needle and syringe assembly is inserted through the chest wall into the pericardial sac, as illustrated here. Electrocardiographic (ECG) monitoring with a leadwire attached to the needle and electrodes placed on the limbs (right arm [RA], right leg [RL], left arm [LA], and left leg [LL]) helps to ensure proper needle placement and to avoid damage to the heart.

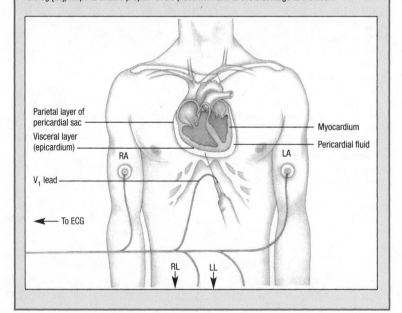

POSTPROCEDURE CARE

◆ Monitor the patient's vital signs, cardiac rhythm, heart sounds, respiratory status, and jugular veins.

⚡ **WARNING** *Be alert for respiratory or cardiac distress. Watch especially for signs of cardiac tamponade, including muffled and distant heart sound, distended jugular veins, paradoxical pulse, and shock. Cardiac tamponade may result from rapid reaccumulation of pericardial fluid or puncture of a coronary vessel, causing bleeding into the pericardial sac.*

PRECAUTIONS

◆ Use specimen tubes with the proper additives to avoid clotting.
◆ Make sure emergency resuscitative equipment is readily available.

⚡ **WARNING** *Watch for grossly bloody aspirate, which may be a sign of inadvertent puncture of a cardiac chamber or blood vessel.*

COMPLICATIONS

◆ Bleeding
◆ Infection
◆ Cardiac arrhythmias
◆ Coronary artery laceration
◆ Myocardial perforation
◆ Respiratory distress
◆ Cardiac tamponade

INTERPRETATION

NORMAL RESULTS

◆ The pericardium contains 10 to 50 ml of sterile fluid.
◆ The fluid is clear and straw-colored, without evidence of pathogens, blood, or malignant cells.
◆ White blood cell (WBC) count in the fluid is usually less than 1,000/µl (SI, $< 1 \times 10^9$/L).
◆ Glucose concentration should approximate the glucose levels in whole blood.

ABNORMAL RESULTS

◆ Effusion suggests pericarditis, neoplasms, acute myocardial infarction, tuberculosis, rheumatoid disease, or systemic lupus erythematosus.
◆ Most exudates containing large amounts of protein suggest inflammation.
◆ An elevated WBC count or neutrophil fraction suggests inflammatory conditions such as bacterial pericarditis.
◆ A high lymphocyte fraction suggests fungal or tuberculosis pericarditis.
◆ Turbid or milky effusions suggest accumulation of lymph or pus in the pericardial sac or from tuberculosis of rheumatoid disease.
◆ Bloody pericardial fluid suggests hemopericardium, hemorrhagic pericarditis, or traumatic tap.
◆ A glucose level below that of whole blood may reflect increased local metabolism because of malignancy, inflammation, or infection.

Peritoneal fluid analysis

DESCRIPTION

- Assesses a specimen of peritoneal fluid obtained by paracentesis
- Requires inserting a trocar and cannula through the abdominal wall while the patient receives a local anesthetic
- In the four-quadrant tap, fluid is aspirated from each quadrant of the abdomen to verify abdominal trauma and confirm the need for surgery

PURPOSE

- To determine the cause of ascites
- To detect abdominal trauma

PREPARATION

- Make sure that the patient or a responsible family member has signed an informed consent form.
- Record baseline vital signs, weight, and abdominal girth.
- No dietary restrictions are required.
- X-rays may be performed before peritoneal analysis.

Teaching points

- Explain that peritoneal fluid analysis helps determine the cause of ascites or detects abdominal trauma.
- Tell the patient who will perform the test and where it'll be done.
- Tell the patient that the test requires a peritoneal fluid specimen and that he'll receive a local anesthetic to minimize discomfort.
- Tell the patient that he need not restrict food or fluids.
- Instruct the patient to void just before the test.
- Tell the patient the test takes about 45 minutes.

DIAGNOSTIC PROCEDURE

KEY STEPS

- Confirm the patient's identity using two patient identifiers according to facility policy.
- Have the patient sit on a bed or in a chair with his feet flat on the floor and his back well-supported. If he can't tolerate being out of bed, place him in high Fowler's position, and make him as comfortable as possible.
- Shave the puncture site, prepare the skin, and drape the area.
- A local anesthetic is injected.
- The physician inserts the needle or trocar and cannula 1″ or 2″ (2.5 to 5 cm) below the umbilicus (or through the flank, iliac fossa, or border of the rectus, or at each quadrant of the abdomen).
- If a trocar and cannula are used, a small incision is made to facilitate insertion. When the needle pierces the peritoneum, a sound can be heard when it "gives." The trocar is removed, and a sample of fluid is aspirated with a 50-ml luer-lock syringe.
- Check the patient's vital signs every 15 minutes during the procedure. Watch for deviations from baseline findings. Observe for dizziness, pallor, perspiration, and increased anxiety.
- If additional fluid is to be drained, assist in attaching one end of an I.V. tube to the cannula and the other end to a collection bag.
- The fluid is then aspirated (no more than 1,500 ml). If aspirating is difficult, reposition the patient.
- After aspiration, the trocar needle is removed, and a pressure dressing is applied. Occasionally, the wound may be sutured first.
- Label the specimens in the order they were drawn. If the patient has received antibiotic therapy, note this on the laboratory request.

POSTPROCEDURE CARE

- Give I.V. infusions and albumin.
- Check the laboratory report for electrolyte and serum protein levels.
- Apply gauze dressing to the puncture site. Check the dressing frequently, and reinforce or apply a pressure dressing if needed.
- Monitor the patient's vital signs until they're stable.
- Weigh the patient and measure his abdominal girth; compare these with his baseline values.
- Monitor the patient's urine output for at least 24 hours, and watch for hematuria, which may indicate bladder trauma.
- Watch the patient for signs of hemorrhage or shock and for increasing pain or abdominal tenderness.
- If a large amount of fluid was aspirated, watch the patient for signs of vascular collapse. Give fluids orally if the patient is alert and can accept them.
- If rapid fluid aspiration induces hypovolemia and shock, reduce the vertical distance between the trocar and the collection bag to slow the drainage rate.
- Monitor the patient's urine output for at least 24 hours, and watch for hematuria, which may indicate bladder trauma.

PRECAUTIONS

- Observe the patient with severe hepatic disease for signs of hepatic coma, which may result from sodium and potassium loss accompanying hypovolemia. Watch him for mental changes, drowsiness, and stupor.

COMPLICATIONS

- Hypovolemia and shock caused by rapid fluid aspiration

INTERPRETATION

NORMAL RESULTS

◆ See *Normal findings in peritoneal fluid analysis.*

ABNORMAL RESULTS

◆ Milk-colored peritoneal fluid may result from chyle or lymph fluid escaping from a thoracic duct that's damaged or blocked by a malignant tumor, lymphoma, tuberculosis, parasitic infestation, adhesion, or hepatic cirrhosis; a pseudochylous condition may result from the presence of leukocytes or tumor cells.

◆ Differential diagnosis of true chylous ascites depends on the presence of elevated triglyceride levels ($\geq$ 400 mg/dl [SI, $\geq$ 4.36 mmol/L]) and microscopic fat globules.

◆ Cloudy or turbid fluid may indicate peritonitis from primary bacterial infection, a ruptured bowel (after trauma), pancreatitis, a strangulated or an infarcted intestine, or an appendicitis.

◆ Bloody fluid may result from a benign or malignant tumor, hemorrhagic pancreatitis, or a traumatic tap; if the fluid fails to clear on continued aspiration, a traumatic tap isn't the cause.

◆ Bile-stained green fluid may indicate a ruptured gallbladder, acute pancreatitis, or a perforated intestine or duodenal ulcer.

◆ A red blood cell count over 100/µl (SI, > 100/L) indicates neoplasm or tuberculosis; a count over 100,000/µl (SI, > 100,000/L) indicates intra-abdominal trauma.

◆ An elevated white blood cell count with more than 25% neutrophils occurs in 90% of patients with spontaneous bacterial peritonitis and in 50% of those with cirrhosis.

◆ A high percentage of lymphocytes suggests tuberculous peritonitis or chylous ascites. Numerous mesothelial cells indicate tuberculous peritonitis.

◆ Protein levels rise above 3 g/dl in malignancy (SI, > 3 g/L) and above 4 g/dl (SI, > 4 g/L) in tuberculosis.

◆ Peritoneal fluid glucose levels fall in the patient with tuberculous peritonitis or peritoneal carcinomatosis.

◆ Amylase levels rise with pancreatic trauma, pancreatic pseudocyst, or acute pancreatitis and may also rise in intestinal necrosis or strangulation.

◆ Peritoneal alkaline phosphatase levels rise to more than twice the normal serum levels in the patient with ruptured or strangulated small intestines.

◆ Peritoneal ammonia levels also exceed twice the normal serum levels in ruptured or strangulated large and small intestines and in a ruptured ulcer or an appendix.

◆ A protein ascitic fluid to serum ratio of 0.5 or greater may suggest a malignancy or tuberculous or pancreatic ascites. The presence of this finding indicates a nonhepatic cause; its absence suggests uncomplicated hepatic disease.

◆ An albumin gradient between ascitic fluid and serum greater than 1 g/dl (SI, > 1 g/L) indicates chronic hepatic disease; a lesser value suggests malignancy.

◆ Cytologic examination of peritoneal fluid accurately detects malignant cells.

◆ Microbiological examination can reveal coliforms, anaerobes, and enterococci, which can enter the peritoneum from a ruptured organ or from infections accompanying appendicitis, pancreatitis, tuberculosis, or ovarian disease.

◆ Gram-positive cocci commonly indicate primary peritonitis; gram-negative organisms, secondary peritonitis.

◆ The presence of fungi may indicate histoplasmosis, candidiasis, or coccidioidomycosis.

Normal findings in peritoneal fluid analysis

Use this table to determine normal findings in peritoneal fluid.

ELEMENT	NORMAL VALUE OR FINDING
Gross appearance	Sterile, odorless, clear to pale yellow color; scant amount (< 50 ml)
Red blood cells	None
White blood cells	< 300/µl (SI, < 300 $\times$ 10^9/L)
Protein	0.3 to 4.1 g/dl (SI, 3 to 41 g/L)
Glucose	70 to 100 mg/dl (SI, 3.5 to 5 mmol/L)
Amylase	138 to 404 units/L (SI, 138 to 404 units/L)
Ammonia	< 50 mcg/dl (SI, < 29 µmol/L)
Alkaline phosphatase	Males over age 18: 90 to 239 units/L (SI, 90 to 239 units/L) Females under age 45: 76 to 196 units/L (SI, 76 to 196 units/L) Females over age 45: 87 to 250 units/L (SI, 87 to 250 units/L)
Cytology	No malignant cells present
Bacteria	None
Fungi	None

Persantine thallium imaging

DESCRIPTION

+ Alternative method of assessing coronary vessel function for patients who can't tolerate exercise or stress electrocardiography (ECG)
+ Dipyridamole (Persantine) infusion: simulates the effects of exercise by increasing blood flow to the collateral circulation and away from the coronary arteries, inducing ischemia
+ Thallium infusion: allows the examiner to evaluate the cardiac vessel response
+ Heart is scanned immediately after thallium infusion and after 2 to 4 hours (diseased vessels can't deliver thallium to the heart, and thallium lingers in diseased areas of the myocardium)

PURPOSE

+ To identify exercise- or stress-induced arrhythmias
+ To assess the presence and degree of cardiac ischemia

PREPARATION

+ Make sure that the patient has signed an informed consent form.
+ The patient must fast before the test.

Teaching points

+ Explain who will perform the test and where it'll be done.
+ Tell the patient that a painless, 5- to 10-minute baseline ECG will precede Persantine thallium imaging.
+ Tell the patient to fast before the test and to avoid caffeine and other stimulants that may cause arrhythmias.
+ Instruct the patient to continue taking his regular medications, with the possible exception of beta-adrenergic blockers.
+ Explain that an I.V. line infuses the medications for the study. Tell the patient who will start the I.V. and when. Explain that he may experience slight discomfort from the tourniquet and the needle puncture.
+ Inform the patient that he may experience mild nausea, headache, dizziness, or flushing after administration of Persantine. Tell him that these reactions are usually temporary and rarely need treatment.
+ If the patient must return for further scanning, tell him to rest and to restrict food and fluids in the interim.
+ Tell the patient that the test may take up to 4 hours to complete.

DIAGNOSTIC PROCEDURE

KEY STEPS

+ Confirm the patient's identity using two patient identifiers according to facility policy.
+ The patient reclines or sits while a resting ECG is performed. Persantine is either given orally or infused I.V. over 4 minutes. Monitor blood pressure, pulse rate, and cardiac rhythm continuously.
+ After Persantine administration, the patient is asked to get up and walk. After it takes effect, thallium is injected.
+ The patient is placed in a supine position for about 40 minutes while the scan is performed. The scan is then reviewed. If necessary, a second scan is performed.

POSTPROCEDURE CARE

+ Inform the practitioner of abnormal results.

PRECAUTIONS

WARNING *The patient may experience arrhythmias, angina, ST-segment depression, or bronchospasm. Make sure resuscitation equipment is readily available.*

COMPLICATIONS

+ Adverse reactions, including nausea, headache, flushing, dizziness, and epigastric pain

INTERPRETATION

NORMAL RESULTS

+ Distribution of the isotope throughout the left ventricle is characteristic and no defects are visible.

ABNORMAL RESULTS

+ The presence of ST-segment depression, angina, and arrhythmias strongly suggests coronary artery disease (CAD).
+ Persistent ST-segment depression usually indicates a myocardial infarction. In contrast, transient ST-segment depression indicates ischemia from CAD.
+ Cold spots usually indicate CAD but may result from sarcoidosis, myocardial fibrosis, cardiac contusion, attenuation because of soft tissue (for example, breast or diaphragm), apical cleft, and coronary spasm.
+ An absence of cold spots in the presence of CAD may result from insignificant obstruction, single-vessel disease, or collateral circulation.

pH test, 24-hour

DESCRIPTION

- Most sensitive indicator of gastric reflux
- Considered the "gold standard" to diagnose gastroesophageal reflux disease
- Also known as a *24-hour ambulatory pH monitoring study*

PURPOSE

- To measure esophageal pH for a total of 24 hours, while a probe is in place
- To determine the presence of gastroesophageal reflux
- To evaluate control of gastroesophageal reflux while on proton pump inhibition
- To determine if reflux episodes correlate with symptoms such as chest pain

PREPARATION

- Make sure the patient has signed an appropriate consent form.
- Note and report allergies.
- The patient should fast before the test and avoid smoking cigarettes.

Teaching points

- Explain the purpose of the test and how it's done.
- Instruct the patient to fast and to avoid cigarette smoking after midnight the night before the test.
- For documenting reflux, explain the need for withholding certain medications including all proton pump inhibitors (PPI) (generally for 7 days before the procedure). It may also be necessary to withhold histamine-2 receptor antagonists, calcium channel blockers, beta-adrenergic blockers, metoclopramide (Reglan), erythromycin (E-Mycin), nitroglycerin (Nitro-Bid), belladonna/phenobarbital (Donnatal), chlordiazepoxide/clidinium (Librax), hyoscyamine sulfate (Levsin), and bethanechol (Urecholine). These medications are generally stopped for at least 48 hours before the test.
- Advise the patient that he may experience slight discomfort and possible gagging or coughing during probe insertion.
- Explain the need for the patient to keep a diary of his symptoms while the probe is in place.

DIAGNOSTIC PROCEDURE

KEY STEPS

- Confirm the patient's identity using two patient identifiers according to facility policy.
- The patient is placed in high Fowler's position.
- A probe, with a pH electrode, is inserted gently into one of the patient's nostrils.
- The probe is advanced to the lower esophageal sphincter.
- After it's appropriately placed, the probe is taped to the patient's cheek and placed behind his ear with the unit attached to the recorder.

POSTPROCEDURE CARE

- Schedule a return visit in 24 hours to remove the probe.
- Instruct the patient to resume his usual diet and medications.

PRECAUTIONS

- If the probe inadvertently enters the trachea, causing respiratory distress or paroxysmal coughing, the catheter is removed immediately.

COMPLICATIONS

- Catheter entering the trachea
- Epistaxis (rare)

INTERPRETATION

NORMAL RESULTS

- pH is 4.0 during 4% or less of the 24 hours.

ABNORMAL RESULTS

- pH of 4.0 occurs during more than 4% of the 24 hours, suggesting gastroesophageal reflux disease.

pH test, urine

DESCRIPTION

- Measures how acidic or alkaline (basic) the urine is; may range from 0 (most acidic) to 14 (most basic)
- Affected by certain types of treatment
- Acidic or alkaline urine: may prevent formation of certain kidney calculi

PURPOSE

- To measure the acidic or alkaline value of urine

PREPARATION

- No dietary restrictions are required.

Teaching points

- Explain to the patient the purpose of the test and how it's done.
- Explain who will perform the test and where it'll be done.
- Tell the patient to avoid foods that will alter pH, such as dairy products and citrus foods.
- Tell the patient to avoid medications such as antacids that will alter pH.
- Tell the patient that the test should take less than 5 minutes.

KEY STEPS

- Confirm the patient's identity using two patient identifiers according to facility policy.
- Collect a urine specimen.
- Test the sample with litmus paper test strips or reagent test strips.

POSTPROCEDURE CARE

- Answer the patient's questions about the test.
- Inform the practitioner of abnormal results.

PRECAUTIONS

- None

COMPLICATIONS

- None

NORMAL RESULTS

- pH is 4.5 to 8.0.

ABNORMAL RESULTS

- pH is less than 4.0 (strongly acidic).
- pH is greater than 9.0 (strongly alkaline).
- Acidic pH may be a sign of severe lung disease (emphysema), uncontrolled diabetes, aspirin overdose, prolonged diarrhea, dehydration, starvation, drinking an excessive amount of alcohol or antifreeze (ethylene glycol), renal tuberculosis, pyrexia, phenylketonuria, alkaptonuria, and acidosis.
- Alkaline pH can be caused by Fanconi's syndrome, metabolic or respiratory alkalosis, prolonged vomiting, kidney disease, urinary tract infection caused by urea-splitting bacteria (*Proteus* and *Pseudomonas*), and asthma.

Phenolsulfonphthalein excretion test

DESCRIPTION

- Evaluates kidney function
- Should be performed in patients with abnormal results in the urine concentration test, an early sign of renal dysfunction
- Also called *PSP*

PURPOSE

- To determine renal plasma flow
- To evaluate tubular function

PREPARATION

- Encourage the patient to drink fluids before and during the test to maintain adequate urine flow.
- No dietary restrictions are needed before the test.
- Notify the laboratory and practitioner of medications the patient is taking that may affect test results; they may be restricted. If the patient must continue them, note this on the laboratory request.
- If the patient is unable to void, place a urinary catheter.

Teaching points

- Explain that this test evaluates kidney function.
- Explain who will perform the test and where it'll be done.
- Tell the patient that he doesn't have to restrict his diet.
- Tell the patient that the test requires an I.V. injection and collection of urine specimens 15 minutes, 30 minutes, 1 hour, and possibly 2 hours after the I.V. injection.
- Tell the patient who will give the I.V. injection and when.
- Explain that the patient may experience slight discomfort from the tourniquet and the needle puncture and that the dye temporarily turns the urine red.
- If the patient can't void and requires catheterization, tell him that he may have the urge to void when the catheter is in place.
- Tell the patient the total test takes about 2½ hours.

DIAGNOSTIC PROCEDURE

KEY STEPS

- Confirm the patient's identity using two patient identifiers according to facility policy.
- Instruct the patient to empty his bladder and discard the urine.
- The physician will give 1 ml of PSP, which equals 6 mg of dye, I.V.
- Collect a urine specimen at 15 minutes, 30 minutes, 1 hour and, possibly 2 hours after the injection.
- Encourage the patient to drink fluids because 40 ml of urine is needed for each specimen.
- Record the PSP dosage on the laboratory request.
- Properly label each specimen and include the collection time.

POSTPROCEDURE CARE

- Monitor the I.V. site for signs of infiltration.
- If the patient had a catheter inserted, make sure he voids within 8 hours after the catheter is removed.
- Keep epinephrine, histamine-1 receptor antagonists (diphenhydramine [Benadryl]), and a glucocorticoid (methylprednisolone [Medrol]) available due to the possibility of allergic reactions to PSP.
- Elevate the arm and apply warm soaks if phlebitis develops at the I.V. site.
- Inform the practitioner of abnormal results.
- Tell the patient to resume his usual medications.

PRECAUTIONS

- Don't use the urine in the drainage bag if the patient already has a catheter in place.
- Empty the bag, and clamp the catheter for 1 hour before the test.
- Send the specimen to the laboratory immediately after collection.
- Refrigerate the specimen if more than 10 minutes will elapse before transport.

COMPLICATIONS

- Phlebitis at the I.V. site
- Allergic reaction to PSP

NORMAL RESULTS

- In adults, 25% of the PSP dose is excreted in 15 minutes, 50% to 60% in 30 minutes, 60% to 70% in 1 hour, and 70% to 80% in 2 hours.
- In children (excluding infants), results should be 5% to 10% higher than those in adults.

ABNORMAL RESULTS

- The 15-minute value is the most sensitive indicator of tubular function and renal plasma flow because depressed excretion at this interval, with normal excretion later, suggests relatively mild or early-stage bilateral renal disease.
- A depressed 2-hour value may reveal moderate to severe renal impairment.
- Depressed PSP excretion is also characteristic in renal vascular disease, urinary tract obstruction, heart failure, and gout.
- Elevated PSP excretion is characteristic in hypoalbuminemia, hepatic disease, and multiple myeloma.

Phenylalanine screening

DESCRIPTION

- Screens infants for elevated serum levels of phenylalanine, a naturally occurring amino acid essential to growth and nitrogen balance; accumulation may indicate phenylketonuria (PKU), a serious enzyme deficiency
- Detects abnormal phenylalanine levels through the growth rate of *Bacillus subtilis,* which needs phenylalanine to thrive
- To ensure accurate results, performed after 3 full days (preferably 4 days) of milk or formula feeding
- Also called the *Guthrie screening test*

PURPOSE

- To screen an infant for PKU

PREPARATION

- No dietary restrictions are required.
- The test requires a blood sample.

Teaching points

- Explain to the parents that this test is a routine screening measure for possible PKU and is required in many states.
- Explain who will perform the test and where it'll be done.
- Tell the parents that a small amount of blood will be drawn from the infant's heel, and that collecting the sample takes only a few minutes.
- Explain that no dietary restriction is needed.
- Reassure the parents of a child who may have PKU that, although this disease is a common cause of congenital mental deficiency, early detection and continuous treatment with a low-phenylalanine diet can prevent permanent mental retardation.

KEY STEPS

- Confirm the patient's identity using two patient identifiers according to facility policy.
- Perform a heelstick, and collect three drops of blood—one in each circle—on the filter paper.
- Note the infant's name and birth date and the date of the first milk or formula feeding on the laboratory request.

POSTPROCEDURE CARE

- Apply direct pressure to the heelstick site until bleeding stops.
- Inform the practitioner of abnormal results.

PRECAUTIONS

- Send the sample to the laboratory immediately.

COMPLICATIONS

- None

NORMAL RESULTS

- A negative test result showing normal phenylalanine levels (< 2 mg/dl [SI, < 121 µmol/L]) suggests no appreciable danger of PKU.

ABNORMAL RESULTS

- A positive test result (> 2 mg/dl [SI, > 121 µmol/L]) may suggest PKU.
- A definitive diagnosis requires exact serum phenylalanine measurement and urine testing. (See *Confirming PKU.*)
- A positive test result may also indicate hepatic disease, galactosemia, or delayed development of certain enzyme systems.

INTERFERING FACTORS *Performing the test before the infant has received at least 3 full days of milk or formula feeding (false-negative results)*

Confirming PKU

If phenylalanine screening detects the possible presence of phenylketonuria (PKU), serum phenylalanine and tyrosine levels are measured to confirm the diagnosis. Phenylalanine hydroxylase is the enzyme that converts phenylalanine to tyrosine. If this enzyme is absent, increasing phenylalanine levels and falling tyrosine levels indicate PKU.

Samples are obtained by venipuncture (femoral or external jugular) and measured by fluorometry. Elevated serum phenylalanine levels (> 4 mg/dl [SI, > 242 µmol/L]) and decreased tyrosine levels — with urinary excretion of phenylpyruvic acid — confirm the diagnosis of PKU.

Phosphate level, serum

DESCRIPTION

- Measures levels of phosphate, the primary anion in intracellular fluid, needed for energy storage and use, calcium level regulation, red blood cell function, acid-base balance, bone formation, and the metabolism of carbohydrates, protein, and fat
- Mostly absorbed by intestines from dietary sources; kidneys excrete phosphates and serve as a regulatory mechanism
- Abnormal levels result of improper excretion rather than faulty ingestion or absorption from dietary sources
- Calcium and phosphate levels normally inversely related: if one is increased, the other is decreased

PURPOSE

- To help diagnose renal disorders and acid-base imbalance
- To detect endocrine, skeletal, and calcium disorders

PREPARATION

- Notify the laboratory and practitioner of medications the patient is taking that may affect test results; they may be restricted.
- No dietary restrictions are required.
- The test requires a blood sample.

Teaching points

- Explain that the serum phosphate test measures phosphate levels in the blood.
- Explain who will perform the test and where it'll be done.
- Inform the patient that he need not restrict food and fluids.
- Tell the patient that the test requires a blood sample and that he may experience slight discomfort from the tourniquet and needle puncture.
- Tell the patient the test takes less than 5 minutes.

KEY STEPS

- Confirm the patient's identity using two patient identifiers according to facility policy.
- Perform a venipuncture without using a tourniquet, if possible, and collect the sample in 3- or 4-ml clot-activator tube.

POSTPROCEDURE CARE

- Apply pressure to the venipuncture site until bleeding stops.
- Inform the practitioner of abnormal results.
- Tell the patient to resume medications.

PRECAUTIONS

- Maintain standard precautions while collecting the sample.
- Handle the sample gently to prevent hemolysis.

COMPLICATIONS

- Hematoma at the venipuncture site

NORMAL RESULTS

- In adults, levels are 2.7 to 4.5 mg/dl (SI, 0.87 to 1.45 mmol/L).
- In children, levels are 4.5 to 6.7 mg/dl (SI, 1.45 to 1.78 mmol/L).

ABNORMAL RESULTS

- Decreased phosphate levels (hypophosphatemia) may result from malnutrition, malabsorption syndromes, hyperparathyroidism, renal tubular acidosis, and treatment of diabetic ketoacidosis (DKA).
- In children, hypophosphatemia can suppress normal growth.
- Symptoms of hypophosphatemia include anemia, prolonged bleeding, bone demineralization, decreased white blood cell count, and anorexia.
- Increased levels (hyperphosphatemia) may result from skeletal disease, healing fractures, hypoparathyroidism, acromegaly, DKA, high intestinal obstruction, lactic acidosis (because of hepatic impairment), and renal failure.
- Hyperphosphatemia is seldom clinically significant, but it can alter bone metabolism in prolonged cases.
- Symptoms of hyperphosphatemia include tachycardia, muscular weakness, diarrhea, cramping, and hyperreflexia.

Phosphate level, urine

OVERVIEW

DESCRIPTION
- Determines if urine phosphate levels parallel serum levels
- Phosphates: absorbed in upper intestine and excreted in feces and urine; help carbohydrate metabolism; and help maintain tissue and fluid pH, electrolyte balance in cells and extracellular fluids, and permeability of cell membranes

PURPOSE
- To evaluate phosphate metabolism and excretion
- To monitor the treatment of phosphate deficiency

PREPARATION
- No dietary restrictions are required.
- Notify the laboratory and practitioner of medications the patient is taking that may affect test results; it may be necessary to restrict them.
- Encourage the patient to be as active as possible before the test.

Teaching points
- Explain that the urine phosphate test measures the amount of phosphate in the urine.
- Tell the patient that the test requires urine collection over a 24-hour period. If the patient will collect the specimen, teach him the proper technique.
- Instruct the patient about medication restrictions.

DIAGNOSTIC PROCEDURE

KEY STEPS
- Confirm the patient's identity using two patient identifiers according to facility policy.
- Collect the patient's urine over a 24-hour period, discarding the first specimen and retaining the last.

POSTPROCEDURE CARE
- Inform the practitioner of abnormal results.
- After the test, tell the patient to resume his usual activities and medications.

PRECAUTIONS
- Tell the patient not to contaminate the specimen with toilet tissue or feces.

COMPLICATIONS
- None

INTERPRETATION

NORMAL RESULTS
- Excretion of phosphate is < 1,000 mg/24 hours.
- Results depend on dietary intake.

ABNORMAL RESULTS
- Excretion of phosphate is > 1,000 mg/24 hours.
- Many disorders may affect phosphate levels.

Phospholipids test

DESCRIPTION

- Quantitative analysis of phospholipids—major form of lipids in cell membranes (aid in cellular membrane composition and permeability; help control enzyme activity within the membrane; help transport fatty acids and lipids across the intestinal barrier and from the liver and other fat stores to other body tissues; and are essential for pulmonary gas exchange)

PURPOSE

- To help evaluate fat metabolism
- To help diagnose hypothyroidism, diabetes mellitus, nephrotic syndrome, chronic pancreatitis, obstructive jaundice, and hypolipoproteinemia

PREPARATION

- Fasting is required overnight before the test.
- Notify the laboratory and practitioner of medications the patient is taking that may affect test results; they may be restricted.
- The test requires a blood sample.

Teaching points

- Explain that the phospholipid test is used to determine how the body metabolizes fats.
- Explain who will perform the test and where it'll be done.
- Instruct the patient to abstain from drinking alcohol for 24 hours before the test and to fast overnight before the test.
- Tell the patient that the test requires a blood sample and that he may experience slight discomfort from the tourniquet and needle puncture.
- Tell the patient the test takes less than 5 minutes.

DIAGNOSTIC PROCEDURE

KEY STEPS

- Confirm the patient's identity using two patient identifiers according to facility policy.
- Perform a venipuncture, and collect the sample in a 10- to 15-ml tube without additives.

POSTPROCEDURE CARE

- Apply direct pressure to the venipuncture site until bleeding stops.
- Inform the practitioner of abnormal results.
- Instruct the patient to resume his usual diet and medications.

PRECAUTIONS

- Send the sample to the laboratory immediately because spontaneous redistribution may occur among plasma lipids.

COMPLICATIONS

- Hematoma at the venipuncture site

INTERPRETATION

NORMAL RESULTS

- Level is 180 to 320 mg/dl (SI, 1.8 to 3.2 g/L).
- Men usually have higher levels than women, unless the woman is pregnant; values in pregnant women exceed those of men.

ABNORMAL RESULTS

- Elevated phospholipid levels may indicate hypothyroidism, diabetes mellitus, nephrotic syndrome, chronic pancreatitis, or obstructive jaundice.
- Decreased levels may indicate primary hypolipoproteinemia.

Plasminogen level, plasma

DESCRIPTION

- Assesses plasminogen level in a plasma sample
- Fibrinolysis: plasmin dissolves fibrin clots to prevent excessive coagulation and impaired blood flow
- Plasmin unable to circulate in active form; can't be directly measured
- Plasminogen, circulating precursor to plasmin, directly measurable and used to evaluate the fibrinolytic system

PURPOSE

- To assess fibrinolysis
- To detect congenital and acquired fibrinolytic disorders

PREPARATION

- Notify the laboratory and practitioner of medications the patient is taking that may affect test results; they may be restricted.
- No dietary restrictions are required.
- The test requires a blood sample.

Teaching points

- Explain that this test is used to evaluate blood clotting.
- Explain who will perform the test and where it'll be done.
- Tell the patient that he doesn't need to restrict his diet.
- Tell the patient that the test requires a blood sample and that he may experience slight discomfort from the tourniquet and needle puncture.
- Tell the patient the test takes less than 5 minutes.

KEY STEPS

- Confirm the patient's identity using two patient identifiers according to facility policy.
- Perform a venipuncture, and collect the sample in a 4.5 ml siliconized tube.

POSTPROCEDURE CARE

- Apply pressure to the venipuncture site until bleeding has stopped.
- Inform the practitioner of abnormal results.

PRECAUTIONS

- Collect the sample as quickly as possible to prevent stasis, which can slow blood flow, causing coagulation and plasminogen activation.
- Avoid excessive probing during venipuncture and rough handling of the sample to prevent hemolysis.
- Invert the tube gently several times, and immediately send the sample to the laboratory. If testing must be delayed, plasma must be separated and frozen at –94° F (–70° C).

COMPLICATIONS

- Hematoma at the venipuncture site

NORMAL RESULTS

- Levels range from 10 to 20 mg/dl (SI, 0.1 to 0.2 g/L) by immunologic methods.

ABNORMAL RESULTS

- Diminished plasminogen levels can result from disseminated intravascular coagulation, tumors, preeclampsia, and eclampsia, which accelerate plasminogen conversion top plasmin and increase fibrinolysis.
- Some liver diseases prevent formation of sufficient plasminogen, decreasing fibrinolysis.

INTERFERING FACTORS *Hormonal contraceptives (may cause slight increases in levels); thrombolytic drugs (may cause decreased levels)*

Platelet count

DESCRIPTION

- Tests function of platelets, or thrombocytes, which promote coagulation and formation of a hemostatic plug in vascular injury
- Determines ability of patient's blood to clot normally

PURPOSE

- To evaluate platelet production
- To assess the effects of chemotherapy or radiation therapy on platelet production
- To diagnose and monitor severe thrombocytosis or thrombocytopenia
- To confirm a visual estimate of platelet number and morphology from a stained blood film

PREPARATION

- Notify the laboratory and practitioner of medications the patient is taking that may affect test results; it may be necessary to restrict them.
- No dietary restrictions are required.
- The test requires a blood sample.

Teaching points

- Explain that the platelet count test determines whether the patient's blood clots normally.
- Explain who will perform the test and where it'll be done.
- Inform the patient that fasting isn't required before the test.
- Tell the patient that the test requires a blood sample, and that he may experience slight discomfort from the tourniquet and needle puncture.
- Tell the patient the test takes less than 5 minutes.

KEY STEPS

- Confirm the patient's identity using two patient identifiers according to facility policy.
- Perform a venipuncture, and collect the sample in a 3- or 4.5-ml EDTA tube.

POSTPROCEDURE CARE

- Make sure that subdermal bleeding has stopped before removing pressure.
- If a large hematoma develops, monitor pulses distal to the venipuncture site.
- Inform the practitioner of abnormal results.
- Tell the patient to resume medications, as ordered.

PRECAUTIONS

- Avoid excessive probing at the venipuncture site, and handle the sample gently to prevent hemolysis.
- Completely fill the collection tube, and invert it gently several times to mix the sample and the anticoagulant thoroughly.

COMPLICATIONS

- Hematoma at the venipuncture site

NORMAL RESULTS

- Adults, 140,000 to 400,000/μl (SI, 140 to 400 $\times$ 10^9/L).
- Children, 150,000 to 450,000/μl (SI, 150 to 450 $\times$ 10^9/L).

ABNORMAL RESULTS

- A count below 50,000/μl can cause spontaneous bleeding; when the count is below 5,000/μl, fatal central nervous system bleeding or massive GI hemorrhage is possible.
- A decreased count (thrombocytopenia, 80 to 100/μl [SI, 0.8 to 1 $\times$ 10^9/L]) can result from aplastic or hypoplastic bone marrow; infiltrative bone marrow disease, such as leukemia, or disseminated infection; megakaryocytic hypoplasia; ineffective thrombopoiesis caused by folic acid or vitamin B_{12} deficiency; pooling of platelets in an enlarged spleen; increased platelet destruction caused by drugs or immune disorders; disseminated intravascular coagulation; Bernard-Soulier syndrome; or mechanical injury to platelets.
- An increased count (thrombocytosis) can result from hemorrhage, infectious disorders, iron deficiency anemia, recent surgery, pregnancy, splenectomy, or inflammatory disorders. In such cases, the platelet count returns to normal after the patient recovers from the primary disorder.
- An increased count remains elevated in primary thrombocythemia, myelofibrosis with myeloid metaplasia, polycythemia vera, and chronic myelogenous leukemia.
- Whenever the platelet count is abnormal, diagnosis usually requires complete blood count, bone marrow biopsy, direct antiglobulin test (direct Coombs' test), and serum protein electrophoresis for confirmation.

Plethysmography, venous

- Reliable, widely used, noninvasive test that measures venous flow in the limbs
- Plethysmograph electrodes applied to the patient's leg to record changes in electrical resistance (impedance) from blood volume variations, which may result from respiration or venous occlusion
- Also called *occlusive impedance phlebography*

PURPOSE

- To detect deep vein thrombosis (DVT) in the proximal deep veins of the leg
- To screen the patient at high risk for thrombophlebitis
- To evaluate the patient with suspected pulmonary embolism (because most pulmonary emboli are complications of DVT in the leg)

PREPARATION

- Keep the room temperature as warm as possible to help prevent the patient's extremities from becoming cold.
- No dietary or medication restrictions are required.

Teaching points

- Explain that plethysmography helps detect DVT.
- Explain who will perform the test and where it'll be done.
- Inform the patient that he need not restrict food, fluids, or medications.
- Explain that both legs will receive the test and that three to five tracings may be made for each leg.
- Assure the patient that the test is painless and safe.
- Just before the test, instruct the patient to void and to put on a hospital gown.
- Reassure the patient that if he experiences pain that interferes with leg relaxation he may receive a mild analgesic.
- Emphasize that accurate testing requires that leg muscles be relaxed and breathing be normal.

- Urge the patient to lie quietly and relax as much as possible.
- Tell the patient the test takes 30 to 45 minutes.

DIAGNOSTIC PROCEDURE

KEY STEPS

- Confirm the patient's identity using two patient identifiers according to facility policy.
- Assist the patient into the supine position, elevating the leg to be tested 30 to 35 degrees. To promote venous drainage, place the calf above the patient's heart level.
- Ask the patient to flex his knee slightly and to rotate his hips by shifting his weight to the same side as the leg being tested.
- After the electrodes (connected to the plethysmograph) have been loosely attached to the calf about 3″ to 4″ (7.5 to 10 cm) apart, the pressure cuff (connected to the air pressure system) is wrapped snugly around the thigh about 2″ (5 cm) above the knee.
- The pressure cuff is inflated to 45 to 60 cm H_2O, allowing full venous distention without interfering with arterial blood flow.
- Pressure is maintained for 45 seconds or until the tracing stabilizes.
- In a patient with reduced arterial blood flow, pressure is maintained for 2 minutes or longer, after which the pressure cuff is rapidly deflated.
- The strip chart tracing, which records the increase in venous volume after cuff inflation and the decrease in venous volume 3 seconds after deflation, is checked.
- The test is repeated for the other leg.
- If necessary, three to five tracings for each leg are obtained to confirm full venous filling and outflow; the tracing showing the greatest rise and fall in venous volume is used as the test result.
- If the result is ambiguous, the position of the patient's leg and placement of the cuff and electrode are checked.

POSTPROCEDURE CARE

- Remove the conductive gel from the patient's skin after the test.
- Inform the practitioner of abnormal results.

PRECAUTIONS

- Decreased peripheral arterial blood flow may interfere with test results.

COMPLICATIONS

- None

NORMAL RESULTS

- Temporary venous occlusion normally produces a sharp rise in venous volume; release of the occlusion produces rapid venous outflow.

ABNORMAL RESULTS

- When clots in a major deep vein obstruct venous outflow, calf vein pressure rises; these veins become distended and can't expand further when more pressure is applied with an occlusive thigh cuff.
- Blockage of major deep veins also decreases the rate at which blood flows from the leg.
- If significant thrombi are present in a major deep vein of the lower leg (such as the popliteal, femoral, or iliac vein), calf vein filling and venous outflow rates are reduced. The practitioner will evaluate the need for further treatment, such as anticoagulant therapy, taking the patient's overall condition into consideration.

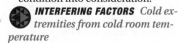 **INTERFERING FACTORS** *Cold extremities from cold room temperature*

Pleural biopsy

OVERVIEW

DESCRIPTION
- Removal of a sample of pleural tissue by needle biopsy or open biopsy for histologic examination
- Percutaneous needle pleural biopsy: performed under local anesthesia using image-guidance
- Open pleural biopsy: performed in the operating room: permits direct visualization of the pleura and the underlying lung

PURPOSE
- To differentiate between nonmalignant and malignant disease
- To diagnose viral, fungal, or parasitic disease
- To diagnose collagen vascular disease of the pleura

PREPARATION
- Make sure the patient has signed an appropriate consent form.
- Note and report all allergies.
- Fasting is required for at least 8 hours before the test.

Teaching points
- Explain the purpose of the test and how it's done.
- Explain who will perform the biopsy and where it'll be done.
- Tell the patient he must fast for 8 hours before the procedure.
- Advise the patient that chest X-rays will be taken before and after the biopsy.
- Provide reassurance that the patient should experience minimal pain.
- Tell him the test takes 30 to 45 minutes.

DIAGNOSTIC PROCEDURE

KEY STEPS
- Confirm the patient's identity using two patient identifiers according to facility policy.
- The skin site is cleaned and prepared.
- A local anesthetic is administered.

- The needle or trocar is inserted into the biopsy site. (See *Using Cope's needle*.)
- The specimen is withdrawn and immediately put into 10% neutral buffered formalin solution in a labeled specimen bottle.
- The skin around the biopsy site is cleaned and dressed.

POSTPROCEDURE CARE
- Obtain a chest X-ray immediately after the biopsy.
- Monitor the patient's vital signs, intake and output, pulse oximetry, respiratory status, breath sounds, and for subcutaneous emphysema.
- Instruct the patient to resume his diet and activity as ordered.
- Have the patient lie on his unaffected side to help promote healing of the biopsy site.

PRECAUTIONS
WARNING *Watch for signs and symptoms of pneumothorax, such as dyspnea, pleuritic chest pain, apprehension, agitation, decreased breath sounds, tracheal deviation, subcutaneous emphysema, or signs of decreased cardiac output.*

COMPLICATIONS
- Pneumothorax
- Hemorrhage
- Vasovagal reaction
- Infection

INTERPRETATION

NORMAL RESULTS
- Pleura consists primarily of mesothelial cells, flattened in a uniform layer.
- Layers of areolar connective tissue contain blood vessels, nerves, and lymphatics.

ABNORMAL RESULTS
- Lesions that are fibrous and epithelial suggest primary neoplasms.
- Specific histologic results from tissue analysis suggest possible disorders including: malignant disease, tuberculosis, viral, fungal, or parasitic disease, and collagen vascular disease.

Using Cope's needle

Cope's needle, which is used to obtain a pleural biopsy specimen, consists of three parts: a sharp obturator (A) and a cannula (B), which when fitted together are called a *trocar,* and a blunt-ended, hooked stylet (C). The trocar is used to gain access to the pleural cavity. The obturator is then removed, leaving the cannula in place. The stylet is passed through the cannula to excise a tissue specimen, as shown below.

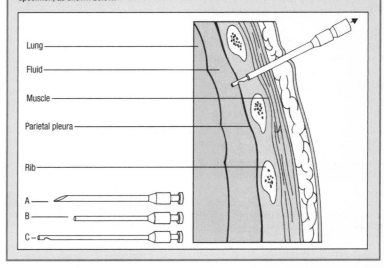

Pleural fluid analysis

DESCRIPTION

- Analyzes a specimen of pleural fluid collected during pleural fluid aspiration (thoracentesis)

PURPOSE

- To determine the cause and nature of pleural effusion
- To permit better radiographic visualization of a lung with large effusions

PREPARATION

- Check the patient's history for hypersensitivity to local anesthetics.
- No dietary restrictions are required.

Teaching points

- Explain that this test assesses the space around the lungs for fluid.
- Explain who will perform the test and where it'll be done.
- Inform the patient that he doesn't need to restrict his diet.
- Warn the patient that he may feel a stinging sensation on injection of the anesthetic and some pressure during withdrawal of the fluid.
- Tell him the test takes about 30 minutes.
- Instruct him not to cough, breathe deeply, or move during the test.

DIAGNOSTIC PROCEDURE

KEY STEPS

- Confirm the patient's identity using two patient identifiers according to facility policy.
- Shave the area around the insertion site.
- Position the patient to widen the intercostal spaces and to allow easier access to the pleural cavity.
- Position the patient at the edge of the bed with a chair or stool supporting his feet, and his head and arms resting on a padded overbed table.
- If he can't sit up, position him on his unaffected side, with the arm on affected side elevated above his head.
- After positioning, the physician disinfects the skin, drapes the area, injects a local anesthetic into the subcutaneous tissue, and inserts the thoracentesis needle.
- When the needle reaches the pocket of fluid, the 50-ml syringe is attached and the stopcock and clamps are opened on the tubing to aspirate the fluid into the container.
- During aspiration, observe for signs of respiratory distress.
- After the needle is withdrawn, apply slight pressure and a small adhesive bandage to the puncture site.
- Label the specimen container, and record the date and time of the test; the amount, color, and character of the fluid; and the exact location from which fluid was removed.
- Note the patient's temperature and whether he's receiving antimicrobial therapy on the laboratory request.

POSTPROCEDURE CARE

- Reposition the patient comfortably on the affected side. Tell him to remain on this side for at least 1 hour.
- Elevate the head of the bed to facilitate breathing.
- Monitor vital signs every 30 minutes for 2 hours and then every 4 hours until stable.
- Tell patient to call a nurse immediately if he experiences difficulty breathing.
- The patient receives a posttest X-ray to detect complications.
- Check puncture site for fluid leakage.

PRECAUTIONS

- Watch for signs of pneumothorax, tension pneumothorax, fluid reaccumulation, and—if a large amount of fluid was withdrawn—pulmonary edema or cardiac distress caused by mediastinal shift.

COMPLICATIONS

- Pneumothorax
- Tension pneumothorax

INTERPRETATION

NORMAL RESULTS

- Pleural cavity pressure is negative, with less than 20 ml of serous fluid.

ABNORMAL RESULTS

- Exudate is a protein-rich fluid leaked from blood vessels with increased permeability.
- Pleural fluid may contain blood (hemothorax), chyle (chylothorax), pus (empyema), or necrotic tissue.
- Blood-tinged fluid may indicate a traumatic tap; the fluid should clear as aspiration progresses.
- Transudative effusion usually results from diminished colloidal pressure, increased negative pressure within the pleural cavity, ascites, systemic and pulmonary venous hypertension, heart failure, hepatic cirrhosis, and nephritis.
- Exudative effusion results from disorders that increase pleural capillary permeability, lymphatic drainage interference, infections, pulmonary infarctions, and neoplasms.
- Exudative effusion with depressed glucose levels, elevated lactate dehydrogenase (LD) isoenzymes, rheumatoid arthritis cells, and negative smears, cultures, and cytologic examination may indicate pleurisy linked to rheumatoid arthritis.
- Cultures are usually positive during the early stages of infection.
- Empyema may result from complications of pneumonia, pulmonary abscess, perforation of the esophagus, or penetration from mediastinitis.
- High percentage of neutrophils suggests septic inflammation.
- Lymphocytes suggest tuberculosis or fungal or viral effusions.
- Serosanguineous fluid suggests pleural extension of a malignant tumor.
- Elevated LD in a nonpurulent, nonhemolyzed, nonbloody effusion may also suggest malignancy.
- Pleural fluid glucose levels 30 to 40 mg/dl lower than blood glucose levels may indicate a malignant tumor, a bacterial infection, nonseptic inflammation, or metastasis.
- Increased amylase levels occur in pleural effusions associated with pancreatitis.

Porphyrin test, urine

DESCRIPTION

- Quantitatively analyzes uroporphyrins and coproporphyrins and their precursors (porphyrinogens)
- Porphyrins: red-orange fluorescent compounds; produced during heme biosynthesis; found in protoplasm and excreted in small amounts
- Increased urine levels of porphyrins or porphyrinogens: may be caused by impaired heme biosynthesis, resulting from inherited enzyme deficiencies or from hemolytic anemia or hepatic disease
- Specific porphyrins and porphyrinogens in urine help identify the impaired metabolic step in heme biosynthesis
- For correct diagnosis of specific porphyria: urine porphyrin levels should be correlated with plasma and fecal porphyrin levels
- Preliminary qualitative screening test is sometimes performed on a random specimen; positive result must be confirmed by the quantitative analysis of a 24-hour specimen

PURPOSE

- To help diagnose congenital or acquired porphyria

PREPARATION

- The test requires urine collection over a 24-hour period.
- No dietary restrictions are required.
- Notify the laboratory and practitioner of medications the patient is taking that may affect test results; they may be restricted.

Teaching points

- Explain that the urine porphyrin test detects abnormal heme formation.
- Tell the patient that the test requires urine collection over a 24-hour period, and teach him the proper collection technique.
- Inform the patient that he need not restrict food and fluids.

DIAGNOSTIC PROCEDURES

KEY STEPS

- Confirm the patient's identity using two patient identifiers according to facility policy.
- Collect the patient's urine over a 24-hour period, discarding the first specimen and retaining the last.
- Put the collection bag in a dark place if an indwelling urinary catheter is in place.
- Send the specimen to the laboratory immediately.

POSTPROCEDURE CARE

- Inform the practitioner of abnormal results.
- Tell the patient to resume his usual medications.

PRECAUTIONS

- Use a light-resistant specimen bottle containing a preservative to prevent degradation of the light-sensitive porphyrins and their precursors.
- Refrigerate the specimen, or keep it on ice during the collection period.

COMPLICATIONS

- None

INTERPRETATION

NORMAL RESULTS

- Uroporphyrin levels are 27 to 52 mcg/24 hours (SI, 32 to 63 nmol/d).
- Coproporphyrin levels are 34 to 230 mcg/24 hours (SI, 52 to 351 nmol/d).

ABNORMAL RESULTS

- Increased urine levels of porphyrins and porphyrin precursors are characteristic of porphyria. (See *Urine porphyrin levels in porphyria*.)
- Infectious hepatitis, Hodgkin's disease, central nervous system disorders, cirrhosis, or heavy metal, benzene, or carbon tetrachloride toxicity may also increase porphyrin levels.

Urine porphyrin levels in porphyria

In porphyria, defective heme biosynthesis increases urine porphyrins and their corresponding precursors.

PORPHYRIA	PORPHYRINS		PORPHYRIN PRECURSORS	
	Uroporphyrins	Coproporphyrins	∂-amino-levulinic acid	Porphobilinogen
Erythropoietic porphyria	Highly increased	Increased	Normal	Normal
Erythropoietic protoporphyria	Normal	Normal	Normal	Normal
Acute intermittent porphyria	Variable	Variable	Highly increased	Highly increased
Variegate porphyria	Normal or slightly increased; may be highly increased during acute attack	Normal or slightly increased; may be highly increased during acute attack	Highly increased during acute attack	Normal or slightly increased; highly increased during acute attack
Coproporphyria	Not applicable	May be highly increased during acute attack	Increased during acute attack	Increased during acute attack
Porphyria cutanea tarda	Highly increased	Increased	Variable	Variable

Positron emission tomography

DESCRIPTION
- Nuclear medicine scan that measures the metabolic process of the organ being observed; also known as *PET*
- Radioactive chemicals administered to patient; positrons emitted from the chemicals in organs are detected by sensors placed around patient during the scan
- Positron counts, with computed tomography, help record the image of the organ in a two- or three-dimensional image
- Scan yields information about anatomy and physiology of an organ by demonstrating glucose metabolism, blood flow, tissue perfusion, and oxygenation of a specific area
- Used mostly in cardiology, neurology, and oncology

PURPOSE
- To detect strokes or aneurysms by decreased blood flow and oxygen consumption
- To diagnose Parkinson's disease and Huntington's disease based on decreased cerebral metabolism
- To evaluate cranial tumor preoperatively and postoperatively to help determine treatment
- To assess the size of myocardial infarcts
- To assess the presence of coronary artery disease as seen by decreased metabolism during ischemia and after angina
- To evaluate the presence or recurrence of cancer or tumors
- To evaluate the presence of metastases of a cancerous tumor
- To monitor the effectiveness of therapy

PREPARATION
- Make sure the patient signs an informed consent form if required.
- Instruct him to void before beginning the test.
- If the patient has diabetes, have him take his insulin at the usual time and eat a meal 4 hours before the test.
- Have all patients fast for 4 hours before the test and avoid alcohol, caffeine, and tobacco for 24 hours before the test.

Teaching points
- Explain that the PET scan will help monitor organ function.
- Explain who will perform the test and where it'll be done.
- Explain that he will have two I.V. access sites.
- Tell the patient to fast for 4 hours before the test.
- Instruct the patient to avoid alcohol, caffeine, and tobacco products for at least 24 hours before the test.
- Warn him not to take a sedative or tranquilizer before the test.
- Reassure him that his exposure to radioactive material will be minimal.
- Tell the patient the test takes 45 to 90 minutes.

KEY STEPS
- Confirm the patient's identity using two patient identifiers according to facility policy.
- Position the patient as appropriate for the organs to be scanned.
- Inject the radioactive material through an I.V. line.
- The gamma rays that are able to penetrate the tissue are recorded outside the body by a series of detectors and are displayed on a computer screen.
- If the patient is having a brain scan done, he may be asked to perform a series of cognitive activities.
- The imagining is done at periodic intervals for up to 1 hour.

POSTPROCEDURE CARE
- Remove the I.V. access, and monitor the site for swelling, hematoma, or redness.
- Inform the practitioner of abnormal results.
- Instruct the patient to increase his fluid intake for 24 to 48 hours to help flush the radionuclide from the body, unless otherwise ordered.

PRECAUTIONS
- Wear gloves while handling the radionuclide.
- Have emergency resuscitation equipment available during the procedure in case the patient has a reaction to the radionuclide.

COMPLICATIONS
- I.V. infiltration
- Reaction to the radionuclide

NORMAL RESULTS
- Normal organ anatomy and physiology, including tissue metabolism, oxygenation, and blood flow, are noted.

ABNORMAL RESULTS
- Abnormalities vary depending on organ being scanned.
- A brain scan will show abnormalities including strokes, metastasis in the brain, dementia, head trauma, migraines, seizure disorders, and tumors.
- Cardiac scan abnormalities may indicate necrotic tissue, hypertrophic left ventricle, myocardial infarction, ischemia, pulmonary edema, and chronic obstructive pulmonary disease.
- Increased radionuclide uptake is seen in abnormal lymph nodes, tumors, and metastasis.

Potassium level, serum

DESCRIPTION

◆ Measures serum levels of potassium (major intracellular cation that helps maintain cellular osmotic equilibrium; regulates muscle activity, enzyme activity, and acid-base balance; and influences renal function)
◆ Potassium deficiency common, developing rapidly (kidneys excrete nearly all ingested potassium, even when body's supply depleted)
◆ Levels affected by variations in secretions of adrenal steroid hormones and by fluctuations in pH, serum glucose levels, and serum sodium levels
◆ Reciprocal relationship between potassium and sodium, substantial intake of one element causing corresponding decrease in the other
◆ Dietary potassium intake of at least 40 mEq/day essential, with average diet usually including 60 to 100 mEq of potassium (see *Dietary sources of potassium;* also see *Treating potassium imbalance,* page 386)

PURPOSE

◆ To evaluate clinical signs of potassium excess (hyperkalemia) or potassium depletion (hypokalemia)
◆ To monitor renal function, acid-base balance, and glucose metabolism
◆ To evaluate neuromuscular and endocrine disorders
◆ To detect the origin of arrhythmias

PREPARATION

◆ Notify the laboratory and practitioner of medications the patient is taking that may affect test results; they may be restricted.
◆ No dietary restrictions are required.
◆ The test requires a blood sample.

Teaching points

◆ Explain that the serum potassium test determines the potassium content of blood.
◆ Explain who will perform the test and where it'll be done.
◆ Inform the patient that he doesn't need to restrict his diet.
◆ Tell the patient that the test requires a blood sample and that he may experience slight discomfort from the tourniquet and needle puncture.
◆ Tell the patient that the test takes less than 5 minutes.

Dietary sources of potassium

A healthy person needs to consume at least 40 mEq of potassium daily. The chart here highlights foods and beverages, their serving sizes, and the amount of potassium each contains.

FOODS AND BEVERAGES	SERVING SIZE	AMOUNT OF POTASSIUM (mEq)
Meats		
Beef	4 oz (112 g)	11.2
Chicken	4 oz	12
Scallops	5 large	30
Veal	4 oz	15.2
Vegetables		
Artichokes	1 large bud	7.7
Asparagus (frozen, cooked)	½ cup (120 g)	5.5
Asparagus (raw)	6 spears	7.7
Beans (dried, cooked)	½ cup	10
Beans (lima)	½ cup	9.5
Broccoli (cooked)	½ cup	7
Carrots (cooked)	½ cup	5.7
Carrots (raw)	1 large	8.8
Mushrooms (raw)	4 large	10.6
Potatoes (baked)	1 small	15.4
Spinach (raw or cooked)	½ cup	8.5
Squash (winter, baked)	½ cup	12
Tomatoes (raw)	1 medium	10.4
Fruits		
Apricots (dried)	4 halves	5
Apricots (raw)	3 small	8
Bananas	1 medium	12.8
Cantaloupe	6 oz	13
Figs (dried)	7 small	17.5
Peaches (raw)	1 medium	6.2
Pears (raw)	1 medium	6.2
Beverages		
Apricot nectar	1 cup (240 ml)	9
Grapefruit juice	1 cup	8.2
Orange juice	1 cup	11.4
Pineapple juice	1 cup	9
Prune juice	1 cup	14.4
Tomato juice	1 cup	11.6
Milk (whole or skim)	1 cup	8.8

(continued)

DIAGNOSTIC PROCEDURE

KEY STEPS

- Confirm the patient's identity using two patient identifiers according to facility policy.
- Perform a venipuncture, and collect the sample in a 3- or 4-ml clot-activator tube.
- Draw the sample immediately after applying the tourniquet because a delay may increase the potassium level by allowing intracellular potassium to leak into the serum.

POSTPROCEDURE CARE

- Apply direct pressure to the venipuncture site until bleeding stops.
- Inform the practitioner of abnormal results.
- Instruct the patient to resume any medications stopped.

PRECAUTIONS

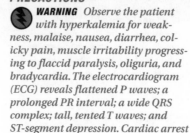 **WARNING** *Observe the patient with hyperkalemia for weakness, malaise, nausea, diarrhea, colicky pain, muscle irritability progressing to flaccid paralysis, oliguria, and bradycardia. The electrocardiogram (ECG) reveals flattened P waves; a prolonged PR interval; a wide QRS complex; tall, tented T waves; and ST-segment depression. Cardiac arrest may occur without warning.*

WARNING *Observe the patient with hypokalemia for decreased reflexes; a rapid, weak, irregular pulse; mental confusion; hypotension; anorexia; muscle weakness; and paresthesia. The ECG shows a flattened T wave, ST-segment depression, and U-wave elevation. In severe cases, ventricular fibrillation, respiratory paralysis, and cardiac arrest can develop.*

- Handle the sample gently to prevent hemolysis.

COMPLICATIONS

- Hematoma at the venipuncture site

INTERPRETATION

NORMAL RESULTS

- Value is 3.5 to 5 mEq/L (SI, 3.5 to 5 mmol/L).

ABNORMAL RESULTS

- Hyperkalemia: when excess potassium enters the blood (possibly indicating burn injury, crush injury, diabetic ketoacidosis, transfusions of large amounts of blood, or myocardial infarction) or when sodium excretion is reduced, possibly because of renal failure (preventing normal exchange of sodium and potassium) or Addison's disease (due to potassium buildup and sodium depletion).
- Hypokalemia: in aldosteronism or Cushing's syndrome, loss of body fluids (such as long-term diuretic therapy, vomiting, or diarrhea), and excessive licorice ingestion.
- Although serum values and clinical symptoms can indicate a potassium imbalance, an ECG allows a definitive diagnosis.

INTERFERING FACTORS *Excessive or rapid potassium infusion, spironolactone (Aldactone) or penicillin G potassium therapy, and renal toxicity from administration of amphotericin B (Amphocin) or tetracycline (Sumycin) (may cause increased values); insulin and glucose administration; diuretic therapy (especially with thiazides but not with triamterene [Dyrenium] or spironolactone); and I.V. infusions without potassium (may cause decreased values)*

Treating potassium imbalance

Hypokalemia and hyperkalemia can cause serious problems if not treated promptly.

HYPOKALEMIA

A patient with a potassium deficiency can be treated with oral potassium chloride replacement and increased dietary intake. In severe cases, potassium can be replaced by I.V. infusion at a rate not exceeding 20 mEq/hour and at a concentration of no more than 80 mEq/L of I.V. fluid. Mix the I.V. solution well because potassium can settle near the neck of the bottle or plastic bag. Failure to mix the solution adequately or to infuse it properly can cause a burning sensation at the I.V. site and possibly even fatal hyperkalemia.

Monitor the electrocardiogram, urine output, and serum potassium levels frequently during the infusion. Never administer I.V. potassium replacement to a patient with inadequate urine flow because diminished excretion can rapidly lead to hyperkalemia.

HYPERKALEMIA

Dangerously high potassium levels may be reduced with sodium polystyrene sulfonate — a potassium-removing resin — administered orally, rectally, or through a nasogastric tube. Hyperkalemia may also be treated with an I.V. infusion of sodium bicarbonate or of glucose and insulin, which lowers blood potassium by causing it to move into cells.

A calcium I.V. infusion provides fast but transient relief from the cardiotoxic effects of hyperkalemia; however, it doesn't directly lower serum potassium levels. In renal failure, dialysis may help remove excess potassium, but this procedure corrects the imbalance much more slowly.

Potassium level, urine

DESCRIPTION

- Quantitative measurement of urine levels of potassium (major intracellular cation that helps regulate acid-base balance and neuromuscular function)
- Potassium imbalance: may cause muscle weakness, nausea, diarrhea, confusion, hypotension, and electrocardiogram changes; severe imbalance may lead to cardiac arrest
- May help evaluate abnormally low potassium levels (hypokalemia) discovered by serum potassium test results, if cause of imbalance is unknown

PURPOSE

- To determine whether hypokalemia is caused by renal or extrarenal disorders

PREPARATION

- No dietary restrictions are required.
- The test requires urine collection over 24 hours.
- Notify the laboratory and practitioner of medications the patient is taking that may affect test results; they may be restricted.

Teaching points

- Explain that the urine potassium test evaluates kidney function.
- Explain who will perform the test and where it'll be done.
- Advise the patient that he doesn't have to restrict his diet.
- Tell the patient that the test requires urine collection over a 24-hour period, and teach him how to collect a 24-hour urine sample.

KEY STEPS

- Confirm the patient's identity using two patient identifiers according to facility policy.
- Collect the patient's urine over a 24-hour period, discarding the first specimen and retaining the last.
- Give the patient potassium supplements, and monitor serum levels as appropriate.
- Instruct the patient not to use a metallic bedpan for collection.
- Tell the patient not to contaminate the specimen with toilet tissue or feces.

POSTPROCEDURE CARE

- Provide dietary supplements and nutritional counseling as necessary.
- Replace fluid volume loss with I.V. or oral fluids as needed.
- Inform the practitioner of abnormal results.
- Tell the patient to resume his usual medications as ordered.

PRECAUTIONS

- Refrigerate the specimen, or place it on ice during the collection period.
- Send the specimen to the laboratory immediately after the collection is complete, or refrigerate it.

COMPLICATIONS

- None

NORMAL RESULTS

- In adults, 25 to 125 mmol/24 hours (SI, 25 to 125 mmol/d) is normal, varying with diet.
- In children, 22 to 57 mmol/24 hours (SI, 22 to 57 mmol/d) is normal.

ABNORMAL RESULTS

- In a patient with hypokalemia, a potassium level less than 10 mmol/24 hours (SI, < 10 mmol/d) suggests normal renal function, indicating that potassium loss is most likely the result of a GI disorder such as malabsorption syndrome.
- In a patient with hypokalemia lasting more than 3 days, urine potassium level above 10 mmol/24 hours (SI, > 10 mmol/d) indicates renal loss of potassium.
- Renal potassium losses may result from such disorders as aldosteronism, renal tubular acidosis, or chronic renal failure.
- Extrarenal disorders, such as dehydration, starvation, Cushing's disease, or salicylate intoxication, may elevate urine potassium levels.

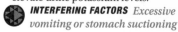 **INTERFERING FACTORS** *Excessive vomiting or stomach suctioning*

Prealbumin test

DESCRIPTION
- Measures protein produced primarily in the liver
- Short half-life (2 days), which makes it a good indicator of nutritional status

PURPOSE
- To evaluate nutritional status

PREPARATION
- Withhold food and fluid for 4 hours before the test.
- The test requires a blood sample.

Teaching points
- Explain that the prealbumin test helps determine his nutritional status.
- Explain who will perform the test and where it'll be done.
- Tell the patient to fast for 4 hours before the test.
- Tell the patient that the test requires a blood sample, and that he may experience slight discomfort from the tourniquet and needle puncture.
- Tell the patient that the test takes less than 5 minutes.

KEY STEPS
- Confirm the patient's identity using two patient identifiers according to facility policy.
- Perform a venipuncture, and collect the sample in a 3- or 4-ml clot-activator tube.

POSTPROCEDURE CARE
- Apply direct pressure to the venipuncture site until bleeding stops.
- Inform the practitioner of abnormal results.

PRECAUTIONS
- Maintain standard precautions while collecting the sample.
- Handle the sample gently to prevent hemolysis.

COMPLICATIONS
- Hematoma at venipuncture site

NORMAL RESULTS
- Value should be 19 to 38 mg/dl (SI, 190 to 380 mg/L).

ABNORMAL RESULTS
- Values of 10 to 15 mg/dl (SI, 100 to 150 mg/L) indicate mild protein depletion.
- Values of 5 to 10 mg/dl (SI, 50 to 100 mg/L) indicate moderate protein depletion.
- Values of 0 to 5 mg/dl (SI, 0 to 50 mg/L) indicate severe protein depletion.
- Decreased values are seen in malnutrition and liver disease that impairs protein synthesis.

Pregnanediol level, urine

OVERVIEW

DESCRIPTION

- Using gas chromatography or radioimmunoassay, measures urine levels of pregnanediol (main metabolite of progesterone)
- Biologically inert; has diagnostic significance because it reflects about 10% of the endogenous production of patent hormone
- Progesterone: produced in nonpregnant females by corpus luteum during latter half of each menstrual cycle; prepares uterus for implantation of a fertilized ovum
- If implantation doesn't occur, progesterone levels decrease sharply; if implantation occurs, corpus luteum secretes more progesterone to further prepare the uterus for pregnancy
- Urine levels reflect variations in progesterone secretion during menstrual cycle and pregnancy

PURPOSE

- To evaluate placental function in pregnant function
- To evaluate ovarian function in nonpregnant patients
- To help diagnose menstrual disorders

PREPARATION

- Notify the laboratory and practitioner of medication the patient is taking that may affect test results; they may be restricted.
- No dietary restrictions are required.

Teaching points

- Explain that this test evaluates placental or ovarian function.
- Explain who will perform the test and where it'll be done.
- Inform the patient that she need not fast before the test.
- Tell the patient that the test requires collection of urine over a 24-hour period, and teach her the proper collection technique.
- Advise the pregnant patient that this test may be repeated several times to obtain serial measurements.

DIAGNOSTIC PROCEDURE

KEY STEPS

- Confirm the patient's identity using two patient identifiers according to facility policy.
- Collect the patient's urine over a 24-hour period, discarding the first specimen and retaining the last.
- If the patient is pregnant, note the approximate week of gestation on the laboratory request.
- For the premenopausal women who aren't pregnant, note the stage of the menstrual cycle on the laboratory request.

POSTPROCEDURE CARE

- Inform the practitioner of abnormal results.
- Instruct the patient that she may resume her usual medications.

PRECAUTIONS

- Refrigerate the specimen, or keep it on ice during the collection period.

COMPLICATIONS

- None

INTERPRETATION

NORMAL RESULTS

- In nonpregnant females, urine pregnanediol values normally range from 0.5 to 1.5 mg/24 hours (SI, 1.49 to 4.5 µmol/d) during the follicular phase of the menstrual cycles.
- In pregnant females, the values at the first trimester are 10 to 30 mg/24 hours (SI, 29.7 to 89.1 µmol/d); at the second trimester, 35 to 70 mg/24 hours (SI, 104 to 207.9 µmol/d); and at the third trimester, 70 to 100 mg/24 hours (SI, 207.9 to 297 µmol/d).
- Normal postmenopausal values range from 0.2 to 1 mg/24 hours (SI, 0.6 to 2.97 µmol/d).
- In males, urine pregnanediol levels are 0 to 1 mg/24 hours (SI, 0 to 2.97 µmol/d).

ABNORMAL RESULTS

- During pregnancy, a marked decrease in urine pregnanediol levels based on a single 24-hour urine specimen or a steady decrease in pregnanediol levels in serial measurements may indicate placental insufficiency and requires investigation.
- A precipitous drop in pregnanediol values may suggest fetal distress or fetal death.
- Pregnanediol measurements aren't reliable indicators of fetal viability because levels can remain normal even after fetal death, as long as maternal circulation to the placenta remains adequate.
- In nonpregnant females, abnormally low levels may occur with anovulation, amenorrhea, or other menstrual abnormalities.
- Low to normal pregnanediol levels may be associated with hydatidiform mole.
- Elevations may indicate luteinized granulosa or theca cella cells tumors, diffuse thecal luteinization, or metastatic ovarian cancer.
- Adrenal hyperplasia or biliary tract obstruction may elevate urine pregnanediol values in males or females.
- Some forms of primary hepatic disease produce abnormally low levels in both sexes.

Pregnant uterus ultrasound

OVERVIEW

DESCRIPTION
* Safest method to evaluate the uterus and fetus in a pregnant female
* May be done with Doppler monitoring of the fetus or monitor fetal heartbeat or respirations
* Used during pregnancy for various monitoring and determinations
* May be performed either by transabdominal or transvaginal route

PURPOSE
* To confirm pregnancy or multiple fetuses by fetal sac determination in the first trimester
* To measure fetal heart rate and body movement
* To determine fetal age and evaluate uterine artery, fetal aorta, and umbilical artery to determine fetal growth
* To evaluate fetal gestational age based on uterine size, crown-rump length measurements, fetal extremities, head, and other anatomical parts at key points in fetal development
* To detect fetal structural abnormalities at gestational week 20 or later
* To determine fetal death, as evidenced by absent fetal heart tones and lack of fetal movement
* To determine cause of bleeding, such as abruptio placentae or placenta previa
* To evaluate placental growth and volume of amniotic fluid
* To determine fetal presentation before birth
* To detect ectopic pregnancies

PREPARATION
* No dietary restrictions are required.

Teaching points
* Explain that this test helps evaluate the fetus and her placenta and uterus.
* Explain who will perform the test and where it'll be done.
* If the patient is to have a transabdominal ultrasound, have her drink 6 glasses of fluid before the procedure and not void.

* Reassure her that there is no risk to her or the fetus.
* Tell her that the test takes 30 to 60 minutes.

DIAGNOSTIC PROCEDURE

KEY STEPS
* Confirm the patient's identity using two patient identifiers according to facility policy.
* Have the patient lay on the examining table with the abdomen exposed.
* Apply conductive gel to the area, and move the transducer over the abdomen.

POSTPROCEDURE CARE
* Allow the patient to void.
* Provide emotional support as needed.
* Wipe off the gel from the patient's skin.

PRECAUTIONS
* Ask the patient to lie as still as possible to obtain the best images.

COMPLICATIONS
* None

INTERPRETATION

NORMAL RESULTS
* The fetus is of normal age, size, position, viability, and functional capacities.
* The placenta is of normal size, position, and structure.
* The volume of amniotic fluid is adequate.

ABNORMAL RESULTS
* Placental variations, including abruptio placentae and placenta previa, are noted.
* The fetus isn't viable.
* Abnormalities in the fetus, such as hydrocephalus, myelomeningocele, cardiac abnormalities, spinal bifida, skeletal defects, and renal defects, are noted.
* An ectopic pregnancy may be noted.
* Malpresentation of fetus in the breech or transverse position may be noted.

Proctosigmoidoscopy

DESCRIPTION

- Endoscopic examination of the lining of the distal sigmoid colon, rectum, and anal canal
- Three steps: digital examination, sigmoidoscopy, and proctoscopy
- Specimens: obtained from suspect areas of the mucosa by biopsy, lavage or cytology brush, or culture swab

PURPOSE

- To help diagnose inflammatory, infectious, and ulcerative bowel disease
- To diagnose hemorrhoids, hypertrophic anal papilla, polyps, fissures, fistulas, and abscesses within the rectum and anal canal
- To evaluate recent changes in bowel habits, lower abdominal and perineal pain, prolapse on defecation, pruritus ani, or passage of mucus, blood, or pus in feces

PREPARATION

- Make sure the patient has signed an appropriate consent form.
- Note and report allergies.
- Check the patient's history for barium tests within the past week.
- A clear liquid diet is required for 24 to 48 hours before the test.
- The patient must fast on the morning of the procedure.
- An enema should be given 3 to 4 hours before the procedure.

Teaching points

- Explain who will perform the test and where it'll be done.
- Instruct the patient to maintain a clear liquid diet for 24 to 48 hours before the test, as ordered, and then to fast the morning of the procedure.
- Explain the need for an enema 3 to 4 hours before the procedure.
- Explain the need for sedation to help the patient relax. Have the patient arrange for someone to drive him home after the procedure.
- Warn the patient that he may have an urge to defecate during insertion of the scope. Tell him that breathing deeply and slowly through his mouth will help reduce this urge.
- Advise the patient that air may be introduced through the endoscope to distend the walls of the intestine. Flatus may escape around the endoscope, and he shouldn't attempt to control it.
- Warn the patient about possible blood in the feces if a biopsy or polypectomy is performed.
- Tell the patient that the test takes 15 to 30 minutes.

KEY STEPS

- Confirm the patient's identity using two patient identifiers according to facility policy.
- Obtain the patient's baseline vital signs and monitor him throughout the procedure.
- The patient is placed in a knee-to-chest or left lateral position with his knees flexed.
- The patient is asked to breathe deeply and slowly through his mouth.
- A well-lubricated, gloved index finger is inserted into the anus.
- Anal canal is palpated for induration and tenderness.
- The rectal mucosa is palpated.
- The sigmoidoscope is inserted into the anus and passed through the anal sphincters, anal canal, and into the rectum.
- At the rectosigmoid junction, a small amount of air may be insufflated to open the bowel lumen.
- The scope is advanced to its full length into the distal sigmoid colon.
- As the sigmoidoscope is slowly withdrawn, air is carefully insufflated, and the intestinal mucosa is thoroughly examined.
- Specimens may be obtained from a suspicious area of the intestinal mucosa.
- Polyps may be removed for histologic examination by insertion of an electrocautery snare through the sigmoidoscope.
- After the sigmoidoscope is withdrawn, the proctoscope is inserted through the anus and gently advanced to its full length.
- After examination, the proctoscope is withdrawn.

POSTPROCEDURE CARE

- Monitor vital signs and intake and output.
- Watch for signs of bowel perforation and for vasovagal reaction.
- When the patient is fully awake, instruct him to resume his previous diet and activities as ordered.

PRECAUTIONS

- Aspirin and most nonsteroidal anti-inflammatory drugs in standard doses don't usually increase the risk of significant bleeding.

COMPLICATIONS

- Rectal bleeding
- Bowel perforation

NORMAL RESULTS

- Mucosa of the sigmoid colon is light pink-orange and marked by semilunar folds and deep tubular pits.
- The rectal mucosa appears redder because of its rich vascular network, deepens to purple at the pectinate line (the anatomic division between the rectum and anus), and has three distinct valves.
- The lower two-thirds of the anus (anoderm) is lined with smooth gray-tan skin and joins with the hair-fringed perianal skin.

ABNORMAL RESULTS

- Biopsy results may suggest the presence of malignant tumors.
- Inflammatory changes suggest possible ulcerative and ischemic colitis.
- Visual examination and palpation may disclose possible abnormalities of the anal canal and rectum, including internal and external hemorrhoids, hypertrophic anal papillae, anal fissures and fistulas, or anorectal abscesses.

Progesterone level, plasma

OVERVIEW

DESCRIPTION
- Quantitative analysis of plasma progesterone levels by radioimmunoassay; provides reliable information about corpus luteum function in fertility studies and placental function in pregnancy
- May perform serial determinations
- Progesterone: ovarian steroid hormone secreted by corpus luteum; causes thickening and secretory development of the endometrium in preparation for implantation of the fertilized ovum
- During midluteal phase of menstrual cycle: progesterone levels peak; if implantation doesn't occur, progesterone (and estrogen) levels drop sharply and menstruation occurs after 2 days
- During pregnancy: placenta releases about 10 times the normal monthly amount of progesterone to maintain the pregnancy; increased secretion begins toward end of first trimester and continues until delivery
- Prevents abortion by decreasing uterine contractions
- With estrogen, helps prepare the breasts for lactation

PURPOSE
- To assess corpus luteum function as part of infertility studies
- To evaluate placental function during pregnancy
- To help confirm ovulation; test results support basal body temperature readings

PREPARATION
- No dietary restrictions are required.
- Check the patient's history to determine if she's taking drugs that may interfere with test results, including progesterone and estrogen. Note findings on the laboratory request.
- The test requires a blood sample.

Teaching points
- Explain that this test helps determine if the patient's female sex hormone secretion is normal.

- Explain who will perform the test and where it'll be done.
- Inform the patient that she doesn't need to restrict her diet.
- Tell the patient that the test requires a blood sample, and that she may experience slight discomfort from the tourniquet and needle puncture.
- Inform the patient that the test may be repeated at specific times coinciding with phases of her menstrual cycle or with each prenatal visit.
- Tell the patient the test takes less than 5 minutes.

DIAGNOSTIC PROCEDURE

KEY STEPS
- Confirm the patient's identity using two patient identifiers according to facility policy.
- Perform a venipuncture, and collect the sample in a 7-ml heparinized tube.
- Completely fill the collection tube; then invert it gently at least 10 times to mix the sample and the anticoagulant adequately.
- Indicate the date of the patient's last menses and the phase of her cycle on the laboratory request. If the patient is pregnant, also indicate the month of gestation.

POSTPROCEDURE CARE
- Apply direct pressure to the venipuncture site until bleeding stops.
- Inform the practitioner of abnormal results.

PRECAUTIONS
- Handle the sample gently to prevent hemolysis.
- Send the sample to the laboratory immediately.

COMPLICATIONS
- Hematoma at the venipuncture site

INTERPRETATION

NORMAL RESULTS
- During menstruation, in the follicular phase, progesterone level is less than 150 ng/dl (SI, < 5 nmol/L); in the luteal phase, the level is 300 to 1,200 ng/dl (SI, 10 to 40 nmol/L).
- During pregnancy, in the first trimester, progesterone level is 1,500 to 5,000 ng/dl (SI, 50 to 160 nmol/L); in the second and third trimesters, the level is 8,000 to 20,000 ng/dl (SI, 250 to 650 nmol/L).
- In menopausal women, progesterone level is 10 to 22 ng/dl (SI, 0 to 2 nmol/L).

ABNORMAL RESULTS
- Elevated progesterone levels may indicate ovulation, luteinizing tumors, ovarian cysts that produce progesterone, or adrenocortical hyperplasia and tumors that produce progesterone along with other steroidal hormones.
- Low progesterone levels are associated with amenorrhea because of several causes (such as panhypopituitarism and gonadal dysfunction), eclampsia, threatened abortion, and fetal death.

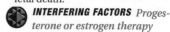 **INTERFERING FACTORS** *Progesterone or estrogen therapy*

Prolactin level test

OVERVIEW

DESCRIPTION

- Quantitative radioimmunoassay to analyze serum levels of prolactin—polypeptide hormone secreted by anterior pituitary gland; levels usually rise 10- to 20-fold during pregnancy, corresponding to accompanying elevations in human placental lactogen levels
- Used in patients who may have pituitary tumors, which secrete excessive amounts of prolactin
- Evaluates hypothalamic dysfunction
- Prolactin: acts directly on tissues; levels rise in response to sleep and physical or emotional stress; essential for developing mammary glands during pregnancy for breast-feeding and for stimulating and maintaining lactation postpartum
- After delivery: prolactin secretion falls to basal levels in mothers who don't breast-feed but increases during breast-feeding in response to suckling trigger, which inhibits the hypothalamus from releasing prolactin-inhibiting factor by the hypothalamus and permits prolactin secretion from the pituitary

---

TRH stimulation test

The thyrotropin-releasing hormone (TRH) test evaluates hypothalamic dysfunction and pituitary tumors by stimulating the release of prolactin. The procedure is as follows: perform a venipuncture in the basal state to obtain a baseline prolactin level, and then place the patient in the supine position. Administer an I.V. bolus dose (500 mcg) of synthetic TRH over 15 to 30 seconds. Take blood samples at 15- and 30-minute intervals to measure prolactin.

A baseline prolactin reading greater than 200 ng/ml (SI, 200 International Units/L) indicates a pituitary tumor, but levels between 30 and 200 ng/ml (SI, 30 to 200 International Units/L) are also consistent with this condition. Normally, patients show at least a twofold increase in prolactin after injection with TRH. If the prolactin level fails to rise, hypothalamic dysfunction or adenoma of the pituitary gland is likely.

PURPOSE

- To facilitate diagnosis of pituitary dysfunction, possibly caused by pituitary adenoma (see *TRH stimulation test*)
- To help diagnose hypothalamic dysfunction regardless of cause
- To evaluate secondary amenorrhea and galactorrhea

PREPARATION

- Withhold drugs that may interfere with test results. If the patient must continue them, note this on the laboratory request.
- Withhold food and fluid and limit physical activity for 12 hours before the test.
- Have the patient relax for about 30 minutes before the test.
- The test requires a blood sample.

Teaching points

- Tell the patient that this test helps evaluate hormonal secretion.
- Explain who will perform the test and where it'll be done.
- Advise the patient to restrict food and fluids and limit physical activity for 12 hours before the test. Encourage her to relax for about 30 minutes before the test.
- Tell the patient that the test requires a blood sample and that she may experience slight discomfort from the tourniquet and needle puncture.
- Tell the patient the test takes less than 5 minutes.

DIAGNOSTIC PROCEDURE

KEY STEPS

- Confirm the patient's identity using two patient identifiers according to facility policy.
- Perform a venipuncture at least 3 hours after the patient wakes; samples collected earlier are likely to show sleep-induced peak levels.
- Collect the sample in a 7-ml clot-activator tube.
- Confirm slight elevations with repeat measurements on two other occasions.

POSTPROCEDURE CARE

- Apply direct pressure to the venipuncture site until bleeding stops.
- Inform the practitioner of abnormal results.
- After the test, instruct the patient that she may resume her usual diet, activities, and medications.

PRECAUTIONS

- Handle the sample gently to prevent hemolysis.

COMPLICATIONS

- Hematoma at the venipuncture site

INTERPRETATION

NORMAL RESULTS

- Levels are undetectable to 23 ng/ml (SI, 23 µg/L) in nonlactating women.
- Levels normally rise 10- to 20-fold during pregnancy and, after delivery, fall to basal levels in mothers who don't breast-feed.
- Prolactin secretion increases during breast-feeding.

ABNORMAL RESULTS

- Abnormally high levels (100 to 300 ng/ml [SI, 100 to 300 µg/L]) suggest autonomous prolactin production by a pituitary adenoma, especially when amenorrhea or galactorrhea is present (Forbes-Albright syndrome).
- Rarely, hyperprolactinemia may also result from severe endocrine disorders such as hypothyroidism.
- Idiopathic hyperprolactinemia may be linked to anovulatory infertility.
- Slight elevations require repeat measurements on two other occasions.
- Decreased prolactin levels in a lactating mother cause failure of lactation and may be associated with postpartum pituitary infarction (Sheehan's syndrome).
- Abnormally low prolactin levels have also occurred in the patient with empty sella syndrome. In these cases, a flattened pituitary gland makes the pituitary fossa look empty.

Prostate gland biopsy

DESCRIPTION

- Needle excision of a prostate tissue specimen for histologic examination
- Three possible approaches: perineal, transrectal, or transurethral
- Transrectal approach usually for high prostatic lesions

PURPOSE

- To confirm prostate cancer
- To determine cause of prostatic hypertrophy

PREPARATION

- Depending on the approach used, the patient may need to fast for 6 to 8 hours before the test.
- Make sure the patient has signed an appropriate consent form.
- Note and report allergies.
- For a transrectal approach, give enemas until the return is clear.
- Give the patient antibiotics, as ordered.
- Give the patient a sedative before the study.

Teaching points

- Explain the purpose of the test and how it's done.
- Explain who will perform the test and where it'll be done.
- Tell the patient about dietary restrictions.
- Explain the need to use a local anesthetic.
- Tell the patient that the test takes less than 30 minutes.

KEY STEPS

- Confirm the patient's identity using two patient identifiers according to facility policy.

Perineal approach

- The patient is placed in the left lateral, knee-chest, or lithotomy position.
- A local anesthetic is given.
- The perineal skin is cleaned and prepared; a 2-mm incision is made into the perineum.
- The biopsy needle is introduced into a prostate lobe.
- Specimens are obtained from several different areas of the prostate.
- Specimens are placed immediately in a labeled specimen bottle containing 10% formalin solution.
- Hemostasis is obtained and a dressing is applied.

Transrectal approach

- The patient is placed in the left lateral position.
- A curved needle guide (or a spring-powered device for cone biopsy) is attached to the finger palpating the rectum.
- The biopsy needle is pushed along the guide, into the prostate.
- The needle is rotated to cut the tissue and is then withdrawn.

Transurethral approach

- An endoscopic instrument with a cutting loop is passed through the urethra.
- The endoscope permits direct viewing of the prostate and passage of a cutting loop.
- Specimens are obtained and placed immediately in a labeled specimen bottle containing 10% formalin solution.

POSTPROCEDURE CARE

- Give the patient an analgesic.
- Monitor vital signs and intake and output.
- Observe the biopsy site for hematoma and for signs and symptoms of infection, such as redness, swelling, and pain. Watch for urine retention, urinary frequency, and hematuria.
- Inform the practitioner of abnormal results.
- Tell the patient to gradually resume his normal diet and activity as tolerated.
- See *Speeding your recovery after prostate surgery.*

PRECAUTIONS

- Observe the biopsy site for and immediately report hematoma and signs of infection, such as redness, swelling, and pain.

COMPLICATIONS

- Bleeding into the prostatic urethra and bladder
- Infection
- Urine retention

NORMAL RESULTS

- A thin, fibrous capsule surrounds the stroma, which is made up of elastic and connective tissues and smooth-muscle fibers.
- Epithelial glands that drain into the chief excreting ducts are evident.
- No cancer cells are found.

ABNORMAL RESULTS

- Increased acid phosphatase levels suggest possible metastatic prostate cancer.
- Low acid phosphatase levels suggest possible cancer that is confined to the prostatic capsule.
- Histologic examination of the tissue reveals various possible disorders, including prostate, rectal, and bladder cancer, benign prostatic hyperplasia, prostatitis, tuberculosis, or lymphomas.

Speeding your recovery after prostate surgery

Dear Patient,

Here's what you can expect after prostate surgery, along with directions for caring for yourself.

EXPECT TROUBLE URINATING

At first, you may have a feeling of heaviness in the pelvic area, burning during urination, a frequent need to urinate, and loss of some control over urination. Don't worry, these symptoms will disappear with time.

If you notice blood in your urine during the first 2 weeks after surgery, drink fluids and lie down to rest. The next time you urinate, the bleeding should decrease.

Let your health care provider know right away if you continue to see blood in your urine or if you can't urinate at all.

Also let your health care provider know immediately if you develop a fever.

PREVENT CONSTIPATION

Eat a well-balanced diet and drink 12 eight-ounce glasses of fluid daily, unless your health care provider directs otherwise. Don't strain to have a bowel movement. If you become constipated, take a mild laxative.

Don't use an enema or place anything, such as a suppository, into your rectum for at least 4 weeks after surgery.

CUT BACK ON ACTIVITIES

Take only short walks, and avoid climbing stairs as much as possible. Don't lift heavy objects. Also, don't drive for at least 2 weeks, and don't exercise strenuously for at least 3 weeks.

STRENGTHEN YOUR PERINEAL MUSCLES

Perform this exercise to strengthen your perineal muscles after surgery: Press your buttocks together, hold this position for a few seconds, and then relax. Repeat this 10 times.

Perform this exercise as many times daily as your health care provider orders.

WAIT TO HAVE SEX

Don't have sex for at least 4 weeks after surgery because sexual activity can cause bleeding.

When you have sex, most of the semen (the fluid that contains sperm) will pass into your bladder rather than out through your urethra. This won't affect your ability to have an erection or an orgasm. However, it will decrease your fertility.

Don't be alarmed if the semen in your bladder causes cloudy urine the first time you urinate after intercourse.

ASK ABOUT WORK

During your next appointment with your health care provider, ask when you can return to work. The timing will vary depending on the type of surgery you had, the kind of work you do, and your general health.

SCHEDULE AN ANNUAL CHECKUP

Continue to have an annual examination so your health care provider can check the prostate area that wasn't removed during surgery.

Prostate-specific antigen test

DESCRIPTION

- Measures level of prostate-specific antigen (PSA), which appears in normal, benign hyperplastic and malignant prostatic tissue, as well as in metastatic prostate cancer
- Measures PSA levels to monitor the spread or recurrence of stage B3 to D1 prostate cancer and evaluate the patient's response to treatment
- PSA level measurement and a digital rectal examination are recommended to screen men older than age 50 for prostate cancer (see *Controversy over PSA screening*)

PURPOSE

- To screen for prostate cancer in men over age 50
- To monitor the course of prostate cancer and evaluate treatment

PREPARATION

- No dietary restrictions are required.
- The test requires a blood sample.

Teaching points

- Explain that this test screens for prostate cancer or, if appropriate, monitors the course of treatment.
- Explain who will perform the test and where it'll be done.
- Tell the patient that the test requires a blood sample and that he may experience slight discomfort from the tourniquet and needle puncture.
- Inform the patient that he need not restrict food and fluids.
- Tell the patient the test takes less than 5 minutes.

DIAGNOSTIC PROCEDURE

KEY STEPS

- Confirm the patient's identity using two patient identifiers according to facility policy.
- Perform a venipuncture, and collect the sample in a 7-ml clot-activator tube.

POSTPROCEDURE CARE

- Apply direct pressure to the venipuncture site until bleeding stops.
- Inform the practitioner of abnormal results.

PRECAUTIONS

- Collect the sample either before digital prostate examination or at least 48 hours after examination to avoid falsely elevated PSA levels.
- Handle the sample gently to prevent hemolysis.
- Immediately put the sample on ice, and send it to the laboratory.

COMPLICATIONS

- Hematoma at the venipuncture site

INTERPRETATION

NORMAL RESULTS

- In men age 40 to 50, the PSA level is 2 to 2.8 ng/ml (SI, 2 to 2.8 mcg/L).
- In men age 51 to 60, the PSA level is 2.9 to 3.8 ng/ml (SI, 2.9 to 3.8 mcg/L).
- In men age 61 to 70, the PSA level is 4 to 5.3 ng/ml (SI, 4 to 5.3 mcg/L).
- In men age 71 and older, the PSA level is 5.6 to 7.2 ng/ml (SI, 5.6 to 7.2 mcg/L).

ABNORMAL RESULTS

- About 80% of patients with prostate cancer have pretreatment PSA values above 4 ng/ml.
- About 20% of patients with benign prostatic hyperplasia also have levels above 4 ng/ml.
- PSA results alone don't confirm a diagnosis of prostate cancer. Further assessment and testing, including tissue biopsy, are necessary to confirm cancer.

Controversy over PSA screening

Measurement of prostate-specific antigen (PSA) allows earlier detection of prostate cancer than does digital rectal examination (DRE) alone. Accordingly, the American Cancer Society and the American Urological Association currently recommend that PSA screening begin at age 40 (with DRE) in black men and any man who has a father or brother with prostate cancer, and at age 50 in all other men.

But does this test actually reduce mortality from prostate cancer? The answer to that question remains unknown. Some specialists question the value of all prostate cancer screening tests because of the costs involved, the uncertain benefits, and the known risks associated with current treatments.

Before undergoing a PSA test, the patient should understand that controversy surrounds nearly every aspect of prostate cancer screening and treatment. The issues he'll face may include:

- Even if cancer is detected, treatment may not be advisable, either because of the patient's advanced age or because the practitioner believes the tumor is so slow growing that it won't result in death.

- The current treatments for prostate cancer — surgery and radiation therapy — may not be as effective as experts formerly believed, and no effective chemotherapy protocol is currently available.
- Surgery and radiation therapy carry a high risk of impotence, incontinence, and other problems, which the patient must weigh against the uncertain benefits of therapy.
- Screening tests sometimes yield false-positive results, requiring transrectal ultrasonography or a biopsy to confirm the diagnosis.
- A mildly elevated PSA level may be the result of normal age-related increases. (Data from a study of more than 9,000 men showed that PSA levels increase about 30% per year in men younger than age 70 and more than 40% per year in men older than age 70.)

In summary, the value of prostate cancer screening in general and PSA testing in particular won't be clearly established until studies show a definitive link between early treatment and reduced mortality.

Protein C level

DESCRIPTION

- Measures level of vitamin K–dependent protein C, which is produced in the liver and circulates in the plasma
- Deficiencies may be acquired or congenital; as a potent anticoagulant, protein C suppresses activated factors V and VIII. Once identified, a deficiency is further investigated to determine its type
- Identifying the role of protein C deficiency in idiopathic venous thrombosis may help prevent thromboembolism

PURPOSE

- To investigate the mechanism of idiopathic venous thrombosis

PREPARATION

- No dietary restrictions are required.
- Notify the laboratory and practitioner of medications the patient is taking that may affect test results; they may be restricted.

Teaching points

- Explain that the protein C test evaluates blood clotting.
- Explain who will perform the test and where it'll be done.
- Tell the patient that the test requires a blood sample and that he may experience slight discomfort from the tourniquet and needle puncture.
- Inform the patient that he need not restrict food and fluids.
- Tell the patient the test takes less than 5 minutes.

KEY STEPS

- Confirm the patient's identity using two patient identifiers according to facility policy.
- Perform a venipuncture. Collect a 3-ml sample in a siliconized vacuum specimen tube or in a special syringe with anticoagulant provided by the laboratory.
- Completely fill the collection tube, and invert it several times to mix the sample and anticoagulant thoroughly; handle the sample gently.

POSTPROCEDURE CARE

- Apply direct pressure to the venipuncture site until bleeding stops.
- Inform the practitioner of abnormal results.
- Tell the patient to resume his usual medications.

PRECAUTIONS

- Send the sample to the laboratory immediately.
- Maintain standard precautions while collecting the sample.

COMPLICATIONS

- Hematoma at the venipuncture site

NORMAL RESULTS

- Level is 70% to 140% (SI, 0.7 to 1.4).

ABNORMAL RESULTS

- Rare, homozygous protein C deficiency is characterized by rapidly fatal thrombosis in the perinatal period, a condition known as purpura fulminans.
- The more common heterozygous deficiency causes genetic susceptibility to venous thromboembolism before age 30 and throughout life. The patient may require long-term treatment with warfarin therapy or protein C supplements from plasma fractions.
- Protein C deficiency is also seen in those with liver cirrhosis and vitamin K deficiency or taking warfarin.

INTERFERING FACTORS *Anticoagulant therapy*

Protein electrophoresis

DESCRIPTION

◆ Used to measure the serum albumin and globulin, the major blood proteins by separating the protein into five distinct fractions: albumin and alpha$_1$, alpha$_2$, beta, and gamma globulin proteins

PURPOSE

◆ To help diagnose hepatic disease, protein deficiency, renal disorders, and GI and neoplastic diseases

PREPARATION

◆ Notify the laboratory and practitioner of medications the patient is taking that may affect test results; they may be restricted.
◆ No dietary restrictions are required.

Teaching points

◆ Explain that this test is used to determine the protein content of blood.
◆ Explain who will perform the test and where it'll be done.
◆ Inform the patient that he need not restrict food or fluids.
◆ Tell the patient that the test requires a blood sample and that he may experience slight discomfort from the tourniquet and needle puncture.
◆ Tell him the test takes less than 5 minutes.

DIAGNOSTIC PROCEDURE

KEY STEPS

◆ Confirm the patient's identity using two patient identifiers according to facility policy.
◆ Perform a venipuncture, and collect the sample in a 7-ml clot-activator tube.

POSTPROCEDURE CARE

◆ Apply direct pressure to the venipuncture site until bleeding stops.
◆ Inform the practitioner of abnormal results.
◆ Tell the patient to resume his usual medications.

PRECAUTIONS

◆ Protein electrophoresis must be performed on a serum sample to avoid measuring the fibrinogen fractions.

COMPLICATIONS

◆ Hematoma

INTERPRETATION

NORMAL RESULTS

◆ The total serum protein levels range from 6.4 to 8.3 g/dl (SI, 64 to 83 g/L).
◆ Albumin fraction ranges from 3.5 to 5 g/dl (SI, 35 to 50 g/L).
◆ Alpha$_1$-globulin fraction ranges from 0.1 to 0.3 g/dl (SI, 1 to 3 g/L).
◆ Alpha$_2$-globulin ranges from 0.6 to 1 g/dl (SI, 6 to 10 g/L).
◆ Beta globulin ranges from 0.7 to 1.1 g/dl (SI, 7 to 11 g/L).
◆ Gamma globulin ranges from 0.8 to 1.6 g/dl (SI, 8 to 16 g/L).

ABNORMAL RESULTS

◆ For common abnormal findings, see *Clinical implications of abnormal protein levels.*

Clinical implications of abnormal protein levels

INCREASED LEVELS

TOTAL PROTEINS	ALBUMIN	GLOBULINS
◆ Chronic inflammatory disease (such as rheumatoid arthritis or early-stage Laënnec's cirrhosis) ◆ Dehydration ◆ Diabetic ketoacidosis ◆ Fulminating and chronic infections ◆ Multiple myeloma ◆ Monocytic leukemia ◆ Vomiting, diarrhea	◆ Multiple myeloma	◆ Chronic syphilis ◆ Collagen diseases ◆ Diabetes mellitus ◆ Hodgkin's disease ◆ Multiple myeloma ◆ Rheumatoid arthritis ◆ Subacute bacterial endocarditis ◆ SLE ◆ Tuberculosis

DECREASED LEVELS

TOTAL PROTEINS	ALBUMIN	GLOBULINS
◆ Benzene and carbon-tetrachloride poisoning ◆ Blood dyscrasias ◆ Essential hypertension ◆ GI disease ◆ Heart failure ◆ Hepatic dysfunction ◆ Hemorrhage ◆ Hodgkin's disease ◆ Hyperthyroidism ◆ Malabsorption ◆ Malnutrition ◆ Nephrosis ◆ Severe burns ◆ Surgical and traumatic shock ◆ Gestational hypertension ◆ Uncontrolled diabetes mellitus	◆ Acute cholecystitis ◆ Collagen diseases ◆ Diarrhea ◆ Essential hypertension ◆ Hepatic disease ◆ Hodgkin's disease ◆ Hyperthyroidism ◆ Hypogamma-globulinemia ◆ Malnutrition ◆ Metastatic carcinoma ◆ Nephritis, nephrosis ◆ Peptic ulcer ◆ Plasma loss from burns ◆ Rheumatoid arthritis ◆ Sarcoidosis ◆ Systemic lupus erythematosus (SLE)	◆ Benzene and carbon-tetrachloride poisoning ◆ Blood dyscrasias ◆ Essential hypertension ◆ GI disease ◆ Heart failure ◆ Hepatic dysfunction ◆ Hemorrhage ◆ Hodgkin's disease ◆ Hyperthyroidism ◆ Malabsorption ◆ Malnutrition ◆ Nephrosis ◆ Severe burns ◆ Surgical and traumatic shock ◆ Gestational hypertension ◆ Uncontrolled diabetes mellitus

---

Protein level, urine

DESCRIPTION

♦ Quantitative test for proteinuria
♦ Usually preceded by qualitative test for proteinuria

PURPOSE

♦ To help diagnose pathologic states characterized by proteinuria, primarily renal disease

PREPARATION

♦ Notify the laboratory and practitioner of medications the patient is taking that may affect test results; they may need to be restricted.
♦ No dietary restrictions are required.
♦ The test requires urine collection over a 24-hour period.

Teaching points

♦ Explain that this test detects protein in the urine.
♦ Explain who will perform the test and where it'll be done.
♦ Inform the patient that he need not restrict food and fluid.
♦ Tell the patient that the test usually requires urine collection over a 24-hour period; a random collection can be done.
♦ Teach the patient how to collect a 24-hour urine specimen if necessary.

KEY STEPS

♦ Confirm the patient's identity using two patient identifiers according to facility policy.
♦ Collect the patient's urine over a 24-hour period, discarding the first specimen and retaining the last. A special specimen container can be obtained from the laboratory.

POSTPROCEDURE CARE

♦ Inform the practitioner of abnormal results.
♦ Tell the patient to resume his usual medications as ordered.

PRECAUTIONS

♦ Tell the patient not to contaminate the sample with toilet tissue or stool.
♦ Refrigerate the specimen or place it on ice during the collection period.

COMPLICATIONS

♦ None

NORMAL RESULTS

♦ At rest, normal urine protein values range from 50 to 80 mg/24 hours (SI, 50 to 80 mg/d).

ABNORMAL RESULTS

♦ Proteinuria is a chief characteristic of renal disease.
♦ Proteinuria can result from glomerular leakage of plasma proteins (a major cause of protein excretion), from overflow of filtered proteins of low molecular weight (when these are present in excessive concentration), from impaired tubular reabsorption of filtered proteins, and from the presence of renal proteins derived from the breakdown of kidney tissue.
♦ Persistent proteinuria indicates renal disease resulting from increased glomerular permeability.
♦ Minimal proteinuria (less than 0.5 g/24 hours) is commonly associated with renal diseases in which glomerular involvement isn't a major factor such as pyelonephritis.
♦ Moderate proteinuria (0.5 to 4 g/24 hours) occurs in several types of renal disease (such as acute or chronic glomerular nephritis, amyloidosis, or toxic neuropathies) or in diseases in which renal failure typically develops as a late condition (such as diabetes or heart failure).
♦ Heavy proteinuria (over 4 g/24 hours) is commonly associated with nephrotic syndrome.
♦ When accompanied by an increased white blood cell count, proteinuria indicates urinary tract infection.
♦ When accompanied by hematuria, proteinuria indicates local or diffuse urinary tract disorders.
♦ Benign proteinuria can result from changes in body position.
♦ Functional proteinuria is associated with exercise as well as emotional or physiological stress and is usually transient.

Prothrombin time

DESCRIPTION

- Measures the time required for a fibrin clot to form in a citrated plasma sample after addition of calcium ions and tissue thromboplastin (factor III)

PURPOSE

- To evaluate the extrinsic coagulation system (factors V, VII, and X and prothrombin and fibrinogen)
- To monitor response to oral anticoagulant therapy

PREPARATION

- Notify the laboratory and practitioner of medications the patient is taking that may affect test results; they may be restricted.
- The test requires a blood sample.
- No dietary restrictions are required.

Teaching points

- Explain that the prothrombin time (PT) test determines whether the blood clots normally.
- Explain who will perform the test and where it'll be done.
- When appropriate, explain that this test monitors the effects of oral anticoagulants; the test will occur daily when therapy begins and will be repeated at longer intervals when medication levels stabilize.
- Inform the patient that he need not restrict food and fluids.
- Tell the patient that the test requires a blood sample and that he may experience slight discomfort from the tourniquet and needle puncture.
- Tell the patient the test takes less than 5 minutes.

KEY STEPS

- Confirm the patient's identity using two patient identifiers according to facility policy.
- Perform a venipuncture, and collect the sample in a 3- or 4.5-ml siliconized tube.
- Completely fill the collection tube, and invert it gently several times to mix the sample and the anticoagulant thoroughly. If the tube isn't filled to the correct volume, an excess of citrate will appear in the sample.

POSTPROCEDURE CARE

- Make sure subdermal bleeding has stopped before removing pressure.
- If a large hematoma develops at the venipuncture site, monitor pulses distal to the site.
- Inform the practitioner of abnormal results.
- Tell the patient to resume his usual diet and medications, as ordered.

PRECAUTIONS

- To prevent hemolysis, avoid excessive probing during venipuncture and handle the sample gently.

COMPLICATIONS

- Hematoma at the venipuncture site

NORMAL RESULTS

- PT should be 10 to 14 seconds (SI, 10 to 14 s), depending on the source of tissue thromboplastin and the type of sensing devices used to measure clot formation.
- In a patient receiving oral anticoagulants, PT should be from 1 to 2½ times the normal control value.

ABNORMAL RESULTS

- Prolonged PT may indicate deficiencies in fibrinogen, prothrombin, factors V, VII, or X (specific assays can pinpoint such deficiencies), or vitamin K. It may also result from ongoing oral anticoagulant therapy.
- A prolonged PT that exceeds 2½ times the control value usually indicates abnormal bleeding.

  INTERFERING FACTORS *Salicylates, more than 1 g/day (may cause increased values)*

Pulmonary angiography

OVERVIEW

DESCRIPTION
- Radiographically examines the pulmonary circulation after injection of a radiopaque contrast medium into the pulmonary artery or one of its branches
- May diagnose pulmonary embolism (PE) when lung ventilation perfusion scans are indeterminate
- May give local thrombolytic therapy in patients with PE
- Also known as *pulmonary arteriography*

PURPOSE
- To detect pulmonary embolism in a symptomatic patient with an equivocal lung scan
- To evaluate pulmonary circulation abnormalities
- To provide accurate preoperative evaluation of patients with shunt physiology caused by congenital heart disease
- To treat identified PE with thrombolysis

PREPARATION
- Make sure the patient has signed an appropriate consent form.
- Note and report allergies.
- Check the patient's history for hypersensitivity to iodine, seafood, or iodinated contrast media.
- Check for and report history of anticoagulation.
- Check for and report history of renal insufficiency.
- Note and inform the practitioner of any abnormal laboratory results.
- Stop heparin infusion 3 to 4 hours before the test.
- Fasting for 8 hours before the test is required.

Teaching points
- Explain the purpose of the study and how it's done.
- Explain who will perform the test and where it'll be done.
- Instruct the patient to fast for 8 hours before the test.
- Explain the need to use a local anesthetic.
- Warn the patient that he may have a possible urge to cough, a flushed feeling, or a salty taste for 3 to 5 minutes after the injection.
- Explain that he will be monitored during the study.
- Tell the patient that the test takes about 1½ to 2 hours.

DIAGNOSTIC PROCEDURE

KEY STEPS
- Confirm the patient's identity using two patient identifiers according to facility policy.
- The patient is placed in the supine position.
- The access site is cleaned and prepared, usually the right groin.
- A local anesthetic is injected.
- The vein is accessed, and a catheter is introduced under image-guidance.
- The catheter is advanced through the right atrium, the right ventricle, and into the pulmonary artery.
- Pulmonary artery pressures are measured, and blood samples may be drawn from various regions of the pulmonary circulation.
- The contrast medium is injected, and images are obtained.
- Thrombolysis is initiated if indicated.
- After the catheter is removed, hemostasis is obtained.
- The access site is cleaned and dressed.

POSTPROCEDURE CARE
- Maintain bed rest for 6 hours.
- Restart anticoagulation, as ordered.
- Check the patient's blood pressure, pulse rate, and catheter insertion site every 15 minutes for 1 hour, every hour for 4 hours, and then every 4 hours for 24 hours.
- Monitor renal function study results and intake and output.
- Monitor the patient for adverse reaction to the contrast medium.
- Tell the patient to resume his usual diet.
- Encourage him to drink fluids, or give I.V. fluids to help eliminate the contrast medium.

PRECAUTIONS
- ⚡ **WARNING** *Observe the site for bleeding and swelling. If these occur, maintain pressure at the insertion site for at least 10 minutes, and notify the practitioner.*
- The test is contraindicated in pregnant patients.
- Monitor the patient for ventricular arrhythmias caused by myocardial irritation from passage of the catheter through the heart chambers.
- Keep emergency resuscitation equipment available in case of a hypersensitivity reaction to the contrast agent.

COMPLICATIONS
- Myocardial perforation or rupture
- Ventricular arrhythmias and conduction defects
- Acute renal failure
- Bleeding and hematoma formation
- Infection
- Adverse reaction to the contrast medium
- Cardiac valve damage
- Right-sided heart failure

INTERPRETATION

NORMAL RESULTS
- The contrast medium flows symmetrically and without interruption through the pulmonary circulation.

ABNORMAL RESULTS
- Interruption of blood flow and filling defects may suggest acute pulmonary embolism.
- Arterial webs, stenoses, irregular occlusions, wall-scalloping, and "pouching" defects (such as a concave edge of thrombus facing the opacified lumen) suggest chronic pulmonary embolism.

Pulmonary artery catheterization

OVERVIEW

DESCRIPTION

- Uses a balloon-tipped, flow-directed catheter to provide intermittent occlusion of the pulmonary artery, permitting measurement of pulmonary artery pressure (PAP) and pulmonary artery wedge pressure (PAWP), which accurately reflects left atrial pressure and left ventricular end-diastolic pressure
- Also known as *Swan-Ganz catheterization*

PURPOSE

- To assess right- and left-sided ventricular function
- To monitor therapy for complications of acute myocardial infarction, shock, pulmonary edema, systolic murmur, and various cardiac arrhythmias
- To monitor fluid status in patients with serious burns, renal disease, noncardiogenic pulmonary edema, or acute respiratory distress syndrome
- To establish baseline pressures preoperatively in patients with existing cardiac disease
- To differentiate between noncardiac and cardiac pulmonary edema
- To monitor the effects of cardiovascular drugs

PREPARATION

- Make sure the patient has signed an appropriate consent form.
- Note and report allergies.

Teaching points

- Explain the purpose of the study and how it's done.
- Explain who will perform the test and where it'll be done.
- Explain the use of a local anesthetic.
- Explain that the catheter will remain in place, causing little or no discomfort, for 48 to 72 hours.
- Tell the patient that catheter insertion takes about 30 minutes.

DIAGNOSTIC PROCEDURE

KEY STEPS

- Confirm the patient's identity using two patient identifiers according to facility policy.
- The patient is placed in a supine position with his head and shoulders slightly lower than his trunk.
- The catheter is introduced into the vein percutaneously.
- The catheter is directed into the right atrium.
- The catheter balloon is partially inflated.
- Venous flow carries the catheter tip through the right atrium and tricuspid valve into the right ventricle and into the pulmonary artery.
- The monitor is observed for characteristic pressure waveform changes as the catheter enters each heart chamber. (See *PA catheterization: Insertion sites and associated waveforms.*)
- As the catheter is passed into the chambers on the right side of the heart, the monitor screen is observed for frequent premature ventricular contractions, ventricular tachycardia, and other arrhythmias. If arrhythmias occur, the catheter may be partially withdrawn or medication given to suppress the arrhythmias.
- For recording PAWP, the catheter balloon is carefully inflated with the specified amount of air (no more than 1.5 cc), until a PAWP waveform is obtained.
- After PAWP is recorded, the air from the balloon is allowed to return to the syringe.
- The monitor screen is observed for a pulmonary artery waveform.
- The catheter may be sutured to the skin and a dressing applied.

⚡ **WARNING** *The balloon catheter shouldn't be overinflated, which could distend the pulmonary artery, causing vessel rupture. If the balloon can't be fully deflated after recording the PAWP, it shouldn't be reinflated unless the practitioner is present; balloon rupture can cause a life-threatening air embolism.*

POSTPROCEDURE CARE

- Obtain a chest X-ray to verify proper catheter placement and to assess for complications such as pneumothorax.
- Monitor the patient's vital signs.
- Watch for cardiac arrhythmias.
- Document PAP waveforms at the beginning of each shift and monitor them frequently throughout the shift and with changes in treatment or condition. Check PAWP and cardiac output, as ordered.
- Watch for infection of the insertion site and bleeding.
- Watch for signs and symptoms of pulmonary emboli, pulmonary artery perforation, and arrhythmias.
- Maintain 300 mm Hg pressure in the pressure bag to permit 3 to 6 ml/ hour fluid flow to flush the system continuously.
- Inform the practitioner of abnormal results.

PRECAUTIONS

- Notify the practitioner if there's difficulty in flushing the system.
- If a damped waveform occurs, it may be necessary to withdraw the catheter slightly; pulmonary infarct can occur if the catheter remains in a wedged position.
- After each PAWP reading, make sure the balloon is completely deflated.
- If the patient shows signs of sepsis, treat the catheter as the source of infection and send it to the laboratory for culture when it's removed.

COMPLICATIONS

- Pulmonary infarction
- Ventricular arrhythmias
- Air emboli
- Infection and sepsis

PA catheterization: Insertion sites and associated waveforms

As the pulmonary artery (PA) catheter is directed through the chambers on the right side of the heart to its wedge position, it produces distinctive waveforms on the oscilloscope screen that are important indicators of the catheter's position in the heart.

RIGHT ATRIAL PRESSURE

When the catheter tip reaches the right atrium from the superior vena cava, the waveform on the oscilloscope screen or readout strip resembles the one shown at right. When this waveform appears, the practitioner inflates the catheter balloon, which floats the tip through the tricuspid valve into the right ventricle.

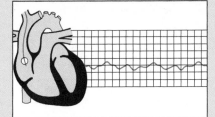

RIGHT VENTRICULAR PRESSURE

When the catheter tip reaches the right ventricle, the waveform looks like the one shown at right.

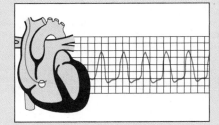

PULMONARY ARTERY PRESSURE

A waveform that resembles the one shown at right indicates that the balloon has floated the catheter tip through the pulmonic valve into the pulmonary artery. A dicrotic notch (see arrow) should be visible in the waveform, indicating the closing of the pulmonic valve.

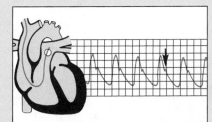

PULMONARY ARTERY WEDGE PRESSURE

Blood flow in the pulmonary artery then carries the catheter balloon into one of the pulmonary artery's many smaller branches. When the vessel becomes too narrow for the balloon to pass through, the balloon wedges in the vessel, occluding it. The monitor then displays a pulmonary artery wedge pressure waveform such as the one shown at right.

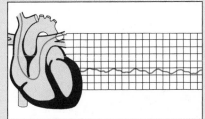

NORMAL RESULTS

- Right atrial (RA) pressure is 1 to 6 mm Hg.
- Right ventricular (RV) systolic pressure is 20 to 30 mm Hg.
- RV end-diastolic pressure is less than 5 mm Hg.
- Systolic PAP is 20 to 30 mm Hg.
- Diastolic PAP is 10 to 15 mm Hg.
- Mean PAWP is less than 20 mm Hg.
- PAWP is 6 to 12 mm Hg.
- Left atrial pressure is 10 mm Hg.

ABNORMAL RESULTS

- High RA pressures may suggest pulmonary disease, right-sided heart failure, fluid overload, or cardiac tamponade.
- High RV pressures may suggest pulmonary hypertension, pulmonary valvular stenosis, right-sided heart failure, pericardial effusion, or ventricular septal defects.
- High PAP may suggest atrial or ventricular septal defects, pulmonary hypertension, mitral stenosis, chronic obstructive pulmonary disease, pulmonary edema or embolus, or left-sided heart failure.
- High PAWP may suggest left-sided heart failure or cardiac tamponade.
- Low PAWP may suggest hypovolemia.

Pulmonary function tests

DESCRIPTION

- Evaluates pulmonary function through a series of spirometric measurements (see *Interpreting pulmonary function tests*)
- Also known as *PFTs*

PURPOSE

- To assess effectiveness of a specific therapeutic regimen
- To determine the cause of dyspnea
- To determine whether a functional abnormality is obstructive or restrictive
- To measure pulmonary dysfunction

PREPARATION

- Make sure the patient has signed an appropriate consent form.
- Note and report allergies.
- The patient should avoid smoking for 12 hours before the tests.
- Withhold bronchodilators for 8 hours, as ordered.
- The patient should avoid having a heavy meal before the tests.

Teaching points

- Explain the purpose of the test and how it's done.
- Explain who will perform the test and where it'll be done.
- Stress the need for the patient to avoid smoking for 12 hours before the tests.
- Instruct the patient not to eat a heavy meal before the tests.
- Tell the patient the test takes 1 or 2 hours.
- Tell the patient to wear loose clothing for the test. (See *Preparing for pulmonary function tests,* page 407.)

Interpreting pulmonary function tests

PULMONARY FUNCTION TEST	METHOD OF CALCULATION	IMPLICATIONS
Tidal volume (V_T)		
Amount of air inhaled or exhaled during normal breathing	Determining the spirographic measurement for 10 breaths and then dividing by 10	Decreased V_T may indicate restrictive disease and requires further testing, such as full pulmonary function studies or chest X-rays.
Minute volume (MV)		
Total amount of air expired per minute	Multiplying V_T by the respiratory rate	Normal MV can occur in emphysema; decreased MV may indicate other diseases such as pulmonary edema. Increased MV can occur with acidosis, increased carbon dioxide (CO_2), decreased partial pressure of arterial oxygen, exercise, and low compliance states.
Carbon dioxide response		
Increase or decrease in MV after breathing various CO_2 concentrations	Plotting changes in MV against increasing inspired CO_2 concentrations	Reduced CO_2 response may occur in emphysema, myxedema, obesity, hypoventilation syndrome, and sleep apnea.
Expiratory reserve volume (ERV)		
Amount of air exhaled after normal expiration	Direct spirographic measurement	ERV varies, even in healthy people, but usually decreases in obese people.
Vital capacity (VC)		
Total volume of air that can be exhaled after maximum inspiration	Direct spirographic measurement or adding V_T, inspiratory reserve volume (IRV), and ERV	Normal or increased VC with decreased flow rates may indicate any condition that causes a reduction in functional pulmonary tissue such as pulmonary edema. Decreased VC with normal or increased flow rates may indicate decreased respiratory effort resulting from neuromuscular disease, drug overdose, or head injury; decreased thoracic expansion; or limited diaphragm movement.
Inspiratory capacity (IC)		
Amount of air that can be inhaled after normal expiration	Direct spirographic measurement or adding IRV and V_T	Decreased IC indicates restrictive disease.
Functional residual capacity (FRC)		
Amount of air remaining in the lungs after normal expiration	Nitrogen washout, helium dilution technique, or adding ERV and residual volume (RV)	Increased FRC indicates overdistention of the lungs, which may result from obstructive pulmonary disease.

Interpreting pulmonary function tests *(continued)*

PULMONARY FUNCTION TEST	METHOD OF CALCULATION	IMPLICATIONS
Total lung capacity (TLC)		
Total volume of the lungs when maximally inflated	Adding V_T, IRV, ERV, and RV; FRC and IC; or VC and RV	Low TLC indicates restrictive disease; high TLC indicates overdistended lungs caused by obstructive disease.
Forced vital capacity (FVC)		
Amount of air exhaled forcefully and quickly after maximum inspiration	Direct spirographic measurement; expressed as a percentage of the total volume of gas exhaled	Decreased FVC indicates flow resistance in the respiratory system from obstructive disease such as chronic bronchitis or from restrictive disease such as pulmonary fibrosis.
Forced expiratory volume (FEV)		
Volume of air expired in the first, second, or third second of an FVC maneuver	Direct spirographic measurement; expressed as a percentage of FVC	Decreased FEV_1 and increased FEV_2 and FEV_3 may indicate obstructive disease; decreased or normal FEV_1 may indicate restrictive disease.
Forced expiratory flow (FEF)		
Average rate of flow during the middle half of FVC	Calculated from the flow rate and the time needed for expiration of the middle 50% of FVC	Low FEF (25% to 75%) indicates obstructive disease of the small and medium-sized airways.
Peak expiratory flow rate (PEFR)		
V_{max} during forced expiration	Calculated from the flow-volume curve or by direct spirographic measurement using a pneumotachometer or electronic tachometer with a transducer to convert flow to electrical output display	Decreased PEFR may indicate a mechanical problem, such as upper airway obstruction, or obstructive disease. PEFR is usually normal in restrictive disease but decreases in severe cases. Because PEFR is effort dependent, it's also low in a person who has poor expiratory effort or doesn't understand the procedure.
Maximal voluntary ventilation (MVV) (also called maximum breathing capacity)		
The greatest volume of air breathed per unit of time	Direct spirographic measurement	Decreased MVV may indicate obstructive disease; normal or decreased MVV may indicate restrictive disease such as myasthenia gravis.
Diffusing capacity for carbon monoxide (DL_{CO})		
Milliliters of CO diffused per minute across the alveolocapillary membrane	Calculated from analysis of the amount of carbon monoxide exhaled compared with the amount inhaled	Decreased DL_{CO} due to a thickened alveolocapillary membrane occurs in interstitial pulmonary diseases, such as pulmonary fibrosis, asbestosis, and sarcoidosis; DL_{CO} is reduced in emphysema because of alveolocapillary membrane loss.

DIAGNOSTIC PROCEDURE

KEY STEPS

- Confirm the patient's identity using two patient identifiers according to facility policy.
- For tidal volume (V_T), the patient breathes normally into the mouthpiece 10 times.
- For expiratory reserve volume (ERV), the patient breathes normally for several breaths and then exhales as completely as possible.
- For vital capacity (VC), the patient inhales as deeply as possible and exhales into the mouthpiece as completely as possible. This is repeated three times, and the largest volume is recorded.
- For inspiratory capacity (IC), the patient breathes normally for several breaths and inhales as deeply as possible.
- For functional residual capacity (FRC), the patient breathes normally into a spirometer. After a few breaths, the levels of gas in the spirometer and in the lungs reach equilibrium. FRC is calculated by subtracting the spirometer volume from the original volume.
- For forced vital capacity (FVC) and forced expiratory volume (FEV), the patient inhales as slowly and deeply as possible and then exhales into the mouthpiece as quickly and completely as possible. This is repeated three times, and the largest volume is recorded. The volume of air expired at 1 second (FEV_1), at 2 seconds (FEV_2), and at 3 seconds (FEV_3) during all three repetitions is recorded.
- For maximal voluntary ventilation, the patient breathes into the mouthpiece as quickly and deeply as possible for 15 seconds.
- For diffusing capacity for carbon monoxide, the patient inhales a gas mixture with a low level of carbon monoxide and holds his breath for 10 to 15 seconds before exhaling.

(continued)

POSTPROCEDURE CARE

◆ Inform the practitioner of abnormal results.
◆ Tell the patient to resume his usual activities, diet, and medications, as ordered.

PRECAUTIONS

⚡ **WARNING** *PFTs may be contraindicated in patients with acute coronary insufficiency, angina, or recent myocardial infarction. Watch for respiratory distress, changes in pulse rate and blood pressure, coughing, and bronchospasm in these patients.*

COMPLICATIONS

◆ Respiratory distress
◆ Bronchospasm
◆ Physical exhaustion

INTERPRETATION

NORMAL RESULTS

◆ Results are based on age, height, weight, and sex; values expressed as a percentage.
◆ V_T is 5 to 7 mg/kg of body weight.
◆ ERV is 25% of VC.
◆ IC is 75% of VC.
◆ FEV_1 is 83% of VC after 1 second.
◆ FEV_2 is 94% of VC after 2 seconds.
◆ FEV_3 is 97% of VC after 3 seconds.

ABNORMAL RESULTS

◆ FEV_1 less than 80% suggests obstructed pulmonary disease.
◆ FEV_1-to-FVC ratio greater than 80% suggests restrictive pulmonary disease.
◆ Low V_T suggests possible restrictive disease.
◆ Low minute volume (MV) suggests possible disorders such as pulmonary edema.
◆ High MV suggests possible acidosis, exercise, or low compliance states.
◆ Low carbon dioxide response suggests possible emphysema, myxedema, obesity, hypoventilation syndrome, or sleep apnea.
◆ Residual volume greater than 35% of total lung capacity after maximal expiratory effort suggests obstructive disease.
◆ Low IC suggests restrictive disease.
◆ High FRC suggests possible obstructive pulmonary disease.
◆ Low total lung capacity (TLC) suggests restrictive disease.
◆ High TLC suggests obstructive disease.
◆ Low FVC suggests flow resistance from obstructive disease or from restrictive disease.
◆ Low forced expiratory flow suggests obstructive disease of the small and medium-sized airways.
◆ Low peak expiratory flow rate suggests upper airway obstruction.
◆ Low diffusing capacity for carbon monoxide suggests possible interstitial pulmonary disease.

Preparing for pulmonary function tests

Dear Patient,

Pulmonary (or lung) function tests have been ordered for you. These tests measure how well your lungs work. Here's what to expect.

HOW THE TESTS WORK

You'll be asked to breathe as deeply as possible into a mouthpiece that's connected to a machine called a *spirometer*. This measures and records the rate and amount of air inhaled and exhaled.

You may also sit in a small, telephone booth–like enclosure for a test called *body plethysmography*. Again, you'll be asked to breathe in and out, and the measurements will be recorded.

BEFORE THE TESTS

Avoid smoking for at least 4 hours before the tests. Eat lightly, and don't drink a lot of fluid. Wear loose, comfortable clothing. Remember to use the bathroom.

To make the tests go quickly, give your full cooperation. Tell the technician if you don't understand the instructions. If you wear dentures, keep them in — they'll help you keep a tight seal around the spirometer's mouthpiece.

DURING THE TESTS

During spirometry, you'll sit upright, and you'll wear a noseclip to make sure you breathe only through your mouth. During body plethysmography, you won't need a noseclip.

If you feel too confined in the small chamber, keep in mind that you can't suffocate. You can talk to the nurse or technician through a window.

The tests have several parts. For each test, you'll be asked to breathe a certain way — for example, to inhale deeply and exhale completely or to inhale quickly. You may need to repeat some tests after inhaling a bronchodilator to expand the airways in your lungs. A blood sample may be obtained from an artery in your arm. This sample will be used to measure how well your body uses the air you breathe.

HOW WILL YOU FEEL?

During the tests, you may feel tired or short of breath. However, you'll be able to take rest breaks between measurements.

Tell the technician right away if you feel dizzy, begin wheezing, or have chest pain, a racing or pounding heart, an upset stomach, or severe shortness of breath. Also tell him if your arm swells or if you're bleeding from the spot where a blood sample was taken or experience weakness or pain in that arm.

AFTER THE TESTS

When the tests are over, rest if you feel like it. Resume your usual activities when you regain your energy.

Pyruvate kinase test

DESCRIPTION

- Assay to confirm pyruvate kinase (PK) deficiency when red blood cell (RBC) enzyme deficiency may cause anemia
- Abnormally low PK level: inherited autosomal recessive trait that may cause an RBC membrane defect resulting in congenital hemolytic anemia
- Helps in anaerobic metabolism of glucose

PURPOSE

- To differentiate PK-deficient hemolytic anemia from other congenital hemolytic anemias or from acquired hemolytic anemia
- To detect PK deficiency in asymptomatic, heterozygous inheritance

PREPARATION

- Check the patient's history for recent blood transfusion, and note it on the laboratory request.
- No dietary restrictions are required.
- The test requires a blood sample.

Teaching points

- Explain that this test detects inherited enzyme deficiencies.
- Explain who will perform the test and where it'll be done.
- Inform the patient that he need not fast.
- Tell the patient that the test requires a blood sample and that he may experience slight discomfort from the tourniquet and needle puncture.
- Tell the patient the test takes less than 5 minutes.

KEY STEPS

- Confirm the patient's identity using two patient identifiers according to facility policy.
- Perform a venipuncture, and collect the sample in a 4-ml EDTA tube.
- Completely fill the collection tube, and invert it gently several times to mix the sample and the anticoagulant.

POSTPROCEDURE CARE

- Apply direct pressure to the venipuncture site until bleeding stops.

PRECAUTIONS

- Handle the sample gently to prevent hemolysis.
- Send the sample to the laboratory immediately; otherwise, refrigerate it.
- Inform the practitioner of abnormal results.

COMPLICATIONS

- Hematoma at the venipuncture site

NORMAL RESULTS

- Level is 9 to 22 units/g of hemoglobin (Hb); in the low substrate assay, it's 1.7 to 6.8 units/g of Hb.

ABNORMAL RESULTS

- Low serum PK levels confirm a diagnosis of PK deficiency and allow differentiation between PK-deficient hemolytic anemia and other inherited disorders.

Quantitative immunoglobulins G, A, and M

DESCRIPTION

- Measures levels of immunoglobulins (Igs) G, A, and M, proteins that function as specific antibodies in response to antigen stimulation, are responsible for the humoral aspects of immunity, and are normally present in serum in predictable percentages
- Detects deviations from normal immunoglobulin percentages, which may occur in many immune disorders, including cancer, hepatic disorders, rheumatoid arthritis, and systemic lupus erythematosus
- Using immunoelectrophoresis, identifies IgG, IgA, and IgM in a serum sample; measures the level of each by radial immunodiffusion or nephelometry (or by indirect immunofluorescence and radioimmunoassay)

PURPOSE

- To diagnose paraproteinemias, such as multiple myeloma and Waldenström's macroglobulinemia
- To detect hypogammaglobulinemia and hypergammaglobulinemia as well as nonimmunologic diseases, such as cirrhosis and hepatitis, that are linked to abnormally high immunoglobulin levels
- To assess the effectiveness of chemotherapy and radiation therapy

PREPARATION

- Check the patient's history for drugs that may affect test results, including alcohol and opioid abuse.
- The test requires a blood sample.
- Restrict food and fluids, except water, for 12 hours before the test.

Teaching points

- Explain that this test measures antibody levels.
- If appropriate, tell the patient that the test evaluates the effectiveness of treatment.
- Explain who will perform the test and where it'll be done.
- Instruct the patient to restrict food and fluids, except for water, for 12 to 14 hours before the test.

- Tell the patient that the test requires a blood sample and that he may experience slight discomfort from the tourniquet and needle puncture.
- Tell the patient the test takes less than 5 minutes.

KEY STEPS

- Confirm the patient's identity using two patient identifiers according to facility policy.
- Perform a venipuncture, and collect the sample in a 7-ml clot-activator tube.
- Send the sample to the laboratory immediately to prevent immunoglobulin deterioration.

POSTPROCEDURE CARE

- Apply direct pressure to the venipuncture site until bleeding stops.
- Inform the practitioner of abnormal results.
- After the test, instruct the patient to resume his usual diet and medications.

PRECAUTIONS

- Advise the patient with abnormally low immunoglobulin levels (especially IgG or IgM) to protect himself against bacterial infection. When caring for such a patient, watch for signs of infection, such as fever, chills, rash, and skin ulcers.
- Instruct patients with abnormally high immunoglobulin levels and symptoms of monoclonal gammopathies to report bone pain and tenderness. Such patients have numerous antibody-producing malignant plasma cells in bone marrow, which hamper production of other blood components. Watch for signs of hypercalcemia, renal failure, and spontaneous pathologic fractures.

COMPLICATIONS

- Hematoma at the venipuncture site

NORMAL RESULTS

- Using nephelometry, in adults, IgG level is 800 to 1,800 mg/dl (SI, 8 to 18 g/L); IgA level is 100 to 400 mg/dl (SI, 1 to 4 g/L); IgM level is 55 to 150 mg/dl (SI, 0.55 to 1.5 g/L).
- IgG is 75% of serum immunoglobulins, including the warm-temperature type; IgA is about 15% of the total; and IgM is about 5%, including cold agglutinins, rheumatoid factor, and ABO blood group isoagglutinins.

ABNORMAL RESULTS

- In congenital and acquired hypogammaglobulinemias, myelomas, and macroglobulinemia, the findings confirm the diagnosis.
- In hepatic and autoimmune diseases, leukemias, and lymphomas, such findings are less important, but they can support the diagnosis based on other tests, such as biopsies and white blood cell differential, and on the physical examination.

Radioactive iodine uptake test

DESCRIPTION

◆ Evaluates thyroid function by measuring the amount of orally ingested iodine-123 (^{123}I) or iodine-131 (^{131}I) that accumulates in the thyroid gland after 2, 6, and 24 hours
◆ Measures the radioactivity in the thyroid as a percentage of the original dose, thus indicating its ability to trap and retain iodine
◆ Accurately diagnoses hyperthyroidism, but is less accurate for hypothyroidism
◆ Performed with radionuclide thyroid imaging and triiodothyronine resin uptake test; differentiates Graves' disease from hyperfunctioning toxic adenoma
◆ Indicated by abnormal results of chemical tests used to evaluate thyroid function
◆ If Hashimoto's disease suspected, may add the perchlorate suppression test to verify diagnosis (see *Perchlorate suppression test*)

PURPOSE

◆ To evaluate thyroid function
◆ To help diagnose hyperthyroidism or hypothyroidism
◆ To help distinguish between primary and secondary thyroid disorders

PREPARATION

◆ Check the patient's history for iodine exposure, which may interfere with test results.
◆ Note previous radiologic tests using contrast media, nuclear medicine procedures, or current use of iodine preparations or thyroid drugs on the film request slip.
◆ Iodine hypersensitivity isn't considered a contraindication because the amount of iodine used is similar to the amount consumed in a normal diet.
◆ Make sure the patient has signed an informed consent form.
◆ The patient should fast overnight before the test.

Teaching points

◆ Explain that this test assesses thyroid function.
◆ Explain who will perform the test and where it'll be done.
◆ Assure the patient that the test is painless and that the small amount of radioactivity is harmless.
◆ Instruct the patient to fast from midnight the night before the test.
◆ Tell the patient that he'll receive radioactive iodine (capsule or liquid) and that he'll then be scanned after 2 hours, 6 hours, and 24 hours.

DIAGNOSTIC PROCEDURE

KEY STEPS

◆ Confirm the patient's identity using two patient identifiers according to facility policy.
◆ After ingesting an oral dose of radioactive iodine, the patient has his thyroid scanned at 2 hours, 6 hours, and 24 hours.
◆ The amount of radioactivity detected by the probe is compared with the amount of radioactivity contained in the original dose to determine the percentage of radioactive iodine retained by the thyroid.

POSTPROCEDURE CARE

◆ Tell the patient to resume a light diet 2 hours after taking the oral dose of radioactive iodine. When the study is complete, instruct the patient to resume his usual diet.

PRECAUTIONS

◆ The test is contraindicated during pregnancy.

COMPLICATIONS

◆ None

INTERPRETATION

NORMAL RESULTS

◆ At 2 hours, 4% to 12% of the radioactive iodine accumulates in the thyroid; after 6 hours, 5% to 20%; at 24 hours, 8% to 29%.
◆ The remaining radioactive iodine is excreted in the urine.

ABNORMAL RESULTS

◆ Below-normal iodine uptake may indicate hypothyroidism, subacute thyroiditis, or iodine overload.
◆ Above-normal uptake may indicate hyperthyroidism, early Hashimoto's thyroiditis, hypoalbuminemia, lithium ingestion, or iodine-deficient goiter.
◆ In hyperthyroidism, the rate of turnover may be so rapid that a falsely normal measurement occurs at 24 hours.

INTERFERING FACTORS *Thyroid hormones, thyroid hormone antagonists, salicylates, penicillins, antihistamines, anticoagulants, corticosteroids, and phenylbutazone (possible decrease)*

Perchlorate suppression test

The perchlorate suppression test is used to evaluate the patient with suspected Hashimoto's disease or to demonstrate an enzyme deficiency within the thyroid gland. Because potassium perchlorate competes with and displaces the iodide ions that aren't organified, this study can identify defects in the iodide organification process within the thyroid.

In this procedure, a small dose of radioactive iodine is administered orally. A radioactive iodine uptake (RAIU) test is performed 1 and 2 hours afterward. After the 2-hour RAIU test, the patient receives 400 mg to 1 g of potassium perchlorate orally. RAIU tests are performed every 15 minutes for the first hour after the dose and then every 30 minutes for the next 2 to 3 hours.

The results of the RAIU tests performed after administration of potassium perchlorate are compared with those of the 2-hour RAIU test performed before perchlorate was administered. In a normal person, the uptake of radioactive iodine won't change significantly after administration of perchlorate. The patient with either Hashimoto's disease or an enzyme deficiency will experience a decrease in uptake. The patient with an enzyme deficiency will experience a drop in his uptake of more than 15% after perchlorate administration.

Radioallergosorbent test

OVERVIEW

DESCRIPTION

♦ Measures immunoglobulin (Ig) E antibodies in serum by radioimmunoassay and identifies specific allergens that cause rash, asthma, hay fever, drug reactions, and other atopic complaints
♦ Compares test results with control values to represent the patient's reactivity to a specific allergen
♦ Easier to perform, more specific, less painful, and less dangerous than skin testing
♦ Careful selection of specific allergens, based on the patient's history, crucial for result effectiveness
♦ May be more useful than skin testing when a skin disorder makes accurate reading of skin tests difficult, when a patient requires continual antihistamine therapy, or when skin test results are negative but the patient's history supports IgE-mediated hypersensitivity
♦ Exposes a sample of the patient's serum to a panel of allergen particle complexes (APCs) on cellulose disks
♦ Works when IgE reacts with APCs to which it's sensitive; radiolabeled anti-IgE antibody then added (binds to IgE-APC complexes); after centrifugation, amount of radioactivity in particulate material directly proportional to amount of IgE antibodies present

PURPOSE

♦ To identify allergens to which the patient has an immediate (IgE-mediated) hypersensitivity
♦ To monitor the patient's response to therapy

PREPARATION

♦ If the patient will receive a radioactive scan, make sure the blood sample is collected before the scan.
♦ No dietary restrictions are required.
♦ The test requires a blood sample.

Teaching points

♦ Explain that this test may detect the cause of allergy or monitor the effectiveness of allergy treatment.
♦ Explain who will perform the test and where it'll be done.
♦ Tell the patient that he doesn't need to restrict his diet.
♦ Tell the patient that the test requires a blood sample, and that he may experience slight discomfort from the tourniquet and needle puncture.
♦ Tell the patient the test takes less than 5 minutes.

DIAGNOSTIC PROCEDURE

KEY STEPS

♦ Confirm the patient's identity using two patient identifiers according to facility policy.
♦ Perform a venipuncture, and collect the sample in a 7-ml clot-activator tube.
♦ Usually, 1 ml of serum is sufficient for five allergen assays.
♦ Note on the laboratory request the specific allergens to be tested.

POSTPROCEDURE CARE

♦ Apply direct pressure to the venipuncture site until bleeding stops.
♦ Inform the practitioner of abnormal results.

PRECAUTIONS

♦ Maintain standard precautions while collecting the sample.

COMPLICATIONS

♦ Hematoma at the venipuncture site

INTERPRETATION

NORMAL RESULTS

♦ Results depend on the relation to a control serum value that differs among laboratories.

ABNORMAL RESULTS

♦ Elevated serum IgE levels suggest hypersensitivity to the specific allergen or allergens used.

Radionuclide renal imaging

DESCRIPTION

◆ Assesses renal blood flow, renal structure, and nephron and collecting system function

PURPOSE

◆ To detect and assess functional and structural renal abnormalities and acute or chronic disease
◆ To assess renal transplantation or renal injury caused by trauma to the urinary tract or obstruction

PREPARATION

◆ Make sure the patient has signed an appropriate consent form.
◆ If the patient receives antihypertensive medication, ask the practitioner if it should be withheld before the test.
◆ No dietary restrictions are required.
◆ A pregnant patient or a young child may receive a supersaturated solution of potassium iodide 1 to 3 hours before the test to block thyroid uptake of iodine.

Teaching points

◆ Explain the purpose of the test and how it's done.
◆ Explain who will perform the test and where it'll be done.
◆ Inform the patient that he'll receive an injection of a radionuclide and that he may experience transient flushing and nausea.
◆ Emphasize that only a small amount of radionuclide is given and that it's usually excreted within 24 hours.
◆ Tell the patient that he doesn't have to restrict his diet.
◆ Tell him that the test lasts about 1 hour.

DIAGNOSTIC PROCEDURE

KEY STEPS

◆ Confirm the patient's identity using two patient identifiers according to facility policy.
◆ The patient is placed prone for posterior views. If the test is to evaluate transplantation, the patient is placed supine for anterior views.
◆ Instruct the patient not to change position.
◆ A perfusion study (radionuclide angiography) is performed first to evaluate renal blood flow.
◆ Next, a function study is performed to measure the transit time of the radionuclide through the kidneys' functional units.
◆ After I.V. iodine-131 (Hippuran) is given, images are obtained at a rate of one per minute for 20 minutes.
◆ Static images are obtained 4 or more hours later, after the radionuclide has drained through the pelvicaliceal system.

POSTPROCEDURE CARE

◆ Monitor the insertion site for signs of hematoma, infection, and discomfort. Apply warm compresses for comfort.
◆ Monitor the patient's intake and output; monitor electrolyte, acid-base, blood urea nitrogen, and creatinine levels as indicated.
◆ Instruct the patient to flush the toilet immediately after each voiding for 24 hours as a radiation precaution.

PRECAUTIONS

◆ The test is contraindicated in breast-feeding patients and in those with a previous allergy to iodine, shellfish, or radioactive tracers.

COMPLICATIONS

◆ Hematoma at the venipuncture site

INTERPRETATION

NORMAL RESULTS

◆ Renal perfusion is seen immediately after uptake of the ^{99m}Tc in the abdominal aorta.
◆ Within 1 or 2 minutes, a normal renal circulation appears.
◆ Kidneys are delineated simultaneously, symmetrically, and with equal intensity.
◆ Kidneys are normal in size, shape, and position.
◆ Maximum counts of the radionuclide in the kidneys occur within 5 minutes after injection (and within 1 minute of each other) and fall to one-third or less of the maximum counts in the same kidney within 25 minutes.
◆ Within this time, kidney function can be evaluated as the level of radionuclide shifts from the cortex to the pelvis and, finally, to the bladder.
◆ In normal total function, the effective renal plasma flow is 420 ml/minute or greater, and more than 66% of the dose is excreted in the urine at 30 to 35 minutes.

ABNORMAL RESULTS

◆ Renal circulation is impeded, such as that caused by trauma and renal artery stenosis or renal infarction.
◆ Renal perfusion is abnormal because of a possible obstruction of the vascular grafts in patients with a kidney transplant.
◆ Abnormalities of the collecting system and urine extravasation are observed.
◆ Reduced radionuclide activity in the collecting system (caused by markedly decreased tubular function) and decreased radionuclide activity in the tubules, with increased activity in the collecting system (caused by outflow obstruction) are noted.
◆ A defined level of ureteral obstruction is evident.
◆ Lesions, congenital abnormalities, and traumatic injury are observed.
◆ Congenital disorders or space-occupying lesions within or surrounding the kidney, such as tumors, infarcts, and inflammatory masses, are noted.
◆ Infarction, rupture, or hemorrhage after trauma are noted.
◆ Lower-than-normal total concentration of the radionuclide is observed, possibly due to diffuse renal disorder, such as acute tubular necrosis, severe infection, or ischemia.
◆ Radionuclide uptake is decreased, indicating organ rejection in a patient with a kidney transplant.
◆ Visualization isn't possible due to possible congenital ectopia or aplasia.

Radionuclide thyroid imaging

DESCRIPTION

- Studies the thyroid by gamma camera after the patient receives iodine-123 (^{123}I), technetium-99m (^{99m}Tc) pertechnetate, or iodine-131 (^{131}I)
- Usually follows discovery of a palpable mass, an enlarged gland, or an asymmetrical goiter and is performed along with thyroid uptake tests and measurements of serum triiodothyronine (T_3) and serum thyroxine (T_4) levels

PURPOSE

- To assess the size, structure, position, and function of the thyroid gland

PREPARATION

- Check the patient's diet and drug history. Drugs, such as thyroid hormones, thyroid hormone antagonists, and iodine preparations may be stopped for 2 to 3 weeks before the test, and phenothiazines, corticosteroids, salicylates, anticoagulants, and antihistamines may be stopped for 1 week before the test.
- Ask the patient if he has undergone tests that used radiographic contrast media within the past 60 days. Note previous radiographic contrast media exposure on the X-ray request.
- Make sure the patient has signed a consent form if required.
- The patient receives ^{123}I or ^{131}I (oral) or ^{99m}Tc pertechnetate (I.V.). Record the date and time of administration.
- If ^{123}I or ^{131}I will be used, the patient should fast after midnight before the procedure.
- The patient receiving an oral radioisotope should fast for another 2 hours after administration.

Teaching points

- Explain that this test helps determine the cause of thyroid dysfunction.
- Explain who will perform the test and where it'll be done.
- Inform the patient that after he receives the radiopharmaceutical, a gamma camera will produce an image of his thyroid.
- Instruct the patient to stop taking drugs, such as thyroid hormones, thyroid hormone antagonists, and iodine preparations (for example, Lugol's solution, some multivitamins, and cough syrups) 2 to 3 weeks before the test. Also, tell him to stop taking phenothiazines, corticosteroids, salicylates, anticoagulants, and antihistamines 1 week before the test.
- Tell the patient not to consume iodized salt, iodinated salt substitutes, and seafood for 14 to 21 days before the test.
- Tell the patient to stop taking T_4 10 days before the test, and to stop taking liothyronine, propylthiouracil, and methimazole 3 days before the test.
- If the patient is to receive ^{123}I or ^{131}I, tell him to fast after midnight the night before the test. Fasting isn't required if he's to receive an I.V. injection of ^{99m}Tc pertechnetate.
- Just before the test, tell the patient to remove dentures, jewelry, and other materials that may interfere with the imaging process.
- Tell the patient that the test takes about 1 hour.

KEY STEPS

- Confirm the patient's identity using two patient identifiers according to facility policy.
- The test is performed 24 hours after oral administration of ^{123}I or ^{131}I or 20 to 30 minutes after I.V. injection of ^{99m}Tc pertechnetate.
- The patient is placed in the supine position with his neck extended; the thyroid gland is palpated.
- The gamma camera is positioned above the anterior portion of his neck.
- Images of the patient's thyroid gland are projected on a monitor and are recorded on X-ray film.
- Three views of the thyroid are obtained: a straight-on anterior view and two bilateral oblique views.

POSTPROCEDURE CARE

- Inform the practitioner of abnormal results.
- Tell the patient to resume his usual diet and medications.

PRECAUTIONS

- The test is contraindicated in pregnant patients and in those with an allergy to iodine, shellfish, or radioactive tracings.

COMPLICATIONS

- Adverse reaction to the radioisotope

(continued)

INTERPRETATION

NORMAL RESULTS

◆ The thyroid gland is about 2″ (5 cm) long and 1″ (2.5 cm) wide, with a uniform uptake of the radioisotope and without tumors.
◆ The gland is butterfly-shaped, with the isthmus located at the midline. Occasionally, a third lobe called the pyramidal lobe may exist.

ABNORMAL RESULTS

◆ Hyperfunctioning nodules (areas of excessive iodine uptake) appear as black regions called *hot spots;* their presence requires a follow-up T_3 thyroid suppression test to determine if the hyperfunctioning areas are autonomous.
◆ Hypofunctioning nodules (areas of little or no iodine uptake) appear as white or light gray regions called *cold spots*. If a cold spot appears, subsequent thyroid ultrasonography may be performed to rule out cysts; in addition, fine-needle aspiration and biopsy of such nodules may be performed to rule out malignancy. (See *Results of thyroid imaging in thyroid disorders*.)

Results of thyroid imaging in thyroid disorders

This chart shows the characteristic findings in radionuclide imaging tests that are associated with various thyroid disorders as well as the possible causes of those disorders.

CONDITION	FINDINGS	CAUSES
Hypothyroidism	◆ Glandular damage or absent gland	◆ Surgical removal of gland ◆ Inflammation ◆ Radiation ◆ Neoplasm (rare)
Hypothyroid goiter	◆ Enlarged gland ◆ Decreased uptake (of radioactive iodine) if glandular destruction is present ◆ Increased uptake possible from congenital error in thyroxine synthesis	◆ Insufficient iodine intake ◆ Hypersecretion of thyroid-stimulating hormone (TSH) caused by thyroid hormone deficiency
Myxedema (cretinism in children)	◆ Normal or slightly reduced gland size ◆ Uniform pattern ◆ Decreased uptake	◆ Defective embryonic development, resulting in congenital absence or underdevelopment of thyroid gland ◆ Maternal iodine deficiency
Hyperthyroidism (Graves' disease)	◆ Enlarged gland ◆ Uniform pattern ◆ Increased uptake	◆ Unknown, but may be hereditary ◆ Production of thyroid-stimulating immunoglobulins
Toxic nodular goiter	◆ Multiple hot spots	◆ Long-standing simple goiter
Hyperfunctioning adenomas	◆ Solitary hot spot	◆ Adenomatous production of triiodothyronine and thyroxine, suppressing TSH secretion and producing atrophy of other thyroid tissue
Hypofunctioning adenomas	◆ Solitary cold spot	◆ Cyst or nonfunctioning nodule
Benign multinodular goiter	◆ Multiple nodules with variable or no function	◆ Local inflammation ◆ Degeneration
Thyroid carcinoma	◆ Usually a solitary cold spot with occasional or no function	◆ Neoplasm

---

Raji cell assay

DESCRIPTION
- Detects the presence of circulating immune complexes; studies the Raji lymphoblastoid cell line
- Identifying these cells (which have receptors for immunoglobulin G complement) helps evaluate autoimmune disease

PURPOSE
- To detect circulating immune complexes
- To help study autoimmune disease

PREPARATION
- No dietary restrictions are required.
- The test requires a blood sample.

Teaching points
- Explain the purpose of the test and how it's done.
- Explain who will perform the test and where it'll be done.
- Tell the patient that he need not restrict food or fluids.
- Tell the patient that the test requires a blood sample and that he may experience slight discomfort from the tourniquet and needle puncture.
- Tell the patient the test takes less than 5 minutes.

KEY STEPS
- Confirm the patient's identity using two patient identifiers according to facility policy.
- Perform a venipuncture, collect a sample in a clot-activator tube, and promptly send it to the laboratory.

POSTPROCEDURE CARE
- Apply direct pressure to the venipuncture site until bleeding stops.
- Inform the practitioner of abnormal results.

PRECAUTIONS
- Maintain standard precautions while collecting the sample.
- Handle the sample gently to prevent hemolysis.

COMPLICATIONS
- Hematoma at the venipuncture site

NORMAL RESULTS
- Raji cells aren't present.

ABNORMAL RESULTS
- A positive result can detect immune complexes, including those found in viral, microbial, and parasitic infections; metastasis; autoimmune disorders; and drug reactions.
- A positive result may also detect immune complexes associated with celiac disease, cirrhosis of the liver, Crohn's disease, cryoglobulinemia, dermatitis herpetiformis, sickle cell anemia, and ulcerative colitis.

Rapid corticotropin test

DESCRIPTION
◆ Gradually replacing the 8-hour corticotropin stimulation test as the most effective diagnostic tool for evaluating adrenal hypofunction
◆ Uses cosyntropin; provides faster results and causes fewer allergic reactions than the 8-hour test (which uses natural corticotropin from animal sources)
◆ Requires prior determination of baseline cortisol levels to evaluate the effect of cosyntropin administration on cortisol secretion
◆ Unequivocally high morning cortisol levels needed to rule out adrenal hypofunction and make further testing unnecessary
◆ Also known as the *cosyntropin test*

PURPOSE
◆ To help identify primary and secondary adrenal hypofunction

PREPARATION
◆ If the patient is an inpatient, withhold corticotropin and all steroid drugs as ordered.
◆ If the patient is an outpatient, tell him to refrain from taking all steroid drugs, if instructed by his practitioner. If he must continue taking them, note this on the laboratory request.
◆ Fasting for 10 to 12 hours before the test is required.
◆ The test requires a blood sample.

Teaching points
◆ Explain that this test helps determine if his condition is caused by a hormonal deficiency.
◆ Explain who will perform the test and where it'll be done.
◆ Inform the patient that he must fast for 10 to 12 hours before the test and must be relaxed and resting quietly for 30 minutes before the test.
◆ Tell the patient that the test requires a blood sample, and that he may experience slight discomfort from the tourniquet and needle puncture.
◆ Tell the patient that the test takes at least 1 hour.

KEY STEPS
◆ Confirm the patient's identity using two patient identifiers according to facility policy.
◆ Draw 5 ml of blood for a baseline value. Collect the sample in a 5-ml heparinized tube. Label this sample "preinjection," and send it to the laboratory.
◆ Inject 250 mcg (0.25 mg) of cosyntropin I.V. or I.M. (I.V. administration provides more accurate results because ineffective absorption after I.M. administration may cause wide variations in response.)
◆ Direct I.V. injection should take about 2 minutes.
◆ Draw another 5 ml of blood at 30 and 60 minutes after the cosyntropin injection.
◆ Collect the samples in 5-ml heparinized tubes. Label the samples "30 minutes postinjection" and "60 minutes postinjection," and send them to the laboratory. Include the collection times on the laboratory request.

POSTPROCEDURE CARE
◆ Apply direct pressure to the venipuncture site until bleeding stops.
◆ Observe the patient for signs of a rare allergic reaction to cosyntropin, such as hives, itching, and tachycardia.
◆ Inform the practitioner of abnormal results.
◆ Tell the patient to resume his usual diet, activities, and medications.

PRECAUTIONS
◆ Handle the samples gently to prevent hemolysis. They require no special precautions other than avoiding stasis.

COMPLICATIONS
◆ Hematoma at the venipuncture site

NORMAL RESULTS
◆ Cortisol levels rise after 30 to 60 minutes to a peak of 18 mg/dl (SI, 500 mmol/L) or more 60 minutes after the cosyntropin injection.
◆ Doubling the baseline value usually indicates a normal response.

ABNORMAL RESULTS
◆ A normal result excludes adrenal hypofunction (insufficiency).
◆ In patients with primary adrenal hypofunction (Addison's disease), cortisol levels remain low.
◆ If test results show subnormal increases in cortisol levels, prolonged stimulation of the adrenal cortex may be needed to differentiate between primary and secondary adrenal hypofunction.

Rapid monoclonal test for cytomegalovirus

DESCRIPTION

◆ Cytomegalovirus (CMV): member of herpes virus group; can cause systemic infection in congenitally infected infants and in immunocompromised patients (for example, transplant recipients, those receiving chemotherapy for neoplastic disease, and those with acquired immunodeficiency syndrome [AIDS])
◆ CMV infections: previously detected in laboratory by recognition of distinctive cytopathic effects (CPE) produced by virus in conventional tube cell cultures in about 9 days
◆ Faster shell vial assay (rapid monoclonal test): based on availability of a monoclonal antibody specific for the 72 kD protein of CMV synthesized during the immediate early stage of viral replication
◆ Indirect immunofluorescence: nuclei of CMV-infected fibroblasts stain densely; readily differentiated from nonspecific background fluorescence of certain specimens

PURPOSE

◆ To obtain rapid laboratory diagnosis of CMV infection, especially in immunocompromised patients who currently have, or are at risk for developing, systemic infections caused by this virus

PREPARATION

◆ No dietary restrictions are required.
◆ The type of specimen to be collected determines the collection method.

Teaching points

◆ Explain the purpose of the test, and describe the procedure for collecting the specimen, which depends on the laboratory used.
◆ Explain who will perform the test and where it'll be done.
◆ Tell the patient that no dietary restrictions are required.

KEY STEPS

◆ Confirm the patient's identity using two patient identifiers according to facility policy.
◆ Specimens should be collected during the prodromal and acute stages of clinical infection to maximize the chances of detecting CMV.
◆ Each type of specimen requires a specific collection device.
◆ For the throat, use a microbiologic transport swab.
◆ For urine or cerebrospinal fluid, use a sterile screw-capped tube or vial.
◆ For bronchoalveolar lavage tissue, use a sterile screw-capped jar.
◆ For blood, use a sterile tube with an anticoagulant (such as heparin).

POSTPROCEDURE CARE

◆ Answer the patient's questions about the test.
◆ Inform the practitioner of abnormal results.

PRECAUTIONS

◆ Transport the specimen to the laboratory as soon as possible after the collection. If the anticipated time between collection and inoculation into shell vial cell cultures is longer than 3 hours, store the specimen at 39.2° F (4° C). Don't freeze the specimen or allow it to become dry.
◆ Use gloves when obtaining and handling all specimens.

COMPLICATIONS

◆ None

NORMAL RESULTS

◆ CMV shouldn't appear in a culture specimen.

ABNORMAL RESULTS

◆ CMV is found in urine and throat specimens from asymptomatic patients. Detection from these sites indicates active, asymptomatic infection, which may herald symptomatic involvement, especially in immunocompromised patients.
◆ Detection of CMV in specimens of blood, tissue, and bronchoalveolar lavage usually indicates systemic infection and disease.

Red blood cell count

OVERVIEW

DESCRIPTION

- Also called an *erythrocyte count*, part of a complete blood count
- Detects the number of red blood cells (RBCs) in a microliter (µl), or cubic millimeter (mm^3), of whole blood
- Doesn't give information about the size, shape, or concentration of hemoglobin (Hb) in the corpuscles but may calculate mean corpuscular volume (MCV) and mean corpuscular hemoglobin (MCH)

PURPOSE

- To provide data for calculating MCV and MCH, which reveal RBC size and Hb content
- To support other hematologic tests for diagnosing anemia or polycythemia

PREPARATION

- No dietary restrictions are required.
- The test requires a blood sample.

Teaching points

- Explain to the patient that the RBC count evaluates the number of blood cells and detects possible blood disorders.
- Explain who will perform the test and where it'll be done.
- Inform the patient that he need not fast.
- Tell the patient that the test requires a blood sample, and that he may experience slight discomfort from the tourniquet and needle puncture.
- Tell the patient the test takes less than 5 minutes.

DIAGNOSTIC PROCEDURE

KEY STEPS

- Confirm the patient's identity using two patient identifiers according to facility policy.
- For adults and older children, draw venous blood into a 3- or 4.5-ml EDTA sodium metabisulfite solution tube.
- For younger children, collect capillary blood in a microcollection device.
- Fill the collection tube completely.
- Invert the tube gently several times to mix the sample and the anticoagulant.

POSTPROCEDURE CARE

- Make sure that subdermal bleeding has stopped before removing pressure.
- Inform the practitioner of abnormal results.

PRECAUTIONS

- Maintain standard precautions while collecting the sample.
- Handle the sample gently to prevent hemolysis.

COMPLICATIONS

- Hematoma at the venipuncture site

INTERPRETATION

NORMAL RESULTS

- In men, RBC count is 4.5 to 5.5 million/µl (SI, 4.5 to 5.5×10^{12}/L) of venous blood.
- In women, RBC count is 4 to 5 million/µl (SI, 4 to 5×10^{12}/L) of venous blood.
- In full-term neonates, RBC count is 4.4 to 5.8 million/µl (SI, 4.4 to 5.8×10^{12}/L) of capillary blood at birth, decreasing to 3 to 3.8 million/µl (SI, 3 to 3.8×10^{12}/L) at age 2 months, and increasing slowly thereafter.
- In children, RBC count is 4.6 to 4.8 million/µl (SI, 4.6 to 4.8×10^{12}/L) of venous blood.
- RBCs may exceed these levels in patients who live at high altitudes or are very active.

ABNORMAL RESULTS

- A high RBC count may indicate absolute or relative polycythemia.
- A low RBC count may indicate anemia, fluid overload, or hemorrhage beyond 24 hours.
- Further tests, such as stained cell examination, hematocrit, Hb, RBC indices, and white blood cell studies, are needed to confirm a diagnosis.

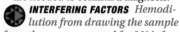 **INTERFERING FACTORS** *Hemodilution from drawing the sample from the same arm used for I.V. infusion of fluids*

Red blood cell indices

DESCRIPTION

- Evaluates mean corpuscular volume (MCV), mean corpuscular hemoglobin (MCH), and mean corpuscular hemoglobin concentration (MCHC)
- Usually done after the red blood cell (RBC) count and hematocrit (HCT) and total hemoglobin (Hb) tests and provides important information about the size, Hb concentration, and Hb weight of an average RBC

PURPOSE

- To help diagnose and classify anemias

PREPARATION

- No dietary restrictions are required.
- The test requires a blood sample.

Teaching points

- Explain to the patient that RBC indices help determine if he has anemia.
- Explain who will perform the test and where it'll be done.
- Tell the patient that the test requires a blood sample and that he may experience slight discomfort from the tourniquet and needle puncture.
- Inform the patient that no dietary restrictions are required.
- Tell the patient the test takes less than 5 minutes.

KEY STEPS

- Confirm the patient's identity using two patient identifiers according to facility policy.
- Perform a venipuncture, and collect the sample in a 3- or 4.5-ml EDTA tube.
- Completely fill the collection tube, and invert it gently several times to adequately mix the sample and the anticoagulant.

POSTPROCEDURE CARE

- Make sure that subdermal bleeding has stopped before removing pressure.
- If a large hematoma develops, monitor distal pulses.
- Inform the practitioner of abnormal results.

PRECAUTIONS

- Maintain standard precautions while collecting the sample.
- Handle the sample gently to prevent hemolysis.

COMPLICATIONS

- Hematoma at the venipuncture site

NORMAL RESULTS

- MCV, the HCT (packed cell volume)-to-RBC count ratio, expresses the average size of the erythrocytes and indicates whether they're undersized (microcytic), oversized (macrocytic), or normal (normocytic).
- MCH (the Hb-to-RBC count ratio) gives the weight of Hb in an average RBC.
- MCHC (the Hb weight-to-HCT ratio) defines the concentration of Hb in 100 ml of packed RBCs. It helps to distinguish normally colored (normochromic) RBCs from paler (hypochromic) RBCs.
- MCV value is 84 to 99 μm^3.
- MCH value is 26 to 32 pg/cell.
- MCHC value is 30 to 36 g/dl.

ABNORMAL RESULTS

- Low MCV and MCHC indicate microcytic, hypochromic anemias caused by iron deficiency anemia, pyridoxine-responsive anemia, or thalassemia.
- A high MCV suggests macrocytic anemias caused by megaloblastic anemias, folic acid or vitamin B_{12} deficiency, inherited disorders of deoxyribonucleic acid synthesis, or reticulocytosis.
- Because the MCV reflects the average volume of many cells, a value within the normal range can encompass RBCs of varying size, from microcytic to macrocytic. (See *Comparative red cell indices in anemias*.)

Comparative red cell indices in anemias

	NORMAL VALUES (Normocytic, normochromic)	IRON DEFICIENCY (Microcytic, hypochromic)	PERNICIOUS ANEMIA (Macrocytic, normochromic)
MCV	84 to 99 μm^3	60 to 80 μm^3	96 to 150 μm^3
MCH	26 to 32 pg/cell	5 to 25 pg/cell	33 to 53 pg/cell
MCHC	30 to 36 g/dl	20 to 30 g/dl	33 to 38 g/dl

Key:
MCV = mean corpuscular volume
MCH = mean corpuscular hemoglobin
MCHC = mean corpuscular hemoglobin concentration

Red blood cell survival time

DESCRIPTION
- Measures the survival time of red blood cells (RBCs) circulating in the blood and identifies sites of their destruction, if RBC survival time is decreased
- RBCs: normally destroyed as they age; in hemolytic diseases, they're destroyed randomly, regardless of age

PURPOSE
- To evaluate unexplained anemias, especially those caused by excessive destruction of RBCs
- To identify the site of abnormal RBC sequestration and destruction

PREPARATION
- No dietary restrictions are required.
- The test requires a blood sample.

Teaching points
- Explain that the test helps identify the cause of anemia.
- Explain who will perform the test and where it'll be done.
- Tell the patient that the test requires a blood sample, and that he may experience slight discomfort from the tourniquet and needle puncture.
- Inform the patient that he need not fast before testing.
- Tell the patient the test takes less than 5 minutes.

KEY STEPS
- Confirm the patient's identity using two patient identifiers according to facility policy.
- Perform a venipuncture, and collect a 30-ml blood sample.
- Blood in the sample is mixed with radioactive chromium (^{51}Cr).
- The mixture is then injected into the patient.
- A blood sample is drawn again in 30 minutes.
- Radioactivity per milliliter of the sample is calculated.
- Gamma camera scans of the patient's chest, back, liver, and spleen detect radioactivity at sites that show an abnormal increase in volume of RBCs in a limited area.

POSTPROCEDURE CARE
- Apply direct pressure to the venipuncture site until bleeding stops.
- Inform the patient that follow-up blood samples are collected every 3 days for 3 to 4 weeks.
- Inform the practitioner of abnormal results.

PRECAUTIONS
- The test is contraindicated during pregnancy because it exposes the fetus to radiation.
- Excess blood loss can invalidate the results, so the test is usually contraindicated in patients with active bleeding or poor clotting function.
- Make sure the patient doesn't receive a blood transfusion during the test period and doesn't have blood samples drawn for other tests.

COMPLICATIONS
- Hematoma at the venipuncture site

NORMAL RESULTS
- The half-life for RBCs labeled with ^{51}Cr is 25 to 30 days.
- Gamma camera scans reveal slight radioactivity in the spleen, liver, and sometimes bone marrow.

ABNORMAL RESULTS
- Decreased RBC survival time indicates a hemolytic disease, such as chronic lymphocytic leukemia, congenital nonspherocytic hemolytic anemia, hemoglobin C disease, hereditary spherocytosis, paroxysmal nocturnal hemoglobinuria, pernicious anemia, sickle cell anemia, elliptocytosis, or idiopathic-acquired hemolytic anemia.
- A gamma camera scan that detects a site of excess RBC sequestration provides direction for treatment.

INTERFERING FACTORS Dehydration, overhydration, blood transfusions during the test period, or blood loss (for example, from severe bleeding or blood samples drawn for other tests)

Refraction

DESCRIPTION

- Enables images to focus on the retina and directly affects visual acuity
- Done routinely during an eye examination or whenever a patient complains of a change in vision; defines refractive error and determines the degree of correction required to improve visual acuity with corrective lenses
- Performed objectively, by using a retinoscope, and subjectively, by asking the patient about his visual acuity while placing trial lenses before his eyes

PURPOSE

- To diagnose refractive error and prescribe corrective lenses, if needed

PREPARATION

- Check the patient's history for angle-closure glaucoma and for previous use of and hypersensitivity to dilating eyedrops. Don't give dilating eyedrops to a patient with either condition.

Teaching points

- Explain that this test helps determine whether the patient needs corrective lenses.
- Explain who will perform the test and where it'll be done.
- Tell the patient that eyedrops may be instilled to dilate his pupils.
- Tell the patient the test takes 10 to 20 minutes.

KEY STEPS

- Confirm the patient's identity using two patient identifiers according to facility policy.
- After short-acting mydriatic eyedrops are given, the ophthalmologist directs the light of the retinoscope at the pupillary opening.
- Through the aperture at the top of the instrument, the ophthalmologist looks for an orange glow—the retinoscope, or red, reflex, which represents the reflection of light from the retinoscope—and notes its brightness, clarity, and uniformity.
- Moving the retinoscope light across the pupil, the ophthalmologist observes the reflex for any movement.
- The ophthalmologist then places trial lenses before the patient's eyes and adjusts the lens power to make the reflex clear, bright, and uniform, and to neutralize its motion. The lens power necessary to make this adjustment is recorded.
- Objective findings can be refined by altering the trial lenses and having the patient read lines on a standardized visual chart. This helps determine which lens or combination of lenses provides the best corrections of his visual acuity.

POSTPROCEDURE CARE

- If corrective lenses are prescribed, advise the patient that images may appear blurred the first time he wears the lenses.
- Instruct the patient to report ocular discomfort or redness immediately.

PRECAUTIONS

- If the patient has worn glasses or contact lenses, he should wear only his new prescription lenses because changing back and forth from the old prescription to the new will prevent his eyes from making the required adjustment to the new lenses.

COMPLICATIONS

- Hypersensitivity reactions
- Ocular discomfort

NORMAL RESULTS

- Refractive poser, measured in diopters, is greatest at the cornea (about 44 diopters) because of its curvature.
- The aqueous humor has the same refractive power as the cornea and is considered to be the same medium.
- The lens, normally a convex structure, has a refractory power of about 10 to 14 diopters but can alter this power by changing its shape. This phenomenon is known as accommodation and occurs when the eye view objects closer than 20' (6 m).
- The vitreous humor, a gelatinous medium, has little refractive power and mainly transmits light.
- In the absence of accommodation, the average refractive power of the human eye is 58 diopters.
- Ideally, the eyes have no refractive error (emmetropia). Parallel light rays emanating from a point source can be focused directly on the retina to produce a clear image.

ABNORMAL RESULTS

- Most patients show some degree of refractive error (ametropia). Hyperopia, or farsightedness, occurs when the eyeball is too short and parallel light rays focus behind the retina.
- Retinoscopic examination shows a red reflex moving in the same direction as the retinoscope's light. A patient with hyperopia sees distant objects clearly but experiences blurring of near objects.
- Myopia, or nearsightedness, occurs when the eyeball is too long and parallel light rays focus in front of the retina.
- Retinoscopic examination shows reflex motion opposite to movement of the retinoscope's light. A patient with myopia sees near objects clearly but experiences blurring of distant objects.
- When light rays entering the eye aren't refracted uniformly and a clear focal point on the retina isn't attained, the patient has astigmatism.

Renal angiography

DESCRIPTION

◆ Permits radiographic examination of the renal vasculature and parenchyma
◆ Requires arterial injection of a contrast medium

PURPOSE

◆ To demonstrate the configuration of total renal vasculature before surgical procedures
◆ To determine the cause of renovascular hypertension
◆ To evaluate chronic renal disease or renal failure
◆ To investigate renal masses and renal trauma
◆ To detect complications following kidney transplantation
◆ To differentiate highly vascular tumors from avascular cysts

PREPARATION

◆ Make sure the patient has signed an appropriate consent form.
◆ Check the patient's history for hypersensitivity to iodine-based contrast media or iodine-containing foods such as shellfish.
◆ Verify adequate renal function and adequate clotting ability.
◆ Evaluate peripheral pulse sites, and mark them for easy access.
◆ Withhold food for 8 hours before the test. Give the patient extra fluid. If the patient isn't able to drink fluid, start an I.V. line.

Teaching points

◆ Explain who will perform the test and where it'll be done.
◆ Instruct the patient to fast for 8 hours before the test and to drink extra fluids the day before the test.
◆ Tell the patient that he may continue oral drugs; a patient with diabetes requires a special order.
◆ Instruct the patient to remove all metallic objects that may interfere with test results.
◆ Tell the patient to void before leaving the unit.

◆ Tell the patient the test takes about 1 hour.

DIAGNOSTIC PROCEDURE

KEY STEPS

◆ Confirm the patient's identity using two patient identifiers according to facility policy.
◆ The patient is placed in the supine position, and a peripheral I.V. infusion is started. The skin over the arterial puncture site is cleaned with antiseptic solution, and a local anesthetic is injected.
◆ The femoral artery is punctured and cannulated under fluoroscopic visualization.
◆ After the flexible guide wire is passed through the artery, the cannula is withdrawn, leaving several inches of wire in the lumen.
◆ A polyethylene catheter is passed over the wire and advanced, under fluoroscopic guidance, up the femoroiliac vessels to the aorta.
◆ The guide wire is removed, and the catheter is flushed with heparin flush solution. The contrast medium is injected, and screening aortograms are taken before proceeding.
◆ When the aortographic study is completed, a renal catheter is exchanged for the vascular catheter.
◆ To determine the position of the renal arteries and ensure that the tip of the catheter is in the lumen, a test bolus (3 to 5 ml) of contrast medium is injected immediately.
◆ If the patient has no adverse reaction to the contrast medium, 20 to 25 ml of the substance is injected just below the origin of the renal arteries.
◆ A series of rapid-sequence X-ray films of the filling of the renal vascular tree is exposed.
◆ If additional selective studies are required, the catheter remains in place. If the films are satisfactory, the catheter is removed.

POSTPROCEDURE CARE

◆ Apply a sterile pad firmly to the puncture site for 15 minutes.
◆ Keep the patient flat in bed, and instruct him to keep the punctured leg straight for at least 6 hours or as otherwise needed.
◆ Check vital signs every 15 minutes for 1 hour, every 30 minutes for 2 hours, and then every hour until they stabilize.
◆ Monitor popliteal and dorsalis pedis pulses for adequate perfusion at least every hour for 4 hours.
◆ Note the color and temperature of the involved extremity, and compare it with the uninvolved extremity.
◆ Watch for signs of pain or paresthesia in the involved limb.
◆ Watch for bleeding or hematomas at the injection site. Keep the pressure dressing in place, and check for bleeding.
◆ Apply cold compresses to the puncture site.
◆ Provide extra fluids (2,000 to 3,000 ml) in the 24-hour period after the test to prevent nephrotoxicity from the contrast medium.

PRECAUTIONS

⚡ **WARNING** *Monitor the patient for signs of anaphylaxis from the contrast medium, such as cardiorespiratory distress, renal failure, and shock.*

◆ Monitor for atrial arrhythmias, and evaluate aspartate aminotransferase and lactate dehydrogenase activity.

COMPLICATIONS

◆ Adverse reaction to the contrast medium
◆ Hematoma at the venipuncture site
◆ Arterial dissection
◆ Infection

NORMAL RESULTS
◆ Normal arborization of the vascular tree and architecture of the renal parenchyma are noted.

ABNORMAL RESULTS
◆ Renal tumors usually show hypervascularity; renal cysts typically appear as clearly delineated, radiolucent masses.
◆ Renal artery stenosis caused by arteriosclerosis produces a noticeable constriction in the blood vessels, usually within the proximal portion of its length.
◆ In renal infarction, blood vessels may appear to be absent or cut off, with the normal tissue replaced by scar tissue.
◆ Triangular areas of infarcted tissue appear near the periphery of the affected kidney. The kidney may appear shrunken.
◆ Renal artery aneurysms (saccular or fusiform) and renal arteriovenous fistula with abnormal widening of and direct passage between the renal artery and renal vein are detected.
◆ Destruction, distortion, and fibrosis of renal tissue with areas of reduced and tortuous vascularity in severe or chronic pyelonephritis may be visible; an increase in capsular vessels with abnormal intrarenal circulation indicates renal abscesses or inflammation.
◆ In renal trauma, intrarenal hematoma, a parenchymal laceration, shattered kidneys, and areas of infarction may be visible.

Renal venography

DESCRIPTION

◆ Allows radiographic examination of the main renal veins and their tributaries
◆ Requires injection of contrast medium by percutaneous catheter passed through the femoral vein and inferior vena cava into the renal vein

PURPOSE

◆ To detect renal vein thrombosis
◆ To evaluate renal vein compression caused by extrinsic tumors or retroperitoneal fibrosis
◆ To assess renal tumors and detect invasion of the renal vein or inferior vena cava
◆ To detect venous anomalies and defects
◆ To differentiate renal agenesis from a small kidney
◆ To collect renal venous blood samples for evaluation of renovascular hypertension

PREPARATION

◆ Make sure the patient has signed an appropriate consent form.
◆ Notify the practitioner of drugs the patient is taking that may affect test results; they may be restricted.
◆ Fasting for 4 hours before the test may be required.
◆ Check the patient's history for hypersensitivity to contrast media, iodine, or iodine-containing foods such as shellfish.
◆ Check the patient's history and any coagulation studies for indications of bleeding disorders.
◆ If the patient will receive renin assays, check his diet and drugs and consult with the practitioner.
◆ Make sure pretest blood urea nitrogen and urine creatinine levels are adequate.

Teaching points

◆ Explain the purpose of the test and how it's done.
◆ Explain who will perform the test and where it'll be done.

◆ If prescribed, instruct the patient to fast for 4 hours before the test.
◆ Tell the patient that the test takes about 1 hour.

DIAGNOSTIC PROCEDURE

KEY STEPS

◆ Confirm the patient's identity using two patient identifiers according to facility policy.
◆ The patient is placed in the supine position on the X-ray table, with his abdomen centered over the film.
◆ The skin over the right femoral vein near the groin is cleaned with antiseptic solution and draped. (The left femoral vein or jugular veins may be used.)
◆ A local anesthetic is injected; the femoral vein is then cannulated.
◆ Under fluoroscopic guidance, a guide wire is threaded a short distance through the cannula, which is then removed. A catheter is passed over the wire into the inferior vena cava.
◆ When catheterization of the femoral vein is contraindicated, the right antecubital vein is punctured, and the catheter is inserted and advanced through the right atrium of the heart into the inferior vena cava.
◆ A test bolus of contrast medium is injected to determine whether the vena cava is patent. If so, the catheter is advanced into the right renal vein, and contrast medium (usually 20 to 40 ml) is injected.
◆ When studies of the right renal vasculature are complete, the catheter is withdrawn into the vena cava, rotated, and guided into the left renal vein.
◆ If visualization of the renal venous tributaries is indicated, epinephrine can be injected into the ipsilateral renal artery by catheter before contrast medium is injected into the renal vein.
◆ Epinephrine temporarily blocks arterial flow and allows filling of distal intrarenal veins. Obstructing the artery briefly with a balloon catheter produces the same effect.

◆ After anteroposterior films are made, the patient lies prone for posteroanterior films.
◆ For renin assays, blood samples are withdrawn under fluoroscopy within 15 minutes after venography.

POSTPROCEDURE CARE

◆ After catheter removal, apply pressure for 15 minutes, and apply a dressing.
◆ Check vital signs and distal pulses every 15 minutes for the first hour, every 30 minutes for the second hour, and then every 2 hours for 24 hours. Keep the patient on bed rest for 2 hours.
◆ Observe the puncture site for bleeding or a hematoma.
◆ Report signs of vein perforation, embolism, and extravasation.
◆ Report complaints of paresthesia or pain in the catheterized limb—symptoms of nerve irritation or vascular compromise.
◆ Instruct the patient to increase fluid intake to clear the contrast medium.
◆ Tell the patient to resume his usual diet and medications, as ordered.

PRECAUTIONS

◆ The test is contraindicated in patients with severe thrombosis of the superior vena cava.

COMPLICATIONS

◆ Hypersensitivity to the contrast medium
◆ Paresthesia, vein perforation, embolism

INTERPRETATION

NORMAL RESULTS

◆ After injection of the contrast medium, immediate opacification of the renal vein and tributaries is seen.
◆ Normal renin content of venous blood in a supine adult is 1.5 to 1.6 ng/ml/hour.

ABNORMAL RESULTS

◆ Renal vein occlusion near the inferior vena cava or the kidney indicates renal vein thrombosis.
◆ A clot is usually identifiable because it's within the lumen and less sharply outlined than a filling defect.
◆ A filling defect of the renal vein may indicate obstruction or compression by an extrinsic tumor or retroperitoneal fibrosis. A renal tumor that invades the renal vein or inferior vena cava usually produces a filling defect with a sharply defined border.
◆ Absence of a renal vein differentiates renal agenesis from a small kidney.
◆ Elevated renin content in renal venous blood usually indicates essential renovascular hypertension when assay results correspond for both kidneys.
◆ Elevated renin levels in one kidney indicate a unilateral lesion and usually require further evaluation by arteriography.

Renin activity test

DESCRIPTION

◆ Screening procedure for renovascular hypertension; doesn't unequivocally confirm diagnosis
◆ Supplemented with other tests, helps establish the cause of hypertension
◆ Can categorize essential hypertension according to renin levels (low, normal, or high) to allow for appropriate therapy
◆ Indexing renin levels against urinary sodium excretion helps identify primary aldosteronism (sodium-depleted result is confirmatory)
◆ Renin: secretion from kidneys is first stage of the renin-angiotensin-aldosterone cycle (controls the body's sodium-potassium balance, fluid volume, and blood pressure); released into renal veins in response to sodium depletion and blood loss; and catalyzes conversion of angiotensinogen to angiotensin I, which is then converted to angiotensin II (vasoconstrictor that stimulates aldosterone production in the adrenal cortex) (see *Renin-angiotensin feedback system*)
◆ Excessive amounts of angiotensin II cause renal hypertension
◆ Plasma renin activity (PRA): measured by radioimmunoassay of a peripheral or renal blood sample; results expressed as rate of angiotensin I formation per unit of time
◆ Preparation critical; may take up to 1 month

PURPOSE

◆ To screen for renal origin of hypertension
◆ To help plan treatment of essential hypertension, a genetic disease commonly aggravated by excess sodium intake
◆ To help identify hypertension linked to unilateral (sometimes bilateral) renovascular disease by renal vein catheterization
◆ To help identify primary aldosteronism (Conn's syndrome) resulting from an aldosterone-secreting adrenal adenoma
◆ To confirm primary aldosteronism (sodium-depleted plasma renin test)

PREPARATION

◆ Notify the laboratory and practitioner of drugs the patient is taking that may affect test results; they may be restricted.
◆ The patient shouldn't receive radioactive treatments for several days before the test.

Renin-angiotensin feedback system

The renin-angiotensin-aldosterone system, sometimes known as the juxtaglomerular apparatus, is an important homeostatic device for regulating the body's sodium and water levels and blood pressure. It works this way:

Juxtaglomerular cells (1) in each of the kidney's glomeruli secrete the enzyme renin into the blood. The rate of renin secretion depends on the rate of perfusion in the afferent renal arterioles (2) and on the amount of sodium in the serum. A low sodium load and low perfusion pressure (as in hypovolemia) increase renin secretion; high sodium and high perfusion pressure decrease it.

Renin circulates throughout the body. In the liver, renin converts angiotensinogen to angiotensin I (3), which passes to the lungs. There it's converted by hydrolysis to angiotensin II (4), a potent vasoconstrictor that acts on the adrenal cortex to stimulate production of the hormone aldosterone (5). Aldosterone acts on the juxtaglomerular cells to stimulate or depress renin secretion, completing the feedback cycle that automatically readjusts homeostasis.

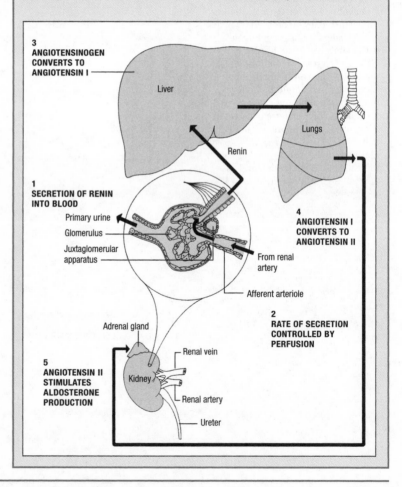

3 ANGIOTENSINOGEN CONVERTS TO ANGIOTENSIN I

Liver

Lungs

Renin

1 SECRETION OF RENIN INTO BLOOD

Primary urine

Glomerulus

Juxtaglomerular apparatus

4 ANGIOTENSIN I CONVERTS TO ANGIOTENSIN II

From renal artery

Afferent arteriole

2 RATE OF SECRETION CONTROLLED BY PERFUSION

Adrenal gland

Renal vein

5 ANGIOTENSIN II STIMULATES ALDOSTERONE PRODUCTION

Kidney

Renal artery

Ureter

- If the patient is to receive renal vein catheterization, make sure he has signed an informed consent form.
- Follow activity and dietary restrictions as ordered.
- The test requires a blood sample.

Teaching points
- Explain that this test helps determine the cause of hypertension.
- Explain who will perform the test and where it'll be done.
- Tell the patient that the procedure will occur in the X-ray department and that he'll receive a local anesthetic.
- Tell the patient to maintain a normal sodium diet (3 g/day) during this period.
- For the sodium-depleted plasma renin test, tell the patient that he'll receive furosemide (Lasix) (or, if he has angina or cerebrovascular insufficiency, chlorothiazide [Diuril]) and will follow a specific low-sodium diet for 3 days.
- If the patient will receive a recumbent sample, instruct him to remain in bed at least 2 hours before the test. (Posture influences renin secretion.)
- If the patient will receive an upright sample, instruct him to stand or sit upright for 2 hours before the test.
- Tell the patient that the test requires a blood sample, and that he may experience slight discomfort from the tourniquet and needle puncture. Collect a morning sample if possible.
- Tell the patient that the test may take several hours to complete.

DIAGNOSTIC PROCEDURE

KEY STEPS
- Confirm the patient's identity using two patient identifiers according to facility policy.
- For a peripheral vein sample, perform a venipuncture, and collect the sample in a 4-ml EDTA tube.
- Note on the laboratory request whether the patient was fasting and whether he was upright or supine during peripheral vein sample collection.

- Completely fill the collection tube, and invert it gently several times to mix the sample and the anticoagulant.
- In renal vein catheterization, a catheter is advanced to the kidneys through the femoral vein under fluoroscopic control, and samples are obtained from the renal veins and vena cava.

POSTPROCEDURE CARE
- Apply direct pressure to the peripheral venipuncture site until bleeding stops.
- After renal vein catheterization, apply pressure to the catheterization site for 10 to 20 minutes to prevent extravasation.

⚡ **WARNING** *Monitor vital signs and check the catheterization site every 30 minutes for 2 hours and then every hour for 4 hours to make sure that the bleeding has stopped. Check the patient's distal pulse for signs of thrombus formation and arterial occlusion (such as cyanosis, loss of pulse, and cool skin).*
- Both methods: After the test, instruct the patient to resume his usual diet and medications.
- Inform the practitioner of abnormal results.

PRECAUTIONS
- Because renin is unstable, the sample must be drawn into a chilled syringe and collection tube, placed on ice, and sent to the laboratory immediately.

COMPLICATIONS
- Hematoma at the venipuncture site

INTERPRETATION

NORMAL RESULTS
- PRA and aldosterone levels decrease with age.

Sodium-depleted, upright, peripheral vein
- For ages 18 to 39, levels are 2.9 to 24 ng/ml/hour; mean, 10.8 ng/ml/hour.

- For age 40 and older, levels are 2.9 to 10.8 ng/ml/hour; mean, 5.9 ng/ml/hour.

Sodium-replete, upright, peripheral vein
- For ages 18 to 39, levels are ≤ 0.6 to 4.3 ng/ml/hour; mean, 1.9 ng/ml/hour.
- For age 40 and older, levels are ≤ 0.6 to 3 ng/ml/hour; mean, 1 ng/ml/hour.

Renal vein catheterization
- The renal venous–renin ratio (renin level in the renal vein compared with the level in the inferior vena cava) is < 1.5 to 1.

ABNORMAL RESULTS
- High renin levels may occur in essential hypertension (uncommon), malignant and renovascular hypertension, cirrhosis, hypokalemia, hypovolemia caused by hemorrhage, renin-producing renal tumors (Bartter syndrome), and adrenal hypofunction (Addison's disease).
- High renin levels may also be found in chronic renal failure with parenchymal disease, end-stage renal disease, and transplant rejection.
- Low renin levels may indicate hypervolemia caused by a high-sodium diet, salt-retaining steroids, primary aldosteronism, Cushing's syndrome, licorice ingestion syndrome, or essential hypertension with low renin levels.
- High serum and urine aldosterone levels with low plasma renin activity help identify primary aldosteronism.
- In the sodium-depleted renin test, low plasma renin level confirms this diagnosis, and differentiates it from secondary aldosteronism (characterized by increased renin).

Respiratory syncytial virus antibodies

DESCRIPTION
- Respiratory syncytial virus (RSV), a paramyxovirus
- Major cause of severe lower respiratory tract disease in infants
- Immunoglobin (Ig) G and IgM class antibodies quantified using indirect immunofluorescence

PURPOSE
- To diagnose infections caused by RSV

PREPARATION
- No dietary restrictions are required.
- The test requires a blood sample.

Teaching points
- Explain the purpose of the RSV antibodies test to the patient or parents.
- Explain who will perform the test and where it'll be done.
- Tell the patient that the test requires a blood sample and that he may experience slight discomfort from the tourniquet and needle puncture.
- Tell the patient that he doesn't need to restrict his diet.
- Tell the patient the test takes less than 5 minutes.

KEY STEPS
- Confirm the patient's identity using two patient identifiers according to facility policy.
- Perform a venipuncture, and collect 5 ml of blood in a clot-activator tube.
- Allow the blood to clot for at least 1 hour at room temperature.

POSTPROCEDURE CARE
- Apply direct pressure to the venipuncture site until bleeding stops.
- Inform the practitioner of abnormal results.

PRECAUTIONS
- Handle the sample gently to prevent hemolysis.
- Transfer the serum to a sterile tube or vial, and send it to the laboratory promptly.
- If transfer must be delayed, store the serum at 39.2° F (4° C) for 1 or 2 days or at –4° F (–20° C) for longer periods to avoid contamination.

COMPLICATIONS
- Hematoma at the venipuncture site

NORMAL RESULTS
- Sera from patients who have never been infected with RSV have no detectable antibodies to the virus (< 1:5).

ABNORMAL RESULTS
- The qualitative presence of IgM or a fourfold or greater increase in IgG antibodies indicates an active RSV infection.
- In infants, serologic diagnosis of RSV infections is difficult because of the presence of maternal IgG antibodies; therefore, the presence of IgM antibodies is most significant.

Reticulocyte count

DESCRIPTION

- Counts reticulocytes in a whole blood sample; value expressed as a percentage of total red blood cell (RBC) count
- Reticulocytes: usually larger than mature RBCs; nonnucleated, immature RBCs that remain in peripheral blood for 24 to 48 hours while maturing
- Values imprecise with manual method of reticulocyte counting using small sample; compared with RBC count or hematocrit
- Useful for evaluating anemia; an index of effective erythropoiesis and bone marrow response to anemia

PURPOSE

- To help distinguish between hypoproliferative and hyperproliferative anemias
- To help assess blood loss, bone marrow response to anemia, and therapy for anemia

PREPARATION

- No dietary restrictions are required.
- Notify the laboratory and practitioner of drugs the patient is taking that may affect test results; it may be necessary to restrict them.
- The test requires a blood sample.

Teaching points

- Explain that the reticulocyte count is used to detect anemia or to monitor its treatment.
- Explain who will perform the test and where it'll be done.
- Inform the patient that he doesn't need to restrict his diet.
- Tell the patient that the test requires a blood sample, and that he may experience slight discomfort from the tourniquet and needle puncture.
- If the patient is an infant or child, explain to the parents that a small amount of blood will be taken from his finger or earlobe.
- Explain that the test takes less than 5 minutes.

KEY STEPS

- Confirm the patient's identity using two patient identifiers according to facility policy.
- Perform a venipuncture, and collect the sample in a 3- or 4.5-ml EDTA tube.
- Completely fill the collection tube, and invert it gently several times to mix the sample and the anticoagulant.

POSTPROCEDURE CARE

- If a hematoma develops at the venipuncture site, apply warm soaks.
- If the hematoma is large, monitor pulses distal to the phlebotomy site.
- Monitor the patient with an abnormal reticulocyte count for trends or significant changes in repeated tests.
- Inform the practitioner of abnormal results.
- Instruct the patient to resume his medications, as ordered.

PRECAUTIONS

- Maintain standard precautions while collecting the sample.
- Handle the sample gently.

COMPLICATIONS

- Hematoma at the venipuncture site

NORMAL RESULTS

- Value is 0.5% to 2.5% (SI, 0.005 to 0.025) of the total RBC count.
- In neonates, the value is 2% to 6% (SI, 0.002 to 0.006) at birth, decreasing to adult levels in 1 or 2 weeks.

ABNORMAL RESULTS

- A low reticulocyte count indicates hypoproliferative bone marrow (hypoplastic anemia) or ineffective erythropoiesis (pernicious anemia).
- A high reticulocyte count indicates a bone marrow response to anemia caused by hemolysis or blood loss.
- The reticulocyte count may also increase after therapy for iron deficiency anemia or pernicious anemia.

Retrograde cystography

DESCRIPTION

♦ Involves the instillation of a contrast medium into the bladder, followed by radiographic examination
♦ Diagnoses bladder rupture without urethral involvement because it can determine the location and extent of the rupture
♦ Suitable for patients with neurogenic bladder; recurrent urinary tract infections (UTIs), especially in children; suspected vesicoureteral reflux; and vesical fistulas, diverticula, and tumors
♦ Done when cystoscopic examination is impractical, such as in male infants, or when excretory urography hasn't adequately shown the bladder

PURPOSE

♦ To evaluate the structure and integrity of the bladder

PREPARATION

♦ Check the patient's history for hypersensitivity to contrast media, iodine, or shellfish; mark it on the chart, and inform the practitioner.
♦ Make sure the patient has signed an appropriate consent form.
♦ No dietary restrictions are required.

Teaching points
♦ Explain that retrograde cystography permits radiographic examination of the bladder.
♦ Explain who will perform the test and where it'll be done.
♦ Tell the patient that he doesn't need to restrict his diet.
♦ Inform the patient that he may experience some discomfort when the catheter is inserted and when the contrast medium is instilled through the catheter.
♦ Tell the patient that he may hear loud, clacking sounds as the X-ray films are made.
♦ Tell the patient the test takes about 1 hour.

DIAGNOSTIC PROCEDURE

KEY STEPS
♦ Confirm the patient's identity using two patient identifiers according to facility policy.
♦ The patient is placed in the supine position on the X-ray table; a preliminary kidney-ureter-bladder X-ray is taken.
♦ The X-ray is developed immediately and scrutinized for renal shadows, calcifications, contours of the bone and psoas muscles, and gas patterns in the lumen of the GI tract.
♦ The bladder is catheterized, and 200 to 300 ml of sterile contrast medium (50 to 100 ml for an infant) is instilled by gravity or gentle syringe injection. The catheter is then clamped.
♦ With the patient in a supine position, an anteroposterior film is taken. The patient is then tilted to one side, then the other, and two posterior oblique (and sometimes lateral) views are taken.
♦ If the patient's condition permits, he's assisted into the jackknife position. A posteroanterior film is taken. A space-occupying vesical lesion may require additional exposures. Rarely, to enhance visualization, 100 to 300 ml of air may be insufflated into the bladder by syringe after removal of the contrast medium (double-contrast technique).
♦ The catheter is then unclamped, the bladder fluid is allowed to drain, and an X-ray is obtained to detect urethral diverticula, reflux into the ureters, fistulous tracts into the vagina, or intraperitoneal or extraperitoneal extravasation of the contrast medium.

POSTPROCEDURE CARE
♦ Monitor the patient's vital signs every 15 minutes for the first hour, every 30 minutes during the second hour, and then every 2 hours for up to 24 hours.
♦ Record the time of the patient's voidings and the color and volume of the urine. Observe for hematuria that persists after the third voiding, and notify the practitioner if necessary.

♦ Watch for signs of urinary sepsis from UTIs or similar signs related to extravasation of contrast medium into the general circulation.
♦ Prepare the patient for surgery and urinary diversion if indicated. Strain urine if calculi are detected.
♦ Monitor for retention or distention if neurogenic bladder is diagnosed and give drugs (baclofen for spasms; bethanechol chloride for hypotonic bladder).
♦ Discuss the use of a percutaneous stimulator if one is being contemplated. Teach self-catheterization if indicated for neurogenic bladder.

PRECAUTIONS
♦ The test is contraindicated in patients with a worsening acute UTI or in those with obstructions that prevent passage of a urinary catheter.
♦ It shouldn't be done in patients with urethral evulsion or transection, unless catheter passage and flow of contrast medium are monitored fluoroscopically.

COMPLICATIONS
♦ Hematuria
♦ Urinary sepsis

INTERPRETATION

NORMAL RESULTS
♦ The bladder appears with normal contours, capacity, integrity, and urethrovesical angle, and no evidence of a tumor, diverticula, or a rupture.
♦ No vesicoureteral reflux is apparent.
♦ The bladder appears without displacement or external compression with a bladder wall that is smooth and not thick.

ABNORMAL RESULTS
♦ Findings may include vesical trabeculae or diverticula, space-occupying lesions (tumors), calculi or gravel, blood clots, high- or low-pressure vesicoureteral reflux, and a hypotonic or hypertonic bladder.

Retrograde ureteropyelography

DESCRIPTION

◆ Allows radiographic examination of the renal collecting system after injection of a contrast medium through a ureteral catheter during cystoscopy

◆ Uses an iodine-based contrast medium; although some may be absorbed through the mucous membranes; test preferred for patients with hypersensitivity to iodine

◆ Not influenced by impaired renal function and, therefore, is indicated when visualization of the renal collecting system by excretory urography is inadequate because of inferior films or marked renal insufficiency

PURPOSE

◆ To assess the structure and integrity of the renal collecting system (see *Sites and types of obstruction indicated by ureteropyelography*)

PREPARATION

◆ Give the patient prescribed premedication just before the procedure.

◆ Withhold food for 8 hours before the test. Make sure the patient is well hydrated for adequate urine flow.

◆ Make sure the patient has signed an appropriate consent form.

Teaching points

◆ Explain that retrograde ureteropyelography shows the urinary collecting system.

◆ Explain who will perform the test and where it'll be done.

◆ If the patient will receive a general anesthetic, instruct him to fast for 8 hours before the test.

◆ If the patient will be awake during the procedure, tell him that he may feel pressure as the catheter is inserted and a pressure sensation in the kidney area when the contrast medium is introduced. Also, he may feel an urgency to void.

◆ Tell the patient the test takes about 1 hour.

KEY STEPS

◆ Confirm the patient's identity using two patient identifiers according to facility policy.

◆ Assist the patient into the lithotomy position.

◆ After the patient is anesthetized, the urologist first performs a cystoscopic examination.

◆ After visual inspection of the bladder, one or both ureters are catheterized with opaque catheters, depending on the condition or abnormality suspected. Radiographic monitoring allows correct positioning of the catheter tip in the renal pelvis.

◆ The renal pelvis is emptied by gravity drainage or aspiration.

◆ About 5 ml of contrast medium is slowly injected through the catheter, using the syringe with the special adapter.

Sites and types of obstruction indicated by ureteropyelography

Ureteropyelography may detect a stricture, neoplasm, blood clot, or calculus that obstructs urine flow in the calyces, pelvis, or ureter. Small calculi may remain in the calyces and pelvis or pass down the ureter. A staghorn calculus (a cast of the calyceal and pelvic collecting system) may form from a calculus that stays in the kidney.

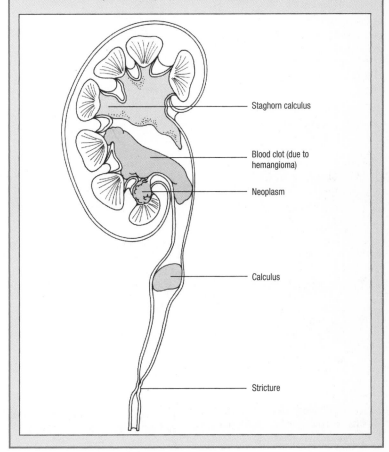

- Staghorn calculus
- Blood clot (due to hemangioma)
- Neoplasm
- Calculus
- Stricture

(continued)

- When adequate filling and opacification have occurred, anteroposterior radiographic films are taken and immediately developed. Lateral and oblique films can be taken, as needed, after the injection of more contrast medium.
- After the X-rays of the renal pelvis are examined, a few more milliliters of contrast medium are injected to outline the ureters as the catheter is slowly withdrawn.
- Delayed films are then taken to check for contrast medium retention, indicating urinary stasis.
- If ureteral obstruction is present, the ureteral catheter may be kept in place and, together with an indwelling urinary catheter, connected to a gravity drainage system until posttest urinary flow is corrected or returns to normal.

POSTPROCEDURE CARE
- Check the patient's vital signs every 15 minutes for the first hour, every 30 minutes for 1 hour, every hour for the next 2 hours, and then every 4 hours for 24 hours.
- Monitor the patient's fluid intake and urine output for 24 hours.
- Observe each specimen for hematuria. Gross hematuria or hematuria after the third voiding is abnormal and should be reported. If the patient doesn't void for 8 hours after the procedure or if the patient immediately feels distress and his bladder is distended, urethral catheterization may be needed.
- Be especially attentive to catheter output if ureteral catheters have been left in place because inadequate output may reflect catheter obstruction, requiring irrigation. Protect ureteral catheters from dislodgment. Note output amounts for each catheter (for example, indwelling, urinary, urethral) separately; this helps determine the location of an obstruction that's causing reduced output.
- Give prescribed analgesics and tub baths, and increase fluid intake for dysuria.

- Watch for and report severe pain in the area of the kidneys as well as any signs of sepsis (such as chills, fever, and hypotension).
- If irrigation is needed, never use more than 10 ml of sterile saline solution.

PRECAUTIONS
- The test must be done carefully in patients with urinary stasis caused by urethral obstruction to prevent further injury to the ureter.
- The test is contraindicated in pregnant patients unless the benefits of the procedure outweigh the risk to the fetus.

COMPLICATIONS
- Hematuria

NORMAL RESULTS
- Opacification of the pelvis and calyces should occur immediately.
- Normal structures should be outlined clearly and should appear symmetrical in bilateral testing.
- Ureters should fill uniformly and appear normal in size and course.
- Inspiratory and expiratory exposures, when superimposed, normally create two outlines of the renal pelvis ¾" (2 cm) apart.

ABNORMAL RESULTS
- Incomplete or delayed drainage reflects an obstruction, most commonly at the ureteropelvic junction.
- Enlargement of the components of the collecting system or delayed emptying of contrast medium may indicate obstruction caused by a tumor, a blood clot, a stricture, or calculi.
- Perinephric inflammation or suppuration commonly causes fixation of the kidney on the same side, resulting in a single sharp radiographic outline of the collecting system when inspiratory and expiratory exposures are superimposed.
- Upward, downward, or lateral renal displacement can result from a renal abscess or tumor or from a perinephric abscess.
- Neoplasms can cause displacement of either pole or the entire kidney.

Retrograde urethrography

DESCRIPTION

◆ Used almost exclusively in men, requires instillation or injection of a contrast medium into the urethra and shows its membranous, bulbar, and penile portions
◆ May be used with voiding cystourethrography if the posterior portion must be viewed more clearly

PURPOSE

◆ To diagnose urethral strictures, diverticula, and congenital anomalies
◆ To assess urethral lacerations or other trauma
◆ To assist with follow-up examination after surgical repair of the urethra

PREPARATION

◆ Check the patient's history for hypersensitivity to iodine-containing foods, such as shellfish, or contrast media.
◆ Give any prescribed sedatives just before the procedure, and have the patient void before leaving the unit.
◆ No dietary restrictions are required.
◆ Make sure the patient has signed an appropriate consent form.

Teaching points

◆ Explain that this procedure helps diagnose urethral structural problems.
◆ Explain who will perform the test and where it'll be done.
◆ Inform the patient that he doesn't need to restrict his diet.
◆ Tell the patient that he may experience some discomfort when the catheter is inserted and when the contrast medium is instilled through the catheter.
◆ Tell the patient that he may hear loud, clacking sounds as the X-ray films are made.
◆ Tell the patient the procedure takes about 30 minutes.

KEY STEPS

◆ Confirm the patient's identity using two patient identifiers according to facility policy.

For men

◆ The patient is placed into a recumbent position on the examining table. Anteroposterior exposures of the bladder and urethra are made, and the resulting films are studied for radiopaque densities, foreign bodies, or calculi.
◆ The glans and meatus are cleaned with an antiseptic solution.
◆ The catheter is filled with the contrast medium before insertion to eliminate air bubbles.
◆ Although no lubricant should be used, the tip of the catheter may be dipped in sterile water to facilitate insertion.
◆ The catheter is inserted until the balloon portion is inside the meatus; the balloon is then inflated with 1 or 2 ml of water, which prevents the catheter from slipping during the procedure.
◆ The patient then assumes the right posterior oblique position, with his right thigh drawn up to a 90-degree angle and the penis placed along its axis. The left thigh is extended.
◆ The contrast medium is injected through the catheter. After three-fourths of the contrast medium has been injected, the first X-ray film is exposed while the remainder of the contrast medium is being injected. Left lateral oblique views may also be taken.
◆ Fluoroscopic control may be helpful, especially for evaluating urethral injury.

For women

◆ The test is used when urethral diverticula are suspected.
◆ A double-balloon catheter is inserted, which occludes the bladder neck from above and the external meatus from below.
◆ The rest of the steps are the same as for men.

For children

◆ The same procedure is used as for adults except with a smaller catheter.

POSTPROCEDURE CARE

◆ Watch for chills and fever related to extravasation of the contrast medium into the general circulation for 12 to 24 hours after retrograde urethrography.
◆ Observe for signs of sepsis and allergic manifestations.
◆ Monitor the patient for a urinary tract infection (UTI).
◆ Inform the practitioner of abnormal results.

PRECAUTIONS

◆ Perform the test cautiously in patients with UTIs.
◆ If urethral trauma is present, watch for stricture, infection, and urinary extravasation.

COMPLICATIONS

◆ Infection
◆ Extravasation of contrast medium

NORMAL RESULTS

◆ The membranous, bulbar, and penile portions of the urethra—and sometimes the prostatic portion—are normal in size, shape, and course.

ABNORMAL RESULTS

◆ X-rays obtained during retrograde urethrography may show urethral diverticula, fistulas, strictures, false passages, calculi, and lacerations; congenital anomalies, such as urethral valves and perineal hypospadias; and, rarely, tumors (in fewer than 1% of cases).

Rhesus blood group system

DESCRIPTION

- Classifies blood according to the presence or absence of rhesus (Rh) antigen, screens all prospective donors for the weak D antigen, and rarely tests for other antigens to establish paternity, determine family studies, or distinguish between heterozygous and homozygous Rh-positive factors
- Rh antigen lacking in red blood cells of 15% or less of population—known as $Rh_o(D)$ factor; blood is typed Rh-negative
- Rh-negative mother and Rh-positive father at risk for having an infant with hemolytic disease of the neonate (HDN)
- Rh immunoglobulin (RhIg) injection given to Rh-negative mother at 28 weeks' gestation; repeated after delivery if baby is Rh positive
- Rh antigen: highly immunogenic (more likely to stimulate antigen formation than other known antigen)
- Rh-positive weak D antigen: less immunogenic than $Rh_o(D)$; may not provoke antibody production in persons who lack it

PURPOSE

- To classify blood according to the presence or absence of Rh antigen
- To screen all prospective donors for the weak D antigen (more common in blacks than in whites)
- To test for other antigens, such as rh8 (C), rh9 (F), hr8 (c), and hr9 (e)—done only in special cases, to establish paternity, determine family studies, or distinguish between heterozygous and homozygous Rh-positive factors
- To prevent HDN in pregnancy or a reaction after a transfusion

PREPARATION

- No dietary restrictions are required.
- The test requires a blood sample.
- For the pregnant patient, at the first prenatal visit, her blood is tested to determine whether she has been previously sensitized to Rh-positive blood. If test results show that the patient wasn't sensitized, a repeat test is scheduled at 28 weeks.

Teaching points

- Explain that this test classifies blood according to the Rh antigen that is found.
- Explain who will perform the test and where it'll be done.
- Tell the patient that the test requires a blood sample and that he may experience slight discomfort from the tourniquet and needle puncture.
- Tell the patient he doesn't have to restrict his diet.
- Explain that the test takes less than 5 minutes.

KEY STEPS

- Confirm the patient's identity using two patient identifiers according to facility policy.
- Perform a venipuncture, and collect the sample in the tube specified by the laboratory.

POSTPROCEDURE CARE

- Apply direct pressure to the venipuncture site until bleeding stops.
- Answer the patient's questions about the test and the results.

PRECAUTIONS

- Maintain standard precautions while collecting the sample.

COMPLICATIONS

- Hematoma at the venipuncture site

NORMAL RESULTS

- If the D antigen is present, that person is Rh-positive.
- If the D antigen is absent, that person is Rh-negative.
- Antibodies to Rh antigens develop only as an immune response after a transfusion or during pregnancy.

ABNORMAL RESULTS

- Rh incompatibility is the most common and severe cause of HDN, possible when an Rh-negative woman and an Rh-positive man produce an Rh-positive baby.

Rheumatoid factor test

DESCRIPTION

- Most useful immunologic test for confirming rheumatoid arthritis (RA)
- Rheumatoid factor (RF): antibody that is measurable in the blood
- Sheep cell agglutination and latex fixation techniques uncover RF, although autoantibody may not be cause of RA
- RA: "renegade" immunoglobulin (Ig) G antibodies, produced by lymphocytes in the synovial joints, react with IgM antibody to produce immune complexes, complement activation, and tissue destruction
- Unknown how IgG molecules become antigenic: may be altered by aggregating with viruses or other antigens

PURPOSE

- To confirm RA when diagnosis is uncertain

PREPARATION

- No dietary restrictions are required.
- The test requires a blood sample.

Teaching points

- Explain that this test helps confirm RA.
- Explain who will perform the test and where it'll be done.
- Inform the patient that he doesn't need to restrict his diet.
- Tell the patient that the test requires a blood sample, and that he may experience slight discomfort from the tourniquet and needle puncture.
- Tell the patient the test takes less than 5 minutes.

KEY STEPS

- Confirm the patient's identity using two patient identifiers according to facility policy.
- Perform a venipuncture, and collect the sample in a 7-ml clot-activator tube.

POSTPROCEDURE CARE

- Apply direct pressure to the venipuncture site until bleeding stops.
- Check regularly for signs of infection.
- Inform the practitioner of abnormal results.

PRECAUTIONS

- Because a patient with RA may be immunologically compromised, keep the venipuncture site clean and dry for 24 hours.

COMPLICATIONS

- Hematoma at the venipuncture site

NORMAL RESULTS

- RF titer is less than 1:20; rheumatoid screening test is nonreactive.

ABNORMAL RESULTS

- Non-RA and RA populations aren't clearly separated regarding the presence of RF: 25% of patients with RA have a nonreactive titer; 8% of non-RA patients are reactive at greater than 39 International Units/ml, and only 3% of non-RA patients are reactive at greater than 80 International Units/ml.
- Patients with various non-RA diseases characterized by chronic inflammation may test positive for RF. These diseases include systemic lupus erythematosus, polymyositis, tuberculosis, infectious mononucleosis, syphilis, viral hepatic disease, and influenza.

Rubella antibody test

DESCRIPTION

- Measurement of immunoglobulin (Ig) G and IgM antibodies produced by rubella (German measles) infection
- Determines present infection and immunity from past infection
- Hemagglutination inhibition test: most commonly used serologic test for rubella antibodies
- Suspected congenital rubella confirmed if rubella-specific IgM antibodies exist in infant's serum
- Immune status in adults confirmed by existing IgG-specific titer
- Exposure risk (when immunity status unknown) evaluated using two serum samples
- First sample drawn in acute phase of symptoms; if symptoms aren't apparent, sample should be drawn promptly after suspected exposure
- Second sample drawn after 3 to 4 weeks during convalescent phase
- Usually mild viral infection in children and young adults; however, can produce severe infection in the fetus, resulting in spontaneous abortion, stillbirth, or congenital rubella syndrome

PURPOSE

- To diagnose rubella infection, especially congenital infection
- To determine susceptibility to rubella in children and in women of childbearing age

PREPARATION

- No dietary restrictions are required.
- The test requires a blood sample.

Teaching points

- Explain that this test diagnoses or evaluates susceptibility to rubella.
- Explain who will perform the test and where it'll be done.
- Inform the patient that he doesn't need to restrict his diet.
- Tell the patient that this test requires a blood sample and that, if a current infection is suspected, a second blood sample will be needed in 2 to 3 weeks to identify a rise in the titer.
- Tell the patient that he may experience slight discomfort from the tourniquet and needle puncture.
- Tell the patient the test takes less than 5 minutes.

DIAGNOSTIC PROCEDURE

KEY STEPS

- Confirm the patient's identity using two patient identifiers according to facility policy.
- Perform a venipuncture, and collect the sample in a 7-ml clot-activator tube.

POSTPROCEDURE CARE

- Apply direct pressure to the venipuncture site until bleeding stops.
- If a woman of childbearing age is found to be susceptible to rubella, advise her that vaccination can prevent rubella. Tell here she must wait at least 3 months after receiving the vaccine to become pregnant or risk permanent damage or death to the fetus.
- If the pregnant patient is found to be susceptible to rubella, instruct her to return for follow-up rubella antibody tests to detect possible subsequent infection.
- If the test confirms rubella in a pregnant patient, provide emotional support. Refer her for appropriate counseling as needed.
- Inform the practitioner of abnormal results.

PRECAUTIONS

- Handle the sample gently to prevent hemolysis.

COMPLICATIONS

- Hematoma at the venipuncture site

INTERPRETATION

NORMAL RESULTS

- A titer of 1:8 or less indicates little or no immunity against rubella; titer more than 1:10 indicates adequate protection against rubella.
- IgM results are reported as positive or negative.

ABNORMAL RESULTS

- Hemagglutination inhibition antibodies normally appear 2 to 4 days after the onset of the rash, peak in 3 to 4 weeks, and then slowly decline but remain detectable for life.
- A fourfold or greater rise from the acute to the convalescent titer indicates a recent rubella infection.
- The presence of rubella-specific IgM antibodies indicates recent infection in an adult and congenital rubella in an infant.

SARS virus tests

DESCRIPTION

◆ Identify infection with severe acute respiratory syndrome (SARS) virus, a coronavirus (CoV) that causes a pneumonia-like infection; incubation period 8 to 10 days
◆ Not done without a high index of suspicion
◆ Three testing methods available:
– *Enzyme-linked immunosorbent assay (ELISA):* identifies antibodies to SARS virus, usually about 20 days after onset of symptoms
– *Immunofluorescence assay:* identifies antibodies to SARS virus as early as 10 days after infection; time-consuming test because it requires virus to be grown in the laboratory
– *Reverse transcriptase-polymerase chain reaction (RT-PCR):* identifies genetic information of ribonucleic acid in the virus
◆ Nasopharyngeal, oropharyngeal, or bronchoalveolar specimens used; serum and blood specimens usually needed for RT-PCR testing

PURPOSE

◆ To identify the SARS CoV as the cause of the infection

PREPARATION

◆ Make sure the patient or a responsible family member has signed an informed consent.
◆ If the specimen will be collected by expectoration, encourage fluid intake the night before collection to help sputum production, unless contraindicated.
◆ If the specimen will be collected by bronchoscopy, the patient will need to fast for 6 hours before the procedure.

Teaching points

◆ Explain that the SARS viral test identifies the organism causing respiratory tract infection.
◆ Explain who will perform the test and where it'll be done.
◆ Tell the patient about the types of specimens that will be collected.
◆ Review dietary restrictions with the patient.
◆ Teach the patient how to expectorate by taking three deep breaths and forcing a deep cough; emphasize that sputum isn't the same as saliva, which is unacceptable for culturing. Tell him to brush his teeth and gargle with water before the specimen collection to reduce contamination with oropharyngeal bacteria.
◆ If the specimen will be collected by swabbing the area, warn the patient that he may feel a slight itching sensation.
◆ If the specimen will be collected by tracheal suctioning, tell the patient that he'll experience discomfort as the catheter passes into the trachea.
◆ If the specimen will be collected by bronchoscopy, instruct the patient to fast for 6 hours before the procedure.

KEY STEPS

◆ Confirm the patient's identity using two patient identifiers according to facility policy.
◆ Put on gloves.

Washing or aspirating of nasopharyngeal area

◆ Have the patient sit with his head tilted slightly back.
◆ Insert a syringe filled with 1 to 1.5 ml of saline (nonbacteriostatic) into one nostril and instill the saline.
◆ Attach a small plastic catheter or tubing to the syringe and flush it with 2 to 3 ml of saline.
◆ Insert the tubing into the nostril and aspirate the secretions; then repeat in the other nostril.

Swabbing of the nasopharyngeal or oropharyngeal area

◆ Obtain sterile swabs that have plastic sticks and Dacron or rayon tips.

⚡ **WARNING** *Never use cotton-tipped applicators or swabs with wooden sticks. Some viruses can become inactivated by the substances contained in these swabs, thus interfering with RT-PCR testing.*

◆ Insert the swab into the nostril and let it remain there for several seconds to absorb the secretions; if swabbing the oropharyngeal area, run the swab along the posterior pharynx and tonsils. Avoid touching the tongue.

(continued)

Expectorating of sputum

◆ Have the patient rinse his mouth with water.
◆ Instruct the patient to cough deeply and expectorate into the sterile dry container.

Collecting of blood and plasma specimens

◆ Perform a venipuncture and collect 5 to 10 ml of whole blood in a serum separator tube (for serum RT-PCR or ELISA antibody testing) or an EDTA tube (for plasma testing).

Collecting of other specimens

◆ Assist with tracheal suctioning, bronchoscopy, or thoracentesis as appropriate.

All tests

◆ Make sure that specimens are placed in the appropriate sterile container for transport.

POSTPROCEDURE CARE

◆ Dispose of equipment properly; seal the container in a biohazard bag before sending it to the laboratory.
◆ Label the container with the patient's name. Include on the test request form the nature and origin of the specimen, the date and time of collection, the initial diagnosis, and any current antimicrobial therapy.
◆ Provide mouth care as indicated.
◆ Inform the practitioner of abnormal results.

PRECAUTIONS

◆ Wear gloves when performing the diagnostic procedure and handling specimens; adhere to your facility's infection control policies at all times.
◆ Because the patient may cough violently during suctioning, also wear a mask and, if necessary, a gown to avoid exposure to pathogens.
◆ Send the specimen to the laboratory immediately after collection.

COMPLICATIONS

◆ Variable, based on collection method

INTERPRETATION

NORMAL RESULTS

◆ No antibodies to the SARS virus are present.

ABNORMAL RESULTS

◆ The specimen tests positive for the SARS virus, indicating infection with SARS.
◆ SARS infection is diagnosed when positive test results occur: in a single specimen that is tested at two distinct times; in two specimens from two different areas; in two specimens for the same area but tested on different days.

Schirmer's tearing test

DESCRIPTION

- Assesses function of the major lacrimal glands (responsible for reflex tearing in response to stressful situations such as the presence of a foreign body); both eyes tested at once
- Stimulates tearing by inserting a strip of filter paper into the lower conjunctival sac; then measuring the amount of moisture absorbed by the paper
- Variation: to evaluate function of the accessory lacrimal glands of Krause and Wolfring by instilling a topical anesthetic before inserting the papers
- Anesthetic: inhibits reflex tearing by the major lacrimal glands, so that only the basic tear film (which maintains adequate corneal moisture) normally produced by the accessory glands is measured

PURPOSE

- To measure tear secretion in patient with suspected tearing deficiency

PREPARATION

- The patient should remove contact lenses before the test.

Teaching points

- Explain that this test requires that a strip of filter paper be placed in the lower part of each eye for 5 minutes.
- Reassure the patient that the procedure is painless.
- Explain who will perform the test and where it will be done.
- If the patient wears contact lenses, ask him to remove them before the test.
- Explain that he doesn't need to diet.
- Tell the patient that the test takes about 15 minutes.
- If a topical anesthetic was instilled, advise the patient not to rub his eyes for at least 30 minutes after instillation because this can cause a corneal abrasion.

DIAGNOSTIC PROCEDURE

KEY STEPS

- Confirm the patient's identity using two patient identifiers according to facility policy.
- Assist the patient into the examining chair with his head against the headrest.
- To remove the test strip from the wrapper, bend the rounded wick end at the indentation and cut open the envelope at the other end.
- Tell the patient to look up, and then gently lower the inferior eyelid.
- Hook the bent end of the strip over the inferior eyelid at the junction of the medial and nasal segments. (See *Proper filter placement in the Schirmer's test.*)
- Insert one strip in each eye and note the time of insertion. Tell the patient not to squeeze or rub his eyes, but to blink normally or to keep his eyes closed lightly.
- After 5 minutes, remove the strips from the patient's eyes and measure the length of the moistened area from the indentation, using the millimeter scale on the envelope.
- Report the results as a fraction: the numerator is the length of the moistened area, and the denominator is the time the strips were left in place. Note which eye was tested — if a strip inserted in the right conjunctival sac for 5 minutes shows 8 mm of moisture, the correct notation is OD

(oculus dexter, or right eye), 8 mm/5 minutes.
- To measure the function of the accessory lacrimal glands of Krause and Wolfring, instill one drop of topical anesthetic into each conjunctival sac before inserting the test strips.

POSTPROCEDURE CARE

- If the patient wears contact lenses, make sure that he doesn't reinsert them for at least 2 hours after the test.

PRECAUTIONS

- To prevent patient discomfort, be careful not to touch the cornea while inserting the test strip.

COMPLICATIONS

- None

NORMAL RESULTS

- The test strip shows at least 15 mm of moisture after 5 minutes. Both eyes usually secrete the same amount of tears.
- Because tear production decreases with age, normal test results in patients older than age 40 range from 10 to 15 mm.

ABNORMAL RESULTS

- Up to 15% of the patients tested have false-positive or false-negative results.
- Because the test is rapid and simple, it may be repeated and findings compared.
- Additional testing, such as a slit-lamp examination with fluorescein or rose Bengal stain, is needed to confirm results.
- A positive result confirmed by additional testing indicates a definite tearing deficiency, which may result from aging or, more seriously, from Sjögren's syndrome, a systemic disease of unknown origin most common in postmenopausal women.
- A tearing deficiency may also occur in lymphoma, leukemia, and rheumatoid arthritis.

Proper filter placement in the Schirmer's test

This illustration shows the proper placement of the filter paper for the Schirmer's test. The filter paper should be inserted into the inferior conjunctival sac of each eye.

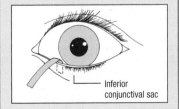

Inferior conjunctival sac

Semen analysis

DESCRIPTION

- Simple, inexpensive, and reasonably definitive test; several uses including evaluating a man's fertility
- Includes measuring seminal fluid volume, performing sperm counts, and microscopically examining spermatozoa
- Sperm: counted in semen similar to method for counting white blood cells, red blood cells, and platelets in a blood sample; motility and morphology studied microscopically after a drop of semen is stained
- Can also detect semen on a rape victim, identify the blood group of an alleged rapist, or prove sterility in a paternity suit (see *Identifying semen for medicolegal purposes*)

PURPOSE

- To evaluate male fertility in an infertile couple
- To substantiate the effectiveness of a vasectomy
- To detect semen on the body or clothing of a suspected rape victim or elsewhere at a crime scene
- To identify blood group substances to exonerate or incriminate a criminal suspect
- To rule out paternity on grounds of complete sterility

PREPARATION

For fertility evaluation

- Give the patient written instructions, and inform him that the most desirable specimen requires masturbation, ideally in a practitioner's office or laboratory.
- If the patient prefers to collect the specimen at home, stress the importance of delivering the specimen to the laboratory within 1 hour after collection. Warn him not to expose the specimen to extreme temperatures or to direct sunlight.

- Ideally, the specimen should remain at body temperature until liquefaction is complete (about 20 minutes). To deliver a semen specimen during cold weather, suggest that the patient keep the specimen container in a coat pocket on the way to the laboratory to protect the specimen from exposure to cold.
- Alternatives to collection by masturbation include coitus interruptus or the use of a condom.
- Fertility can also be determined by collecting semen from the woman after coitus to assess the ability of the spermatozoa to penetrate the cervical mucus and remain active.

For rape victim

- Prepare the victim for insertion of the speculum just as you would a patient scheduled for postcoital examination.

- Handle the victim's clothes as little as possible. If her clothes are moist, put them in a paper bag — not a plastic bag (which causes seminal stains and secretions to mold). Label the bag properly, and send it to the laboratory immediately.
- Provide emotional support by speaking to the patient calmly and reassuringly. Encourage her to express fears and anxieties. Listen sympathetically.
- If she's scheduled for vaginal lavage, tell her to expect a cold sensation when saline solution is instilled to wash out the specimen.
- Help the patient relax by instructing her to breathe deeply and slowly through her mouth.

Teaching points

- Tell the patient to follow the written instructions regarding the period of sexual continence before the test because this may increase his sperm count.
- Review the proper collection methods with the patient.
- Inform a patient undergoing infertility studies that test results should be available in 24 hours.

Identifying semen for medicolegal purposes

Spermatozoa (or their fragments) persist in the vagina for more than 72 hours after intercourse. This allows detection and positive identification of semen from vaginal aspirates or smears or from stains on clothing, other fabrics, skin, or hair, which is usually necessary for medicolegal purposes, most often in connection with rape or homicide investigations. Identification of spermatozoa taken from the vagina of an exhumed body is also possible if the body has been properly embalmed and remains reasonably intact.

To determine which stains or fluids require further investigation, clothing or other fabrics can be scanned with ultraviolet light to detect the typical green-white fluorescence of semen. Soaking appropriate samples of clothing, fabric, or hair in physiologic saline solution extracts the semen and spermatozoa. Deposits of dried semen can be gently sponged from the victim's skin.

The two most common ways to identify semen are testing for *acid phosphatase* concentration (the more sensitive test) and a *microscopic examination* for the presence of spermatozoa. Acid phosphatase appears in semen in significantly greater levels than in other body fluids. In microscopic examination, spermatozoa or head fragments can be identified or stained smears prepared directly from vaginal scrapings or aspirates or from the concentrated sediment of eluates or lavages.

Like other body fluids, semen contains the soluble A, B, and H blood group substance in about 80% of men who are genetically determined secretors (men who have the dominant secretor gene in a homonozygous or heterozygous state). Thus, the man who has group A blood and is a secretor has soluble blood group A substance in his seminal fluid and group A substance on the surface of his red blood cells. This fact can be of considerable medicolegal importance. Semen analysis can demonstrate that the semen of a rape or homicide investigation suspect is different from or consistent with semen found in or on the victim's body.

For postcoital cervical mucus test

◆ Instruct the patient to report for examination 1 or 2 days before ovulation as determined by basal temperature records.
◆ Instruct the couple to abstain from intercourse for 2 days and then to have sexual intercourse 2 to 8 hours before the examination. Remind them to avoid using lubricants.
◆ Explain to the patient that she'll be placed in the lithotomy position and that a speculum will be inserted into the vagina to collect the specimen. Tell her that she may feel some pressure but no pain.

For collection by coitus interruptus

◆ Instruct the patient to withdraw immediately before ejaculation and to deposit the ejaculate in a suitable specimen container.

For collection by condom

◆ Tell the patient to first wash the condom with soap and water, rinse it thoroughly, and allow it to dry completely. (Powders or lubricants applied to the condom may be spermicidal.) Special sheaths that don't contain spermicide are also available for semen collection.
◆ Instruct the patient to tie the condom after collection, place it in a glass jar, and promptly deliver it to the laboratory.

For semen collection from a rape victim

◆ Instruct the victim to urinate just before the test, but warn her not to wipe the vulva afterward because this may remove semen.
◆ Tell the patient that the examiner will try to obtain a semen specimen from her vagina.

DIAGNOSTIC PROCEDURE

KEY STEPS

◆ Confirm the patient's identity using two patient identifiers according to facility policy.

◆ Obtain a semen specimen for a fertility study by asking the patient to collect semen in a clean plastic specimen container.
◆ Before postcoital examination, the examiner wipes excess mucus from the external cervix and collects the specimen by direct aspiration of the cervical canal using a 1-ml tuberculin syringe without a cannula or needle.
◆ A specimen is obtained from the vagina of a rape victim by direct aspiration, saline lavage, or a direct smear of vaginal contents using a Pap stick or, less desirably, a cotton applicator stick.
◆ Dried smears are usually collected from the suspected rape victim's skin by gently washing the skin with a small piece of gauze moistened with physiologic saline solution.
◆ Prepare direct smears on glass microscopic slides after labeling the frosted end. Immediately place smeared slides in Coplin jars containing 95% ethanol.

POSTPROCEDURE CARE

◆ Refer the patient to an appropriate specialist for counseling.

PRECAUTIONS

◆ If the patient prefers to collect the specimen during coitus interruptus, tell him he must prevent any loss of semen during ejaculation.
◆ Deliver all specimens to the laboratory within 1 hour.
◆ Protect semen specimens for fertility studies for extremes of temperature and direct sunlight during delivery to the laboratory.
◆ Never lubricate the vaginal speculum. Oil or grease hinders examination of spermatozoa by interfering with smear preparation and staining and by inhibiting sperm motility through toxic ingredients. Instead, moisten the speculum with water or physiologic saline solution.

COMPLICATIONS

◆ None

INTERPRETATION

NORMAL RESULTS

◆ Semen volume is 0.7 to 6.5 ml.
◆ The semen volume of many men in infertile couples is increased compared with the normal range.
◆ Abstinence for 1 week or more increases semen volume. (With abstinence of up to 10 days, sperm counts increase, sperm motility progressively decreases, and sperm morphology stays the same.)
◆ Liquefied semen is generally highly viscid, translucent, and gray-white, with a musty or acrid odor. After liquefaction, specimens of normal viscosity can be poured in drops.
◆ Normally, semen is slightly alkaline with a pH of 7.3 to 7.9.
◆ Semen coagulates immediately and liquefies within 20 minutes; the normal sperm count is 20 to 150 million/ml and can be greater; 40% of spermatozoa have normal morphology; and 20% or more of spermatozoa show progressive motility within 4 hours of collection.
◆ The normal postcoital cervical mucus test shows 10 to 20 motile spermatozoa per microscopic high-power field and spinnbarkeit (a measurement of the tenacity of the mucus) of at least 4″ (10 cm). These findings indicate adequate spermatozoa and receptivity of the cervical mucus. Shaking or dead sperm may indicate antisperm antibodies.

ABNORMAL RESULTS

◆ Abnormal semen isn't synonymous with infertility.
◆ Only one viable spermatozoon is needed to fertilize an ovum.
◆ Only men who can't deliver any viable spermatozoa in their ejaculate during sexual intercourse are absolutely sterile.
◆ Subnormal sperm counts, decreased sperm motility, and abnormal morphology usually indicate decreased fertility.

Sex chromosome test

DESCRIPTION

- Indicated for abnormal sexual development, ambiguous genitalia, amenorrhea, and suspected chromosomal abnormalities
- Screens for abnormalities in the number of sex chromosomes; test replaced by faster, simpler, more accurate full karyotype (chromosome analysis)

PURPOSE

- To quickly screen for abnormal sexual development (X and Y chromatin tests)
- To help assess an infant with ambiguous genitalia (X chromatin test)
- To determine the number of Y chromosomes in an individual (Y chromatin test)

PREPARATION

- No dietary restrictions are required.
- The test requires a specimen from the inside of the patient's cheek.

Teaching points

- Explain to the patient or his parents, if appropriate, why the sex chromosome test is required.
- Explain who will perform the test and where it'll be done.
- Tell the patient that this test requires that the inside of his cheek be scraped to obtain a specimen.
- Assure the patient that the test takes only a few minutes but may require a follow-up chromosome analysis.
- Advise the patient that the laboratory needs up to 4 weeks to complete the analysis.

Sex chromosome anomalies

DISORDER AND CHROMOSOMAL ANEUPLOIDY	CAUSE AND INCIDENCE	PHENOTYPIC FEATURES
Klinefelter's syndrome		
◆ 47,XXY ◆ 48,XXXY ◆ 49,XXXXY ◆ 48,XXYY ◆ 49,XXXYY	◆ Nondisjunction or improper chromatid separation during anaphase I or II of oogenesis or spermatogenesis results in abnormal gamete ◆ 1 per 1,000 male births	◆ Syndrome usually inapparent until puberty ◆ Small penis and testes ◆ Sparse facial and abdominal hair; feminine distribution of pubic hair ◆ Somewhat enlarged breasts (gynecomastia) ◆ Sexual dysfunction ◆ Truncal obesity ◆ Sterility ◆ Possible mental retardation (greater incidence with increased X chromosomes)
Polysomy Y		
◆ 47,XYY	◆ Nondisjunction during anaphase II of spermatogenesis causes both Y chromosomes to pass to the same pole and results in a YY sperm ◆ 1 per 1,000 male births	◆ Above-average stature (commonly over 72″ [182.9 cm]) ◆ Increased incidence of severe acne ◆ May display aggressive, psychopathic, or criminal behavior ◆ Normal fertility ◆ Learning disabilities
Turner's syndrome		
◆ 45,XO ◆ Mosaics: XO/XX or XO/XXX ◆ Aberrations of X chromosomes, including deletion of short arm of one X chromosome, presence of a ring chromosome, or presence of an isochromosome on the long arm of an X chromosome	◆ Nondisjunction during anaphase I or II of spermatogenesis results in sperm without any sex chromosomes ◆ 1 per 3,500 female births (most common chromosome complement in first-trimester abortions)	◆ Short stature (usually under 57″ [144.8 cm]) ◆ Webbed neck ◆ Low posterior hairline ◆ Broad chest with widely spaced nipples ◆ Underdeveloped breasts ◆ Juvenile external genitalia ◆ Primary amenorrhea common ◆ Congenital heart disease (30% with coarctation of the aorta) ◆ Renal abnormalities ◆ Sterility from underdeveloped internal reproductive organs (ovaries are only strands of connective tissue) ◆ No mental retardation, but possible problems with space perception and orientation

Sex chromosome anomalies (continued)

DISORDER AND CHROMOSOMAL ANEUPLOIDY	CAUSE AND INCIDENCE	PHENOTYPIC FEATURES
Other X polysomes		
◆ 47,XXX	◆ Nondisjunction at anaphase I or II of oogenesis	
	◆ 1 per 1,400 female births	◆ Commonly, no obvious anatomic abnormalities ◆ Normal fertility
◆ 48,XXXX	◆ Rare ◆ Rare	◆ Mental retardation ◆ Ocular hypertelorism ◆ Reduced fertility
◆ 49,XXXXX		◆ Severe mental retardation ◆ Ocular hypertelorism with unco-ordinated eye movement ◆ Abnormal sexual organ development ◆ Various skeletal anomalies

DIAGNOSTIC PROCEDURE

KEY STEPS
◆ Confirm the patient's identity using two patient identifiers according to facility policy.
◆ Scrape the buccal mucosa firmly with a wooden or metal spatula at least twice to obtain a specimen of healthy cells (vaginal mucosa is occasionally used in young women).
◆ Rub the spatula over the glass slide, making sure the cells are evenly distributed.
◆ Spray the slide with a cell fixative and send it to the laboratory with a brief patient history and indications for the test.

POSTPROCEDURE CARE
◆ Answer the patient's questions.
◆ Refer the patient or his parents for genetic counseling after identification of the cause of chromosomal abnormal sexual development, as appropriate.

PRECAUTIONS
◆ Scrape the buccal mucosa firmly to ensure a sufficient number of cells.

COMPLICATIONS
◆ None

INTERPRETATION

NORMAL RESULTS
◆ A normal female (XX) has only one X chromatin mass (the number of X chromatin masses discernible is one less than the number of X chromosomes in the cells examined).
◆ An X chromatin mass is ordinarily discernible in only 20% to 50% of the buccal mucosal cells of a normal woman.
◆ A normal male (XY) has only one Y chromatin mass (the number of Y chromatin masses equals the number of Y chromosomes in the cells examined).

ABNORMAL RESULTS
◆ If less than 20% of the cells in a buccal smear contain an X chromatin mass, some cells are presumed to contain only one X chromosome, necessitating full karyotyping.
◆ A person with a female phenotype and a positive Y chromatin mass runs a high risk of developing a malignancy in the intra-abdominal gonads. In such cases, removal of these gonads is indicated and should be performed before age 5.
◆ A medical team of physicians, psychologists, psychiatrists, and educators must decide the child's sex if a child is phenotypically of one sex and genotypically of the other. This careful evaluation should be made early to prevent developmental problems related to incorrect gender identification. (See *Sex chromosome anomalies*.)

Sexual assault assessment

DESCRIPTION

- Uses specific specimen collection protocol for sexual assault cases, which varies at each facility
- Specimens collected from sources including blood, hair, nails, tissues, and body fluids, such as urine, semen, saliva, and vaginal secretion
- Accurate and precise specimen collection critical; information often used as evidence in legal proceedings

PURPOSE

- To obtain a specimen for testing after a sexual assault

PREPARATION

- Assess the patient's ability to undergo the specimen collection procedure.
- Make sure that the patient or family has consented to specimen collection.
- Ensure patient privacy during the collection procedure.
- Ask the patient if she would like someone, such as a family member, friend, or other person to stay with her during the specimen collection.

Teaching points

- Explain the procedures that the patient will undergo, what specimens will be collected and from where, and provide emotional support.
- Explain what will be done with the specimen and test results.

KEY STEPS

- Confirm the patient's identity using two patient identifiers according to facility policy.
- When possible, use a special Sexual Assault Evidence Collection Kit.
- Before obtaining any specimens, inspect the genital area using a Wood's lamp. This device uses long wave ultraviolet light to scan the area for secretions and helps identify areas of trauma.
- Include the victim's clothing as part of the collection procedure.
- Obtain photographs of all injuries for documentation.
- Include written documentation of the victim's physical and psychological condition on first encounter, during specimen collection, and afterwards.
- If available, have a sexual assault nurse examiner care for the patient.

Clothing for specimen collection

- Ask the patient to stand on a clean piece of examination paper if she's able to stand; if she can't stand, then have her remain on the examination table or bed.
- Have the patient remove each article of clothing, one at a time, and place each article in a separate, clean paper bag.
- If the clothing is wet, allow it to dry before placing it in the paper bag.

  WARNING *Never use plastic bags to collect clothing. Plastic promotes bacterial growth and can destroy DNA.*
- Fold the examination paper onto itself and place it into a clean paper bag.
- Fold over, seal, label, and initial each bag.

Vaginal or cervical secretion collection

- Swab the vaginal area thoroughly with four swabs; swab the cervical area with two swabs, making sure to keep the vaginal swabs separate from the cervical swabs.

- Run the vaginal swabs over a slide (supplied in the kit) and allow the slide and swabs to air-dry; do the same for the cervical swabs.
- Place the vaginal swabs in the swab container and close it; place the slide in the cardboard sleeve, close it and tape it shut; repeat this procedure for the cervical swabs.
- Place the swab container and cardboard sleeve into the envelope, and seal it securely.
- Complete the information as provided on the front of the envelope; if both vaginal and cervical swabs are obtained, use a separate envelope for each.

Anal secretion collection

- Moisten a single swab with sterile water.
- Insert the swab gently into the patient's rectum about $1\frac{1}{4}''$ (3 cm).
- Rotate the swab gently and then remove it.
- Allow the swab to air-dry and then place it in an envelope.
- Seal and label the envelope appropriately.

Penile secretion collection

- Moisten a single swab with sterile water.
- Swab the entire external surface of the penis.
- Repeat this at least once (so that at least two swabs are obtained).
- Allow the swab to air-dry and then place it in an envelope.
- Seal and label the envelope appropriately.

Pubic hair collection

- Use the comb provided in the kit and comb through the pubic hair.
- Collect about 20 to 30 pubic hairs and place them in the envelope; or, obtain 20 to 30 plucked hairs from the patient; allow the patient the option of plucking her own pubic hair.
- Place the hair in the envelope, seal and label it appropriately.

Blood samples

- After performing a venipuncture, obtain at least 5 ml of blood in an EDTA tube.
- Write the patient's name and date on the label of the tube.
- Remove the DNA stain card from the kit and label it with the patient's name.
- Using the blood collected in the tube, withdraw 1 ml of blood and apply blood to each of the four circles on the card, completely filling each circle if possible.
- Let the card air-dry and then place the card in the envelope.
- Seal and label the envelope appropriately.
- Place the blood tube into the tube holder supplied in the kit and seal the holder with tape supplied in the kit (may be referred to as evidence tape).
- Place the tube and holder in the zippered bag provided.
- Collect additional blood samples to test for pregnancy; sexually transmitted disease, such as gonorrhea, chlamydia, and syphilis; or toxicology as appropriate and send to the laboratory immediately.

Urine specimens

- Obtain a random urine specimen from the patient; if needed, obtain the urine specimen via catheterization.

POSTPROCEDURE CARE

- Refrigerate blood samples obtained.
- Place all other specimens in the specimen kit and keep the kit at room temperature.
- Follow the directions in the kit precisely to make sure that the chain of evidence is followed.
- Provide follow-up counseling and support to the patient.
- Administer ordered medications, such as tetanus or antibiotics, as needed.
- Make sure the patient has a support person to accompany her home.
- Arrange for referral to a local support group or follow-up with a trained counselor.

- Give all the specimens to the police when they arrive.

PRECAUTIONS

- Be knowledgeable about your facility's policies and procedures for specimen collection in sexual assault cases.
- When obtaining specimens, be sure to collect them from the victim and, if possible, from the suspect.
- Check with local law enforcement agencies about additional specimens that may be needed; for example, trace evidence, such as soot, grass, gravel, glass, or other debris.
- Wear gloves and change them frequently; use disposable equipment and instruments if possible.
- Avoid coughing, sneezing, talking over specimens, and touching your face, nose, or mouth when collecting specimens.
- Place all items collected in a paper bag.

  WARNING *Never allow a specimen or item considered as evidence to be left unattended.*

- Document each item or specimen collected; have another person witness each collection and document it.

COMPLICATIONS

- None

- This test is done for specimen collection only, and the specimen is then passed on to law enforcement for legal purposes.

NORMAL RESULTS
- Not applicable

ABNORMAL RESULTS
- Not applicable

Sickle cell test

OVERVIEW

DESCRIPTION

◆ Also known as the *hemoglobin (Hb) S test*
◆ Detects sickle cells (severely deformed, rigid erythrocytes that may slow blood flow)
◆ Sickle cell trait (characterized by heterozygous Hb S): occurs almost exclusively in blacks — 0.2% of blacks born in the United States have sickle cell disease (see *Inheritance patterns in sickle cell anemia*)
◆ Used as a rapid screening procedure; may produce erroneous results
◆ If sickle cell disease is suspected, diagnosis confirmed by Hb electrophoresis

PURPOSE

◆ To identify sickle cell disease and sickle cell trait

PREPARATION

◆ Check the patient's history for a blood transfusion within the past 3 months.
◆ No dietary restrictions are required.
◆ The test requires a blood sample.

Teaching points

◆ Explain that the sickle cell test detects sickle cell disease.
◆ Explain who will perform the test and where it'll be done.
◆ Tell the patient that the test requires a blood sample and that he may experience slight discomfort from the tourniquet and needle puncture.
◆ If the patient is an infant or child, explain to his parents that a small amount of blood will be taken from the finger or earlobe.
◆ Inform the patient that he need not restrict food or fluids.
◆ Tell the patient that the test takes less than 5 minutes.

DIAGNOSTIC PROCEDURE

KEY STEPS

◆ Confirm the patient's identity using two patient identifiers according to facility policy.
◆ Perform a venipuncture and collect the sample in a 3- or 4.5-ml EDTA tube.
◆ For young children, collect capillary blood in a microcollection device.
◆ Completely fill the collection tube and invert it gently several times to thoroughly mix the sample and the anticoagulant.

POSTPROCEDURE CARE

◆ Apply direct pressure to the venipuncture site until bleeding stops.
◆ Provide genetic counseling referral to the parents if needed.
◆ Inform the practitioner of abnormal results.

PRECAUTIONS

◆ Maintain standard precautions while collecting the sample.

COMPLICATIONS

◆ Hematoma at the venipuncture site; if large, monitor pulses distal to the phlebotomy site

INTERPRETATION

NORMAL RESULTS

◆ A negative result suggests the absence of Hb S.

ABNORMAL RESULTS

◆ A positive result may indicate the presence of sickle cells, but Hb electrophoresis is needed to further diagnose the sickling tendency of cells.
◆ Rarely, in the absence of Hb S, other abnormal Hb may cause sickling.

Inheritance patterns in sickle cell anemia

When both parents have sickle cell anemia (left), childbearing — if possible at all — is dangerous for the mother, and all offspring will have sickle cell anemia. When one parent has sickle cell anemia and one does not (right), all offspring will be carriers of sickle cell anemia.

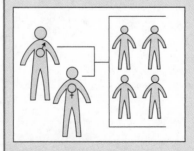
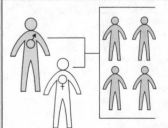

■ Sickle cell anemia
■ Sickle cell trait
□ Normal

Sigmoidoscopy, flexible

OVERVIEW

DESCRIPTION

- Endoscopic examination of the lining of the descending colon, sigmoid colon, rectum, and anal canal, using a flexible sigmoidoscope
- Allows several methods for obtaining specimens from suspicious areas of the mucosa: biopsy, cytology brush, or aspirate
- Used in colorectal screening (starting at age 50 for normal-risk individuals without family history of colorectal cancer or adenomatous colon polyps)

PURPOSE

- To help diagnose acute or chronic diarrhea and rectal bleeding
- To evaluate changes in bowel habits or feces characteristics
- To help assess known ulcerative colitis

PREPARATION

- Note and report allergies.
- Check the patient's history for barium tests within the last week because barium in the colon makes accurate examination impossible.
- Withhold food and fluid, as ordered.

Teaching points

- Explain the purpose of the test and how it's done.
- Explain who will perform the test and where it'll be done.
- Tell the patient if fasting is needed before the procedure.
- Discuss the possible use of sedation to help the patient relax.
- Warn the patient about a possible urge to defecate during the procedure.
- Advise the patient that air may be introduced through the endoscope to distend the walls of the colon, which causes flatus.
- Tell the patient that he may receive a laxative or enema before the test.
- Tell the patient that the test takes 10 to 30 minutes.
- See *Preparing for a sigmoidoscopy,* page 448.

DIAGNOSTIC PROCEDURE

KEY STEPS

- Confirm the patient's identity using two patient identifiers according to facility policy.
- The patient is placed in the Sims' position on the examination table.
- Before the procedure, the endoscopist visually inspects the anus and perineum.
- Digital rectal examination is performed.
- The flexible sigmoidoscope is slowly advanced to the splenic flexure, if possible, or as far as the patient can tolerate with only mild discomfort.
- Specimens may be obtained from any suspicious area of the intestinal mucosa.
- Polyps may be biopsied for histologic diagnosis or removed by the insertion of an electrocautery snare through the endoscope and submitted for histologic examination.
- Feces aspirate may be obtained if indicated for laboratory analysis.
- Before withdrawal of the scope, retroflexion is performed, allowing examination of the internal anal verge and the adjacent rectal mucosa.
- The scope is withdrawn, the lining of the colon is thoroughly examined, and air is removed.

POSTPROCEDURE CARE

- If the patient has received sedation, don't have him resume his diet and activity until he's fully awake.
- Encourage the patient to expel flatus.
- Monitor the patient's vital signs.
- Monitor feces and bowel sounds.
- Observe the patient for bleeding.
- Observe closely for any signs of bowel perforation (such as abdominal distention and pain, nausea, vomiting, and fever).
- Observe for vasovagal reaction (such as hypotension, pallor, diaphoresis, and bradycardia).
- Tell the patient to resume his previous diet, as ordered.

- If the patient received a biopsy or polypectomy, tell him that he may notice a small amount of blood in his feces.

PRECAUTIONS

- The procedure is contraindicated when patient has a perforated viscus or acute diverticulitis.

COMPLICATIONS

- Rectal bleeding
- Bowel perforation
- Vasovagal reaction
- Adverse reaction to sedation

INTERPRETATION

NORMAL RESULTS

- Mucosa of the anal canal is pearly white or pigmented, depending on the patient's race.
- Mucosa of the rectum is pink and may appear velvety because of the prevalence of lymphoid tissue.
- The rich vascular network becomes less prominent at the rectosigmoid junction.
- Three semilunar valves (Houston's valves) are present in the proximal half of the rectum.
- Mucosa of the sigmoid and descending colon is light pink-orange.

ABNORMAL RESULTS

- Biopsy results suggest possible benign, precancerous, or malignant polyps or tumors and various forms of colitis.
- Visual inspection of the anus and perineum may disclose abnormalities, such as external hemorrhoids, anal fissure, anorectal cellulitis or abscess, and perirectal skin tag.
- Digital rectal examination may disclose rectal mass, internal hemorrhoids, or anorectal abscess.
- Inflammatory change suggests possible diverticulitis.
- Melanosis coli (a brownish discoloration of the colon) suggests possible chronic laxative use.

(continued)

Preparing for a sigmoidoscopy

Dear Patient,

Your health care provider wants you to undergo a flexible sigmoidoscopy. A sigmoidoscopy allows the health care provider to see inside the *lower* part of the large bowel, which includes the sigmoid colon, rectum, and anus. To do this, the health care provider will gently insert a flexible fiber-optic tube called an *endoscope* into the rectum.

WHY IS THIS TEST NECESSARY?

Sigmoidoscopy allows for careful examination of the lower bowel and rectum for disease. (These areas are difficult to visualize in X-rays.) If needed, this test will also enable the health care provider to take a biopsy specimen for further testing or to remove polyps.

WILL I NEED TO PREPARE FOR THE TEST?

Yes. Be sure to follow your health care provider's directions for diet and bowel preparation. Stay on a liquid diet for 48 hours beforehand. You may drink clear juices without pulp, broth, tea, gelatin, and water, and you may continue to take prescription medicine.

Take a laxative the evening before the test and give yourself an enema the morning of the test or as directed by your health care provider. If the test is scheduled for early morning, don't consume anything past midnight.

Just before the test, you'll take off your clothes and put on a hospital gown. Leave your socks on for warmth. Also,

empty your bladder.

WHAT CAN I EXPECT DURING THE TEST?

The test is done by the health care provider and an assistant in an office or a special procedures room. It will last about 15 to 30 minutes. Before the test begins, the assistant will help you lie on your left side with your knees flexed and drape you with a sheet.

When you're in position, the health care provider will gently insert a well-lubricated, gloved finger into the anus to examine the area and dilate the rectal sphincter.

Next, the health care provider will gently insert the endoscope through the anus into the rectum. As it passes through the rectal sphincter, you may feel some lower abdominal discomfort and the urge to move your bowels. Bear down gently when the endoscope is first inserted. Also, breathe slowly and deeply through your mouth to help you relax. This will help ease the passage of the endoscope through the sphincter. The health care provider will gradually

advance the endoscope through the rectum into the lower bowel.

Sometimes air is blown through the endoscope into the bowel to distend it and permit better viewing. If you feel the urge to expel some air, don't try to control it or be embarrassed. The passing of air is expected. You may hear and feel a suction machine removing liquid that obscures the health care provider's view during the test. This machine causes no pain.

The health care provider will advance the endoscope slowly about 24 inches into the lower bowel. Continue to breathe slowly and deeply through your mouth to help the test go smoothly.

The health care provider may remove biopsy specimens or polyps from the lining of the bowel at any time during the test. These procedures are also painless because the bowel lining doesn't sense pain.

Toward the end of the test, the health care provider may insert a rigid ano-scope into the lower rectum. This instrument will provide a clearer view of the anal wall, revealing any abnormalities that the endoscope might miss.

WHAT CAN I EXPECT AFTERWARD?

The assistant will monitor your vital signs for about 1 hour afterward. You'll begin to pass large amounts of gas. You may also have slight rectal bleeding if the health care provider removed tissue specimens. Immediately report heavy, bright red bleeding; fever; abdominal swelling; or tenderness.

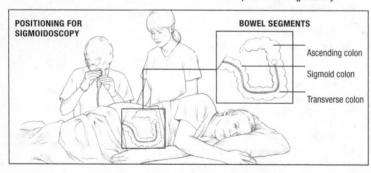

POSITIONING FOR SIGMOIDOSCOPY

BOWEL SEGMENTS

Ascending colon

Sigmoid colon

Transverse colon

Site-of-lesion tests

DESCRIPTION

◆ Identify location of a lesion suggested by patient history or pure tone audiometry

◆ Indicated in patients having difficulty understanding speech, disproportionate to the degree of pure tone loss; dizziness, tinnitus, or sudden or fluctuating hearing loss; or other neural symptoms; or a difference between sensorineural components in each ear

◆ Distinguish cochlear from retrocochlear lesions and localize lesions in the retrocochlear system at the eighth nerve, in the extra-axial (peripheral) or intra-axial brain stem, and in the cortex

PURPOSE

◆ To distinguish cochlear from retrocochlear hearing loss

◆ To localize lesions in the retrocochlear component of the auditory system

PREPARATION

◆ Note and report all allergies.

◆ No dietary restrictions are required.

Teaching points

◆ Explain to the patient the purpose of the test and how it's done.

◆ Explain who will perform the test and where it'll be done.

◆ Tell the patient that he doesn't need to restrict his diet.

◆ Tell the patient that the test takes about 90 minutes.

KEY STEPS

◆ Confirm the patient's identity using two patient identifiers according to facility policy.

◆ Earphones are applied to the patient.

Alternate binaural loudness

◆ A tone is presented to one ear and then the other. The tone in one ear is held at a constant intensity of 90 dB hearing level (HL); the other tone is varied.

◆ The patient indicates when the tones sound equally loud to both ears.

Simultaneous binaural midplane localization

◆ A 90-dB HL tone is presented to one ear, and tones of varying intensity are presented simultaneously to the other ear.

◆ The patient indicates when he perceives a single tone in the center of his head.

Rosenburg tone decay

◆ A tone is presented at or near threshold; the patient indicates how long he can hear it.

◆ If the tone becomes inaudible or changes to a buzzing or hissing sound, the tone is raised 5 dB to produce a tone that the patient should again be able to hear.

◆ The process is repeated until the patient hears the tone continuously for 60 seconds.

Suprathreshold adaptation test

◆ A tone is presented at 110 dB sensation level, rounded to 100 dB HL at 500 and 2,000 Hz and to 105 dB HL at 1,000 Hz.

Békésy audiometry

◆ The patient controls the tone intensity by depressing a response button whenever he hears a tone. When the tone softens and disappears, he releases the button; the tone then becomes louder.

◆ The patient repeats this procedure for several minutes, and the resulting audiometric tracing shows excursions above and below the actual threshold.

◆ Tracings are obtained for pulsed and continuous tones. The relationship between these two categories can be grouped into diagnostic patterns.

Masking level differences

◆ A 500-Hz tone and a narrow-band masking noise are presented to both ears at the same time. The noise is held at a constant intensity, and the patient's threshold for the tonal stimulus in that noise is determined. Then the phase of the tone is changed to one ear by 180 degrees, and the difference is tested.

Difficult speech discrimination tasks

◆ To gauge the patient's ability to discriminate speech in white noise, a speech stimulus is presented to one ear; the result is scored.

◆ White noise and a speech stimulus are presented simultaneously to the same ear, and the result is scored. The two scores are then compared.

◆ The task is repeated for the other ear and the scores are compared. Finally, each ear's score is compared with the other and with normal range.

(continued)

Auditory brain stem electrical response measures

- Electrodes are placed at the vertex of the patient's scalp (active), the mastoid process or earlobe of the stimulated ear (reference), and the mastoid process or earlobe of the opposite ear (ground).
- Stimuli are presented in the form of clicks or rapid rise time (1 millisecond) tone pips at 10 per second until 2,000 time-locked responses are collected and averaged. This tests mainly the 1,000- to 4,000-Hz frequency.

Competing message tasks

- A different message is presented to each ear, and the patient is asked to discriminate between the messages.
- In a gross measure test, such as the Northwestern University Test #20, speech discrimination words are presented to one ear, and the patient is asked to repeat them. Then speech discrimination words are presented to the same ear, and short sentences are simultaneously presented to the other ear; the patient is asked to repeat the words and ignore the sentences. The patient's scores on each task are then compared.

Precise message test

- An example of this type of test is the dichotic nonsense syllables test.
- Carefully aligned nonsense syllables are presented to both ears at once, and the patient is asked to repeat or write both syllables. The number of syllables correctly identified in one ear is compared with the number of syllables correctly identified in the other ear, as well as with a normal range.

POSTPROCEDURE CARE

- Answer the patient's questions about the tests.
- Inform the practitioner of abnormal results.

PRECAUTIONS

- None

COMPLICATIONS

- None

INTERPRETATION

NORMAL RESULTS

- Sensory and neural deficits are absent.

ABNORMAL RESULTS

- Sensory deficits suggest lesions of the auditory portions of the inner ear (cochlea).
- Neural deficits suggest lesions beyond the inner ear (retrocochlear).
- Abnormal adaptation to a continuous tone in tone decay tests suggests the presence of retrocochlear lesions.

Skin biopsy

DESCRIPTION
- Removal of a small piece of tissue, under local anesthesia, from lesion suspected of being malignant
- For histologic examination: specimen obtained by shave, punch, or excision biopsy
- Fully developed lesions preferred for biopsy; they provide more diagnostic information than resolving lesions or those in early developing stages

PURPOSE
- To allow differential diagnosis of basal cell carcinoma, squamous cell carcinoma, malignant melanoma, and benign growths
- To diagnose chronic bacterial or fungal skin infections

PREPARATION
- Make sure the patient has signed an appropriate consent form.
- No dietary restrictions are required.
- Note and report all allergies.
- A local anesthetic will be given before the procedure.

Teaching points
- Explain to the patient the purpose of the test and how it's done.
- Explain who will perform the test and where it'll be done.
- Tell the patient that fasting isn't required.
- Inform the patient that he will receive a local anesthetic to minimize pain during the procedure.
- Tell the patient that the test takes about 15 minutes.
- Instruct the patient with adhesive strips to leave them in place for 14 to 21 days or until they fall off.
- Advise the patient with sutures to keep the area clean and as dry as possible. Facial sutures are removed in 3 to 5 days; trunk sutures, in 7 to 14 days.

DIAGNOSTIC PROCEDURE

KEY STEPS
- Confirm the patient's identity using two patient identifiers according to facility policy.
- Position the patient comfortably and clean the biopsy site.
- The patient is given a local anesthetic.

Shave biopsy
- The protruding growth is cut off at the skin line with a #15 scalpel, and the tissue placed immediately in a properly labeled specimen bottle containing 10% formalin solution.
- Pressure is applied to the area to stop the bleeding.

Punch biopsy
- The skin surrounding the lesion is pulled taut, and the punch is firmly introduced into the lesion and rotated to obtain a tissue specimen.
- The plug is lifted with forceps or a needle and is severed as deeply into the fat layer as possible.
- The specimen is placed in a properly labeled specimen bottle containing 10% formalin solution or, if indicated, in a sterile container.
- The method used to close the wound depends on the size of the punch.

Excision biopsy
- A #15 scalpel is used to excise the lesion completely; the incision is made as wide and as deep as necessary.
- The practitioner removes the tissue specimen and places it immediately in a properly labeled specimen bottle containing 10% formalin solution.
- Pressure is applied to the site to stop the bleeding. The wound is closed, and if the incision is large, a skin graft may be required.

POSTPROCEDURE CARE
- If the patient experiences pain at the biopsy site, give an analgesic.
- Monitor the patient for bleeding and infection.

PRECAUTIONS
- Maintain standard precautions during the biopsy.
- Send the specimen to the laboratory immediately.

COMPLICATIONS
- Bleeding
- Infection

INTERPRETATION

NORMAL RESULTS
- Normal skin consists of squamous epithelium (epidermis) and fibrous connective tissue (dermis).

ABNORMAL RESULTS
- Histologic examination of the tissue specimen suggests possible benign lesions such as dermatofibromas, or malignant lesions such as malignant melanoma.
- Cultures can be used to detect chronic bacterial and fungal infections.

Skull radiography

DESCRIPTION

- Noninvasive neurologic test; use has declined with increased use of other diagnostic studies, such as computed tomography and magnetic resonance imaging
- Provides complete skull examination (because bones of the skull form a complex anatomic structure, requires several radiologic views of each area)
- For head injuries: offers limited information about skull fractures
- Used to study abnormalities of the base of the skull and the cranial vault, neoplasms, congenital and perinatal anomalies, and many metabolic and endocrinologic diseases that produce bone defects of the skull

PURPOSE

- To detect fractures in patients with head trauma
- To help diagnose pituitary tumors
- To detect congenital anomalies
- To detect metabolic and endocrinologic disorders

PREPARATION

- Note and report all allergies.
- No dietary restrictions are required.

Teaching points

- Explain to the patient the purpose of the test and how it's done.
- Explain who will perform the test and where it'll be done.
- Tell the patient that the procedure causes no discomfort.
- Tell the patient that he need not restrict food or fluids.
- Instruct the patient to remove his glasses, dentures, jewelry, and metal objects in the radiographic field.
- Tell the patient that the test takes about 15 minutes.

KEY STEPS

- Confirm the patient's identity using two patient identifiers according to facility policy.
- The patient is placed in the supine position on an X-ray table or seated in a chair. Instruct him to keep still while the X-rays are taken.
- A headband, foam pads, or sandbags are used to immobilize the patient's head and increase his comfort.
- Routinely, five views of the skull are taken: left and right lateral, anteroposterior Towne's, posteroanterior Caldwell's, and axial (or base).

POSTPROCEDURE CARE

- Answer the patient's questions.
- Inform the practitioner of abnormal results.

PRECAUTIONS

- None

COMPLICATIONS

- None

NORMAL RESULTS

- Size, shape, thickness, and position of cranial bones and vascular markings, sinuses, and sutures are normal.

ABNORMAL RESULTS

- Structural abnormalities suggest possible fractures of the vault or base of the skull or congenital anomalies.
- Erosion, enlargement, or decalcification of the sella turcica suggests possible increased intracranial pressure.
- Areas of calcification suggest possible conditions, such as osteomyelitis, or the presence of neoplasms within the brain substance that contain calcium, such as oligodendrogliomas or meningiomas.
- Midline shifting of a calcified pineal gland suggests a possible space-occupying lesion.
- Changes in bone structure suggest possible metabolic disorders, such as acromegaly or Paget's disease.

Sleep studies

DESCRIPTION

- Helps in the differential diagnosis of sleep-disordered breathing
- Parameters evaluated for sleep disorder: cardiac rate and rhythm, chest and abdominal wall movement, nasal and oral airflow, oxygen saturation, muscle activity, retinal function, and brain activity during the sleep phase
- Also known as *polysomnography*

PURPOSE

- To diagnose a breathing disorder in patients with history of excessive snoring, narcolepsy, excessive daytime sleepiness, insomnia, cardiac rhythm disorders, or restless leg spasms

PREPARATION

- Make sure the patient has signed an appropriate consent form.
- Note and report all allergies.
- Caffeine-containing products and naps should be avoided for 2 to 3 days before the test.
- Schedule the tests for the evening and night hours, usually from 10 p.m. to 6 a.m.

Teaching points

- Explain to the patient who will perform the test and where it'll be done.
- Instruct the patient to avoid caffeine-containing products and taking naps for 2 to 3 days before the test.
- Advise the patient to maintain a normal sleep schedule so that he's neither deprived of sleep nor overrested.
- Tell the patient that he may bathe or shower before the test.

KEY STEPS

- Confirm the patient's identity using two patient identifiers according to facility policy.
- Electrodes are secured to the patient's skin, depending on the type of monitoring being used.
- The patient is made comfortable and told that normal body movements won't interfere with the electrodes.
- The lights are turned off and the EEG monitored for a baseline reading before the patient falls asleep.
- The recording and video equipment record the sleep events as they occur.
- Monitoring of the patient during sleep continues until the test is complete.

POSTPROCEDURE CARE

- Monitor the patient for respiratory distress during the study.

PRECAUTIONS

- For the patient with known sleep apnea, split-night studies may be required, such as monitoring the patient for the first half of the night, then using continuous positive airway pressure or nasal ventilation to open the obstructed airway during the second half of the night.

COMPLICATIONS

- Respiratory distress

NORMAL RESULTS

- Respiratory disturbance index (or apnea-hypopnea index) of fewer than 5 to 10 episodes per study period.
- No ischemic change or arrhythmia (electrocardiogram) is noted.
- Normal impedance (chest and abdominal wall motion).
- Normal airway (nasal and oral airflow).
- Normal arterial oxygen saturation (oximetry).
- Normal leg electromyogram (for muscle activity).
- Normal electro-oculogram (for retinal function).
- Normal EEG (for brain activity).

ABNORMAL RESULTS

- Abnormal recordings suggest possible obstructive sleep apnea syndrome.
- Abnormal movement during sleep suggests a possible seizure or movement disorder.

Slit-lamp examination

OVERVIEW

DESCRIPTION

- Examines the eye using an instrument comprising a special lighting system and a binocular microscope (see *Understanding biomicroscopic examination*)
- Allows ophthalmologist to view the anterior segment of the eye, including eyelids, eyelashes, conjunctiva, sclera, cornea, tear film, anterior chamber, iris, crystalline lens, and vitreous face
- Evaluates transparent ocular fluids and tissues

PURPOSE

- To detect and evaluate abnormalities of the anterior segment tissues and structures

PREPARATION

- Make sure the patient has signed an appropriate consent form.
- Note and report all allergies.
- Mydriatics aren't used for a routine eye examination because the slit lamp's bright light hurt the dilated eyes.
- Some diseases, such as iritis, require pupillary dilation to alleviate pain and allow the ophthalmologist to examine the eyes with adequate illumination.

Teaching points

- Explain the purpose of the test and how it's done.
- Explain who will perform the test and where it'll be done.
- Instruct the patient to remove his contact lenses before the test, unless the test is to evaluate the fit of the contact lenses.
- Stress the need to remain still during the test.
- Tell the patient that the examination is painless.
- Tell him that the test takes 5 to 10 minutes.

DIAGNOSTIC PROCEDURE

KEY STEPS

- Confirm the patient's identity using two patient identifiers according to facility policy.
- The patient is placed into the examining chair with both feet on the floor.
- The patient is assessed before the examination for the presence of obvious signs, such as different corneal diameters or heterochromia.
- The patient is asked to place his chin on the rest and his forehead against the bar.
- The room lights are dimmed.
- The ophthalmologist examines the patient's eyes — starting with the lids and lashes and progressing to the vitreous face — altering light and magnification as needed.
- A special camera may be attached to the slit lamp to photograph portions of the eye.
- If a corneal abrasion or ulcer is detected, a fluorescein stain allows better visualization.
- If a tearing deficiency is suspected, the ophthalmologist may examine the eye after applying a fluorescein or rose Bengal stain; he may also perform the Schirmer's tearing test.

POSTPROCEDURE CARE

- If dilating drops were instilled, tell the patient that his near vision will be blurred for 40 minutes to 2 hours after the test.

PRECAUTIONS

- Don't instill mydriatic drops into the eyes of patients with angle-closure glaucoma or in those who have a hypersensitivity reaction to the drops.

COMPLICATIONS

- Increased intraocular pressure (when mydriatic drops are used in patients with angle-closure glaucoma)
- Hypersensitivity reaction to eyedrops

INTERPRETATION

NORMAL RESULTS

- Normal anterior segment tissues and structures are noted.

ABNORMAL RESULTS

- Irregular corneal shape suggests possible keratoconus.
- A parchment-like consistency of the lid skin, with redness, minor swelling, and moderate itching, suggests a possible hypersensitivity reaction.
- Early-stage lens opacities suggest the possible development of cataracts.

Understanding biomicroscopic examination

The patient shown here is undergoing a slit-lamp biomicroscopic examination. The slit lamp directs an intense, narrow beam of light on optic tissue, allowing the ophthalmologist to see the patient's cornea and lens as layers of different optical densities, not transparent structures. This method permits accurate detection of pathologic conditions in the eye's anterior segment.

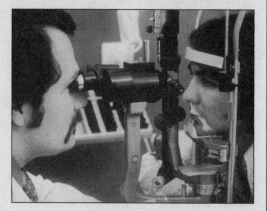

Small-bowel biopsy

DESCRIPTION
- Uses a capsule to obtain larger tissue samples for histologic analysis than in endoscopic biopsy
- Allows removal of tissue from areas beyond the reach of an endoscope (see *Endoscopic biopsy of the GI tract*)
- Causes little pain and few complications

PURPOSE
- To evaluate diseases of the intestinal mucosa that may cause malabsorption or diarrhea
- To confirm the diagnosis of some diseases, such as Whipple's disease and tropical sprue

PREPARATION
- Make sure the patient has signed an appropriate consent form.
- Note and report all allergies.
- Make sure that the patient received coagulation tests and that abnormal results were reported to the practitioner.
- Withhold aspirin and anticoagulants.
- Fasting is required for 8 hours before the test.

Teaching points
- Explain the purpose of the test and how it's done.
- Explain who will perform the test and where it'll be done.
- Tell the patient to fast for at least 8 hours before the test.
- Tell the patient that the biopsy takes 45 to 60 minutes.

DIAGNOSTIC PROCEDURE

KEY STEPS
- Confirm the patient's identity using two patient identifiers according to facility policy.
- Check the tubing and the weight bag for leaks.
- The tubing and capsule are lightly lubricated with a water-soluble lubricant and the weight bag moistened with water.
- The back of the patient's throat is sprayed with a local anesthetic to decrease gagging during passage of the tube.
- With the patient seated upright, the capsule is placed in his pharynx, and he is asked to flex his neck and swallow as the practitioner advances the tube about 20″ (50 cm). (If a local anesthetic is used to control the gag reflex, the patient must not receive any fluids to help him swallow the capsule.)
- The patient is positioned on his right side; the tube is advanced another 20″.
- The tube position is checked by fluoroscopy or by instilling air through the tube and listening with a stethoscope for air to enter the stomach.
- Next, the tube is advanced 2″ to 4″ (5 to 10 cm) at a time to pass the capsule through the pylorus.
- Talk to the patient about food to stimulate the pylorus and help the capsule pass.
- When fluoroscopy confirms that the capsule has passed the pylorus, the patient is kept on his right side to allow the capsule to move into the second and third portions of the small bowel.
- The patient is instructed that he may hold the tube loosely to one side of his mouth if it makes him more comfortable.

Endoscopic biopsy of the GI tract

Endoscopy allows direct visualization of the GI tract and any site that requires biopsy of tissue specimens for histologic analysis. This relatively painless procedure helps detect, support diagnosis of, or monitor GI tract disorders. Its complications, notably hemorrhage, perforation, and aspiration, are rare.

Endoscopic biopsy of the GI tract can be used to diagnose cancer, lymphoma, amyloidosis, candidiasis, and gastric ulcers; to support a diagnosis of Crohn's disease, chronic ulcerative colitis, gastritis, esophagitis, and melanosis coli in laxative abuse; and to monitor progression of Barrett's esophagus, multiple gastric polyps, colon cancer and polyps, and chronic ulcerative colitis.

PREPARING THE PATIENT

Careful patient preparation is vital for this procedure. Describe the procedure to the patient, and reassure him that he'll be able to breathe with the endoscope in place. Tell him to fast for at least 8 hours before the procedure. For lower GI biopsy, clean the bowel. Make sure the patient or a responsible family member has signed an informed consent form.

Just before the procedure, administer the prescribed sedative to the patient. He should be relaxed but not asleep because his cooperation is necessary to promote smooth passage of the endoscope. Spray the back of his throat with a local anesthetic to suppress his gag reflex. Have suction equipment and bipolar cauterization electrodes available to prevent aspiration and excessive bleeding.

OBTAINING THE SAMPLE

After the endoscope is passed into the upper or lower GI tract and a lesion, node, or other abnormal area is visualized, a biopsy forceps is pushed through a channel in the endoscope until this, too, can be seen. The forceps are then opened, positioned at the biopsy site, and closed on the tissue. The closed forceps and tissue specimen are removed from the endoscope, and the tissue is taken from the forceps. Then the forceps may be used to cauterize any remaining abnormal tissue to stop bleeding.

The specimen is placed mucosal side up on fine-mesh gauze or filter paper and then placed in a labeled biopsy bottle containing fixative. When all specimens have been collected, the endoscope is removed. Specimens are sent to the laboratory immediately.

(continued)

- Capsule position is rechecked by fluoroscopy, and the biopsy site determined.
- The patient is placed in the supine position so the capsule position can be verified fluoroscopically.
- A glass syringe is placed on the end of the tube, and steady suction is applied to close the capsule and cut off a tissue specimen.
- Suction is maintained on the syringe as the tube and capsule are removed; then the suction is released.
- The specimen is gently removed with forceps, placed mucosal side up on a piece of mesh, and placed in a biopsy bottle with the required fixative.
- The specimen is sent to the laboratory immediately.

POSTPROCEDURE CARE
- Tell the patient to resume his normal diet after his gag reflex returns.
- Tell the patient to report abdominal pain or bleeding.
- Monitor vital signs.
- Observe the patient for infection, aspiration, and abdominal distention.
- Monitor bowel sounds.
- Inform the practitioner of abnormal results.

PRECAUTIONS
WARNING *Watch for and immediately report signs and symptoms of hemorrhage, bacteremia, and bowel perforation.*
- Keep suction equipment nearby in case aspiration occurs.

COMPLICATIONS
- Hemorrhage
- Bacteremia
- Bowel perforation

INTERPRETATION

NORMAL RESULTS
- Normal small-bowel biopsy specimen consists of fingerlike villi, crypts, columnar epithelial cells, and round cells.

ABNORMAL RESULTS
- Histologic changes in cell structure suggest Whipple's disease, abetalipoproteinemia, lymphoma, lymphangiectasia, eosinophilic enteritis, parasitic infections (such as giardiasis and coccidiosis), celiac disease, tropical sprue, infectious gastroenteritis, intraluminal bacterial overgrowth, folate and vitamin B_{12} deficiency, radiation enteritis, or malnutrition, requiring further investigation.

Sodium level, serum

OVERVIEW

DESCRIPTION
◆ Measures serum levels of sodium in relation to the amount of water in the body
◆ Sodium: major extracellular cation; affects body water distribution, maintains osmotic pressure of extracellular fluid, helps promote neuromuscular function, helps maintain acid-base balance, and influences chloride and potassium levels
◆ Extracellular sodium level: helps kidneys to regulate body water (decreased sodium levels promote water excretion and increased levels promote retention); serum sodium levels evaluated in relation to the amount of water in the body (see *Fluid imbalances*)

◆ Sodium-water balance: regulated through aldosterone, which inhibits sodium excretion and promotes its resorption (with water) by the renal tubules to maintain balance
◆ Low sodium levels: stimulate aldosterone secretion; elevated sodium levels depress it

PURPOSE
◆ To evaluate fluid-electrolyte and acid-base balance and related neuromuscular, renal, and adrenal functions

PREPARATION
◆ Notify the laboratory and practitioner of drugs the patient is taking that may affect test results; they may be restricted.
◆ No dietary restrictions are required.
◆ The test requires a blood sample.

Teaching points
◆ Explain to the patient that the serum sodium test determines the sodium content of the blood.
◆ Explain who will perform the test and where it'll be done.
◆ Tell the patient that the test requires a blood sample and that he may experience slight discomfort from the tourniquet and needle puncture.
◆ Inform the patient that he need not restrict food or fluids.
◆ Tell the patient that the test takes less than 5 minutes.

DIAGNOSTIC PROCEDURE

KEY STEPS
◆ Confirm the patient's identity using two patient identifiers according to facility policy.
◆ Perform a venipuncture and collect the sample in a 3- or 4-ml clot-activator tube.

POSTPROCEDURE CARE
◆ Apply direct pressure to the venipuncture site until bleeding stops.
◆ If increased total body sodium causes water retention, observe for hypertension, dyspnea, edema, and heart failure.
◆ Inform the practitioner of abnormal results.
◆ Instruct the patient to resume his medications, as ordered.

Fluid imbalances

This chart lists the causes, signs and symptoms, and laboratory findings associated with hypervolemia (increased fluid volume) and hypovolemia (decreased fluid volume).

CAUSES	SIGNS AND SYMPTOMS	LABORATORY FINDINGS
Hypervolemia		
◆ Increased water intake ◆ Decreased water output due to renal disease ◆ Heart failure ◆ Excessive ingestion or infusion of sodium chloride ◆ Long-term administration of adrenocortical hormones ◆ Excessive infusion of isotonic solutions	◆ Increased blood pressure, pulse rate, body weight, and respiratory rate ◆ Bounding peripheral pulses ◆ Moist pulmonary crackles ◆ Moist mucous membranes ◆ Moist respiratory secretions ◆ Edema ◆ Weakness ◆ Seizures and coma due to swelling of brain cells	◆ Decreased red blood cell (RBC) count, hemoglobin concentration, packed cell volume, serum sodium concentration (dilutional decrease), and urine specific gravity
Hypovolemia		
◆ Decreased water intake ◆ Fluid loss due to fever, diarrhea, or vomiting ◆ Systemic infection ◆ Impaired renal concentrating ability ◆ Fistulous drainage ◆ Severe burns ◆ Hidden fluid in body cavities	◆ Increased pulse and respiratory rates ◆ Decreased blood pressure and body weight ◆ Weak and thready peripheral pulses ◆ Thick, slurred speech ◆ Thirst ◆ Oliguria ◆ Anuria ◆ Dry skin	◆ Increased RBC count, hemoglobin concentration, packed cell volume, serum sodium concentration, and urine specific gravity

(continued)

PRECAUTIONS

◆ Handle the sample gently to prevent hemolysis.
◆ In patients with increased sodium levels (hypernatremia) and loss of water, observe for signs of thirst, restlessness, dry and sticky mucous membranes, flushed skin, oliguria, and diminished reflexes.
◆ In patients with decreased sodium levels (hyponatremia), watch for apprehension, lassitude, headache, decreased skin turgor, abdominal cramps, and tremors that may progress to seizures.

COMPLICATIONS

◆ Hematoma at the venipuncture site

INTERPRETATION

NORMAL RESULTS

◆ Level is 135 to 145 mEq/L (SI, 135 to 145 mmol/L).

ABNORMAL RESULTS

◆ Increased or decreased sodium level or altered state of hydration may be found.
◆ Hypernatremia may be caused by excessive sodium intake, inadequate water intake, water loss in excess of sodium (such as diabetes insipidus, impaired renal function, prolonged hyperventilation and, occasionally, severe vomiting or diarrhea), and sodium retention (such as aldosteronism).
◆ Hyponatremia may be caused by inadequate sodium intake or excessive sodium loss because of profuse sweating, GI suctioning, diuretic therapy, diarrhea, vomiting, adrenal insufficiency, burns, and chronic renal insufficiency with acidosis.

Sodium level, urine

DESCRIPTION

- Determines urine levels of sodium, the major extracellular cation
- Less significant than serum sodium levels; test performed less often
- Evaluates renal conservation of sodium and chloride and confirms their levels in the serum

PURPOSE

- To help evaluate fluid and electrolyte imbalance
- To monitor the effects of a low-salt diet
- To help evaluate renal and adrenal disorders

PREPARATION

- Notify the laboratory and practitioner of drugs the patient is taking that may affect test results; they may be restricted.
- No dietary restrictions are required.
- The test requires urine collection over a 24-hour period.

Teaching points

- Explain to the patient that the urine sodium and chloride test helps determine the balance of salt and water in the body.
- Advise the patient that he need not restrict food or fluids.
- Tell the patient that the test requires urine collection over a 24-hour period.
- If the specimen will be collected at home, teach the patient about the proper collection technique. Advise the patient not to contaminate the specimen with toilet tissue or feces.

KEY STEPS

- Confirm the patient's identity using two patient identifiers according to facility policy.
- Collect the patient's urine over a 24-hour period, discarding the first specimen and retaining the last.

POSTPROCEDURE CARE

- Inform the practitioner of abnormal results.
- Tell the patient to resume his usual medications, as ordered.

PRECAUTIONS

- The specimen shouldn't be contaminated with toilet tissue or feces.
- Don't use a metallic bedpan for specimen collection.

COMPLICATIONS

- None

NORMAL RESULTS

- Results depend on dietary salt intake and perspiration.
- In adults, 40 to 220 mEq/L/24 hours (SI, 40 to 220 mmol/d).
- In children, 41 to 115 mEq/L/24 hours (SI, 41 to 115 mmol/d).

ABNORMAL RESULTS

- Abnormal levels indicate the need for more specific testing.
- Elevated urine sodium levels may reflect increased salt intake, adrenal failure, salicylate toxicity, diabetic acidosis, salt-losing nephritis, and water-deficient dehydration.
- Decreased urine sodium levels suggest decreased salt intake, primary aldosteronism, acute renal failure, and heart failure.
- To evaluate fluid-electrolyte imbalance, results must be correlated with findings of serum electrolyte studies.

Soluble amyloid beta protein precursor test

OVERVIEW

DESCRIPTION

♦ Assesses the extracellular deposition of amyloid beta-peptide (in the form of cerebrovascular amyloid and extracellular plaques), a major neuropathologic sign of Alzheimer's disease (AD)

♦ Amyloid beta-peptide generated proteolytically from the large beta-amyloid precursor protein (APP)

♦ APP: major protein subunit of the vascular and plaque amyloid filaments in patients with AD and in elderly patients with trisomy 21 (Down syndrome)

PURPOSE

♦ To diagnose AD
♦ To monitor the progression of AD and the effectiveness of its treatment

PREPARATION

♦ No dietary restrictions are required.

Teaching points

♦ Explain the purpose of the test to the patient and his family.
♦ Explain who will perform the test and where it'll be done.
♦ Tell the patient that he doesn't need to restrict his diet.
♦ Tell him the test should take less than 5 minutes.

DIAGNOSTIC PROCEDURE

KEY STEPS

♦ Confirm the patient's identity using two patient identifiers according to facility policy.
♦ Check with the laboratory for the appropriate tube.
♦ Perform a venipuncture and collect 5 ml of blood in the tube.

POSTPROCEDURE CARE

♦ Answer the patient's questions.
♦ Provide referral for counseling and support groups.
♦ Inform the practitioner of abnormal results.

PRECAUTIONS

♦ Maintain standard precautions while collecting the sample.

COMPLICATIONS

♦ Hematoma at the venipuncture site

INTERPRETATION

NORMAL RESULTS

♦ Establish the patient's baseline level; then track his levels over time to help determine if he will develop AD.

ABNORMAL RESULTS

♦ Mutations in the beta-amyloid precursor protein gene on chromosome 21 cause a small proportion of AD cases.
♦ Abnormal cerebrovascular levels of beta-amyloid protein (low level for the patient's age) and tau protein (high level for the patient's age) confirm the diagnosis of AD; this measurement isn't reliable for asymptomatic patients.

Speech test

DESCRIPTION

- Uses speech signals to determine the lowest level at which a patient can hear words and his ability to correctly recognize words presented above the threshold level
- Degrades speech signal by using interfering speech, filtered speech that removes frequencies, and speech that's delivered at a faster rate
- Stresses the auditory processing system to determine the patient's function in challenging conditions

PURPOSE

- To determine the degree of hearing loss for speech recognition

PREPARATION

- Review any educational materials given to the patient by the audiologist.
- Remove significant cerumen accumulation from the patient's ear canals.

Teaching points

- Explain the purpose of the test and how it's done.
- Explain who will perform the test and where it'll be done.
- Tell the patient the test should take about 1 hour.

DIAGNOSTIC PROCEDURE

KEY STEPS

- Confirm the patient's identity using two patient identifiers according to facility policy.
- To obtain the threshold of speech reception, the audiologist presents two-syllable words (spondee words) to the patient, decreasing the intensity until the threshold is obtained.
- Threshold testing results are reported as spondee thresholds, or speech reception thresholds (SRTs).
- Children may be asked to point to pictures representing the words. Very young children who lack the vocabulary to identify pictures are asked to point to body parts, such as eyes, nose, and mouth.
- Speech awareness thresholds are used in lieu of SRTs to assess the lowest level at which a patient can detect speech (usually 10 dB below the SRT).
- Speech awareness threshold testing may substitute for the SRT test in young children and for patients who speak a foreign language.
- To estimate the patient's ability to understand speech, lists of one-syllable words are presented, typically in quiet and at an intensity that's comfortable for the patient.
- The speech discrimination test or word recognition test assesses word understanding. Given at the level of typical conversational speech (40 to 50 dB hearing level [HL]), this test estimates the impact of hearing loss on communication in ideal environments. Given at an intensity level that's comfortable for the patient, it provides limited prognostic information about probable benefit from amplification. A percentage correct score is obtained.
- When there's a suspicion of cranial nerve VIII or other retrocochlear involvement, the speech understanding testing may be repeated at a very high intensity. This form of testing is referred to as *rollover testing*.

POSTPROCEDURE CARE

- Answer questions for the patient or his parents.
- Inform the practitioner of abnormal results.

PRECAUTIONS

- None

COMPLICATIONS

- None

INTERPRETATION

NORMAL RESULTS

- A normal speech threshold (spondee threshold, SRT) is −10 to 15 dB HL for children ages 2 and older and −10 to 25 dB HL for adults.
- Word recognition scores are 100%. Speech tests for auditory processing are interpreted by comparing the patient's score to age-appropriate norms.

ABNORMAL RESULTS

- Abnormal auditory processing test results are those significantly below the expected level when compared with age-appropriate norms.
- SRTs higher than 25 dB HL indicate that the patient can't hear a whispered sound.
- Thresholds that range up to 40 dB HL suggest that the patient has difficulty hearing faint or distant speech.
- If the person doesn't wear a hearing aid and has an SRT of 30 to 40 dB HL, speak to the patient in a quiet environment from a distance of no more than 6' (1.8 m).
- Speech reception thresholds above 40 dB HL indicate increasing difficulty understanding speech.
- When thresholds exceed 50 dB HL, the patient can't be expected to understand you without amplification.
- The audiologist will compare the SRT with the pure tone average to cross-check test reliability.
- The patient whose SRT and pure tone average differ by 10 dB may have misunderstood test instructions.
- The patient with nonorganic loss (exaggeration of hearing thresholds) commonly has a better SRT than pure tone testing would predict.
- Word understanding scores below 90% indicate that the patient has some degree of communication difficulty.
- The audiologist uses the score, interpreted in conjunction with the presentation level and the audiometric configuration, as a prognostic indicator of potential for success with amplification.
- The audiologist's finding of decreased word understanding at a high-intensity level indicates rollover, which, if significant, is an indicator of possible retrocochlear involvement.

Sputum culture

DESCRIPTION

- Bacteriologic examination of sputum, collected by expectoration or tracheal suctioning
- Acid-fast sputum smear: may disclose evidence of mycobacterial infection such as tuberculosis (TB)

PURPOSE

- To isolate and identify causes of pulmonary infections
- To help diagnose respiratory diseases, such as bronchitis, TB, lung abscess, and pneumonia

PREPARATION

- No dietary restrictions are required.
- The test requires a sputum specimen.

Teaching points

- Explain that specimens may be collected on at least three consecutive mornings if the suspected organism is *Mycobacterium tuberculosis.*
- Explain who will perform the test and where it'll be done.
- Inform the patient that this test requires a sputum specimen.
- Inform him that results for TB cultures take up to 2 months.
- Tell him that results for all other cultures are usually available in 48 to 72 hours.

DIAGNOSTIC PROCEDURE

KEY STEPS

- Confirm the patient's identity using two patient identifiers according to facility policy.
- Maintain asepsis; wear personal protective equipment.

Expectoration

- Instruct the patient to cough deeply and expectorate into the container.
- A Gram stain of expectorated sputum must be examined to make sure that it's a representative specimen of secretions from the lower respiratory tract (many white blood cells [WBCs], few epithelial cells) rather than one contaminated by oral flora (few WBCs, many epithelial cells).
- If the cough is nonproductive, use chest physiotherapy or nebulization to induce sputum.
- Don't use more than 20% propylene glycol with water as an inducer for a specimen scheduled for TB culturing because higher concentrations inhibit the growth of *M. tuberculosis.* (If propylene glycol isn't available, use 10% to 20% acetylcysteine with water or sodium chloride.)
- Close the container securely.
- Dispose of equipment properly; seal the container in a leakproof bag before sending it to the laboratory.

Tracheal suctioning

- Give oxygen to the patient before and after the procedure as needed.
- Attach the sputum trap to the suction catheter. (See *Using an in-line trap.*)
- Lubricate the catheter with normal saline solution and pass the catheter through the patient's nostril without suction.
- Advance the catheter into the trachea; apply suction while withdrawing the catheter, not during catheter insertion.
- Suction for only 5 to 10 seconds at a time.
- Stop suction and remove the catheter.
- Discard the catheter in the proper receptacle.

- Detach the in-line sputum trap from the suction apparatus and cap the opening.
- Label the container with the patient's name, the nature and origin of the specimen, the date and time of collection, the initial diagnosis, and any current antimicrobial therapy.
- Send the specimen to the laboratory immediately after collection.

POSTPROCEDURE CARE

- Provide mouth care for the patient.
- Monitor the patient's vital signs and respiratory status.
- Monitor oxygen saturations with a pulse oximeter.
- Inform the practitioner of abnormal results.

PRECAUTIONS

WARNING *If the patient becomes hypoxic or cyanotic during suctioning, remove the catheter immediately and give oxygen while monitoring pulse oximetry.*

- During passage through the throat and oropharynx, sputum specimens are commonly contaminated with indigenous bacterial flora.

COMPLICATIONS

- Hypoxemia
- Cardiac arrhythmias
- Laryngospasm
- Bronchospasm
- Pneumothorax
- Perforation of the trachea or bronchus
- Trauma to respiratory structures
- Bleeding

Using an in-line trap

Push the suction tubing onto the male adapter of the in-line trap.

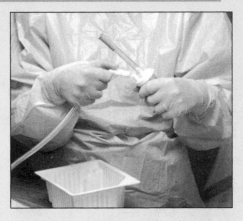

With one hand, insert the suction catheter into the rubber tubing of the trap. Then suction the patient.

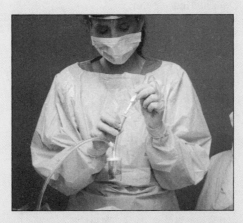

After suctioning, disconnect the in-line trap from the suction tubing and catheter. To seal the container, connect the rubber tubing to the female adapter of the trap.

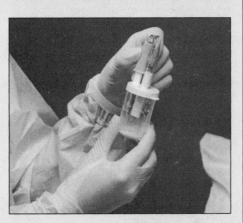

NORMAL RESULTS

◆ Common flora includes alpha-hemolytic streptococci, *Neisseria* species, and diphtheroid.
◆ Presence of common flora doesn't rule out infection.

ABNORMAL RESULTS

◆ Because sputum is invariably contaminated with normal oropharyngeal flora, a culture isolate must be interpreted in light of the patient's overall clinical condition.
◆ Isolation of *M. tuberculosis* suggests TB.
◆ Isolation of pathogenic organisms most often includes *Streptococcus pneumoniae*, *M. tuberculosis*, *Klebsiella pneumoniae* (and other *Enterobacteriaceae*), *Haemophilus influenzae*, *Staphylococcus aureus*, and *Pseudomonas aeruginosa*.

Stool culture

DESCRIPTION

- Bacteriologic examination of the feces
- Identifies organisms, prevents possible fatal complication (especially in debilitated patients), and confines infectious diseases
- Detects viruses, such as enterovirus, which can cause aseptic meningitis
- May require sensitivity testing following isolation of pathogen

PURPOSE

- To identify pathogenic organisms causing GI disease, such as typhus and dysentery
- To identify carrier states

PREPARATION

- Obtain the patient's history for dietary patterns, recent antimicrobial therapy, and recent travel that may suggest an endemic infection or infestation.
- Collect specimens before starting antimicrobial therapy.
- No dietary restrictions are required.

Teaching points

- Explain to the patient the purpose of the study and how it's done.
- Advise the patient that testing may require the collection of a stool specimen on 3 consecutive days.
- Tell the patient that he doesn't have to restrict his diet.

DIAGNOSTIC PROCEDURE

KEY STEPS

- Confirm the patient's identity using two patient identifiers according to facility policy.
- Wear personal protective equipment.
- Collect stool specimen directly in the container.
- If the patient isn't ambulatory, collect the stool specimen in a clean, dry bedpan; use a tongue blade to transfer the specimen.
- If the specimen is to collected by rectal swab, insert the swab beyond the anal sphincter, rotate it gently, and withdraw it. Place the swab in the appropriate container.
- Check with the laboratory for the proper collection procedure before obtaining a specimen for a virus test.
- Label the specimen with the patient's name, practitioner's name, hospital number, and date and time of collection.

POSTPROCEDURE CARE

- Ensure perirectal skin integrity.
- Inform the practitioner of abnormal results.

PRECAUTIONS

- Send the specimen to the laboratory immediately; be sure to include blood and mucoid portions.
- If specimens can't be transported within 1 hour, refrigerate or place it in transport media.
- Put the specimen in a leakproof bag before sending it to the laboratory.

COMPLICATIONS

- None

INTERPRETATION

NORMAL RESULTS

- More than 95% of normal fecal flora consists of anaerobes, including non-spore-forming bacilli, clostridia, and anaerobic streptococci. The rest consists of aerobes, including gram-negative bacilli (predominantly *Escherichia coli* and other *Enterobacteriaceae,* plus small amounts of *Pseudomonas*), gram-positive cocci (mostly enterococci), and a few yeasts.

ABNORMAL RESULTS

- Isolation of some pathogens (such as *Salmonella, Shigella, Campylobacter, Yersinia,* and *Vibrio*) suggests bacterial infection in patients with acute diarrhea. (See *Pathogens of the GI tract.*)
- Because normal fecal flora may include *Clostridium difficile, E. coli,* and other organisms, isolation of these may require further tests to demonstrate invasiveness or toxin production.
- Isolation of pathogens such as *C. botulinum* suggests food poisoning, although the pathogens must also be isolated from the contaminated food.
- In patients undergoing long-term antimicrobial therapy and those with acquired immunodeficiency syndrome or who're taking immunosuppressant drugs, isolation of large numbers of *Staphylococcus aureus* or such yeasts and *Candida* suggests possible infection.
- Isolation of enteroviruses suggests possible aseptic meningitis.
- A highly increased polymorphonuclear leukocyte count in fecal material suggests a possible invasive pathogen.

Pathogens of the GI tract

The presence of the following pathogens in a stool culture may indicate certain disorders:

Aeromonas hydrophila: gastroenteritis, which causes diarrhea, especially in children

Campylobacter jejuni: gastroenteritis

Clostridium botulinum: food poisoning and infant botulism (a possible cause of sudden infant death syndrome)

Toxin-producing *Clostridium difficile:* pseudomembranous enterocolitis

Clostridium perfringens: food poisoning

Enterotoxigenic *Escherichia coli:* gastroenteritis (resembles cholera or shigellosis)

Salmonella: gastroenteritis, typhoid fever, nontyphoidal salmonellosis, paratyphoid fever, enteric fever

Shigella: shigellosis, bacillary dysentery

Staphylococcus aureus: food poisoning, suppression of normal bowel flora from antimicrobial therapy

Vibrio cholerae: cholera

Vibrio parahaemolyticus: food poisoning, especially seafood

Yersinia enterocolitica: gastroenteritis, enterocolitis (resembles appendicitis), mesenteric lymphadenitis, ileitis.

Stool examination for ova and parasites

DESCRIPTION
◆ Examines a stool specimen to assess for intestinal parasites (nonpathogenic and disease causing)
◆ May reveal roundworms *Ascaris lumbricoides* and *Necator americanus* (hookworm); tapeworms *Diphyllobothrium latum, Taenia saginata,* and, rarely, *T. solium;* amoeba *Entamoeba histolytica;* flagellate *Giardia lamblia,* or *Cyclospora*

PURPOSE
◆ To confirm or rule out intestinal parasitic infection and disease

PREPARATION
◆ If the patient has diarrhea, record recent dietary and travel history.
◆ Check the patient's history for use of antiparasitic drugs, such as tetracycline, paromomycin, metronidazole, and iodoquinol, within 2 weeks of the test.
◆ No dietary restrictions are required.
◆ Treatment with castor or mineral oil, bismuth, magnesium or antidiarrheal compounds, barium enemas, and antibiotics should be avoided for 7 to 10 days before the test.
◆ The test requires three stool specimens — one every other day or every third day. Up to six specimens may be needed to confirm the presence of *E. histolytica.*

Teaching points
◆ Explain that this test detects intestinal parasitic infection.
◆ Explain who will perform the test and where it'll be done.
◆ Instruct the patient to avoid treatments with castor or mineral oil, bismuth, magnesium or antidiarrheal compounds, barium enemas, and antibiotics for 7 to 10 days before the test.
◆ Tell him that the test requires three stool specimens — one every other day or every third day. Up to six specimens may be needed to confirm the presence of *E. histolytica.*
◆ Explain that the patient doesn't need to restrict his diet, but review medication restrictions.

KEY STEPS
◆ Confirm the patient's identity using two patient identifiers according to facility policy.
◆ Put on gloves and collect a stool specimen directly in the container.
◆ If the patient is bedridden, collect the specimen in a clean, dry bedpan; then, using a tongue blade, transfer it into a properly labeled container.
◆ If the entire stool can't be sent to the laboratory, include macroscopic worms or worm segments as well as bloody and mucoid portions of the specimen.
◆ Note on the laboratory request the date and time of collection and the specimen consistency. Also record recent or current antimicrobial therapy and any pertinent travel or dietary history.

POSTPROCEDURE CARE
◆ Inform the practitioner of abnormal results.
◆ Tell the patient to resume his usual medications, as ordered.

PRECAUTIONS
◆ Send the specimen to the laboratory immediately. If a liquid or soft stool specimen can't be examined within 30 minutes of passage, place some of it in a preservative; if a formed stool specimen can't be examined immediately, refrigerate it or place it in preservative.

COMPLICATIONS
◆ None

NORMAL RESULTS
◆ No parasites or ova are present in stool.

ABNORMAL RESULTS
◆ *E. histolytica* confirms amebiasis; *G. lamblia,* giardiasis (extent of infection depends on degree of tissue invasion).
◆ If amebiasis is suspected but stool examination result is negative, specimen collection after saline catharsis using buffered sodium biphosphate or during sigmoidoscopy may be needed.
◆ If giardiasis is suspected but stool examination result is negative, examination of duodenal contents may be required.
◆ Because injury to the host is difficult to detect — even when helminth ova or larvae appear — the number of worms is usually correlated with the patient's clinical symptoms to distinguish between helminth infestation and helminth diseases.
◆ Eosinophilia may also indicate parasitic infection.
◆ Helminths may migrate from the intestinal tract, producing pathologic changes in other parts of the body. For example, *Ascaris* may perforate the bowel wall (causing peritonitis) or may migrate to the lungs (causing pneumonitis).
◆ Hookworms can cause hypochromic microcytic anemia secondary to bloodsucking and hemorrhage, especially in the patient with an iron-deficient diet.
◆ The tapeworm *D. latum* may cause megaloblastic anemia by removing vitamin B_{12}.

✦ **INTERFERING FACTORS** *Stool collected from a toilet bowl (water is toxic to trophozoites and may contain organisms that interfere with results)*

Stool examination for rotavirus antigen

OVERVIEW

DESCRIPTION
- Detects human rotaviruses using sensitive, specific enzyme immunoassays that yield results within minutes or hours (depending on assay); human rotaviruses don't replicate efficiently in laboratory cell cultures
- *Rotavirus infection:* common cause of infectious diarrhea (with vomiting, fever, and abdominal pain) in infants (especially those in group settings such as hospitals, preschools, and day-care centers) and young children ages 3 months to 2 years, occurs usually in winter; can infect all age-groups but is often more severe in young children
- Transmission likely by fecal-oral route, from person to person; in a facility setting, nosocomial spread of this viral infection causes significant harm

PURPOSE
- To obtain a laboratory diagnosis of rotavirus gastroenteritis

PREPARATION
- No dietary restrictions are required.
- The test requires a stool specimen.

Teaching points
- Explain the purpose of the test to the patient or his parents if the patient is a child.
- Inform the patient that the test requires a stool specimen.
- Explain that he doesn't need to restrict his diet.

DIAGNOSTIC PROCEDURE

KEY STEPS
- Confirm the patient's identity using two patient identifiers according to facility policy.
- Collect the specimens during the prodromal and acute stages of clinical infection to ensure detection of the viral antigens by enzyme immunoassay.
- Usually, a stool specimen (1 g in a screw-capped tube or vial) is used to detect rotaviruses. If a microbiological transport swab is used, it must be heavily stained with stool to be diagnostically productive for rotavirus.
- Avoid using collection containers with preservatives, metal ions, detergents, and serum, which may interfere with the assay.

POSTPROCEDURE CARE
- Monitor the patient's intake and output and provide him with fluids to avoid dehydration caused by vomiting and diarrhea.
- Inform the practitioner of abnormal results.

PRECAUTIONS
- Store feces specimens for up to 24 hours at 35.6° to 46.4° F (2° to 8° C). If a longer period of storage or shipment is necessary, freeze specimens at –4° F (–20° C) or colder. Repeated freezing and thawing will cause the specimen to deteriorate and yield misleading results.
- Don't store the specimen in a self-defrosting freezer.

COMPLICATIONS
- None

INTERPRETATION

NORMAL RESULTS
- No rotavirus is present in the specimen.

ABNORMAL RESULTS
- Rotavirus detected by enzyme immunoassay confirms current infection with the organism.

Sweat test

DESCRIPTION
- Quantitative measurement of electrolyte concentrations (primarily sodium and chloride) in sweat, usually through pilocarpine iontophoresis (pilocarpine is a sweat inducer)
- Used mainly in children to confirm cystic fibrosis (CF) — congenital condition that increases sodium and chloride electrolyte levels in sweat
- Genetic testing for CF available (see *Tag-It Cystic Fibrosis Kit*)

PURPOSE
- To confirm CF
- To exclude the diagnosis in siblings of those with CF

PREPARATION
- Make sure a consent form is signed.
- Note and report all allergies.
- No restrictions are required before the test.

Teaching points
- Explain the purpose of the study and how it's done.
- Explain who will perform the test and where it'll be done.
- Tell the patient that the test takes 20 to 45 minutes and that he may experience a slight tickling sensation during the procedure.

DIAGNOSTIC PROCEDURE

KEY STEPS
- Confirm the patient's identity using two patient identifiers according to facility policy.
- The area to be tested (flexor surface of the right forearm or, as with an infant, the right thigh) is cleaned using distilled water and dried thoroughly.
- A gauze pad saturated with premeasured pilocarpine solution is placed on the positive electrode; another pad saturated with normal saline solution is placed on the negative electrode. Both electrodes are applied to the area to be tested and secured with straps.

- Leadwires to the analyzer are given a current of 4 mA in 15 to 20 seconds. This process (iontophoresis) is continued at 15- to 20-second intervals for 5 minutes.
- After iontophoresis, both electrodes are removed, the pads are discarded, and the patient's skin is cleaned with distilled water and dried.
- Using forceps, a dry gauze pad or filter paper (previously weighed on a gram scale) is placed on the area where the pilocarpine was used.
- Cover the pad or filter paper with a slightly larger piece of plastic and seal the edges of the plastic with waterproof adhesive tape.
- The gauze pad or filter paper is left in place for about 45 minutes. (The appearance of droplets on the plastic usually indicates induction of an adequate amount of sweat.)
- Remove the pad or filter paper with the forceps and place it immediately in the weighing bottle.
- Carefully seal the gauze pad or filter paper in the weighing bottle and send the bottle to the laboratory.
- The difference between the first and second weights indicates the weight of the sweat specimen collected.
- Make sure at least 100 mg of sweat is collected in 45 minutes.

POSTPROCEDURE CARE
- Wash the tested area with soap and water, and dry it thoroughly.
- If the area looks red, explain that this is normal and that the redness will disappear in a few hours.

PRECAUTIONS
WARNING *Never perform iontophoresis on the chest, especially in a child, because the current can induce cardiac arrest.*
- Stop the test immediately if the patient complains of a burning sensation, which usually indicates that the positive electrode is exposed or positioned improperly. Adjust the electrode and continue the test.

COMPLICATIONS
- Electric shock if improperly performed

NORMAL RESULTS
- Sodium level is 10 to 30 mEq/L (SI, 10 to 30 mmol/L).
- Chloride level is 10 to 35 mEq/L (SI, 10 to 35 mmol/L).
- In women, sweat electrolyte levels fluctuate cyclically. Chloride levels peak 5 to 10 days before menses.

ABNORMAL RESULTS
- Sodium and chloride levels of 50 to 60 mEq/L (SI, 50 to 60 mmol/L) strongly suggest CF.
- Levels greater than 60 mEq/L (SI, > 60 mmol/L) with typical signs and symptoms confirm the diagnosis.
- Elevated sweat electrolyte levels may also suggest untreated adrenal insufficiency, type I glycogen storage disease, vasopressin-resistant diabetes insipidus, meconium ileus, and renal failure.

Tag-It Cystic Fibrosis Kit

The U.S. Food and Drug Administration approved the use of a deoxyribonucleic acid (DNA) test for diagnosing cystic fibrosis (CF). The test, called the *Tag-It Cystic Fibrosis Kit*, is a blood test that screens for genetic mutations and variations in the cystic fibrosis transmembrane conductance regulator (CFTR) gene. This test identifies 23 genetic mutations and 4 variations in the CFTR gene. It also screens for 16 additional mutations in the gene that are involved in many cases of CF.

The test is recommended for use in detecting and identifying these mutations and variations in the gene as a means for determining carrier status in adults, screening neonates, and for confirming diagnostic testing in neonates and children. There are over 1,300 genetic variations in the CFTR gene responsible for causing CF. Therefore, the test isn't recommended as the only means for diagnosing CF. Test results need to be viewed with the patient's condition, ethnic background, and family history. Additionally, genetic counseling is suggested to help patients understand the results and their implications.

Synovial fluid analysis

DESCRIPTION

◆ Insertion of a sterile needle into a joint space, most commonly the knee, to obtain a fluid specimen for analysis

◆ Performed in patients with undiagnosed articular effusion, a condition marked by the excessive accumulation of synovial fluid

PURPOSE

◆ To aid differential diagnosis or arthritis, particularly septic or crystal-induced arthritis

◆ To identify the cause and nature of joint effusion

◆ To relieve the pain and distention resulting from the accumulation of fluid within the joint

◆ To give a drug locally (usually corticosteroids)

PREPARATION

◆ Make sure the patient or a responsible family member has signed an informed consent form.

◆ Check the patient's history for hypersensitivity to iodine compounds (such as povidone-iodine), procaine, lidocaine, or other local anesthetics.

◆ Give a sedative as ordered.

◆ Withhold food and fluids as ordered.

Teaching points

◆ Explain that the test helps determine the cause of joint inflammation and swelling and also helps relieve the associated pain.

◆ Explain the procedure to the patient and answer his questions.

◆ Explain who will perform the test and where it'll be done.

◆ Instruct the patient to fast for 6 to 12 hours before the test if glucose testing of synovial fluid is ordered; otherwise, inform him that he need not restrict food or fluids.

◆ Warn the patient that although he'll receive a local anesthetic, he may still feel slight pain when the needle penetrates the joint capsule.

◆ Tell the patient the test takes about 30 minutes.

DIAGNOSTIC PROCEDURE

KEY STEPS

◆ Confirm the patient's identity using two patient identifiers according to facility policy.

◆ Position the patient and explain that he'll need to maintain this position during the procedure.

◆ Clean the skin over the puncture site with surgical detergent and alcohol.

◆ Paint the site with tincture of povidone-iodine and allow it to air-dry for 2 minutes.

◆ Know that after the local anesthetic is administered, the aspirating needle is quickly inserted through the skin, subcutaneous tissue, and synovial membrane into the joint space.

◆ Be aware that as much fluid as possible is aspirated into the syringe; at least 15 ml should be obtained, although a smaller amount is usually adequate for analysis.

Synovial fluid findings in various disorders

DISEASE	COLOR	CLARITY	VISCOSITY	MUCIN CLOT	NEUTROPHILS
Group I noninflammatory					
Traumatic arthritis	Straw to bloody to yellow	Transparent to cloudy	Variable	Good to fair	1,000; 25%
Osteoarthritis	Yellow	Transparent	Variable	Good to fair	700; 15%
Group II inflammatory					
Systemic lupus erythematosus	Straw	Clear to slightly cloudy	Variable	Good to fair	2,000; 30%
Rheumatic fever	Yellow	Slightly cloudy	Variable	Good to fair	14,000; 50%
Pseudogout	Yellow	Slightly cloudy (if acute)	Low (if acute)	Fair to poor	15,000; 70%
Gout	Yellow to milky	Cloudy	Low	Fair to poor	20,000; 70%
Rheumatoid arthritis	Yellow to green	Cloudy	Low	Fair to poor	20,000; 70%
Group III septic					
Tuberculous arthritis	Yellow	Cloudy	Low	Poor	20,000; 60%
Septic arthritis	Gray or bloody	Turbid, purulent	Low	Poor	90,000; 90%

Assist as appropriate to maintain the joint (except for the area around the puncture site) wrapped with an elastic bandage to compress the free fluid into this portion of the sac, ensuring maximal fluid collection.

If a corticosteroid is being infected, prepare the dose as necessary. For instillation, the syringe is detached, leaving the needle in the joint, and the syringe containing the steroid is attached to the needle instead.

After the steroid is injected and the needle withdrawn, wipe the puncture site with an alcohol pad.

Apply pressure to the puncture site for about 2 minutes to prevent bleeding, and then apply a sterile dressing.

If synovial fluid glucose levels are being measured, perform a venipuncture to obtain a specimen for blood glucose analysis.

For cultures

Obtain 2 to 5 ml of synovial fluid and, if possible, inoculate the medium immediately. Otherwise, add one or two drops of heparin to the specimen.

For cytologic analysis

Add 5 mg of EDTA or one or two drops of heparin to 2 to 5 ml of synovial fluid.

For glucose analysis

Add potassium oxalate, as specified by the laboratory, to 3 to 5 ml of fluid.

For crystal examination

Add heparin, as specified by the laboratory.

For other studies

For general appearance and clot evaluation, obtain 2 to 5 ml of synovial fluid, but don't add an anticoagulant.

Send the properly labeled specimens to the laboratory immediately after collection — gonococci are particularly labile. If a white blood cell (WBC) count is also being obtained, clearly label the specimen SYNOVIAL FLUID and CAUTION: DON'T USE ACID DILUENTS.

POSTPROCEDURE CARE

Apply ice or cold packs to the affected joint for 24 to 36 hours after aspiration to decrease pain and swelling. Use pillows for support. If a large quantity of fluid was aspirated, apply an elastic bandage to stabilize the joint.

Watch for increased pain or fever; these signs and symptoms may indicate joint infection.

Be careful when handling the dressing and linens of the patient with drainage from the joint space, especially if septic arthritis is confirmed or suspected.

If the patient's condition permits, tell him that he may resume his usual activity immediately. However, warn him to avoid excessive use of the affected joint for a few days even if pain and swelling subside.

Tell the patient to resume his usual diet.

PRECAUTIONS

Wear gloves when handling specimens.

Don't perform the test in areas of skin or wound infections.

Use strict sterile technique throughout the aspiration to prevent contamination of the joint space of the synovial fluid specimen.

COMPLICATIONS

Infections

Accumulation of blood in the joint

WBC COUNT/ DEBRIS	CARTILAGE CRYSTALS	ARTHRITIS CELLS	RHEUMATOID BACTERIA
None	None	None	None
Usually present	None	None	None
None	None	Lupus erythematosus (LE) cells	None
None	None	Possibly LE cells	None
Usually present	Calcium pyrophosphate	None	None
None	Urate	None	None
None	Occasionally, cholesterol	Usually present	None
None	None	None	Usually present
None	None	None	Usually present

(continued)

NORMAL RESULTS

♦ Routine examination includes gross analysis for color, clarity, quantity, viscosity, pH, and the presence of a mucin clot as well as microscopic analysis for WBC count and differential. (See *Normal findings in synovial fluid*.)

♦ Special examination includes microbiologic analysis for formed elements (including crystals) and bacteria, serologic analysis, and chemical analysis for such components as glucose, protein, and enzymes.

ABNORMAL RESULTS

♦ Synovial fluid examination may reveal various joint diseases, including noninflammatory disease (for example, traumatic arthritis and osteoarthritis), inflammatory disease (such as systemic lupus erythematosus, rheumatic fever, pseudogout, gout, and rheumatoid arthritis), and septic disease (such as tuberculous and septic arthritis). (See *Synovial fluid findings in various disorders*, pages 468 and 469.)

Normal findings in synovial fluid

FEATURE	RESULTS
Gross	
Color	Colorless to pale yellow
Clarity	Clear
Quantity (in knee)	0.3 to 3.5 ml
Viscosity	5.7 to 1,160
pH	7.2 to 7.4
Mucin clot	Good
Microscopic	
White blood cell (WBC) count	0 to 200/µl
WBC differential:	
♦ Lymphocytes	♦ 0 to 78/µl
♦ Monocytes	♦ 0 to 71/µl
♦ Clasmatocytes	♦ 0 to 26/µl
♦ Polymorphonuclear lymphocytes	♦ 0 to 25/µl
♦ Other phagocytes	♦ 0 to 21/µl
♦ Synovial lining cells	♦ 0 to 12/µl
Microbiological	
Formed elements	Absence of crystals and cartilage debris
Bacteria	None
Serologic	
Complement:	
♦ For 10 mg protein/dl	♦ 3.7 to 33.7 units/ml
♦ For 20 mg protein/dl	♦ 7.7 to 37.7 units/ml
Rheumatoid arthritis cells	None
Lupus erythematosus cells	None
Chemical	
Total protein	10.7 to 21.3 mg/dl
Fibrinogen	None
Glucose	70 to 100 mg/dl
Uric acid	2 to 8 mg/dl (men), 2 to 6 mg/dl (women)
Hyaluronate	0.3 to 0.4 g/dl
Partial pressure of arterial carbon dioxide	40 to 60 mm Hg
Partial pressure of arterial oxygen	40 to 80 mm Hg

Synovial membrane biopsy

DESCRIPTION

◆ Needle excision of a tissue specimen of the thin epithelial layer lining the diarthrodial joint capsules for histologic examination
◆ Performed when analysis of synovial fluid (a viscous, lubricating fluid contained within the synovial membrane) is nondiagnostic or fluid is absent
◆ Preliminary arthroscopy to help select biopsy site in a large joint such as the knee

PURPOSE

◆ To diagnose gout, pseudogout, bacterial infections and lesions, and granulomatous infections
◆ To help diagnose rheumatoid arthritis, systemic lupus erythematosus, or Reiter syndrome
◆ To monitor joint pathology

PREPARATION

◆ Make sure the patient has signed an appropriate consent form.
◆ Note and report all allergies.
◆ Give the patient a sedative if needed.
◆ No dietary restrictions are required.

Teaching points

◆ Explain to the patient who will perform the test and where it'll be done.
◆ Tell the patient that he doesn't need to restrict food or fluids.
◆ Assure the patient that he'll receive a local anesthetic to minimize discomfort.
◆ Warn the patient about transient pain when the needle enters the joint.
◆ Explain which site was selected for biopsy (usually, the most symptomatic joint): knee (most common), elbow, wrist, ankle, or shoulder.
◆ Tell the patient the test takes about 30 minutes and results are available within 1 or 2 days.

KEY STEPS

◆ Confirm the patient's identity using two patient identifiers according to facility policy.
◆ The patient is positioned properly.
◆ The biopsy site is prepared and draped.
◆ Local anesthetic is injected into the joint space.
◆ The trocar is forcefully thrust into the joint space, away from the site of anesthetic infiltration.
◆ The biopsy needle is inserted through the trocar.
◆ Although the trocar is held stationary, the biopsy needle is twisted to cut off a tissue segment.
◆ The needle is then withdrawn, and the specimen is placed in a properly labeled sterile container or a specimen bottle containing heparin or absolute ethyl alcohol.
◆ It's possible to obtain several specimens without reinserting the trocar.
◆ After the trocar is removed, the biopsy site is cleaned and a dressing applied.

POSTPROCEDURE CARE

◆ Instruct the patient to rest the joint from which the tissue specimen was removed for 1 day before resuming normal activities.
◆ Give the patient analgesics.
◆ Monitor vital signs.
◆ Watch the patient for bleeding into the joint.
◆ Observe the biopsy site for infection.
◆ Inform the practitioner of abnormal results.

PRECAUTIONS

◆ The test is contraindicated in areas of skin or wound infection.

COMPLICATIONS

◆ Bleeding into the joint
◆ Infection

NORMAL RESULTS

◆ Synovial membrane contains cells identical to those found in other connective tissue and is relatively smooth, except for villi, folds, and fat pads that project into the joint cavity.
◆ Synovial membrane tissue produces synovial fluid and contains a capillary network, lymphatic vessels, and a few nerve fibers.

ABNORMAL RESULTS

◆ Histologic examination of synovial tissue can diagnose coccidioidomycosis, gout, pseudogout, hemochromatosis, tuberculosis, sarcoidosis, amyloidosis, pigmented villonodular synovitis, or synovial tumors.

T- and B-lymphocyte assays

DESCRIPTION

◆ Lymphocytes: key cells in immune system; recognize antigens through special receptors on their surfaces
◆ T and B cells: two primary kinds of lymphocytes that originate in bone marrow and mature either under thymus gland influence (T cells) or without such influence (B cells)
◆ Cell separation: isolates lymphocytes from other cellular blood elements through a procedure in which a whole blood sample is layered on Ficoll-Hypaque in a narrow tube that's centrifuged, allowing granulocytes and erythrocytes to form sediment at the bottom of the tube and lymphocytes, monocytes, and platelets to forma distinct band at the Ficoll-Hypaque plasma interface
◆ Recovers about 80% of the lymphocytes but doesn't differentiate between T and B cells; percentage of T and B cells determined by attaching a label or marker and by using different identification techniques
◆ E rosette test: identifies T cells, which tend to form unstable clusterlike shapes (or rosettes) after exposure to sheep red blood cells at 39.2° F (4° C)
◆ Direct immunofluorescence: detects B cells, which have monoclonal immunoglobulin on their surfaces; unlike T cells, B cells present receptors for complement and for Fc portions of immunoglobulin

PURPOSE

◆ To help diagnose primary and secondary immunodeficiency diseases
◆ To distinguish between benign and malignant lymphocytic proliferative diseases
◆ To monitor the patient's response to therapy

PREPARATION

◆ No dietary restrictions are required.
◆ The test requires a blood sample.

Teaching points

◆ Explain the purpose of the test and how it's done.
◆ Explain who will perform the venipuncture and where it'll be done.
◆ Tell the patient that the test requires a blood sample and that he may experience slight discomfort from the tourniquet and needle puncture.
◆ Inform the patient that he doesn't have to restrict his diet.
◆ Tell the patient that the test takes less than 5 minutes.

KEY STEPS

◆ Confirm the patient's identity using two patient identifiers according to facility policy.
◆ Perform a venipuncture and collect the sample in a 7-ml green-top tube.
◆ Fill the collection tube completely and invert it gently several times to mix the sample and the anticoagulant adequately.
◆ If antilymphocyte antibodies are suspected, as in autoimmune disease, notify the laboratory.

POSTPROCEDURE CARE

◆ Apply direct pressure to the venipuncture site until bleeding stops.
◆ Because the patient may have a compromised immune system, keep the venipuncture site clean and dry.
◆ Inform the practitioner of abnormal results.

PRECAUTIONS

◆ Maintain standard precautions while collecting the sample.
◆ Send the sample to the laboratory immediately to make sure you have viable lymphocytes.

COMPLICATIONS

◆ Hematoma at the venipuncture site

NORMAL RESULTS

◆ T-cell and B-cell values may vary with laboratories, depending on test technique.
◆ T cells usually constitute 68% to 75% of total lymphocytes; B cells, 10% to 20%; and null cells, 5% to 20%.
◆ In adults, the total lymphocyte count is 1,500 to 3,000/μl, the T-cell count is 1,400 to 2,700/μl, and the B-cell count is 270 to 640/μl; these counts are higher in children.
◆ Normal T-cell and B-cell counts don't necessarily ensure a competent immune system. In autoimmune diseases, such as systemic lupus erythematosus and rheumatoid arthritis, T and B cells may be present in normal numbers but may not be functionally competent.

ABNORMAL RESULTS

◆ An abnormal T-cell or B-cell count suggests, but doesn't confirm, specific diseases.
◆ The B-cell count remains normal in many immunoglobulin deficiency diseases, especially if only one immunoglobulin class is deficient.
◆ The B-cell count decreases in acute lymphocytic leukemia and in some congenital or acquired immunoglobulin deficiency diseases.
◆ The B-cell count increases in chronic lymphocytic leukemia (believed to be a B-cell malignancy), multiple myeloma, Waldenström's macroglobulinemia, and DiGeorge syndrome (a congenital T-cell deficiency).
◆ The T-cell count may increase in infectious mononucleosis, multiple myeloma, and acute lymphocytic leukemia.
◆ The T-cell count decreases in congenital T-cell deficiency diseases, such as DiGeorge, Nezelof, and Wiskott-Aldrich syndromes, and in some B-cell proliferative disorders, such as chronic lymphocytic leukemia, Waldenström's macroglobulinemia, and acquired immunodeficiency syndrome.

Tangent screen examination

OVERVIEW

DESCRIPTION
- Evaluates central visual field in each eye by moving an object across a tangent screen, usually a piece of black felt with concentric circles and lines radiating from a central fixation point, like a spider web
- Detects and follows the progression of ocular diseases, such as glaucoma and optic neuritis, and detects and evaluates neurologic disorders, such as brain tumors and strokes
- Localizes a specific visual field defect, usually indicating the underlying pathology

PURPOSE
- To detect central visual field loss and evaluate its progression or regression

PREPARATION
- If the patient usually wears corrective lenses, tell him to wear them during the test.

Teaching points
- Explain the purpose of the test and how it's done.
- Explain who will perform the test and where it'll be done.
- Reassure the patient that the test causes no pain but requires his full cooperation.
- Tell the patient that the test takes about 30 minutes.

DIAGNOSTIC PROCEDURE

KEY STEPS
- Confirm the patient's identity using two patient identifiers according to facility policy.
- Have the patient sit comfortably about 3′ (1 m) from the tangent screen so that the eye being tested is directly in line with the central fixation target on the screen.
- Occlude the patient's left eye, and tell him that while he fixates on the central target, you'll move a test object into his visual field.
- The test object is white on one side and black on the other; its diameter varies in size from 1 to 10 mm, depending on the patient's visual acuity (for example, if he has 20/20 vision, the test object should have a diameter of 1 mm).
- Tell the patient not to look for the test object but to wait for it to appear and then to signal when he sees it. Stand to the side of the eye being tested.
- Move the test object inward from the periphery of the screen at 30-degree intervals, as represented by the radiating lines on the screen.
- Using black-tipped straight pins, plot the points on the screen at which the patient can see the object. When connected, this becomes the boundary of the areas of equal visual acuity (called an isopter).
- To guarantee the adequacy of fixation, the physiologic blind spot should be clearly identified.
- After plotting the boundaries of the patient's central visual field, test how well he can see within his visual field by turning the test object to the black side. Then turn it over within each 30-degree interval, and ask the patient to signal when he sees the test object.
- Plot suspicious areas — those in which the patient has failed to identify the test object — for size, shape, and density.
- Record the patient's visual field on the recording chart, marked in degrees, and note any abnormal areas within the field.
- Because isopters vary with the patient's age, visual acuity, and pupil size; the size and color of the test object; and the distance between the patient and the screen, carefully record all measurements.
- Occlude the patient's right eye and repeat the test.

POSTPROCEDURE CARE
- Explain that repeat tangent screen examinations can help evaluate progression or regression of a diagnosed disorder.
- Inform the practitioner of abnormal results.

PRECAUTIONS
- Remind the patient that he must maintain fixation on the central target in the tangent screen.
- The test measures only the central 30 degrees on visual field.

COMPLICATIONS
- None

INTERPRETATION

NORMAL RESULTS
- The central visual field normally forms a circle, extending 25 degrees superiorly, nasally, inferiorly, and temporally.
- The physiologic blind spot lies 12 to 15 degrees temporal to the central fixation point, about 1.5 degrees below the horizontal meridian. It extends about 7.5 degrees in height and 5.5 degrees in width.
- The test object should be visible throughout the patient's entire central visual field, except within the physiologic blind spot.

ABNORMAL RESULTS
- The inability to see the test object within the temporal half of the central visual field may indicate bitemporal hemianopsia, resulting from lesions of the optic chiasm, stroke, craniopharyngiomas in young patients, and meningiomas or an aneurysm of the circle of Willis in adults.
- Bilateral homonymous hemianopsia is uncommon but may follow multiple thrombi in the posterior cerebral circulation. Plotting visual fields after a stroke helps locate cerebrovascular lesions.
- An enlarged blind spot, a central scotoma, or a centrocecal scotoma may be caused by diseases that involve the optic nerve such as glaucoma.
- Retinitis pigmentosa, a slowly progressive disease that leads to night blindness, causes a ring 10 or more degrees away from the fixation point. The peripheral area beyond this ring is usually spared. Retinal detachment can be outlined as well.

Technetium-99m pyrophosphate scanning

OVERVIEW

DESCRIPTION
- Detects and determines the extent of recent myocardial infarction (MI)
- I.V. tracer isotope (technetium-99m pyrophosphate): accumulates in damaged myocardial tissue (perhaps by combining with calcium in the damaged myocardial cells), where it forms a hot spot on a scan made with a scintillation camera
- Used when serum cardiac enzyme tests are unreliable or when patients have equivocal electrocardiograms (ECGs) such as in left bundle-branch block
- Also known as *hot spot myocardial imaging* and *infarct avid imaging*

PURPOSE
- To confirm a recent MI
- To define the size and location of a recent MI
- To assess prognosis after an acute MI

PREPARATION
- Make sure the patient has signed an appropriate consent form.
- Note and report all allergies.
- No dietary restrictions are required.

Teaching points
- Explain the purpose of the test and how it's done.
- Explain who will perform the test and where it'll be done.
- Tell the patient that he need not restrict food or fluids.
- Reassure the patient that he will feel only transient discomfort during isotope injection and that the scan itself is painless.
- Stress the need to remain quiet and motionless during scanning.
- Tell the patient that the test takes 30 to 60 minutes.

DIAGNOSTIC PROCEDURE

KEY STEPS
- Confirm the patient's identity using two patient identifiers according to facility policy.
- Inject technetium-99m pyrophosphate into the antecubital vein.
- After 2 to 3 hours, assist the patient into a supine position.
- Attach ECG electrodes for continuous monitoring during the test.
- Scans are usually taken with the patient in several positions, including anterior, left anterior oblique, right anterior oblique, and left lateral.
- Each scan takes about 10 minutes.

POSTPROCEDURE CARE
- Answer the patient's questions.
- Inform the practitioner of abnormal results.

PRECAUTIONS
- Although rare, watch for adverse reactions to the isotope.

COMPLICATIONS
- None

INTERPRETATION

NORMAL RESULTS
- No isotope found in the myocardium.

ABNORMAL RESULTS
- Isotope is taken up by the sternum and ribs, and their activity is compared with that of the heart; 2+, 3+, and 4+ activity (equal to or greater than bone) suggest a positive myocardial scan.
- Areas of isotope accumulation, or hot spots, suggest damaged myocardium.

Tensilon test

OVERVIEW

DESCRIPTION
◆ Involves I.V. administration of edrophonium chloride (Tensilon) — a rapid, short-acting anticholinesterase that improves strength of muscles by increasing their response to nerve impulses

PURPOSE
◆ To help diagnose myasthenia gravis
◆ To differentiate myasthenic from cholinergic crises
◆ To monitor oral anticholinesterase therapy

PREPARATION
◆ Make sure the patient has signed the appropriate consent form.
◆ Note and report all allergies.
◆ Check the patient's history for use of drugs that affect muscle function.
◆ If the patient is receiving anticholinesterase therapy, note this on the requisition form with the last dose received and time it was given.
◆ Withhold drugs.
◆ Start an I.V. infusion of dextrose 5% in water or normal saline solution.
◆ No dietary restrictions are required.

Teaching points
◆ Explain the purpose of the test, how it's done, who will perform it, and where it will be done.
◆ Tell the patient that he need not restrict food or fluids.
◆ Warn the patient about possible transient unpleasant effects from the Tensilon, including nausea, dizziness, and blurred vision.
◆ Reassure the patient that someone will stay with him at all times.
◆ Inform the patient that the test takes 15 to 30 minutes and may be repeated several times.

DIAGNOSTIC PROCEDURE

KEY STEPS
◆ Confirm the patient's identity using two patient identifiers according to facility policy.

◆ Give atropine during the test to patients with respiratory disorders such as asthma to minimize Tensilon's adverse effects.

To diagnose myasthenia gravis
◆ Give the patient 2 mg of Tensilon initially. Adjust dosage for infants and children.
◆ Before giving the rest of the dose, the practitioner may want to tire the muscles by asking the patient to perform various exercises, such as looking up until ptosis develops or holding his arms above his shoulders until they drop.
◆ When the muscles are fatigued, give the remaining 8 mg of Tensilon over 30 seconds.
◆ If a placebo is used (to evaluate the patient's muscle response more accurately), observe the patient after its administration.
◆ After giving the Tensilon, ask the patient to perform repetitive muscular movements, such as crossing and uncrossing his legs.
◆ Observe the patient closely for improved muscle strength.
◆ If muscle strength doesn't improve within 3 to 5 minutes, repeat the test.

To differentiate between myasthenic crisis and cholinergic crisis
◆ Infuse 1 or 2 mg of Tensilon.
◆ After infusion, monitor vital signs continuously.
◆ Watch the patient closely for respiratory distress.
◆ If muscle strength doesn't improve, infuse more Tensilon cautiously — 1 mg at a time, up to 5 mg — and watch the patient for signs of distress.
◆ Give the patient neostigmine immediately if the test demonstrates myasthenic crisis; give atropine for cholinergic crisis.

To evaluate oral anticholinesterase therapy
◆ Infuse 2 mg of Tensilon 1 hour after the patient's last dose of the anticholinesterase.
◆ Watch for adverse reactions and muscle response.

◆ After giving the patient Tensilon, keep I.V. line open at 20 ml/hour until all responses are evaluated.

POSTPROCEDURE CARE
◆ When the test is complete, stop the I.V. infusion.
◆ Monitor vital signs and respiratory status.
◆ Monitor muscle strength.
◆ Watch for adverse effects of Tensilon.
◆ Tell the patient to resume his medications, as ordered.

PRECAUTIONS
◆ Because of the systemic adverse reactions Tensilon may produce, this test may be contraindicated in patients with hypotension, bradycardia, apnea, or mechanical obstructions of the intestine or urinary tract.

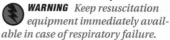 **WARNING** *Keep resuscitation equipment immediately available in case of respiratory failure.*

COMPLICATIONS
◆ Seizures
◆ Bradycardia, heart block, cardiac arrest
◆ Paralysis of respiratory muscles
◆ Bronchospasm, laryngospasm
◆ Respiratory depression
◆ Respiratory arrest

INTERPRETATION

NORMAL RESULTS
◆ Fasciculations develop.

ABNORMAL RESULTS
◆ Improvement in muscle strength (a positive response) suggests myasthenia gravis, motor neuron disease, some neuropathies, and myopathies.
◆ Patients in myasthenic crisis briefly have more muscle strength after receiving Tensilon.
◆ Patients in cholinergic crisis have more muscle weakness after receiving Tensilon.

Terminal deoxynucleotidyl transferase level test

DESCRIPTION

◆ Measures levels of terminal deoxynucleotidyl transferase (TdT), using indirect immunofluorescence

PURPOSE

◆ To help differentiate acute lymphocytic leukemia (ALL) from acute non-lymphocytic leukemia
◆ To help differentiate lymphoblastic lymphomas from malignant lymphomas
◆ To monitor the patient's response to therapy, help determine his prognosis, or obtain early diagnosis of a relapse

PREPARATION

◆ Give a mild sedative 1 hour before the bone marrow aspiration.
◆ Check the patient's history for hypersensitivity to the local anesthetic.
◆ A blood sample may be needed for the test.

Teaching points

◆ Explain that this test detects an enzyme that can help classify tissue origin.

For blood test

◆ Tell the patient to fast for 12 to 14 hours before the test.
◆ Tell the patient who will perform the venipuncture and when it'll be done.
◆ Explain that he may experience slight discomfort from the tourniquet and the needle puncture.

For bone marrow aspiration

◆ Tell the patient which bone will be the biopsy site.
◆ Inform the patient that he need not restrict food or fluids.
◆ Tell the patient that the biopsy usually takes 5 to 10 minutes.
◆ Make sure the patient or a responsible family member has signed an informed consent form.
◆ Inform the patient that although he'll receive a local anesthetic, he'll feel pressure on insertion of the biopsy needle and a brief, pulling pain when the marrow is withdrawn.

DIAGNOSTIC PROCEDURE

KEY STEPS

◆ Confirm the patient's identity using two patient identifiers according to facility policy.
◆ If the patient is to receive a blood test, perform a venipuncture and collect the sample in one 10-ml heparinized blood tube and one EDTA tube.
◆ If assisting with bone marrow aspiration, inject 1 ml of bone marrow into a 7-ml heparinized tube and dilute it with 5 ml of normal saline solution, or submit four air-dried marrow smears.

POSTPROCEDURE CARE

◆ Because a patient with leukemia may bleed excessively, apply pressure to the venipuncture site until bleeding stops.
◆ Check the bone marrow aspiration site for bleeding and inflammation, and observe the patient for signs of hemorrhage and infection.
◆ Inform the practitioner of abnormal results.

PRECAUTIONS

◆ Send the sample to the laboratory immediately.
◆ Because the patient may have a compromised immune system, take special care to keep the venipuncture site clean and dry.

COMPLICATIONS

◆ Hematoma at the venipuncture site
◆ Infection at the bone marrow aspiration site

INTERPRETATION

NORMAL RESULTS

◆ TdT is present in less than 2% of marrow cells and undetectable in normal peripheral blood.

ABNORMAL RESULTS

◆ Positive cells are present in more than 90% of patients with ALL, in 33% of patients with chronic myelogenous leukemia in blast crisis, and in 5% of patients with nonlymphocytic leukemias.
◆ TdT-positive cells are absent in patients with ALL who are in remission.

Testosterone level test

DESCRIPTION

- Competitive protein-binding test that measures level of testosterone in the blood
- Testosterone: main androgen secreted by interstitial cells of the testes (Leydig cells), which induces puberty in the male and maintains male secondary sex characteristics
- Evaluates gonadal dysfunction; performed along with plasma gonadotropin level measurement (follicle-stimulating hormone and luteinizing hormone)
- Low prepubertal levels; increased secretion during puberty stimulates growth of seminiferous tubules and sperm production; also leads to enlargement of external genitalia, accessory sex organs (such as prostate glands), and voluntary muscles and to the growth of facial, pubic, and axillary hair
- Production rises at onset of puberty and continues in adulthood; tapers at about age 40 and eventually drops to about one-fifth of peak level by age 80
- In women, small amounts secreted by adrenal glands and ovaries

PURPOSE

- To facilitate in the differential diagnosis of male sexual precocity in boys under age 10 (distinguishing true precocious puberty from pseudoprecocious puberty)
- To aid in the differential diagnosis of hypogonadism (distinguishing primary from secondary hypogonadism)
- To evaluate male infertility or other sexual dysfunction
- To evaluate hirsutism and virilization in women

PREPARATION

- No dietary restrictions are required.
- The test requires a blood sample.

Teaching points

- Explain that this test helps determine if male sex hormone secretion is adequate.
- Explain who will perform the test and where it'll be done.
- Tell the patient that the test requires a blood sample and that he may experience slight discomfort from the tourniquet and needle puncture.
- Inform the patient that he need not restrict food or fluids.
- Tell the patient that the test takes less than 5 minutes.

DIAGNOSTIC PROCEDURE

KEY STEPS

- Confirm the patient's identity using two patient identifiers according to facility policy.
- Perform a venipuncture and collect a serum sample in a 7-ml clot-activator tube.
- If plasma is to be collected, use a heparinized tube.
- Indicate the patient's age, sex, and history of hormone therapy on the laboratory request.

POSTPROCEDURE CARE

- Apply direct pressure to the venipuncture site until bleeding stops.
- Inform the practitioner of abnormal results.

PRECAUTIONS

- Maintain standard precautions while collecting the sample.
- Handle the sample gently to prevent hemolysis, and send it to the laboratory promptly.

COMPLICATIONS

- Hematoma at the venipuncture site

NORMAL RESULTS

- In men, 300 to 1,200 ng/dl (SI, 10.4 to 41.6 nmol/L).
- In women, 20 to 80 ng/dl (SI, 0.7 to 2.8 nmol/L).
- In prepubertal children, lower values than adults.

ABNORMAL RESULTS

- Increased testosterone levels may occur with a benign adrenal tumor or cancer, hyperthyroidism, and incipient puberty.
- Increased testosterone levels in women with ovarian tumors or polycystic ovary syndrome may rise, leading to hirsutism.
- Increased testosterone levels in prepubertal boys may indicate true sexual precocity caused by excessive gonadotropin secretion or pseudoprecocious puberty caused by male hormone production by a testicular tumor.
- Decreased testosterone levels can indicate primary hypogonadism (as in Klinefelter's syndrome), secondary hypogonadism (hypogonadotropic eunuchoidism) from hypothalamic-pituitary dysfunction.
- Decreased testosterone levels may also follow orchiectomy, testicular or prostate cancer, delayed male puberty, estrogen therapy, and cirrhosis of the liver.
- Decreased testosterone levels may also indicate congenital adrenal hyperplasia, which results in precocious puberty in boys (from ages 2 to 3) and pseudohermaphroditism and milder virilization in girls.

INTERFERING FACTORS *Exogenous sources of estrogens and androgens, thyroid and growth hormones, and other pituitary-based hormones (may affect test results)*

Thallium imaging

DESCRIPTION

◆ Evaluates blood flow after I.V. injection of the radioisotope thallium-201 or Cardiolite

Cardiolite

◆ Has a better energy spectrum for imaging
◆ Requires living myocardial cells for uptake and allows for imaging the myocardial blood flow both before and after reperfusion

Thallium

◆ Concentrates in healthy myocardial tissue but not in necrotic or ischemic tissue; taken up rapidly in areas of the heart with normal blood supply and intact cells; fails to be taken up by areas with poor blood flow and ischemic cells, which appear as cold spots on a scan

Rest imaging

◆ Can disclose acute myocardial infarction (MI) within the first few hours of symptoms but doesn't distinguish an old from a new infarct

Stress imaging

◆ Performed after exercise stress testing or after pharmacologic stress testing
◆ Also known as *cardiac nuclear imaging, cold spot myocardial imaging,* or *myocardial perfusion scan*

PURPOSE

◆ To assess myocardial scarring and perfusion
◆ To demonstrate the location and extent of an MI
◆ To diagnose CAD (stress imaging)
◆ To evaluate coronary artery patency following surgical revascularization
◆ To evaluate effectiveness of antianginal therapy or percutaneous revascularization interventions (stress imaging)

PREPARATION

◆ Make sure the patient has signed the appropriate consent form.

◆ Note and report all allergies.
◆ Withhold food and fluids for 3 hours before the test.

Teaching points

◆ Explain the purpose of the test and how it's done.
◆ Explain who will perform the test and where it'll be done.
◆ For the patient undergoing stress imaging, instruct him to wear comfortable walking shoes.
◆ Inform the patient that he must restrict his use of alcohol, tobacco, and nonprescription medications for 24 hours before the test.
◆ Tell the patient to fast for 3 hours before the test.
◆ Tell the patient to report fatigue, pain, shortness of breath, or other anginal symptoms immediately.
◆ Tell the patient that the test takes 45 to 90 minutes and that additional scans may be needed.

KEY STEPS

◆ Confirm the patient's identity using two patient identifiers according to facility policy.
◆ Stress imaging: the patient walks on a treadmill at a regulated pace that's gradually increased while his electrocardiogram (ECG), blood pressure, and heart rate are monitored.
◆ When the patient reaches peak stress, give him 1.5 to 3 mCi of thallium.
◆ The patient exercises an additional 45 to 60 seconds to permit circulation and uptake of the isotope.

⚡ **WARNING** *Stop the stress imaging immediately if the patient develops chest pain, dyspnea, fatigue, syncope, hypotension, ischemic ECG changes, significant arrhythmias, or other signs or symptoms (such as confusion, staggering, or diaphoresis).*

◆ Disconnect the patient from monitoring equipment as long as he's clinically stable, and position him on his back under the nuclear medicine camera.
◆ Additional scans may be taken after the patient rests and occasionally after 24 hours.

◆ Resting imaging: Give the patient an injection of thallium I.V. or Cardiolyte.
◆ Scanning is performed as in stress imaging.

POSTPROCEDURE CARE

◆ If further scanning is required, have the patient rest and restrict foods and beverages other than water.
◆ Monitor vital signs and ECGs.
◆ Watch for cardiac arrhythmias and anginal symptoms.
◆ Inform the practitioner of abnormal results.

PRECAUTIONS

◆ The test is contraindicated in pregnant patients and in those with impaired neuromuscular function, acute MI, myocarditis, critical aortic stenosis, acute infection, unstable metabolic conditions (such as diabetes), digoxin toxicity, and recent pulmonary infarction.

COMPLICATIONS

◆ Cardiac arrhythmias
◆ Myocardial ischemia, MI
◆ Respiratory distress
◆ Cardiac arrest
◆ Hypotension or hypertension

NORMAL RESULTS

◆ Normal distribution of the isotope throughout the left ventricle without defects (cold spots) is observed.
◆ After coronary artery bypass surgery, improved regional perfusion suggests graft patency.
◆ The results may be normal if the patient has narrowed coronary arteries but adequate collateral circulation.
◆ Improved perfusion after nonsurgical revascularization interventions suggests increased coronary flow.

ABNORMAL RESULTS

◆ Persistent defects suggest MI.
◆ Transient defects (those that disappear after a 3- to 6-hour rest) suggest myocardial ischemia caused by CAD.

Thoracentesis

DESCRIPTION

- Obtains specimens of pleural fluid for analysis, or therapeutically relieves respiratory symptoms caused by the accumulation of excess pleural fluid
- Examines specimens for color, consistency, pH, glucose and protein content, cellular composition, and the enzymes lactate dehydrogenase (LD) and amylase; also examined cytologically for malignant cells and cultured for pathogens
- Also known as *pleural fluid aspiration*

PURPOSE

- To provide pleural fluid specimens to determine the cause and nature of pleural effusion
- To provide symptomatic relief with large pleural effusion

PREPARATION

- Make sure the patient has signed the appropriate consent form.
- Note and report all allergies.
- Record the patient's baseline vital signs.
- If the patient will receive sedation, restrict food and fluids.

Teaching points

- Explain that pleural fluid may be located by chest X-ray or ultrasound study.
- Explain who will perform the test and where it'll be done.
- Tell the patient that he'll receive a local anesthetic.
- Instruct the patient to avoid coughing, deep breathing, or moving during the test.
- Tell the patient that the test takes about 1 hour.

DIAGNOSTIC PROCEDURE

KEY STEPS

- Confirm the patient's identity using two patient identifiers according to facility policy.

- Position the patient to widen the intercostal spaces and allow easier access to the pleural cavity.
- If the patient can't sit up, position him on his unaffected side with the arm on the affected side elevated.
- After the patient is in the proper position, prepare and drape the site.
- Inject a local anesthetic into the subcutaneous tissue; the thoracentesis needle is then inserted.
- When the needle reaches the pocket of fluid, it's attached to a 50-ml syringe or a vacuum bottle and the fluid is removed.
- During aspiration, the patient is monitored for signs of respiratory distress and hypotension.
- Monitor the patient for reexpansion pulmonary edema (RPE), a rare but serious complication of thoracentesis. Stop the test if the patient has sudden chest tightness or coughing.
- Pleural fluid characteristics and total volume are noted.
- After the needle is withdrawn, apply pressure until hemostasis is obtained and a small dressing is applied.
- Place specimens in proper containers, label appropriately, and send to the laboratory immediately.
- Pleural fluid for pH determination must be collected anaerobically, heparinized, kept on ice, and analyzed promptly.

POSTPROCEDURE CARE

- Elevate the head of the bed to facilitate breathing.
- Obtain a chest X-ray.
- Immediately report signs and symptoms of pneumothorax, tension pneumothorax, and pleural fluid reaccumulation.
- Monitor vital signs, pulse oximetry, and breath sounds.
- Observe the puncture site and dressings.
- Watch for subcutaneous emphysema.
- Monitor pleural pressure.
- Tell the patient to immediately report difficulty breathing.

PRECAUTIONS

- Supplemental oxygen is administered and close pulse oximetry is monitored during thoracentesis.
- The test is contraindicated in patients with uncorrected bleeding disorders or anticoagulant therapy.

COMPLICATIONS

- Laceration of intercostal vessels
- Pneumothorax
- Mediastinal shift
- RPE
- Bleeding, infection

INTERPRETATION

NORMAL RESULTS

- Negative pressure in the pleural cavity with less than 50 ml serous fluid is noted.

ABNORMAL RESULTS

- Bloody fluid suggests possible hemothorax, malignancy, or traumatic tap.
- Milky fluid suggests chylothorax.
- Fluid with pus suggests empyema.
- Transudative effusion suggests heart failure, hepatic cirrhosis, or renal disease.
- Exudative effusion suggests lymphatic drainage abstraction, infections, pulmonary infarctions, and neoplasms.
- Positive cultures suggest infection.
- Predominating lymphocytes suggest tuberculosis or fungal or viral effusions.
- Elevated LD levels in a nonpurulent, nonhemolyzed, nonbloody effusion suggest possible malignant tumor.
- Pleural fluid glucose levels that are 30 to 40 mg/dl lower than blood glucose levels may indicate cancer, bacterial infection, or metastasis.
- Increased amylase suggests pleural effusions associated with pancreatitis.

INTERFERING FACTORS *Improper collection of the specimen (may affect test results)*

Thoracoscopy

DESCRIPTION

- Insertion of an endoscope directly into the chest wall allowing visualization of the pleural space
- Used for diagnostic and therapeutic purposes; can replace traditional thoracotomy
- Reduces morbidity (avoids open-chest surgery) and postoperative pain, decreases surgical and anesthesia time, and allows faster recovery

PURPOSE

- To diagnose pleural disease
- To obtain biopsy specimens from the mediastinum, lung, or pericardium
- To facilitate treatment of pleural conditions, such as cysts, blebs, and effusions
- To allow resection such as wedge biopsy

PREPARATION

- Make sure the patient has signed an appropriate consent form.
- Note and report all allergies.
- Fasting for at least 10 hours before the test is required.

Teaching points

- Make sure appropriate preoperative tests (such as pulmonary function and coagulation tests, electrocardiogram, and chest X-ray) are complete; report abnormal results to the practitioner.
- Explain that it's common to use general anesthesia for this test.
- Explain who will perform the test and where it'll be done.
- Instruct the patient to fast for 10 to 12 hours before the procedure.
- Tell the patient pain medication will be available after the procedure.

DIAGNOSTIC PROCEDURE

KEY STEPS

- Confirm the patient's identity using two patient identifiers according to facility policy.
- The patient is anesthetized and a double-lumen endobronchial tube is inserted.
- The lung on the operative side is collapsed and a small intercostal incision is made, through which a trocar is inserted.
- A lens is inserted to view the area and assess thoracoscopy access.
- Two or three more small incisions are made, and trocars are placed for insertion of suctioning and dissection instruments.
- The camera lens and instruments are moved from site to site as needed.
- After thoracoscopy, the lung is reexpanded, and a chest tube is placed through one incision site.
- The other incisions are closed with adhesive strips and dressed.
- A water-seal drainage system is attached to the chest tube.

POSTPROCEDURE CARE

- Give the patient analgesics.
- Monitor vital signs and respiratory status.
- Monitor the patient's intake and output.
- Observe patency of the chest tube and drainage system.
- Monitor the patient for bleeding and infection.
- Tell the patient to resume his normal diet and activity, as ordered.

PRECAUTIONS

- Send specimens to the laboratory immediately.
- The test is contraindicated in patients with coagulopathies or lesions near major blood vessels or with extensive pleural disease or pleural adhesion and in those who can't be adequately oxygenated with one lung.

  WARNING *Be alert for complications, although rare, including hemorrhage, nerve injury, perforation of the diaphragm, air emboli, and tension pneumothorax.*

COMPLICATIONS

- Hemorrhage
- Nerve injury
- Perforation of the diaphragm
- Air emboli
- Tension pneumothorax

INTERPRETATION

NORMAL RESULTS

- The pleural cavity contains a small amount of lubricating fluid that facilitates movement of the lung and chest wall.
- The parietal and visceral layers are lesion-free and able to separate from each other.

ABNORMAL RESULTS

- Lesions adjacent to or involving the pleura or mediastinum suggest possible malignancy; will be biopsied for diagnosis and determination of treatment.
- Blebs suggest possible presence of chronic lung disease; can be removed by wedge resection to reduce the risk of spontaneous pneumothorax.
- The presence of increased pleural fluid indicates pleural effusion; specimens can be obtained for analysis and diagnosis of the cause.

Throat and nose culture

OVERVIEW

DESCRIPTION
- Requires swabbing the throat, streaking a culture plate, and allowing organisms to grow for isolation and identification of pathogens
- Obtains preliminary identification through a Gram-stained smear, which guides clinical management and determines the need for further tests
- Rapid nonculture antigen-tests: detect group A streptococcal antigen in about 5 minutes; all negative specimens should be cultured

PURPOSE
- To isolate and identify pathogens, especially group A beta-hemolytic streptococci
- To screen asymptomatic carriers of pathogens, especially *Neisseria meningitides*

PREPARATION
- Note and report all allergies.
- Maintain asepsis during all procedures.
- Wear personal protective equipment during the procedure.
- Check the patient's history for recent antimicrobial therapy.
- Determine immunization history if pertinent to the preliminary diagnosis.
- Obtain a specimen before beginning antimicrobial therapy.

Teaching points
- Explain the purpose of the test and how it's done.
- Explain who will perform the test and where it'll be done.
- Tell the patient that he doesn't need to restrict his diet.
- Warn the patient that he may gag during the swabbing.
- Tell the patient that the test takes less than 1 minute and results are available in 2 to 3 days.

DIAGNOSTIC PROCEDURE

KEY STEPS
- Confirm the patient's identity using two patient identifiers according to facility policy.
- Ask the patient to tilt his head back and close his eyes.
- With the throat well illuminated, check for inflamed areas, using a tongue blade.
- Swab the tonsillar areas from side to side; include any inflamed or purulent sites. Don't touch the tongue, cheeks, or teeth with the swab.
- Immediately place the swab in the culture tube. If a commercial sterile collection and transport system is used, crush the ampule and force the swab into the medium to keep it moist.
- Note recent antimicrobial therapy on the laboratory request.
- Label the specimen with the patient's name, practitioner's name, date and time of collection, and origin of the specimen. Also indicate the suspected organism, especially *Corynebacterium diphtheriae* (requires two swabs and a special growth medium) and *N. meningitidis* (requires enriched selective media).

POSTPROCEDURE CARE
- Answer the patient's questions.
- Inform the practitioner of abnormal results.

PRECAUTIONS
- Maintain standard precautions while collecting the sample.

COMPLICATIONS
- None

INTERPRETATION

NORMAL RESULTS
- The presence of usual or normal flora: nonhemolytic and alpha-hemolytic streptococci, *Neisseria* species, staphylococci, diphtheroids, some *Haemophilus* species, pneumococci, yeasts, enteric gram-negative organisms, spirochetes, *Veillonella* species, and *Micrococcus* species.

ABNORMAL RESULTS
- Group A beta-hemolytic streptococci (*Streptococcus pyogenes*) suggest possible scarlet fever or pharyngitis.
- *Candida albicans* suggests thrush.
- *C. diphtheriae* suggests diphtheria.
- *Bordetella pertussis* suggests whooping cough.
- *Legionella* species and *Mycoplasma pneumoniae* suggest bacterial pneumonia.
- *Histoplasma capsulatum, Coccidioides immitis,* and *Blastomyces dermatitidis* suggest fungal infections.
- Adenovirus, enterovirus, herpesvirus, rhinovirus, influenza virus, and parainfluenza virus suggest viral infections.

Thrombin time test

DESCRIPTION

◆ Measures how quickly a clot forms when a standard amount of bovine thrombin is added to a platelet-poor plasma sample from the patient and to a normal plasma control sample
◆ Allows a quick but imprecise estimation of plasma fibrinogen levels, which are a function of clotting time
◆ Also called *thrombin clotting time test*

PURPOSE

◆ To detect a fibrinogen deficiency or defect
◆ To help diagnose disseminated intravascular coagulation (DIC) and hepatic disease
◆ To monitor the effectiveness of treatment with heparin or thrombolytic agents

PREPARATION

◆ Notify the laboratory and practitioner of drugs the patient is taking that may affect test results; they may be restricted.
◆ No dietary restrictions are required.
◆ The test requires a blood sample.

Teaching points

◆ Explain that the plasma thrombin time test determines whether blood clots normally.
◆ Explain who will perform the test and where it'll be done.
◆ Tell the patient that the test requires a blood sample and that he may experience slight discomfort from the tourniquet and needle puncture.
◆ Inform the patient that he need not restrict food or fluids.
◆ Tell the patient that the test takes less than 5 minutes.

DIAGNOSTIC PROCEDURE

KEY STEPS

◆ Confirm the patient's identity using two patient identifiers according to facility policy.
◆ Perform a venipuncture and collect the sample in a 3- to 4.5-ml siliconized tube.
◆ Completely fill the collection tube and invert it gently several times to mix the sample and the anticoagulant thoroughly. If the tube isn't filled to the correct volume, an excess of citrate appears in the sample.

POSTPROCEDURE CARE

◆ Make sure that bleeding has stopped before removing pressure.
◆ If a large hematoma develops at the venipuncture site, monitor pulses distal to the site.
◆ Inform the practitioner of abnormal results.
◆ Tell the patient to resume taking his medications, as ordered.

PRECAUTIONS

◆ To prevent hemolysis, avoid excessive probing during venipuncture and rough handling of the sample.
◆ Immediately put the sample on ice and send it to the laboratory.

COMPLICATIONS

◆ Hematoma at the venipuncture site

INTERPRETATION

NORMAL RESULTS

◆ Thrombin time is 10 to 15 seconds (SI, 10 to 15 s).

ABNORMAL RESULTS

◆ A prolonged thrombin time may indicate heparin therapy, hepatic disease, DIC, hypofibrinogenemia, or dysfibrinogenemia.
◆ Patients with a prolonged thrombin time may require measurement of fibrinogen levels; in suspected DIC, the test for fibrin split products is also needed.

INTERFERING FACTORS *Heparin, fibrinogen, or fibrin degradation products (possible prolonged thrombin time)*

Thyroid biopsy

OVERVIEW

DESCRIPTION

- Excision of a thyroid tissue specimen for histologic examination
- May be performed in patients with thyroid enlargement or nodules; breathing and swallowing difficulties; vocal cord paralysis, weight loss, hemoptysis, or a sensation of fullness in the neck
- Performed when noninvasive tests, such as thyroid ultrasonography and scans, are abnormal or inconclusive
- Specimens obtained with hollow needle under local anesthesia or during open (surgical) biopsy under general anesthesia

PURPOSE

- To differentiate between benign and malignant thyroid disease
- To help diagnose Hashimoto's disease, hyperthyroidism, and nontoxic nodular goiter

PREPARATION

- Make sure the patient has signed an appropriate consent form.
- Note and report all allergies.
- Give the patient a sedative.
- Obtain results of coagulation studies and report abnormal results to the practitioner.

Teaching points

- Explain the purpose of the test and how it's done.
- Explain who will perform the test and where it'll be done.
- Tell the patient that he doesn't need to fast unless he's to receive a general anesthetic.
- Explain the use of a local anesthetic.
- Warn the patient that he might experience some pressure when the tissue specimen is obtained.
- Tell the patient that the test takes 15 to 30 minutes and results are available within 48 to 72 hours.

DIAGNOSTIC PROCEDURE

KEY STEPS

- Confirm the patient's identity using two patient identifiers according to facility policy.
- For needle biopsy, assist the patient into a supine position with a pillow under his shoulder blades. This position pushes the trachea and thyroid forward and allows the jugular veins to fall backward.
- The biopsy site is prepared.
- The patient is given a local anesthetic.
- The carotid artery is palpated, and the biopsy needle is inserted parallel to and about 1″ (2.5 cm) from the thyroid cartilage to prevent damage to the deep structures and the larynx.
- After the specimen is obtained, the needle is removed and the specimen is immediately placed in formalin.
- Apply pressure to the biopsy site until hemostasis is obtained.
- Clean and dress the biopsy site.

POSTPROCEDURE CARE

- Place the patient in semi-Fowler's position.
- Explain that a sore throat is possible the day after the test.
- Keep the biopsy site clean and dry.
- Monitor the patient's vital signs and voice quality.
- Measure neck circumference.
- Monitor the patient's swallowing ability.
- Watch for signs of infection.
- Teach the patient to avoid undue strain on the biopsy site by putting both hands behind his neck when he sits up.
- Observe for difficulty breathing associated with edema or hematoma, with resultant tracheal compression. Also check the back of the patient's neck and his pillow for bleeding every hour for 8 hours. Report bleeding immediately.

PRECAUTIONS

- Bleeding may persist in a patient with abnormal prothrombin time or abnormal activated partial thromboplastin time or in a patient with a large, vascular thyroid and distended jugular veins.

COMPLICATIONS

- Bleeding
- Infection
- Respiratory compromise

INTERPRETATION

NORMAL RESULTS

- Fibrous networks divide the gland into pseudolobules that consist of follicles and capillaries.
- Cuboidal epithelium lines the follicle walls and contains the protein thyroglobulin, which stores triiodothyronine and thyroxine.

ABNORMAL RESULTS

- Well-encapsulated, solitary nodules of uniform but abnormal structure suggest possible malignant tumors.
- Hypertrophy, hyperplasia, and hypervascularity suggest possible benign conditions such as nontoxic nodular goiter.
- Characteristic histologic patterns suggest possible subacute granulomatous thyroiditis, Hashimoto's disease, and hyperthyroidism.

Thyroid-stimulating hormone level, serum

OVERVIEW

DESCRIPTION

◆ Radioimmunoassay that measures serum levels of thyroid-stimulating hormone (TSH), also called thyrotropin, which promotes increases in the size, number, and activity of thyroid cells and stimulates release of triiodothyronine and thyroxine, which affect total body metabolism and are essential for normal growth and development
◆ Detects primary hypothyroidism and determines if hypothyroidism results from thyroid gland failure or from pituitary or hypothalamic dysfunction

PURPOSE

◆ To confirm or rule out primary hypothyroidism and distinguish it from secondary hypothyroidism
◆ To monitor drug therapy in the patient with primary hypothyroidism

PREPARATION

◆ Withhold steroids, thyroid hormones, aspirin, and other drugs that may influence test results. If the patient must continue taking them, note this on the laboratory request.
◆ Keep the patient relaxed and recumbent for 30 minutes before the test.
◆ The test requires a blood sample.

Teaching points

◆ Explain that this test helps assess thyroid gland function.
◆ Explain who will perform the test and where it'll be done.
◆ Tell the patient that the test requires a blood sample and that he may experience slight discomfort from the tourniquet and needle puncture.
◆ Tell him that the test takes less than 5 minutes.

DIAGNOSTIC PROCEDURE

KEY STEPS

◆ Confirm the patient's identity using two patient identifiers according to facility policy.
◆ Between 6 a.m. and 8 a.m., perform a venipuncture and collect the sample in a 5-ml clot-activator tube.

POSTPROCEDURE CARE

◆ Apply direct pressure to the venipuncture site until bleeding stops.
◆ Inform the practitioner of abnormal results.
◆ Tell the patient to resume his medications, as ordered.

PRECAUTIONS

◆ Maintain standard precautions while collecting the sample.
◆ Handle the sample gently to prevent hemolysis.

COMPLICATIONS

◆ Hematoma at the venipuncture site

INTERPRETATION

NORMAL RESULTS

◆ TSH levels are undetectable to 15 µIU/ml (SI, 15 mU/L).
◆ Normal levels rule out primary hypothyroidism.

ABNORMAL RESULTS

◆ TSH levels may be slightly increased in euthyroid patients with thyroid cancer.
◆ Levels greater than 20 µIU/ml (SI, > 20 mU/L) suggest primary hypothyroidism or, possibly, endemic goiter.
◆ Decreased or undetectable TSH levels may be normal but occasionally indicate secondary hypothyroidism (with inadequate secretion of TSH or thyrotropin-releasing hormone [TRH]).
◆ Decreased TSH levels may also result from hyperthyroidism (Graves' disease) and thyroiditis; both are marked by hypersecretion of thyroid hormones, which suppresses TSH release. Provocative testing with TRH is needed to confirm the diagnosis. (See *TRH challenge test*.)
◆ Low-normal and low levels may be indistinguishable, especially in secondary hypothyroidism.

TRH challenge test

The thyrotropin-releasing hormone (TRH) challenge test, which evaluates thyroid function and is the first direct test of pituitary reserve, is a reliable diagnostic tool in thyrotoxicosis (Graves' disease). The challenge test requires an injection of TRH.

PROCEDURE

After a venipuncture is performed to obtain a baseline thyroid-stimulating hormone (TSH) reading, synthetic TRH (protirelin) is administered by I.V. bolus in a dose of 200 to 500 mcg. As many as five samples (5 ml each) are then drawn at 5, 10, 15, 20, and 60 minutes after the TRH injection to assess thyroid response. To facilitate blood collection, an indwelling catheter can be used to obtain the required samples.

TEST RESULTS

A sudden spike above the baseline TSH reading indicates a normally functioning pituitary, but suggests hypothalamic dysfunction. If the TSH level fails to rise or remains undetectable, pituitary failure is likely. In thyrotoxicosis and thyroiditis, TSH levels fail to rise when challenged by TRH.

Thyroid-stimulating immunoglobulin level test

OVERVIEW

DIAGNOSTIC PROCEDURE

INTERPRETATION

OVERVIEW

DESCRIPTION

◆ Detects thyroid-stimulating immunoglobulin (TSI; formerly called *long-acting thyroid stimulator*), which appears in the blood of most patients with Graves' disease

◆ TSI: reacts with the cell-surface receptors that combine with thyroid-stimulating hormone (TSH), activates intracellular enzymes, and promotes epithelial cell activity that functions outside the normal feedback regulation mechanism for TSH

◆ Also stimulates the thyroid gland to produce and excrete excessive amounts of thyroid hormone

◆ Elevated TSH levels in 90% of people with Graves' disease; positive test results suggest Graves' disease, despite normal routine thyroid tests in those still suspected of having Graves' disease or progressive exophthalmos

PURPOSE

◆ To help evaluate suspected thyroid disease

◆ To help diagnose suspected thyrotoxicosis, especially in patients with exophthalmos

◆ To monitor treatment of thyrotoxicosis

PREPARATION

◆ No dietary restrictions are required.

◆ The test requires a blood sample.

Teaching points

◆ Explain that this test evaluates thyroid function, as appropriate.

◆ Explain who will perform the test and where it'll be done.

◆ Tell the patient that the test requires a blood sample and that he may experience slight discomfort from the tourniquet and needle puncture.

◆ Tell him that the test takes less than 5 minutes.

DIAGNOSTIC PROCEDURE

KEY STEPS

◆ Confirm the patient's identity using two patient identifiers according to facility policy.

◆ Perform a venipuncture and collect the sample in a 5-ml clot-activator tube.

◆ If the patient had a radioactive iodine scan within 48 hours of the test, note this on the laboratory request.

POSTPROCEDURE CARE

◆ Apply direct pressure to the venipuncture site until bleeding stops.

◆ Inform the practitioner of abnormal results.

PRECAUTIONS

◆ Handle the sample gently to prevent hemolysis and send it to the laboratory immediately.

COMPLICATIONS

◆ Hematoma at the venipuncture site

INTERPRETATION

NORMAL RESULTS

◆ TSI doesn't normally appear in serum, but it's considered normal at less than 130% of basal activity.

ABNORMAL RESULTS

◆ Increased TSI levels are linked to exophthalmos, Graves' disease (thyrotoxicosis), and recurrence of hyperthyroidism.

Thyroxine-binding globulin level, serum

DESCRIPTION

◆ Measures serum thyroxine-binding globulin (TBG) level, the predominant protein carrier for circulating thyroxine (T_4) and triiodothyronine (T_3)
◆ TBG: sample saturated with radioactive T_4, then electrophoresed; radioimmunoassay measures amount of TBG by amount of radioactive T_4
◆ Amount of free T_4 (FT_4) in circulation affected by conditions affecting TBG levels
◆ TBG abnormality: renders tests for total T_3 and T_4 inaccurate; doesn't affect accuracy of tests for free T_3 (FT_3) and FT_4

PURPOSE

◆ To evaluate abnormal thyrometabolic states that don't correlate with thyroid hormone (T_3 or T_4) values (for example, a patient with overt signs of hypothyroidism and a low FT_4 level with a high total T_4 level caused by a marked increase of TBG secondary to hormonal contraceptives)
◆ To identify TBG abnormalities

PREPARATION

◆ Withhold drugs that may affect the accuracy of test results, such as estrogens, anabolic steroids, phenytoin, salicylates, or thyroid preparations. If the patient must continue taking them, note this on the laboratory request.
◆ Drugs may be continued to determine if prescribed drugs are affecting TBG levels.
◆ The test requires a blood sample.

Teaching points
◆ Explain that this test helps evaluate thyroid function.
◆ Explain who will perform the test and where it'll be done.
◆ Tell the patient that the test requires a blood sample and that he may experience slight discomfort from the tourniquet and needle puncture.
◆ Tell him that the test takes less than 5 minutes.
◆ Review medication restrictions with the patient.

DIAGNOSTIC PROCEDURE

KEY STEPS

◆ Confirm the patient's identity using two patient identifiers according to facility policy.
◆ Perform a venipuncture and collect the sample in a 7-ml clot-activator tube.

POSTPROCEDURE CARE

◆ Apply direct pressure to the venipuncture site until bleeding stops.
◆ Inform the practitioner of abnormal results.
◆ Tell the patient to resume his medications, as ordered.

PRECAUTIONS

◆ Handle the sample gently to prevent hemolysis.

COMPLICATIONS

◆ Hematoma at the venipuncture site

INTERPRETATION

NORMAL RESULTS

◆ TBG level by immunoassay is 16 to 32 mcg/dl (SI, 120 to 180 mg/ml).

ABNORMAL RESULTS

◆ Elevated TBG levels may indicate hypothyroidism or congenital (genetic) excess, some forms of hepatic disease, or acute intermittent porphyria.
◆ TBG levels rise during pregnancy and are high in neonates.
◆ Suppressed levels may indicate hyperthyroidism or congenital deficiency and can occur in active acromegaly, nephrotic syndrome, and malnutrition associated with hypoproteinemia, acute illness, or surgical stress.
◆ Patients with TBG abnormalities require additional testing, such as the serum FT_3 and T_4 tests, to evaluate thyroid function more precisely.

Thyroxine level, serum

DESCRIPTION

- Measures total circulating thyroxine (T_4) level by immunoassay when thyroxine-binding globulin (TBG) is normal; common thyroid diagnostic tool
- T_4: amine secreted by thyroid gland in response to thyroid-stimulating hormone (TSH) and, indirectly, thyrotropin-releasing hormone
- Secretion regulated by negative and positive feedback system that involve the thyroid, anterior pituitary, and hypothalamus
- T_4: suspected precursor (prohormone) of triiodothyronine (T_3); believed to convert to T_3 by monodeiodination (occurs in liver and kidneys)
- Minute fraction of T_4 (0.05%) circulating freely in blood; rest binds to plasma proteins, primarily TBG; responsible for clinical effects of thyroid hormone
- TBG: binds so tenaciously that T_4 survives in plasma for a long time; half-life about 6 days

PURPOSE

- To evaluate thyroid function
- To help diagnose hyperthyroidism and hypothyroidism
- To monitor the patient's response to antithyroid medication in hyperthyroidism or to thyroid replacement therapy in hypothyroidism (TSH estimates needed to confirm hypothyroidism)

PREPARATION

- Withhold drugs that may interfere with test results. If they must be continued, note this on the laboratory request.
- If this test is to monitor thyroid therapy, the patient should continue to receive daily thyroid supplements.
- The test requires a blood sample.

Teaching points

- Explain that this test helps evaluate thyroid gland function.
- Explain who will perform the test and where it'll be done.
- Inform the patient that he need not fast or restrict activity before the test.
- Tell the patient that the test requires a blood sample and that he may experience slight discomfort from the tourniquet and needle puncture.
- Review medication restrictions with the patient.
- Tell him that the test takes less than 5 minutes.

KEY STEPS

- Confirm the patient's identity using two patient identifiers according to facility policy.
- Perform a venipuncture and collect the sample in a 7-ml clot-activator tube.

POSTPROCEDURE CARE

- Apply direct pressure to the venipuncture site until bleeding stops.
- Inform the practitioner of abnormal results.
- Tell the patient to resume his medications, as ordered.

PRECAUTIONS

- Handle the sample gently to prevent hemolysis.
- Send the sample to the laboratory immediately so that the serum can be separated.

COMPLICATIONS

- Hematoma at the venipuncture site

NORMAL RESULTS

- Total T_4 level is 5 to 13.5 mcg/dl (SI, 60 to 165 mmol/L).

ABNORMAL RESULTS

- Increased T_4 levels are consistent with primary and secondary hyperthyroidism, including excessive T_4 (levothyroxine) replacement therapy (factitious or iatrogenic hyperthyroidism).
- Subnormal levels suggest primary or secondary hypothyroidism or may be caused by T_4 suppression by normal, elevated, or replacement T_3 levels.
- When hypothyroidism can't be confirmed, TSH levels may need to be measured.
- Normal T_4 levels don't guarantee euthyroidism; for example, normal readings occur in T_3 toxicosis.
- Overt signs of hyperthyroidism require further testing.

INTERFERING FACTORS *Estrogens, progestins, levothyroxine, and methadone (may cause increased levels); high doses of free fatty acids, heparin, iodides, liothyronine sodium, lithium, methylthiouracil, phenylbutazone, phenytoin, propylthiouracil, and salicylates (decreased levels); steroids, sulfonamides, and sulfonylureas (decreased levels)*

Tonometry

DESCRIPTION

◆ Indirectly measures intraocular pressure (IOP) to screen for glaucoma (occurs in 2% of people over age 40 and is common cause of blindness); uses one of two procedures
◆ Indentation tonometry: observes how deeply a known weight depresses the cornea
◆ Applanation tonometry: observes how much force is required to flatten an area of the cornea
◆ Requires cornea to be anesthetized; follow careful examination technique
◆ If indentation tonometry shows elevated IOP, confirm diagnosis with other tests (such as applanation tonometry, visual field testing, or ophthalmoscopy)
◆ Portable tonometer used by patients with increased IOP to self-monitor

PURPOSE

◆ To measure IOP
◆ To help diagnose and follow-up evaluation of glaucoma

PREPARATION

◆ Contact lenses should be removed before the test and not reinserted until the anesthetic has worn off.
◆ Have the patient lie supine. Make sure he's relaxed, and have him loosen restrictive clothing around his neck.

Teaching points

◆ Explain that tonometry measures the pressure within his eyes.
◆ Explain who will perform the test and where it'll be done.
◆ If the patient wears contact lenses, tell him to remove them before the test and not to reinsert them until the anesthetic wears off completely, or at least 2 hours.
◆ Instruct the patient not to cough or squeeze his eyelids together.
◆ Tell the patient that the test takes only a few minutes and requires that his eyes be anesthetized; reassure him that the procedure is painless.

◆ Tell the patient not to rub his eyes for at least 20 minutes after the test to prevent corneal abrasion.

DIAGNOSTIC PROCEDURE

KEY STEPS

◆ Confirm the patient's identity using two patient identifiers according to facility policy.
◆ Ask the patient to look down. Raise his superior eyelid with your thumb, place one drop of the topical anesthetic at the top of the sclera, and have the patient blink.
◆ Check the tonometer for a zero reading on the steel test block that comes with the instrument. Make sure the plunger moves freely. The first measurement on each eye is obtained with the 5.5-g weight.
◆ Have the patient look up and stare at a spot on the ceiling. Then ask him to open his mouth, take a deep breath, and exhale slowly for distraction.
◆ With the thumb and forefinger of one hand, hold the lids of his right eye open against the orbital rim.
◆ Hold the tonometer vertically with the thumb and forefinger of the other hand, and rest the footplate on the apex of the cornea.
◆ With the footplate in place, check the indicator needle for a rhythmic transmission caused by the ocular pulse, and then record the calibrated scale reading that converts to a measurement of IOP.
◆ If the reading doesn't exceed 4, add an additional weight (7.5, 10, or 15 g) to obtain a reliable result.
◆ Repeat the procedure on the left eye and record the time the test is performed.

POSTPROCEDURE CARE

◆ Tell the patient that if he feels a scratching sensation on his eye, it should disappear within 24 hours.

PRECAUTIONS

◆ Avoid the test in patients with corneal ulcer or infection, except by skilled examiner and only in an emergency such as suspected acute angle-closure glaucoma.

COMPLICATIONS

◆ Resting your fingers on the cornea or pressing on the cornea (increases IOP)
◆ Touching the patient's lashes (may trigger a blink response or Bell's phenomenon: upward movement of the eyes with forced closure of the lids, which can cause the footplate to move and scratch the cornea)

NORMAL RESULTS

◆ IOP is 12 to 20 mm Hg, with diurnal variations: the highest point is upon waking; the lowest point, in the evening.

ABNORMAL RESULTS

◆ Increased IOP requires further testing for glaucoma.
◆ Because IOP varies diurnally, findings must be supplemented with serial measurements obtained at different times on different days.

TORCH test

DESCRIPTION
- Detects exposure to pathogens from toxoplasmosis, rubella, cytomegalovirus, and herpes simplex antibodies (TORCH)
- TORCH: pathogens often linked to asymptomatic congenital and neonatal infections that may severely impair the central nervous system
- Detects specific immunoglobulin M–associated antibodies in infant blood

PURPOSE
- To help diagnose acute, congenital, and intrapartum infections

PREPARATION
- No dietary restrictions are required.
- The test requires a blood sample.

Teaching points
- Explain to the parents the purpose of the test.
- Tell the parents that the test requires a blood sample and that the patient may experience slight discomfort from the tourniquet and needle puncture.
- Tell the parents that the test should take less than 5 minutes.

DIAGNOSTIC PROCEDURE

KEY STEPS
- Confirm the patient's identity using two patient identifiers according to facility policy.
- Obtain a 3-ml sample of venous or cord blood.
- Send the sample to the laboratory immediately.

POSTPROCEDURE CARE
- Apply direct pressure to the venipuncture site until bleeding stops.
- Inform the practitioner of abnormal results.

PRECAUTIONS
- Handle the sample gently to prevent hemolysis.
- Don't freeze the sample.

COMPLICATIONS
- Hematoma at the venipuncture site

INTERPRETATION

NORMAL RESULTS
- Results are negative for TORCH pathogens.

ABNORMAL RESULTS
- Toxoplasmosis is diagnosed by sequential examination that shows rising antibody titers, changing titers, and serologic conversion from negative to positive; a titer of 1:256 suggests recent *Toxoplasma* infection.
- In infants younger than age 6 months, rubella infection is linked to a marked and persistent rise in complement-fixing antibody titer over time.
- Persistence of rubella antibody in an infant after age 6 months strongly suggests congenital infection, which may lead to cardiac anomalies, neurosensory deafness, growth retardation, and encephalitic symptoms.
- In infants, a screen for congenital infections may show the presence of antibodies, which may indicate diseases such as cytomegalovirus and syphilis.
- Detection of herpes antibodies in cerebrospinal fluid with signs of herpetic encephalitis and persistent herpes simplex virus type 2 antibody levels confirms herpes simplex infection in a neonate without obvious herpetic lesions.

Total carbon dioxide content test

DESCRIPTION

- Measures total concentration of all forms of carbon dioxide (CO_2) in serum, plasma, or whole blood samples
- Assesses bicarbonate levels because 90% of CO_2 appears in the serum as bicarbonate
- Reflects adequacy of gas exchange in the lungs and efficiency of the carbonic acid–bicarbonate buffer system, which maintains acid-base balance and normal pH
- Performed in patients with respiratory insufficiency; usually included in assessment of electrolyte balance
- Results most significant when considered with pH and arterial blood gas values

PURPOSE

- To help evaluate acid-base balance

PREPARATION

- Notify the laboratory and practitioner of drugs the patient is taking that may affect test results; they may be restricted.
- The test requires a blood sample.
- No dietary restrictions are required.

Teaching points

- Explain that the total CO_2 content test measures the amount of CO_2 in his blood.
- Explain who will perform the test and where it'll be done.
- Tell the patient that the test requires a blood sample and that he may experience slight discomfort from the tourniquet and needle puncture.
- Inform him that he doesn't need to restrict food or fluids.
- Tell the patient that the test takes less than 5 minutes.

KEY STEPS

- Confirm the patient's identity using two patient identifiers according to facility policy.
- Perform a venipuncture.
- When CO_2 content is measured along with electrolytes, use a 3- or 4-ml clot-activator tube.
- When this test is performed alone, use a heparinized tube.

POSTPROCEDURE CARE

- Apply direct pressure to the venipuncture site until bleeding stops.
- Inform the practitioner of abnormal results.
- Tell the patient to resume his medications, as ordered.

PRECAUTIONS

- Fill the tube completely to prevent diffusion of CO_2 into the vacuum.

COMPLICATIONS

- Hematoma at the venipuncture site

NORMAL RESULTS

- Total CO_2 level is 22 to 26 mEq/L (SI, 22 to 26 mmol/L).
- Levels vary, depending on the patient's sex and age.

ABNORMAL RESULTS

- CO_2 pressure in red blood cells over 40 mm Hg causes CO_2 to spill out of the cells and dissolve in plasma; may combine with water to form carbonic acid, which may dissociate into hydrogen and bicarbonate ions.
- High CO_2 levels may occur in metabolic alkalosis, respiratory acidosis, primary aldosteronism, and Cushing's syndrome.
- Levels may also increase after excessive loss of acids, such as severe vomiting and continuous gastric drainage.
- Decreased CO_2 levels are common in metabolic acidosis, possibly from loss of bicarbonate, and in respiratory alkalosis.

INTERFERING FACTORS *Excessive use of corticotropin, cortisone, or thiazide diuretics and excessive ingestion of alkali or licorice (may increase levels); salicylates, paraldehyde, methicillin, dimercaprol, ammonium chloride, and acetazolamide and ingestion of ethylene glycol or methyl alcohol (may decrease levels)*

Total cholesterol level test

DESCRIPTION

- Quantitative analysis of serum cholesterol that measures circulating levels of free cholesterol and cholesterol esters; reflects level of two forms in which this biochemical compound appears in body
- High serum cholesterol levels: may be linked to an increased risk of coronary artery disease (CAD)
- Three-minute skin test: available for use in practitioner's office (see *Skin test for cholesterol*)

PURPOSE

- To assess the risk of CAD
- To evaluate fat metabolism
- To help diagnose nephrotic syndrome, pancreatitis, hepatic disease, hypothyroidism, and hyperthyroidism
- To assess the efficacy of lipid-lowering drug therapy

PREPARATION

- Notify the laboratory and practitioner of drugs the patient is taking that may affect test results; they may be restricted.
- Withhold food and fluid, except water, for 12 hours before the test.
- The test requires a blood sample.

Teaching points

- Explain that the total cholesterol test assesses the body's fat metabolism.
- Explain who will perform the test and where it'll be done.
- Tell the patient that the test requires a blood sample and that he may experience slight discomfort from the tourniquet and needle puncture.
- Instruct the patient to fast for 12 hours before the test; tell him he can drink water.
- Tell the patient that the test takes less than 5 minutes.

DIAGNOSTIC PROCEDURE

KEY STEPS

- Confirm the patient's identity using two patient identifiers according to facility policy.
- The patient should be in a sitting position for 5 minutes before the blood is drawn.
- Perform a venipuncture and collect the sample in a 4-ml EDTA tube.
- Fingersticks may also be used for initial screening when using an automated analyzer.

POSTPROCEDURE CARE

- Apply direct pressure to the venipuncture site until bleeding stops.
- Inform the practitioner of abnormal results.
- Tell the patient to resume his usual diet and medications, as ordered.

PRECAUTIONS

- Maintain standard precautions while collecting the sample.
- Send the sample to the laboratory immediately.

COMPLICATIONS

- Hematoma at the venipuncture site

INTERPRETATION

NORMAL RESULTS

- In men, less than 205 mg/dl (SI, < 5.3 mmol/L).
- In women, less than 190 mg/dl (SI, < 4.9 mmol/L).
- In children ages 12 to 18, less than 170 mg/dl (SI, < 4.4 mmol/L).

ABNORMAL RESULTS

- Increased serum cholesterol levels (hypercholesterolemia) may indicate a risk of CAD, incipient hepatitis, lipid disorders, bile duct blockage, nephrotic syndrome, obstructive jaundice, pancreatitis, and hypothyroidism.
- Decreased serum cholesterol levels (hypocholesterolemia) are usually linked to malnutrition, cellular necrosis of the liver, and hyperthyroidism.
- Abnormal cholesterol levels usually require further testing to determine the cause.

Skin test for cholesterol

A 3-minute test that measures the amount of cholesterol in the skin rather than in the blood is available. It measures how much cholesterol is present in other tissues in the body and provides additional data about a person's risk of heart disease.

The test, which doesn't require patients to fast, involves placing a bandagelike applicator pad on the palm of the hand. Drops of a special solution that reacts to skin cholesterol are then added to the pad; 3 minutes later, a handheld computer translates the information into a skin cholesterol reading.

Because the test measures the amount of cholesterol that has accumulated in the tissues over time, results don't correlate with blood cholesterol levels, so the test isn't meant to be a substitute or surrogate for a blood cholesterol test. In addition, the Food and Drug Administration cautions that the test isn't intended for use as a screening tool for heart disease in the general population. Instead, it has been approved for use among adults with severe heart disease — those with at least a 50% blockage of two or more heart arteries.

Total hemoglobin level test

DESCRIPTION

- Measures the amount of hemoglobin (Hb) in a deciliter (dl, or 100 ml) of whole blood

PURPOSE

- To measure the severity of anemia or polycythemia and to monitor response to therapy
- To obtain data for calculating the mean corpuscular hemoglobin (MCH) and mean corpuscular hemoglobin concentration (MCHC)

PREPARATION

- No dietary restrictions are required.
- The test requires a blood sample.

Teaching points

- Explain that the total Hb test detects anemia or polycythemia or assesses the patient's response to therapy.
- Explain who will perform the test and where it'll be done.
- Tell the patient that the test requires a blood sample and that he may experience slight discomfort from the tourniquet and needle puncture.
- Tell him that he doesn't need to fast.
- Tell the patient that the test takes less than 5 minutes.

KEY STEPS

- Confirm the patient's identity using two patient identifiers according to facility policy.
- Perform a venipuncture and collect the sample in a 3- or 4.5-ml EDTA tube.

POSTPROCEDURE CARE

- Apply pressure until the bleeding stops.
- If a hematoma develops at the venipuncture site, apply pressure.
- Inform the practitioner of abnormal results.

PRECAUTIONS

- Completely fill the collection tube and invert it several times to thoroughly mix the sample and the anticoagulant.
- Handle the sample gently to prevent hemolysis.

COMPLICATIONS

- Hematoma at venipuncture site

NORMAL RESULTS

- Hb concentration varies depending on the type of sample drawn and the patient's sex and age.
- Adult males, 14 to 17.4 g/dl (SI, 140 to 174 g/L).
- Adult females, 12 to 16 g/dl (SI, 120 to 160 g/L).
- Neonates, 17 to 22 g/dl (SI, 170 to 220 g/L).
- Up to age 1 week, 15 to 20 g/dl (SI, 150 to 200 g/L).
- Up to age 1 month, 11 to 15 g/dl (SI, 110 to 150 g/L).
- Ages 2 months to 6 months, 10.7 to 17.3 g/dl (SI, 107 to 173 g/L).
- Ages 6 months to 1 year, 9.9 to 14.5 g/dl (SI, 99 to 145 g/L).
- Ages 1 to 6, 9.5 to 14.1 g/dl (SI, 95 to 141 g/L).
- Ages 6 to 16, 10.3 to 14.9 g/dl (SI, 103 to 149 g/L).
- Ages 16 to 18, 11.1 to 15.7 g/dl (SI, 111 to 157 g/L).
- Persons who are more active or who live in high altitudes may have higher values.

ABNORMAL RESULTS

- Low Hb concentration may indicate anemia, recent hemorrhage, or fluid retention, causing hemodilution.
- Elevated Hb suggests hemoconcentration from polycythemia or dehydration.

Transcranial Doppler studies

OVERVIEW

DESCRIPTION
◆ Provide information about the presence, quality, and changing nature of circulation to an area of the brain by measuring the velocity of blood flow through cerebral arteries
◆ Advantageous because studies provide diagnostic information noninvasively
◆ After transcranial Doppler studies and before surgery: patients may undergo cerebral angiography to further define cerebral blood flow patterns and to locate the exact vascular abnormality

PURPOSE
◆ To measure the velocity of blood flow through certain cerebral vessels
◆ To detect and monitor the progression of cerebral vasospasm
◆ To determine the presence of collateral blood flow before surgical ligation or radiologic occlusion of diseased blood vessels

PREPARATION
◆ No dietary restrictions are required.

Teaching points
◆ Explain the purpose of the test and how it's done.
◆ Explain who will perform the test and where it'll be done.
◆ Tell the patient that he doesn't need to fast before the test.
◆ Explain that the test usually takes less than 1 hour, depending on the number of vessels to be examined and any interfering factors.

DIAGNOSTIC PROCEDURE

KEY STEPS
◆ Confirm the patient's identity using two patient identifiers according to facility policy.
◆ The patient reclines in a chair or on a stretcher or bed.
◆ A small amount of gel is applied to the transcranial "window" (temporal, transorbital, and through the fora-

men magnum), where bone is thin enough to allow the Doppler signal to enter and be detected.
◆ The technician directs the signal toward the artery being studied and then records the velocities detected.
◆ In a complete study, the middle cerebral arteries, anterior cerebral arteries, ophthalmic arteries, carotid siphon, vertebral arteries, and basilar artery are studied.
◆ The Doppler signal can be transmitted to varying depths.
◆ Waveforms may be printed for later analysis.

POSTPROCEDURE CARE
◆ Remove any remaining gel from the patient's skin.
◆ Inform the practitioner of abnormal results.

PRECAUTIONS
◆ Dressing over the test site may affect the accuracy of results.

COMPLICATIONS
◆ None

INTERPRETATION

NORMAL RESULTS
◆ Normal waveforms and velocities are observed.

ABNORMAL RESULTS
◆ High velocities suggest that blood flow is too turbulent or the vessel is too narrow; or possible stenosis, vasospasm, or arteriovenous malformation. (See *Comparing velocity waveforms*.)

Comparing velocity waveforms

A normal transcranial Doppler signal is usually characterized by mean velocities that fall within the normal reported values. Additional information can be gathered by evaluating the shape of the velocity waveform.

EFFECT OF SIGNIFICANT PROXIMAL VESSEL OBSTRUCTION
A delayed systolic upstroke can be seen in a waveform when significant proximal vessel obstruction is present.

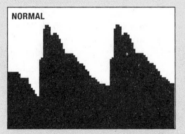
NORMAL

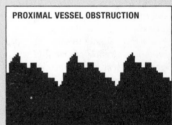
PROXIMAL VESSEL OBSTRUCTION

EFFECT OF INCREASED CEREBROVASCULAR RESISTANCE
Changes in cerebrovascular resistance, as occur with increased intracranial pressure, cause a decrease in diastolic flow.

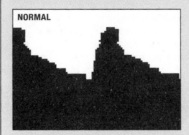
NORMAL

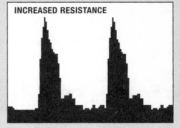
INCREASED RESISTANCE

Transesophageal echocardiography

DESCRIPTION
◆ Combines ultrasonography with endoscopy to provide a better view of the heart's structures
◆ Involves a small transducer attached to the end of a gastroscope and inserted into the esophagus, allowing images to be taken from the posterior aspect of the heart
◆ Causes less tissue penetration and interference from chest wall structures and produces high-quality images of the thoracic aorta, except for the superior ascending aorta, which is shadowed by the trachea

PURPOSE
◆ To visualize and evaluate thoracic and aortic disorders, such as dissection and aneurysm; valvular disease (especially of the mitral valve); endocarditis; and congenital heart disease
◆ To visualize and evaluate intracardiac thrombi, cardiac tumors, cardiac tamponade, and ventricular dysfunction

PREPARATION
◆ Make sure the patient has signed an appropriate consent form.
◆ Note and report all allergies.
◆ Review the patient's medical history and report possible contraindications to the test, such as esophageal obstruction or varices, GI bleeding, previous mediastinal radiation therapy, or severe cervical arthritis.
◆ Note and report any loose teeth.
◆ Fasting for 6 hours before the test is needed.

Teaching points
◆ Explain who will perform the test and where it'll be done.
◆ Explain the need for I.V. sedation and continuous monitoring during the study.
◆ Tell the patient to fast for 6 hours before the procedure.
◆ Instruct the patient to remove dentures or oral prostheses.
◆ Explain the use of a topical anesthetic throat spray.

◆ Warn the patient that he may gag when the tube is inserted.
◆ Tell the patient that the study takes about 2 hours, including preparation and recovery.
◆ If the procedure is done on an outpatient basis, advise the patient to have someone drive him home.

DIAGNOSTIC PROCEDURE

KEY STEPS
◆ Confirm the patient's identity using two patient identifiers according to facility policy.
◆ Connect the patient to monitors for continual blood pressure, heart rate, and pulse oximetry assessment.
◆ Assist the patient into a supine position on his left side and give him a sedative.
◆ Spray the back of his throat with a topical anesthetic.
◆ Place a bite block in the patient's mouth and instruct him to close his lips around it.
◆ The endoscope is inserted and advanced 12″ to 14″ (30 to 36 cm) to the level of the right atrium.

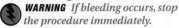 **WARNING** *If bleeding occurs, stop the procedure immediately.*

◆ To visualize the left ventricle, the scope is advanced 16″ to 18″ (41 to 46 cm).
◆ Ultrasound images are obtained and reviewed.

POSTPROCEDURE CARE
◆ Ensure the patient's safety and a patent airway until the sedative wears off.
◆ Withhold food and water until his gag reflex returns.
◆ Monitor the patient's level of consciousness and vital signs.
◆ Monitor the patient's respiratory status and cardiac arrhythmias.
◆ Watch for bleeding.
◆ Observe for gag reflex.
◆ Use pulse oximetry to detect hypoxia.

PRECAUTIONS
◆ Keep resuscitation and suction equipment immediately available.

◆ Observe closely for a vasovagal response, which may occur with gagging.
◆ Laryngospasm, arrhythmias, or bleeding increases the risk of complications. Postpone the test if these occur.

COMPLICATIONS
◆ Adverse reaction to sedation
◆ Bleeding
◆ Cardiac arrhythmias
◆ Laryngospasm

NORMAL RESULTS
◆ The heart is without structural abnormalities.
◆ No vegetations or thrombi are visible.
◆ No tumors are visible.

ABNORMAL RESULTS
◆ Structural thoracic and aortic abnormalities suggest possible endocarditis, congenital heart disease, intracardiac thrombi, or tumors.
◆ Congenital defects suggest possible patent ductus arteriosus.

Transferrin level test

DESCRIPTION

◆ Quantitatively analyzes serum levels of transferrin (siderophilin), a glycoprotein formed in the liver; evaluates iron metabolism; and simultaneously obtains serum iron level
◆ Transports circulating iron obtained from dietary sources or the breakdown of red blood cells by reticuloendothelial cells to bone marrow for use in hemoglobin synthesis or to the liver, spleen, and bone marrow for storage

PURPOSE

◆ To determine the iron-transporting capacity of the blood
◆ To evaluate iron metabolism in iron-deficiency anemia

PREPARATION

◆ Notify the laboratory and practitioner of drugs the patient is taking that may affect test results; they may be restricted.
◆ No dietary restrictions are required.
◆ The test requires a blood sample.

Teaching points

◆ Explain that the transferrin test determines the cause of anemia.
◆ Explain who will perform the test and where it'll be done.
◆ Tell the patient that the test requires a blood sample and that he may experience slight discomfort from the tourniquet and needle puncture.
◆ Tell him that he doesn't need to restrict food and fluids.
◆ Explain that the test takes less than 5 minutes.

DIAGNOSTIC PROCEDURE

KEY STEPS

◆ Confirm the patient's identity using two patient identifiers according to facility policy.
◆ Perform a venipuncture and collect the sample in a 4-ml clot-activator tube.

POSTPROCEDURE CARE

◆ Apply direct pressure to the venipuncture site until bleeding stops.
◆ Inform the practitioner of abnormal results.
◆ Tell the patient to resume his medications, as ordered.

PRECAUTIONS

◆ Handle the sample gently to prevent hemolysis.
◆ Send the sample to the laboratory immediately.

COMPLICATIONS

◆ Hematoma at the venipuncture site

INTERPRETATION

NORMAL RESULTS

◆ Level is 200 to 400 mg/dl (SI, 2 to 4 g/L).

ABNORMAL RESULTS

◆ Inadequate transferrin levels may lead to impaired hemoglobin synthesis and, possibly, anemia.
◆ Low serum levels may indicate inadequate transferrin production caused by hepatic damage or excessive protein loss from renal disease.
◆ Decreased transferrin levels may also result from acute or chronic infection and cancer.
◆ Increased serum transferrin levels may indicate severe iron deficiency.

INTERFERING FACTORS *Hormonal contraceptives and late pregnancy (possible increase in level)*

Transvaginal ultrasonography

OVERVIEW

DESCRIPTION

◆ Uses high-frequency sound waves to produce images of the pelvic structures
◆ Allows evaluation of pelvic anatomy and diagnosis of pregnancy at an earlier gestational age
◆ Eliminates need for a full bladder and circumvents difficulties encountered with obese patients
◆ Also known as *endovaginal ultrasound*

PURPOSE

◆ To establish early pregnancy with fetal heart motion as early as the 5th to 6th week of gestation
◆ To identify ectopic pregnancy
◆ To monitor follicular growth during infertility treatment
◆ To evaluate abnormal pregnancy (such as blighted ovum, missed or incomplete abortion, or molar pregnancy)
◆ To visualize retained products of conception
◆ To diagnose fetal abnormalities, placental location, and cervical length
◆ To evaluate adnexal pathology, such as tubo-ovarian abscess, hydrosalpinx, and ovarian masses
◆ To evaluate the uterine lining (in patients with dysfunctional uterine bleeding and postmenopausal bleeding)

PREPARATION

◆ Note and report all allergies.
◆ If the sonographer is a man, assure the patient that a female assistant will be present during the examination.
◆ No dietary restrictions are required.

Teaching points

◆ Explain that the test requires insertion of a vaginal probe and that self-insertion may be possible.
◆ Explain the purpose of the test and how it's done.
◆ Tell the patient she doesn't need to restrict her diet.
◆ Tell her that the test takes about 30 minutes.

DIAGNOSTIC PROCEDURE

KEY STEPS

◆ Confirm the patient's identity using two patient identifiers according to facility policy.
◆ Assist the patient into the lithotomy position.
◆ Water-soluble gel is placed on the transducer tip to allow better sound transmission, and a protective sheath is placed over the transducer.
◆ Additional lubricant is placed on the sheathed transducer tip, which is gently inserted into the vagina by the patient or the sonographer.
◆ The pelvic structures are observed by rotating the probe 90 degrees to one side and then the other.

POSTPROCEDURE CARE

◆ Help the patient remove residual gel.

PRECAUTIONS

◆ Make sure the patient has privacy during the examination.

COMPLICATIONS

◆ None

INTERPRETATION

NORMAL RESULTS

◆ The uterus and ovaries are normal in size and shape.
◆ The body of the uterus lies on the superior surface of the bladder; the uterine tubes are attached laterally.
◆ The ovaries are located on the lateral pelvic walls with the external iliac vessels above and the ureters posteroinferior, and are covered by the fimbria of the uterine tubes medially.
◆ In pregnancy, the gestational sac and fetus are of normal size for the gestational period.

ABNORMAL RESULTS

◆ Free peritoneal fluid in the pelvic cavity suggests possible peritonitis.
◆ A tubal mass suggests possible ectopic pregnancy.
◆ Structural abnormalities in a nonpregnant woman may indicate cancer of the uterus, ovaries, vagina, and other pelvic structures; noncancerous growths of the uterus and ovaries; ovarian torsion; areas of infection, including pelvic inflammatory disease; and congenital malformations.
◆ Structural abnormalities in a pregnant woman may suggest threatened abortion; multiple pregnancies; fetal death; placental abnormalities, including placenta previa and placental abruption; and tumors of pregnancy, including gestational trophoblastic disease.

Triglycerides level test

DESCRIPTION
- Provides quantitative analysis of triglycerides — main storage form of lipids — which constitute about 95% of fatty tissue
- Allows early identification of hyperlipidemia and the risk of coronary artery disease (CAD)

PURPOSE
- To screen for hyperlipidemia or pancreatitis
- To help identify nephrotic syndrome and the individual with poorly controlled diabetes mellitus
- To assess the risk of CAD
- To calculate the low-density lipoprotein cholesterol level using the Friedewald equation

PREPARATION
- Notify the laboratory and practitioner of drugs the patient is taking that may affect test results; they may be restricted.
- The test requires a blood sample.

Teaching points
- Explain that the triglyceride test is used to detect fat metabolism disorders.
- Explain who will perform the test and where it'll be done.
- Instruct the patient to fast for at least 12 hours before the test and to abstain from alcohol for 24 hours. Tell him that he may drink water.
- Tell the patient that the test requires a blood sample and that he may experience slight discomfort from the tourniquet and needle puncture.
- Tell him that the test takes less than 5 minutes.

KEY STEPS
- Confirm the patient's identity using two patient identifiers according to facility policy.
- Perform a venipuncture and collect the sample in a 4-ml EDTA tube.

POSTPROCEDURE CARE
- Apply direct pressure to the venipuncture site until bleeding stops.
- Inform the practitioner of abnormal results.
- Tell the patient to resume his usual diet and medications, as ordered.

PRECAUTIONS
- Send the sample to the laboratory immediately.
- Avoid prolonged venous occlusion; remove the tourniquet within 1 minute of application.

COMPLICATIONS
- Hematoma at the venipuncture site

NORMAL RESULTS
- In men, levels are 44 to 180 mg/dl (SI, 0.44 to 2.01 mmol/L).
- In women, levels are 10 to 190 mg/dl (SI, 0.11 to 2.21 mmol/L).

ABNORMAL RESULTS
- An increased or decreased serum triglyceride level is abnormal; additional tests are required for a definitive diagnosis.
- A mild to moderate increase in serum triglyceride levels indicates biliary obstruction, diabetes mellitus, nephrotic syndrome, endocrinopathies, or overconsumption of alcohol.
- Markedly increased levels without an identifiable cause reflect congenital hyperlipoproteinemia and require lipoprotein phenotyping to confirm the diagnosis.
- Decreased serum triglyceride levels are rare and occur mainly in malnutrition and abetalipoproteinemia.

Triiodothyronine level, serum

OVERVIEW

DESCRIPTION
- Highly specific radioimmunoassay that measures total (bound and free) serum triiodothyronine (T_3); used to investigate clinical indications of thyroid dysfunction
- T_3: amine derived primarily (50% to 90%) from thyroxine (T_4) through monodeiodination; more potent thyroid hormone than T_4
- Rest of T_3 secreted by thyroid gland in response to thyroid-stimulating hormone (TSH) and thyrotropin-releasing hormone
- Minute amounts of T_3 in blood; although T_3 is metabolically active for only a short time, its impact on body metabolism dominates that of T_4
- T_3 bond less firm to thyroxine-binding globulin

PURPOSE
- To help diagnose T_3 toxicosis
- To help diagnose hypothyroidism and hyperthyroidism
- To monitor the patient's response to thyroid replacement therapy in hypothyroidism

PREPARATION
- Withhold drugs, such as steroids, propranolol, cholestyramine, and thyroid preparations, which may influence thyroid function. If the patient must continue them, record this information on the laboratory request. (See *Drugs that interfere with T_3 tests*.)
- The test requires a blood sample.

Teaching points
- Explain that this test helps evaluate thyroid gland function and determine the cause of his symptoms.
- Explain who will perform the test and where it'll be done.
- Tell the patient that the test requires a blood sample and that he may experience slight discomfort from the tourniquet and needle puncture.
- Inform the patient of any medication restrictions.

- Tell the patient that the test takes less than 5 minutes.

DIAGNOSTIC PROCEDURE

KEY STEPS
- Confirm the patient's identity using two patient identifiers according to facility policy.
- Perform a venipuncture and collect the sample in a 7-ml clot-activator tube.

POSTPROCEDURE CARE
- Apply direct pressure to the venipuncture site until bleeding stops.
- Inform the practitioner of abnormal results.
- Instruct the patient to resume his medications, as ordered.

PRECAUTIONS
- Send the sample to the laboratory as soon as possible.

COMPLICATIONS
- Hematoma at the venipuncture site

INTERPRETATION

NORMAL RESULTS
- T_3 level is 80 to 200 ng/dl (SI, 1.2 to 3 nmol/L).
- In pregnant patients, increased serum T_3 levels are noted.
- Serum T_3 and T_4 levels rise and fall in tandem.

ABNORMAL RESULTS
- T_3 level is usually a more accurate diagnostic indicator of hyperthyroidism than T_4 levels.
- In T_3 toxicosis, T_3 levels rise, whereas total and free T_4 levels remain normal. T_3 toxicosis occurs in patients with Graves' disease, toxic adenoma, or toxic nodular goiter.
- T_3 levels also surpass T_4 levels in patients receiving thyroid replacement therapy containing more T_3 than T_4.

- In iodine-deficient areas, the thyroid may produce larger amounts of T_3 than of T_4 to try to maintain the euthyroid state.
- Although T_3 and T_4 levels are increased in about 90% of patients with hyperthyroidism, there's a disproportionate increase in T_3.
- In some patients with hypothyroidism, T_3 levels may fall within the normal range and not be diagnostically significant.
- Low T_3 levels may appear in euthyroid patients with systemic illness (especially hepatic or renal disease), during severe acute illness, and after trauma or major surgery; in such cases, TSH levels are within normal limits.
- Low T_3 levels are sometimes found in the euthyroid patient with malnutrition.

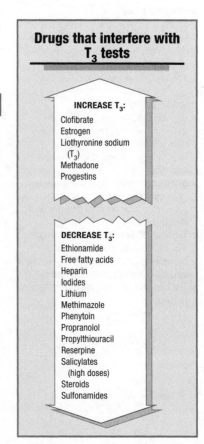

Drugs that interfere with T_3 tests

INCREASE T_3:
Clofibrate
Estrogen
Liothyronine sodium (T_3)
Methadone
Progestins

DECREASE T_3:
Ethionamide
Free fatty acids
Heparin
Iodides
Lithium
Methimazole
Phenytoin
Propranolol
Propylthiouracil
Reserpine
Salicylates (high doses)
Steroids
Sulfonamides

Triiodothyronine uptake test

DESCRIPTION

- Indirectly measures free thyroxine (FT_4) levels by demonstrating the availability of serum protein-binding sites for thyroxine (T_4)
- Results combined with a T_4 radioimmunoassay or $T_4(D)$ (competitive protein-binding test) to calculate the FT_4 index — reflects FT_4 levels by correcting for thyroxine-binding globulin (TBG) abnormalities
- Less popular because rapid tests for T_3, T_4, and thyroid-stimulating hormone are readily available
- Also called the *T_3 uptake test*

PURPOSE

- To help diagnose hypothyroidism and hyperthyroidism when TBG is normal
- To help diagnose primary disorders of TBG levels

PREPARATION

- Withhold drugs that may interfere with test results, such as estrogens, androgens, phenytoin, salicylates, and thyroid preparations. If the patient must continue them, note this on the laboratory request.
- The test requires a blood sample.

Teaching points

- Explain that this test helps evaluate thyroid function.
- Explain who will perform the test and where it'll be done.
- Tell the patient that the test requires a blood sample and that he may experience slight discomfort from the tourniquet and needle puncture.
- Review medication restrictions with the patient.
- Tell the patient that the test takes less than 5 minutes and the laboratory requires several days to complete the analysis.

KEY STEPS

- Confirm the patient's identity using two patient identifiers according to facility policy.
- Perform a venipuncture and collect the sample in a 7-ml clot-activator tube.

POSTPROCEDURE CARE

- Apply direct pressure to the venipuncture site until bleeding stops.
- Inform the practitioner of abnormal results.
- Tell the patient to resume his medications, as ordered.

PRECAUTIONS

- Maintain standard precautions while collecting the sample.
- Handle the sample gently to avoid hemolysis.

COMPLICATIONS

- Hematoma at the venipuncture site

NORMAL RESULTS

- T_3 uptake value is 25% to 35%.

ABNORMAL RESULTS

- A high T_3 uptake percentage with increased T_4 levels indicates hyperthyroidism.
- A low T_3 uptake percentage with decreased T_4 levels indicates hypothyroidism.
- A high T_3 uptake percentage with a decreased or normal FT_4 level suggests decreased TBG levels. Such decreased levels may be caused by protein loss (as in nephrotic syndrome), decreased production (caused by androgen excess or genetic or idiopathic causes), or competition for T_4 binding sites by certain drugs (salicylates, phenylbutazone, and phenytoin).
- A low T_3 uptake percentage and an increased or normal FT_4 level suggest increased TBG levels; such levels may result from exogenous or endogenous estrogen levels (pregnancy) or from idiopathic causes.
- In primary disorders of TBG levels, measured T_4 and free sites change in the same direction.
- In primary thyroid disease, T_4 and T_3 uptake vary in the same direction; availability of binding sites varies inversely.
- Discordant variance in T_4 and T_3 uptake suggests a TBG abnormality.

INTERFERING FACTORS *Antithyroid agents, clofibrate, estrogen, hormonal contraceptives, and thiazide diuretics (may decrease T_3 uptake)*

Troponin level test

DESCRIPTION

- Detects cardiac troponin I (cTnI) and cardiac troponin T (cTnT), proteins in the striated cells that are extremely specific markers of cardiac damage
- Proteins released when injury occurs to myocardial tissue
- Elevations in troponin levels detectable within 1 hour of myocardial infarction (MI); persist for 1 week or longer

PURPOSE

- To detect and diagnose acute MI and reinfarction
- To evaluate the possible causes of chest pain

PREPARATION

- No dietary restrictions are required.
- The test requires a blood sample.

Teaching points

- Explain that this test helps assess myocardial injury and that multiple samples may be drawn to detect fluctuations in serum levels.
- Explain who will perform the test and where it'll be done.
- Inform the patient that he doesn't need to restrict food and fluids.
- Tell the patient that the test requires a blood sample and that he may experience slight discomfort from the tourniquet and needle puncture.
- Tell the patient that the test takes less than 5 minutes.

KEY STEPS

- Confirm the patient's identity using two patient identifiers according to facility policy.
- Perform a venipuncture and collect the specimen in a 7-ml clot-activator tube.

POSTPROCEDURE CARE

- Apply direct pressure to venipuncture site until bleeding stops.

PRECAUTIONS

- Maintain standard precautions while collecting the sample.
- Obtain each specimen on schedule and note the date and collection time on each.
- Inform the practitioner of abnormal results.

COMPLICATIONS

- Hematoma at the venipuncture site

NORMAL RESULTS

- cTnI level is less than 0.35 mcg/L (SI, < 0.35 µg/L).
- cTnT level is less than 0.1 mcg/L (SI, < 0.1 µg/L).

ABNORMAL RESULTS

- Some laboratories may call a test positive if it shows any detectable levels, and others may give a range for abnormal results.
- cTnI levels over 2 mcg/L (SI, > 2 µg/L) and cTnT rapid immunoassay results over 0.1 mcg/L (SI, > 0.1 µg/L) suggest cardiac injury. If tissue injury continues, the troponin levels remain high.
- Troponin levels rise rapidly and are detectable within 1 hour of myocardial cell injury.

INTERFERING FACTORS *Cardiotoxic drugs such as doxorubicin (may increase levels)*

Tuberculin skin tests

DESCRIPTION

- Screen for previous infection by the tubercle bacillus
- Performed when radiographic findings suggest tuberculosis (TB)
- Purified protein derivative (PPD) test: intradermal injection of tuberculin antigen causes a delayed hypersensitivity reaction in patients with active or dormant TB
- Mantoux test: uses a single-needle intradermal injection of PPD, permitting precise dose measurement
- Multipuncture tests (such as the tine test, Mono-Vacc tests, and Aplitest): used for screening; intradermal injections with tines impregnated with PPD; require less skill and are more rapidly given; positive result confirmed by follow-up Mantoux test

PURPOSE

- To distinguish TB from blastomycosis, coccidioidomycosis, and histoplasmosis
- To identify people who need diagnostic investigation for TB because of possible exposure

PREPARATION

- Check the patient's history for active TB, the results of previous skin tests, and hypersensitivities.
- If the patient has had TB, don't perform a skin test.
- If the patient has had a positive reaction to previous skin tests, consult the practitioner or follow facility policy.

Teaching points

- Explain that this test helps detect TB.
- Explain who will perform the test and where it'll be done.
- Tell the patient that the test requires an intradermal injection, which may cause him discomfort.
- Inform the patient that a positive reaction to a skin test appears as a red, hard, raised area at the injection site. Although the area may itch, instruct him not to scratch it.
- Tell the patient when to return to have the results read, as necessary.

- If performing a tuberculin test on an outpatient, instruct him to return at the specified time so that test results can be read.
- Stress that a positive reaction doesn't always indicate active TB.

KEY STEPS

- Confirm the patient's identity using two patient identifiers according to facility policy.
- Ask the patient to sit and support his extended arm on a flat surface.
- Clean the volar surface of the upper forearm with alcohol and allow the area to dry completely.
- Mantoux test: Perform an intradermal injection.
- Multipuncture test: Remove the protective cap on the injection device to expose the four tines.
- Hold the patient's forearm in one hand, stretching the skin of the forearm tightly. Then, with your other hand, firmly depress the device into the patient's skin without twisting it.
- Hold the device in place for at least 1 second before removing it.
- If you've applied sufficient pressure, you'll see four puncture sites and a circular depression made by the device on the patient's skin.

POSTPROCEDURE CARE

- Both tests: Record where the test was given, the date and time, and when the results are to be read. Tuberculin skin tests are generally read 48 to 72 hours after injection; the Mono-Vacc tests can be read 48 to 96 hours after the test.
- If an ulceration or necrosis develops at the injection site, apply cold soaks or a topical steroid.
- Inform the practitioner of abnormal results.

PRECAUTIONS

- Have epinephrine available to treat a possible anaphylactic or acute hypersensitivity reaction.
- Don't perform a skin test in areas with excessive hair, acne, or insufficient subcutaneous tissue, such as over a tendon or bone.

COMPLICATIONS

- Ulceration or necrosis at the injection site
- Anaphylactic or acute hypersensitivity reaction

NORMAL RESULTS

- In tuberculin skin tests, negative or minimal reactions.
- In the Mantoux test, no induration or induration less than 5 mm in diameter.
- In the tine test and Aplitest, no vesiculation or induration or induration less than 2 mm in diameter.
- In the Mono-Vacc tests, no induration.

ABNORMAL RESULTS

- A positive tuberculin reaction indicates previous infection by tubercle bacilli. It doesn't distinguish between an active and a dormant infection or provide a definitive diagnosis.
- If a positive reaction occurs, sputum smear and culture and chest radiography are needed.
- In the Mantoux test, induration 5 to 9 mm in diameter indicates a borderline reaction; larger induration, a positive reaction.
- Because patients infected with atypical mycobacteria other than tubercle bacilli may have borderline reactions, repeat testing is needed.
- In the tine test or Aplitest, vesiculation indicates a positive reaction; induration 2 mm in diameter without vesiculation requires confirmation by the Mantoux test. Any induration in the Mono-Vacc tests indicates a positive reaction; this reaction should be confirmed by the Mantoux test.

INTERFERING FACTORS *Corticosteroids, other immunosuppressants, and live vaccine viruses (such as measles, mumps, rubella, and polio within 4 to 6 weeks before the test) (may suppress skin reaction)*

Two-hour postprandial plasma glucose level test

OVERVIEW

DESCRIPTION
◆ Screens for diabetes mellitus
◆ Done when patient shows symptoms of diabetes (such as polydipsia and polyuria) or when results of the fasting plasma glucose test suggest diabetes
◆ Also called the *2-hour postprandial blood sugar test*

PURPOSE
◆ To help diagnose diabetes mellitus
◆ To monitor drug or diet therapy in the patient with diabetes mellitus

PREPARATION
◆ Notify the laboratory and practitioner of drugs the patient is taking that may affect test results; they may be restricted.
◆ The test requires a blood sample.

Teaching points
◆ Explain that the 2-hour postprandial plasma glucose test evaluates glucose metabolism and detects diabetes.

◆ Explain who will perform the test and where it'll be done.
◆ Tell the patient to eat a balanced meal or one containing 100 g of carbohydrates before the test and then to fast for 2 hours. Instruct him to avoid smoking and exercising strenuously after the meal.
◆ Tell the patient that the test requires a blood sample and that he may experience slight discomfort from the tourniquet and needle puncture.

DIAGNOSTIC PROCEDURE

KEY STEPS
◆ Confirm the patient's identity using two patient identifiers according to facility policy.
◆ Perform a venipuncture and collect the sample in a 5-ml clot-activator tube.

POSTPROCEDURE CARE
◆ Apply direct pressure to the venipuncture site until bleeding stops.
◆ Inform the practitioner of abnormal results.

◆ Tell the patient to resume his usual diet, medications, and activity.

PRECAUTIONS
◆ Send the sample to the laboratory immediately or refrigerate it.
◆ Specify on the laboratory request when the patient last ate, the time of the sample collection, and when the last pretest dose of insulin or oral antidiabetic drug was given.

COMPLICATIONS
◆ Hematoma at the venipuncture site

INTERPRETATION

NORMAL RESULTS
◆ In patients who don't have diabetes, postprandial glucose values are below 145 mg/dl (SI, < 8 mmol/L) by the glucose oxidase or hexokinase method.
◆ Levels are slightly higher in patients older than age 50. (See *Two-hour postprandial plasma glucose levels by age.*)

ABNORMAL RESULTS
◆ Two-hour postprandial blood glucose values of 200 mg/dl (SI, 11.1 mmol/L) or above indicate diabetes mellitus.
◆ High glucose levels (hyperglycemia) occur with pancreatitis, Cushing's syndrome, acromegaly, pheochromocytoma, hyperlipoproteinemia (especially type III, IV, or V), chronic hepatic disease, nephrotic syndrome, brain tumor, sepsis, gastrectomy with dumping syndrome, eclampsia, anoxia, and seizure disorders.
◆ Low glucose levels (hypoglycemia) occur in hyperinsulinism, insulinoma, von Gierke's disease, functional and reactive hypoglycemia, myxedema, adrenal insufficiency, congenital adrenal hyperplasia, hypopituitarism, malabsorption syndrome, and hepatic insufficiency.

⬢ **INTERFERING FACTORS** *Recent illness, infection, or pregnancy (may increase glucose levels); strenuous exercise or stress (may decrease levels)*

Two-hour postprandial plasma glucose levels by age

The greatest difference in normal and diabetic insulin responses, and thus in plasma glucose concentration, occurs about 2 hours after a glucose challenge. Test values can fluctuate according to the patient's age. After age 50, for example, normal levels rise markedly and steadily, sometimes reaching 160 mg/dl (SI, 8.82 mmol/L) or higher. In a younger patient, a glucose concentration of more than 145 mg/dl (SI > 8 mmol/L) suggests incipient diabetes and requires further evaluation.

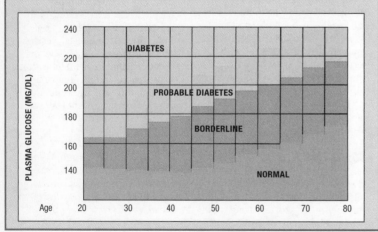

Ultrasonography

OVERVIEW

DESCRIPTION

- Transmits high-frequency sound waves into the targeted tissue; resultant echoes are converted to electrical impulses, amplified by a transducer, and displayed on a monitor
- Sound waves: travel at varying speeds depending on density of tissue they're passing through; difference reflected as images on the display screen

PURPOSE

- To measure organ size and evaluate structure
- To detect foreign bodies and differentiate between a cyst and solid tumor
- To monitor tissue response to radiation or chemotherapy

PREPARATION

- Make sure the patient has signed an appropriate consent form.
- Note and report allergies.

Teaching points

- Explain the purpose of the test and how it's done.
- Explain who will perform the test and where it'll be done.
- Inform the patient that the procedure is painless and safe and that no radiation exposure is involved.
- Stress the importance of remaining still during scanning to prevent a distorted image.
- Review dietary restrictions required.
- Tell the patient how long the test will take.

DIAGNOSTIC PROCEDURE

KEY STEPS

- Confirm the patient's identity using two patient identifiers according to facility policy.
- Assist the patient into a supine position; use pillows to support the area to be examined.
- Coat the target area with a water-soluble jelly. The transducer is used to scan the area, projecting the images on the oscilloscope screen. The image on the screen is photographed for subsequent examination.
- The patient may need assistance into right or left lateral positions for subsequent views.

POSTPROCEDURE CARE

- Remove the contact jelly from the patient's skin.
- Inform the practitioner of abnormal results.

PRECAUTIONS

- None

COMPLICATIONS

- None

INTERPRETATION

NORMAL RESULTS

- See "Normal results" for a specific type of ultrasonography (for example, abdominal aorta, gallbladder and biliary system, kidney and perirenal structures, liver, pancreas, pelvic area, spleen, and thyroid).

ABNORMAL RESULTS

- See "Abnormal results" for a specific type of ultrasonography (for example, abdominal aorta, gallbladder and biliary system, kidney and perirenal structures, liver, pancreas, pelvic area, spleen, and thyroid).

Ultrasonography, abdominal aorta

OVERVIEW

DESCRIPTION

◆ Method of choice for measuring diameter of aortic aneurysm
◆ Performed every 6 months to monitor changes in a patient's status
◆ Transducer: directs focused beam of high-frequency sound waves into the abdomen over a wide area from the xiphoid process to the umbilical region; creates echoes that vary with changes in tissue density
◆ Sound waves: transmitted as electrical impulses and displayed on a monitor to show the size and course of the abdominal aorta and other major vessels

PURPOSE

◆ To detect and measure a suspected abdominal aortic aneurysm
◆ To monitor expansion of a known abdominal aortic aneurysm

PREPARATION

◆ Make sure the patient has signed an appropriate consent form.
◆ Note and report allergies.
◆ Withhold food and fluids for 12 hours before the test.
◆ Give the patient simethicone to reduce bowel gas if necessary.

Teaching points

◆ Explain the purpose of the test and how it's done.
◆ Explain who will perform the test and where it'll be done.
◆ Tell the patient to fast for 12 hours before the test to minimize bowel gas and motility.
◆ Inform the patient that he will feel slight pressure in the area being tested.
◆ Instruct the patient to remain still during scanning and to hold his breath when asked.
◆ Tell the patient that the test takes 30 to 45 minutes.

DIAGNOSTIC PROCEDURE

KEY STEPS

◆ Confirm the patient's identity using two patient identifiers according to facility policy.
◆ Assist the patient into a supine position.
◆ Apply acoustic coupling gel or mineral oil to the abdomen.
◆ Longitudinal scans are then made at 0.5- to 1-cm intervals to the left and right of midline until the entire abdominal aorta is outlined.
◆ Transverse scans are made at 1- to 2-cm intervals from the xiphoid process to the bifurcation at the common iliac arteries.
◆ It may be necessary to place the patient in right and left lateral positions.
◆ Appropriate views are photographed or videotaped.

POSTPROCEDURE CARE

◆ Remove residual gel from the patient's skin.
◆ Inform the practitioner of abnormal results.
◆ Tell the patient to resume his usual diet and medications, as ordered.

PRECAUTIONS

WARNING *Remember that sudden onset of constant abdominal or back pain accompanies rapid expansion of the aneurysm; sudden, excruciating pain with weakness, sweating, tachycardia, and hypotension signals rupture.*

COMPLICATIONS

◆ None

INTERPRETATION

NORMAL RESULTS

◆ The abdominal aorta tapers from about ½″ to 1″ (1 to 2.5 cm) in diameter along its length from the diaphragm to the bifurcation.
◆ The abdominal aorta descends through the retroperitoneal space, anterior to the vertebral column and slightly left of the midline.
◆ Four of the abdominal aorta's major branches are usually well visualized: the celiac trunk, the renal arteries, the superior mesenteric artery, and the common iliac arteries.

ABNORMAL RESULTS

◆ Luminal diameter of the abdominal aorta greater than 1½″ (4 cm) indicates an aneurysm.
◆ Luminal diameter of the abdominal aorta greater than 2⅓″ (6 cm) indicates an aneurysm with a high risk of rupture.

Ultrasonography, gallbladder and biliary system

DESCRIPTION

- Focused beam of high-frequency sound waves passed into right upper quadrant of the abdomen; creates echoes that vary with changes in tissue density
- Reveals the size, shape, structure, and position of gallbladder and biliary system
- Procedure of choice for evaluating jaundice and for emergency diagnosis of patient with signs of acute cholecystitis with or without local tenderness
- When site of biliary obstruction isn't clearly defined: need for percutaneous transhepatic cholangiography or endoscopic retrograde cholangiopancreatography

PURPOSE

- To confirm diagnosis of cholelithiasis
- To diagnose acute cholecystitis
- To distinguish between obstructive and nonobstructive jaundice

PREPARATION

- Make sure the patient has signed an appropriate consent form.
- Note and report allergies.
- Provide a fat-free meal in the evening before the test.
- Fasting is required for 8 to 12 hours before the procedure.

Teaching points

- Explain the purpose of the test.
- Explain who will perform the test and where it'll be done.
- Tell the patient to fast for 8 to 12 hours before the procedure.
- Instruct the patient to remain as still as possible during the procedure and to hold his breath when requested; this ensures that the gallbladder is in the same position for each scan.
- Tell him that a darkened room aids visualization.
- Tell him that the test takes about 15 to 30 minutes.

DIAGNOSTIC PROCEDURE

KEY STEPS

- Confirm the patient's identity using two patient identifiers according to facility policy.
- Place the patient in a supine position.
- A water-soluble lubricant is applied to the face of the transducer, and transverse scans of the gallbladder are taken at 1-cm intervals.
- Longitudinal oblique scans are taken at 5-mm intervals parallel to the long axis of the gallbladder marked on the patient's skin.
- During each scan the patient is asked to exhale deeply and hold his breath.
- If the gallbladder is positioned deeply under the right costal margin, a scan may be taken through the intercostal spaces, while the patient inhales deeply and holds his breath.
- The patient is placed in a left lateral decubitus position and scanned beneath the right costal margin. This allows for displacing stones lodged in the cystic duct region, which escape detection in the supine position.
- Scanning with the patient erect helps demonstrate mobility or fixation of suspicious echogenic areas.
- Oscilloscopic views are obtained and photographed for later study.

POSTPROCEDURE CARE

- Remove the lubricating jelly from the patient's skin.
- Inform the practitioner of abnormal results.
- Instruct the patient to resume his normal diet, as ordered.

PRECAUTIONS

- Fasting before the test prevents excretion of bile in the gallbladder.

COMPLICATIONS

- None

INTERPRETATION

NORMAL RESULTS

- The normal gallbladder is sonolucent; it appears circular on transverse scans and pear-shaped on longitudinal scans.
- Although the gallbladder's size varies, its outer walls normally appear sharp and smooth.
- Intrahepatic radicles seldom appear because the flow of sonolucent bile is very fine.
- The cystic duct may be indistinct because folds known as Heister's valves line the cystic duct lumen.
- When visualized, the cystic duct has a serpentine appearance.
- The common bile duct has a linear appearance but is sometimes obscured by overlying bowel gas.

ABNORMAL RESULTS

- Mobile, echogenic areas, usually associated with an acoustic shadow, suggests gallstones within the gallbladder lumen or the biliary system.
- When the gallbladder is shrunken or fully impacted with gallstones, inadequate bile may make gallstone detection difficult and the gallbladder itself may fail to be visualized. In this case, the presence of an acoustic shadow at the gallbladder fossa suggests cholelithiasis.
- An acoustic shadow in the cystic and common bile ducts suggests possible choledocholithiasis.
- Fixed echogenic areas within the gallbladder lumen suggests possible polyps or tumors; polyps usually appear as sharply defined, echogenic areas; carcinoma appears as a poorly defined mass commonly associated with a thickened gallbladder wall.
- A fine layer of echoes that slowly gravitate to the dependent portion of the gallbladder as the patient changes position suggests biliary sludge within the gallbladder lumen.
- An enlarged gallbladder with thickened, double-rimmed walls, accompanied by gallstones within the lumen, suggests acute cholecystitis.
- A contracted gallbladder with thickened walls suggests chronic cholecystitis.
- A dilated biliary system and, usually, a dilated gallbladder suggest obstructive jaundice.

Ultrasonography, kidney and perirenal structures

OVERVIEW

DESCRIPTION

- High-frequency sound waves (1 to 5 million cycles/second): transmitted from transducer and through the kidneys and perirenal structures; resulting echoes are amplified and converted into electrical impulses and displayed on an oscilloscope screen as anatomic images
- Usually done with other urologic tests to detect abnormalities or provide more information about abnormalities detected by other tests
- Safe, painless procedure; especially useful when excretory urography is ruled out (for example, hypersensitivity to contrast medium or need for serial examinations)
- Doesn't require adequate renal function (unlike excretory urography); useful in patients with renal failure
- May also include ultrasonography of ureter, bladder, and gonads

PURPOSE

- To determine the size, shape, and position of the kidneys, their internal structures, and perirenal tissues
- To evaluate and localize urinary obstruction and abnormal accumulation of fluid
- To assess and diagnose complications after kidney transplantation
- To detect renal or perirenal masses
- To differentiate between renal cysts and solid masses
- To verify placement of a nephrostomy tube

PREPARATION

- No dietary restrictions are required.

Teaching points

- Explain that the test is used to detect abnormalities in the kidneys.
- Explain who will perform the test and where it'll be done.
- Tell the patient he doesn't need to restrict his diet before the test.
- Tell the patient that the test takes about 30 minutes.

DIAGNOSTIC PROCEDURE

KEY STEPS

- Confirm the patient's identity using two patient identifiers according to facility policy.
- The patient is placed in the prone position and the area to be scanned is exposed.
- Ultrasound jelly is applied to the area before the scanning begins.
- The longitudinal axis of the kidneys is located using measurements from excretory urography or by performing transverse scans through the upper and lower renal poles.
- These points are marked on the skin and connected with straight lines.
- Sectional images (1 or 2 cm apart) can be obtained by moving the transducer longitudinally and transversely or at any other angle required.
- During the test, the patient may be asked to breathe deeply to visualize upper portions of the kidney.

POSTPROCEDURE CARE

- After the procedure, remove the conduction jelly from the patient's skin.
- If bladder abnormalities are found, prepare the patient for further testing.
- If rejection of a transplanted kidney is suspected or diagnosed, monitor intake and output, blood pressure, blood urea nitrogen and creatinine levels, and vital signs.
- If an adrenal tumor is detected, monitor for adrenal dysfunction (such as hypotension, decreased urine output, and electrolyte imbalances).
- If a nephrostomy tube has been placed in the patient, monitor the amount and characteristics of drainage and tube patency.
- Inform the practitioner of abnormal results.

PRECAUTIONS

- None

COMPLICATIONS

- None

INTERPRETATION

NORMAL RESULTS

- The kidneys are located between the superior iliac crests and the diaphragm.
- The renal capsule should be outlined sharply; the cortex should produce more echoes than the medulla.
- In the center of each kidney, the renal collecting systems appear as irregular areas of higher density than surrounding tissue.

ABNORMAL RESULTS

- Fluid-filled, circular structures that don't reflect sound waves suggest cysts.
- Multiple echoes appearing as irregular shapes suggest tumor.
- Fluid-filled structures with slightly irregular boundaries that don't reflect sound waves well suggest abscesses.
- A renal capsule that appears irregular and a kidney that appears smaller than normal and is associated with an increased number of echoes arising from the parenchyma because of fibrosis may suggest acute pyelonephritis and glomerulonephritis.
- A large, echo-free, central mass that compresses the renal cortex may indicate hydronephrosis.
- After kidney transplantation, compensatory hypertrophy is normal but an acute increase in size indicates rejection of the transplant.
- Abnormal accumulation of fluid within or around the kidneys may suggest an obstruction.
- Increased urine volume or residual urine postvoiding may indicate bladder dysfunction.

Ultrasonography, liver

DESCRIPTION
- Cross-sectional images of the liver produced by channeling high-frequency sound waves into right upper quadrant of the abdomen; resultant echoes converted to electrical energy, amplified by a transducer, and displayed on a monitor
- Various tissue densities depicted as shades of gray
- Shows intrahepatic structures as well as organ size, shape, and position
- Suitable for patients with jaundice of unknown etiology, unexplained hepatomegaly and abnormal biochemical test results, suspected metastatic tumors and elevated serum alkaline phosphatase levels, and recent abdominal trauma
- To complement liver-spleen scanning: can define cold spots — focal defects that fail to pick up the radionuclide — such as tumors, abscesses, or cysts; also provides better views of the periportal and perihepatic spaces than liver-spleen scanning

PURPOSE
- To distinguish between obstructive and nonobstructive jaundice
- To screen for hepatocellular disease
- To detect hepatic metastases and hematoma
- To define cold spots as tumors, abscesses, or cysts

PREPARATION
- Note and report all allergies.
- The patient needs to fast for 8 to 12 hours before the test.

Teaching points
- Explain the purpose of the test and how it's done.
- Explain who will perform the test and where it'll be done.
- Tell the patient to fast for 8 to 12 hours before the test.
- Warn the patient that he may feel mild pressure as the transducer presses against his skin.
- Stress the need to remain as still as possible during the procedure and hold his breath when asked.
- Tell the patient that the test takes 15 to 30 minutes.

KEY STEPS
- Confirm the patient's identity using two patient identifiers according to facility policy.
- The patient is placed in a supine position.
- A water-soluble lubricant is applied to the face of the transducer, and transverse scans are taken at $\frac{3}{8}''$ (1 cm) intervals, using a single-sweep technique between the costal margins
- Sector scans are taken through the intercostal spaces to view the remainder of the right lobe.
- Scans are taken longitudinally, from the right lobe of the liver to the left.
- Oblique cephalad-angled scans may be taken beneath the right costal margin for better demonstration of the right lateral dome.
- Scans are then taken parallel to the hepatic portal, at a 45-degree angle toward the superior right lateral dome, to examine the peripheral anatomy, portal venous system, common bile duct, and biliary tree.
- During each scan, the patient is asked to hold his breath briefly in deep inspiration.
- Clear images are photographed for later study.

POSTPROCEDURE CARE
- Remove lubricating jelly from the patient's skin.
- Inform the practitioner of abnormal results.
- Tell the patient to resume his usual diet, as ordered.

PRECAUTIONS
- None

COMPLICATIONS
- None

NORMAL RESULTS
- The liver demonstrates a homogenous, low-level echo pattern, interrupted only by the different echo patterns of its vascular channels.
- Intrahepatic biliary radicles and hepatic arteries aren't apparent, but portal and hepatic veins, the aorta, and the inferior vena cava appear on ultrasound.
- Hepatic veins appear completely sonolucent; portal veins have margins that are high echogenic.

ABNORMAL RESULTS
- Dilated intrahepatic biliary radicles and extrahepatic ducts suggest obstructive jaundice.
- Variable liver size; dilated, tortuous portal branches associated with portal hypertension; and an irregular echo pattern with increased echo amplitude causing overall increased attenuation suggest possible cirrhosis.
- Hepatomegaly and a regular echo pattern that, although greater in echo amplitude than that of normal parenchyma, don't alter attenuation suggest possible fatty infiltration of the liver.
- Hypoechoic or echogenic and poorly defined or well-defined areas suggest possible metastasis in the liver.
- Sonolucent masses with ill-defined, slightly thickened borders and accentuated posterior wall transmission suggest possible abscesses.
- The presence of fluid lacking internal echoes with a more regular border suggests possible ascitic fluid.
- Spherical, sonolucent areas with ill-defined borders and accentuated posterior wall transmission suggest possible cysts.
- Poorly defined, relatively sonolucent masses, with possible scattered internal echoes caused by clotting suggest possible intrahepatic hematomas.
- A focal, sonolucent mass on the periphery of the liver or a diffuse, sonolucent area surrounding part of the liver suggests possible subcapsular hematoma.

Ultrasonography, pancreas

DESCRIPTION

- Cross-sectional images of the pancreas produced by channeling high-frequency sound waves into the epigastric region; converts resultant echoes to electrical impulses, and displays them as real-time images on a monitor
- Shows size, shape, and position of the pancreas and surrounding viscera; pattern varies with tissue density
- Can't provide a sensitive measure of pancreatic function; useful in detecting anatomic abnormalities, such as pancreatic carcinoma and pseudocysts, and to guide the insertion of biopsy needles
- Doesn't expose the patient to radiation; procedure has replaced hypotonic duodenography, endoscopic retrograde cholangiopancreatography, radioisotope studies, and arteriography

PURPOSE

- To aid diagnosis of pancreatitis, pseudocysts, and pancreatic carcinoma

PREPARATION

- Note and report all allergies.
- Fasting is required for 8 to 12 hours before the test to reduce bowel gas, which hinders transmission of ultrasound.

Teaching points

- Explain the purpose of the test and how it's done.
- Explain who will perform the test and where it'll be done.
- Instruct the patient to avoid smoking before the test.
- Provide reassurance that although the test isn't harmful or painful, he may feel mild pressure.
- Tell the patient to fast for 8 to 12 hours before the test.
- Instruct him to inhale deeply during the scanning, when requested.
- Stress the need to remain as still as possible during imaging.
- Tell the patient that the test takes 30 minutes.

DIAGNOSTIC PROCEDURE

KEY STEPS

- Confirm the patient's identity using two patient identifiers according to facility policy.
- The patient is placed in a supine position.
- A water-soluble lubricant or mineral oil is applied to the abdomen and, with the patient at full inspiration, transverse scans are taken at ⅜" (1-cm) intervals, starting from the xiphoid and moving caudally.
- Other scanning techniques include the longitudinal scan to view the head, body, and tail of the pancreas in sequence; the right anterior oblique view for the head and body of the pancreas; the oblique sagittal view for the portal vein and the sagittal view for the vena cava.
- Good oscilloscopic views are photographed for later study.

POSTPROCEDURE CARE

- Remove the lubricating jelly from the patient's skin.
- Inform the practitioner of abnormal results.
- Tell the patient to resume his usual diet, as ordered.

PRECAUTIONS

- None

COMPLICATIONS

- None

NORMAL RESULTS

- The pancreas demonstrates a coarse, uniform echo pattern (reflecting tissue density) and usually appears more echogenic than the adjacent liver.

ABNORMAL RESULTS

- Alterations in the size, contour, and parenchymal texture of the pancreas suggest possible pancreatic disease.
- An enlarged pancreas with decreased echogenicity and distinct borders suggests pancreatitis.
- A well-defined mass with an essentially echo-free interior suggests pseudocyst.
- An ill-defined mass with scattered internal echoes or a mass in the head of the pancreas (obstructing the common bile duct) and a large non-contracting gallbladder suggests pancreatic carcinoma.

Ultrasonography, pelvic area

OVERVIEW

DESCRIPTION
- Transmits high-frequency sound waves into the interior pelvic region; resultant echoes converted to electrical impulses, amplified by a transducer, and displayed on a monitor
- A-mode: records distances between interfaces
- B-mode (brightness modulation): creates a two-dimensional or cross-sectional image
- Gray-scale: represents organ texture in shades of gray on a screen
- Real-time imaging: creates instant images of tissues in motion, similar to fluoroscopic examination
- Photographed views: may be examined later and kept as record of test
- Used to evaluate symptoms that suggest pelvic disease, to confirm a tentative diagnosis, and to determine fetal growth during pregnancy
- May be needed in pregnant women with a history or signs of fetal anomalies or multiple pregnancies, a history of bleeding, inconsistency of fetal size and conception date, or indications for amniocentesis

PURPOSE
- To detect foreign bodies and distinguish between cysts and solid masses (tumors)
- To measure organ size
- To evaluate fetal viability, position, gestational age, and growth rate
- To detect multiple pregnancy
- To confirm fetal abnormalities (such as molar pregnancy, and abnormalities of the arms and legs, spine, heart, head, kidneys, and abdomen)
- To confirm maternal abnormalities (such as posterior placenta and placenta previa)
- To guide amniocentesis by determining placental location and fetal position

PREPARATION
- Note and report all allergies.
- Review dietary requirements with the patient.

Teaching points
- Explain the purpose of the test and how it's done.
- Explain who will perform the test and where it'll be done.
- Instruct the patient to drink fluids and avoid voiding before the test because pelvic ultrasonography requires a full bladder as a landmark to define pelvic organs.
- Explain that the test won't harm the fetus.
- Explain that the test will take from a few minutes to several hours.

DIAGNOSTIC PROCEDURE

KEY STEPS
- Confirm the patient's identity using two patient identifiers according to facility policy.
- With the patient in a supine position, coat the lower abdomen with mineral oil or water-soluble jelly to increase sound wave conduction.
- The transducer crystal is guided over the area, images are observed on the oscilloscope screen, and good images are photographed.

POSTPROCEDURE CARE
- Allow the patient to empty her bladder immediately after the test.
- Remove ultrasound jelly from the patient's skin.

PRECAUTIONS
- When the bladder is empty, the uterus is more difficult to see because it's farther down inside the pelvis. Bones disrupt ultrasound signals. Failure to keep the bladder full will interfere with the test results, making interpretation difficult.

COMPLICATIONS
- None

INTERPRETATION

NORMAL RESULTS
- The uterus is normal in size and shape.
- The ovaries are normal in size, shape, and sonographic density.
- The body of the uterus lies on the superior surface of the bladder; the uterine tubes are attached laterally.
- The ovaries are located on the lateral pelvic walls, with the external iliac vessels above and the ureters posteroinferior, and are covered by the fimbria of the uterine tubes medially.
- No other masses are visible.
- If the patient is pregnant, the gestational sac and fetus are of normal size for date; the placenta is located in the fundus of the uterus.

ABNORMAL RESULTS
- Homogeneous densities suggest both cysts and solid masses; however, solid masses (such as fibroids) appear more dense on ultrasonography.
- Inappropriate fetal size suggests possible miscalculation of conception or delivery date.
- Abnormal echo patterns suggest possible foreign bodies (such as an intrauterine device), multiple pregnancy, placenta previa or abruptio placentae, or fetal abnormalities (such as molar pregnancy or abnormalities of the arms and legs, spine, heart, head, kidneys, and abdomen).
- Fetal abnormalities suggest possible malpresentation (such as breech or shoulder presentation) and cephalopelvic disproportion.

Ultrasonography, spleen

OVERVIEW

DESCRIPTION
- High-frequency sound waves focused into left upper quadrant of the abdomen; creates echoes that vary with changes in tissue density, converted to electrical energy, amplified by a transducer, and displayed on a monitor
- Shows series of real-time images representing size, shape, and position of spleen and surrounding viscera
- Indicated for patients with left upper quadrant mass of unknown origin, with known splenomegaly to evaluate changes in the spleen's size, with left upper quadrant pain and local tenderness, and with recent abdominal trauma
- Can show splenomegaly but usually doesn't identify the cause

PURPOSE
- To demonstrate splenomegaly
- To monitor progression of primary and secondary splenic disease
- To evaluate the effectiveness of therapy
- To evaluate the spleen after abdominal trauma
- To detect splenic cysts and subphrenic abscess

PREPARATION
- Note and report allergies.
- Fasting is required for 8 to 12 hours before the procedure.

Teaching points
- Explain the purpose of the test and how it's done.
- Explain who will perform the test and where it'll be done.
- Tell the patient to fast for 8 to 12 hours before the procedure.
- Inform the patient that he will feel only mild pressure during the procedure.
- Instruct him to remain as still as possible during the test and to hold his breath when requested.
- Tell him that the test takes about 15 to 30 minutes.

DIAGNOSTIC PROCEDURE

KEY STEPS
- Confirm the patient's identity using two patient identifiers according to facility policy.
- Because the procedure for ultrasonography varies, depending on the size of the spleen of the patient's body habitus, the patient is usually repositioned several times; the transducer scanning angle or path is also changed.
- A water-soluble lubricant is applied to the face of the transducer, and transverse scans of the spleen are taken at 1- or 2-cm intervals, beginning at the level of the diaphragm and moving posteriorly.
- After the patient is placed in right lateral decubitus position, additional transverse scans are taken through the intercostal spaces using a sectoring motion.
- A pillow may be placed under the patient's right side to help separate the intercostal spaces, making it easier to position the transducer face between them.
- For longitudinal scans, the patient remains in the right lateral decubitus position and scans are taken from the axilla toward the iliac crest.
- To prevent rib artifacts, oblique scans are taken by passing the transducer face along the intercostal spaces; this scan provides the best view of the splenic parenchyma.
- During each scan, the patient may be asked to hold his breath briefly at varying stages of inspiration.

POSTPROCEDURE CARE
- Remove the lubricating jelly from the patient's skin.
- Inform the practitioner of abnormal results.
- Tell the patient to resume his usual diet, as ordered.

PRECAUTIONS
- Patients with a splenic injury may be unable to tolerate the procedure because of pain.

COMPLICATIONS
- None

INTERPRETATION

NORMAL RESULTS
- The splenic parenchyma demonstrates a homogeneous, low-level echo pattern.
- The superior and lateral splenic borders are clearly defined, each having a convex margin.
- The undersurface and medial borders, in contrast, show indentation from surrounding organs (for example, stomach, left kidney, and pancreas).
- The hilar region, where the vascular pedicle enters the spleen, usually produces an area of highly reflected echoes.
- The medial surface is usually concave, a characteristic particularly useful when differentiating between left upper quadrant masses and an enlarged spleen.
- Even when splenomegaly is present, the spleen usually remains concave medially, unless a space-occupying lesion distorts this contour.

ABNORMAL RESULTS
- Increased echogenicity and enlarged vascular channels, especially in the hilar region, suggest splenomegaly.
- Splenomegaly and an irregular, sonolucent area (the presence of free intraperitoneal fluid) suggest splenic rupture.
- Splenomegaly as well as the presence of a double contour (blood accumulation between the splenic parenchyma and the intact splenic capsule), altered splenic position, and a relatively sonolucent area on the periphery of the spleen suggest subcapsular hematoma.
- A sonolucent area beneath the diaphragm suggests possible subphrenic abscess.
- Spherical, sonolucent areas with well-defined, regular margins, with acoustic enhancement behind them, suggest cysts.

Ultrasonography, thyroid

DESCRIPTION

- Emits pulses from a piezoelectric crystal in a transducer, directed at the thyroid gland, and reflected back to the transducer; pulses converted electronically to produce structural visualization on an oscilloscope screen
- Differentiates between a cyst and a tumor larger than 1 cm with about 85% accuracy when the mass is located by palpation or by thyroid imaging
- Useful in evaluating thyroid nodules during pregnancy because it doesn't expose the fetus to radioactive iodine
- Can be performed on parathyroid glands (see *Parathyroid ultrasonography*)

PURPOSE

- To evaluate the thyroid structure
- To differentiate between a cyst and a solid tumor
- To monitor the size of the thyroid gland during suppressive therapy
- To allow accurate measurement of a nodule
- To aid in the performance of thyroid needle biopsy

PREPARATION

- Note and report all allergies.
- No dietary restrictions are required.

Teaching points

- Explain the purpose of the test and how it's done.
- Explain who will perform the test and where it'll be done.
- Tell the patient that he doesn't need to restrict food and fluids before the test.
- Inform the patient that the test is painless and safe.
- Tell the patient that the test takes about 10 minutes.

KEY STEPS

- Confirm the patient's identity using two patient identifiers according to facility policy.
- Assist the patient into a supine position with a pillow under his shoulder blades to hyperextend his neck.
- Coat the patient's neck with water-soluble gel.
- The transducer scans the thyroid, projecting its echographic image on the oscilloscope screen.
- The image on the screen is photographed for subsequent examination.

POSTPROCEDURE CARE

- Thoroughly clean the patient's neck to remove the contact solution.
- Inform the practitioner of abnormal results.

PRECAUTIONS

- None

COMPLICATIONS

- None

Parathyroid ultrasonography

On ultrasonography, the parathyroid glands appear as solid masses, 5 mm or smaller in size, with an echo pattern of less amplitude than thyroid tissue. Glandular enlargement is usually characteristic of tumor growth or of hyperplasia. Normally, on a scan, the parathyroid glands are indistinguishable from the nearby neurovascular bundle.

NORMAL RESULTS

- A uniform echo pattern throughout the gland is observed.

ABNORMAL RESULTS

- Smooth-bordered, echo-free areas with enhanced sound transmission suggest cysts.
- Solid and well-demarcated areas with identical echo patterns suggest adenomas and carcinomas.

Unstable hemoglobin test

OVERVIEW

DESCRIPTION
◆ Detects presence of unstable hemoglobin (Hb), a rare, congenital defect caused by amino acid substitutions in the Hb structure causing it to decompose easily
◆ Detected by precipitation tests (using heat stability or isopropanol solubility)
◆ Unstable Hb: may lead to formation of small masses (Heinz bodies) that may accumulate on red blood cell membranes and cause mild to severe hemolysis (see *Signs and symptoms of unstable hemoglobin*)

PURPOSE
◆ To detect unstable Hb

PREPARATION
◆ Notify the laboratory and practitioner of drugs the patient is taking that may affect test results; they may be restricted.
◆ No dietary restrictions are required.
◆ The test requires a blood sample.

Teaching points
◆ Explain that the unstable Hb test detects abnormal Hb in the blood.
◆ Explain who will perform the test and where it'll be done.
◆ Inform the patient that he doesn't need to restrict food and fluids.
◆ Tell the patient that the test requires a blood sample and that he may experience slight discomfort from the tourniquet and needle puncture.
◆ Tell the patient that the test takes less than 5 minutes.

DIAGNOSTIC PROCEDURE

KEY STEPS
◆ Confirm the patient's identity using two patient identifiers according to facility policy.
◆ Perform a venipuncture and collect the sample in a 3- or 4.5-ml EDTA tube.
◆ Completely fill the collection tube and invert it gently several times to mix the sample and anticoagulant thoroughly.

POSTPROCEDURE CARE
◆ Make sure that subdermal bleeding has stopped before removing pressure.
◆ If a large hematoma develops at the venipuncture site, monitor pulses distal to the site.
◆ Inform the practitioner of abnormal results.
◆ Tell the patient to resume his medications.

PRECAUTIONS
◆ To avoid hemolysis, don't shake the tube vigorously.

COMPLICATIONS
◆ Hematoma at the venipuncture site

INTERPRETATION

NORMAL RESULTS
◆ Heat stability test result is negative; isopropanol solubility test result is stable.

ABNORMAL RESULTS
◆ A positive heat stability test result or unstable solubility test result, especially with hemolysis, strongly suggests the presence of unstable Hb.

Signs and symptoms of unstable hemoglobin

More than 60 varieties of unstable hemoglobin (Hb) exist, each named after the city in which it was discovered. Their effects vary according to their number, the degree of instability, the condition of the spleen, and the oxygen-binding abilities of the unstable Hb.

Patients with unstable Hb typically exhibit pallor, jaundice, splenomegaly, and — with severely unstable Hb — cyanosis, pigmenturia, and hemoglobinuria. Thalassemia commonly causes similar signs and symptoms, but the molecular bases of the two diseases differ greatly.

Upper GI and small-bowel series

DESCRIPTION

◆ Fluoroscopically examines the esophagus, stomach, and small intestine after ingestion of barium sulfate, a contrast agent
◆ Shows peristalsis and mucosal contours of organs; spot films record significant findings
◆ Suitable for patients with upper GI symptoms (such as difficulty swallowing, regurgitation, burning, or gnawing epigastric pain), signs of small-bowel disease (for example, diarrhea or weight loss), or signs of GI bleeding (such as hematemesis and melena)
◆ Detects mucosal abnormalities; biopsy may be needed later to rule out cancer or distinguish specific inflammatory diseases
◆ For suspected GI tract perforation, Gastrografin (water-soluble contrast medium) used

PURPOSE

◆ To detect hiatal hernia, diverticula, and varices
◆ To help diagnose strictures, ulcers, tumors, regional enteritis, and malabsorption syndrome
◆ To detect motility disorders

PREPARATION

◆ Make sure the patient has signed an appropriate consent form.
◆ Note and report all allergies.
◆ Withhold oral medications after midnight and anticholinergics and opioids for 24 hours because these drugs affect small intestine motility.
◆ Withhold antacids, histamine-2 receptor antagonists, and proton pump inhibitors if gastric reflux is suspected.

Teaching points

◆ Explain the purpose of the test and how it's done.
◆ Explain who will perform the test and where it'll be done.
◆ Instruct the patient to maintain a low-residue diet for 2 or 3 days before the test. Also tell him to fast and avoid smoking after midnight the night before the test.
◆ Instruct the patient to remove all jewelry and metal objects.
◆ Inform the patient that the barium mixture has a milkshake consistency and chalky taste; although flavored, the patient may find the taste unpleasant. Tell him that he will need 16 to 20 oz (475 to 600 ml) for a complete examination.
◆ Warn the patient that the abdomen may be compressed to ensure proper coating of the stomach or intestinal walls with barium or to separate overlapping bowel loops.
◆ Tell the patient the test may take up to 6 hours, so he should bring something to read or otherwise pass the time.
◆ Inform the patient that his feces will be light-colored for 24 to 72 hours after the test.

KEY STEPS

◆ Confirm the patient's identity using two patient identifiers according to facility policy.
◆ After securing the patient in a supine position on the X-ray table, the table is tilted until the patient is erect, and the heart, lungs, and abdomen are examined fluoroscopically.
◆ The patient is then instructed to take several swallows of the barium suspension; its passage through the esophagus is observed.
◆ Occasionally, the patient is given a thick barium suspension, especially when esophageal pathology is strongly suspected.
◆ During fluoroscopic examination, spot films of the esophagus are taken from lateral angles and from right and left posteroanterior angles.
◆ When barium enters the stomach, the patient's abdomen is palpated or compressed to ensure adequate coating of the gastric mucosa with barium.
◆ To perform a double-contrast examination, the patient is instructed to sip the barium through a perforated straw. As he does so, a small amount of air is also introduced into the stomach to allow detailed examination of the gastric rugae, and spot films of significant findings are taken.
◆ The patient is instructed to ingest the remaining barium suspension, and the filling of the stomach and emptying into the duodenum are observed fluoroscopically.
◆ Two series of spot films of the stomach and duodenum are taken from posteroanterior, anteroposterior, oblique, and lateral angles, with the patient erect and then in a supine position.

(continued)

- The passage of barium into the remainder of the small intestine is then observed fluoroscopically, and spot films are taken at 30- to 60-minute intervals until the barium reaches the ileocecal valve and the region around it.
- If abnormalities in the small intestine are detected, the area is palpated and compressed to help clarify the defect, and a spot film is taken.
- When barium enters the cecum, the examination is complete.

POSTPROCEDURE CARE
- Make sure additional X-rays aren't needed before allowing the patient food, fluids, and oral drugs.
- Give a cathartic or enema.
- Because barium retention in the intestine may cause obstruction or fecal impaction, notify the practitioner if the patient doesn't pass barium within 2 to 3 days.
- Monitor the patient's vital signs, intake and output, and bowel movements.
- Watch for abdominal distention.
- Monitor bowel sounds.
- Inform the practitioner of abnormal results.
- Tell the patient to drink plenty of fluid (unless contraindicated) to help eliminate the barium.
- Tell him to notify the practitioner if he experiences abdominal fullness or pain or a delay in return to brown feces.

PRECAUTIONS
- The test is contraindicated in patients with obstruction or GI tract perforation because barium may intensify the obstruction or seep into the abdominal cavity. The test is also contraindicated in pregnant patients because of the possible teratogenic effects of radiation.

COMPLICATIONS
- Bowel obstruction
- Fecal impaction

INTERPRETATION

NORMAL RESULTS
- After the patient swallows the barium suspension, it pours over the base of the tongue into the pharynx and is propelled by a peristaltic wave through the entire length of the esophagus in about 2 seconds.
- The bolus evenly fills and distends the lumen of the pharynx and esophagus, and the mucosa appears smooth and regular.
- When the peristaltic wave reaches the base of the esophagus, the cardiac sphincter opens, allowing the bolus to enter the stomach; this is followed by closing of the cardiac sphincter.
- As barium enters the stomach, it outlines the characteristic longitudinal folds called rugae, which are best observed using the double-contrast technique.
- When the stomach is completely filled with barium, its outer contour appears smooth and regular without evidence of flattened, rigid areas suggesting intrinsic or extrinsic lesions.
- After barium enters the stomach, it quickly empties into the duodenal bulb through relaxation of the pyloric sphincter.
- Although the mucosa of the duodenal bulb is relatively smooth, circular folds become apparent as barium enters the duodenal loop; these folds deepen and become more numerous in the jejunum.
- Barium temporarily lodges between these folds, producing a speckled pattern on the X-ray film.
- As barium enters the ileum, the circular folds become less prominent and, except for their broadness, resemble those in the duodenum.
- The diameter of the small intestine tapers gradually from the duodenum to the ileum.

ABNORMAL RESULTS
- Structural abnormalities of the esophagus suggest possible strictures, tumors, hiatal hernia, diverticula, varices, and ulcers.
- Dilatation of the esophagus suggests possible benign strictures.
- Erosive changes in the esophageal mucosa suggest possible malignant strictures.
- Filling defects in the column of barium suggest possible esophageal tumors; malignant esophageal tumors change the mucosal contour.
- Narrowing of the distal esophagus strongly suggests achalasia (cardiospasm).
- Backflow of barium from the stomach into the esophagus suggests gastric reflux.
- Filling defects in the stomach, which usually disrupt peristalsis, suggest malignant tumors, usually adenocarcinomas.
- Outpouchings of the gastric mucosa that usually don't affect peristalsis suggest benign tumors, such as adenomatous polyps and leiomyomas.
- Evidence of partial or complete healing, characterized by radiating folds extending to the edge of the ulcer crater, suggests benign ulcers.
- Radiating folds that extend beyond the ulcer crater to the edge of the mass suggest malignant ulcers.
- Edematous changes in the mucosa of the antrum or duodenal loop, or dilation of the duodenal loop suggests possible pancreatitis or pancreatic carcinoma.
- Edematous changes, segmentation of the barium column, and flocculation in the small intestine suggest possible malabsorption syndrome.
- Filling defects of the small intestine suggest possible Hodgkin's disease and lymphosarcoma.

Urea clearance test

DESCRIPTION

◆ Quantitative analysis of urine levels of urea, the main nitrogenous component in urine and end product of protein metabolism (see *How urea is formed*)

◆ Urea clearance: blood urea content and total amount of urea excreted in urine are proportional only when rate of urine flow is 2 ml/minute or higher

◆ Accuracy decreased at lower flow rates

PURPOSE

◆ To assess overall renal function

PREPARATION

◆ Check the patient's medication history for drugs that may affect urea clearance. Review your findings with the laboratory and then notify the practitioner; the medications may be restricted.

◆ Withhold food and fluid for 8 hours before the test.

◆ The test requires two timed urine specimens and one blood sample.

Teaching points

◆ Explain that the test evaluates kidney function.

◆ Explain who will perform the test and where it'll be done.

◆ Instruct the patient to fast from midnight before the test and to abstain from exercise before and during the test.

◆ Tell the patient that the test requires two timed urine specimens and one blood sample.

◆ Tell him how the urine specimens will be collected.

◆ Inform the patient that he may experience slight discomfort from the tourniquet and the needle puncture.

◆ Tell the patient the test takes about 90 minutes.

KEY STEPS

◆ Confirm the patient's identity using two patient identifiers according to facility policy.

◆ Instruct the patient to empty his bladder and discard the urine. Then give him water to drink to ensure adequate urine output.

◆ Collect two specimens 1 hour apart, and mark the collection time on the laboratory request.

◆ Perform a venipuncture anytime during the collection period, and collect the sample in a 7-ml red-top tube.

POSTPROCEDURE CARE

◆ Apply pressure at the venipuncture site until bleeding stops.

◆ Inform the practitioner of abnormal results.

◆ After the test, tell the patient to resume his usual diet, medications, and activity.

PRECAUTIONS

◆ Send each specimen to the laboratory promptly.

◆ If the patient is catheterized, empty the drainage bag before beginning the sample collection.

◆ Handle the blood sample gently to prevent hemolysis.

◆ If the urine flow rate is less than 1 ml/minute, don't perform the test.

NORMAL RESULTS

◆ Urea clearance ranges from 64 to 99 ml/minute with maximal clearance.

◆ If the flow rate is less than 2 ml/minute, normal clearance is 41 to 68 ml/minute.

ABNORMAL RESULTS

◆ Low values may indicate decreased renal blood flow (due to shock or renal artery obstruction), acute or chronic glomerulonephritis, advanced bilateral chronic pyelonephritis, acute tubular necrosis, or nephrosclerosis.

◆ Low clearance rates may also result from advanced bilateral renal lesions (such as polycystic kidney disease, renal tuberculosis, or cancer), bilateral ureteral obstruction, heart failure, or dehydration.

◆ High urea clearance rates aren't diagnostically significant.

How urea is formed

Urea, the main nitrogenous component in urine, is the final product of protein metabolism. Amino acids are absorbed by the intestinal villi and pass from the portal vein into the liver. Because the liver stores only small amounts of amino acids — which are later returned to the blood for use in the synthesis of enzymes, hormones, or new protoplasm — the excess is converted into other substances, such as glucose, glycogen, and fat.

Before this conversion, the amino acids are deaminated — they lose their nitrogenous amino groups. These amino groups are then converted to ammonia. Because ammonia is extremely toxic, especially to the brain, it must be removed as quickly as it's formed. (Serious liver disease causes elevated blood ammonia levels and eventually leads to hepatic coma.)

In the liver, ammonia combines with carbon dioxide to form urea, which is released into the blood and ultimately secreted in urine.

Uric acid level test

OVERVIEW

DESCRIPTION
◆ Measures serum levels of uric acid, the major end metabolite of purine
◆ Helps detect disorders of purine metabolism, rapid destruction of nucleic acids, and conditions marked by impaired renal excretion, which typically raise serum uric acid levels

PURPOSE
◆ To confirm the diagnosis of gout
◆ To help detect renal dysfunction

PREPARATION
◆ Notify the laboratory and practitioner of drugs the patient is taking that may affect test results; they may be restricted.
◆ The patient should fast for 8 hours before the test.
◆ The test requires a blood sample.

Teaching points
◆ Explain that the uric acid test detects gout and kidney dysfunction.
◆ Explain who will perform the test and where it'll be done.
◆ Instruct the patient to fast for 8 hours before the test.
◆ Tell the patient that the test requires a blood sample and that he may experience slight discomfort from the tourniquet and needle puncture.
◆ Tell him the test takes less than 5 minutes.

DIAGNOSTIC PROCEDURE

KEY STEPS
◆ Confirm the patient's identity using two patient identifiers according to facility policy.
◆ Perform a venipuncture and collect the sample in a 3- or 4-ml clot-activator tube.

POSTPROCEDURE CARE
◆ Apply direct pressure to the venipuncture site until bleeding stops.
◆ Inform the practitioner of abnormal results.
◆ Tell the patient to resume his usual diet and medications, as ordered.

PRECAUTIONS
◆ Maintain standard precautions while collecting the sample.

COMPLICATIONS
◆ Hematoma at the venipuncture site

INTERPRETATION

NORMAL RESULTS
◆ In men, 3.4 to 7 mg/dl (SI, 202 to 416 µmol/L).
◆ In women, 2.3 to 6 mg/dl (SI, 143 to 357 µmol/L).

ABNORMAL RESULTS
◆ Increased uric acid levels may indicate gout or impaired kidney function.
◆ Levels may also rise in heart failure, glycogen storage disease (such as type I, von Gierke's disease), infections, hemolytic and sickle cell anemia, polycythemia, neoplasms, and psoriasis.
◆ Low uric acid levels may indicate defective tubular absorption (such as Fanconi's syndrome) or acute hepatic atrophy.

INTERFERING FACTORS Loop diuretics, ethambutol, vincristine, pyrazinamide, thiazides, and low doses of aspirin (may cause increased levels); aspirin in high doses (may cause decreased levels)

Urinalysis

DESCRIPTION

- Evaluates physical characteristics of urine; determines specific gravity and pH; detects and measures protein, glucose, and ketone bodies; examines sediment for blood cells, casts, and crystals
- Includes visual examination, reagent strip screening, refractometry for specific gravity, and microscopic inspection of centrifuged sediment

PURPOSE

- To screen the patient's urine for renal or urinary tract disease
- To help detect metabolic or systemic disease unrelated to renal disorders
- To detect substances (drugs)

PREPARATION

- Notify the laboratory and practitioner of drugs the patient is taking that may affect laboratory results.
- No dietary restrictions are required.

Teaching points

- Explain that this analysis helps to diagnose renal or urinary tract disease and to evaluate overall body function.
- Explain who will perform the test and where it'll be done.
- Inform the patient that he doesn't need to restrict food and fluids.
- Tell the patient that the test takes less than 5 minutes.

KEY STEPS

- Confirm the patient's identity using two patient identifiers according to facility policy.
- Collect a random urine specimen of at least 15 ml. Obtain a first-voided morning specimen if possible.
- Strain the specimen to catch calculi or calculus fragments if the patient is being evaluated for renal colic. Carefully pour the urine through an unfolded 4″ × 4″ gauze pad or a fine-mesh sieve placed over the specimen container.

POSTPROCEDURE CARE

- Inform the practitioner of abnormal results.
- Tell the patient to resume his usual medications, as ordered.

PRECAUTIONS

- Refrigerate the specimen if analysis will be delayed by 1 hour or greater.

COMPLICATIONS

- None

NORMAL RESULTS

- Color of urine is straw to dark yellow.
- Odor is slightly aromatic.
- Specimen appears clear.
- Specific gravity is 1.005 to 1.035.
- pH is 4.5 to 8.0.
- Red blood cells (RBCs) are 0 to 2 per high-power field.
- White blood cells (WBCs) or epithelial cells are 0 to 5 per high-power field.
- 1 to 2 hyaline casts/low-power field are found.
- Crystals are present.

ABNORMAL RESULTS

- Nonpathologic variations in normal values may result from diet, nonpathologic conditions, specimen collection time, and other factors.
- An alkaline pH (above 7.0) — characteristic of a vegetarian diet — causes turbidity and the formation of phosphate, carbonate, and amorphous crystals.
- An acid pH (below 7.0) — typical of a high-protein diet — produces turbidity and the formation of oxalate, cystine, leucine, tyrosine, amorphous urate, and uric acid crystals.
- Protein may be present in a benign condition known as orthostatic (postural) proteinuria.
- Most common in patients ages 10 to 20, proteinuria is intermittent, appears after prolonged standing, and disappears after recumbency.
- Transient benign proteinuria may also occur with fever, exposure to cold, emotional stress, or strenuous exercise.
- Systemic diseases that may cause proteinuria include lymphoma, hepatitis, diabetes mellitus, toxemia, hypertension, lupus erythematosus, and febrile illnesses.
- Proteinuria suggests renal failure or disease or multiple myeloma.
- Sugars may appear under normal conditions; most common sugar in urine is glucose.

(continued)

- Transient nonpathologic glycosuria may result from emotional stress or pregnancy and may follow ingestion of a high-carbohydrate meal.
- Centrifuged urine sediment contains cells, casts, crystals, bacteria, yeast, and parasites. RBCs commonly don't appear in urine without pathologic significance; however, strenuous exercise can cause hematuria.
- Color change can result from diet, drugs, and diseases.
- In diabetes mellitus, starvation, and dehydration, a fruity odor accompanies formation of ketone bodies.
- In urinary tract infections (UTIs), a fetid odor commonly is associated with *Escherichia coli.*
- Maple syrup urine disease and phenylketonuria also cause distinctive odors.
- Other abnormal odors include those similar to a brewery, sweaty feet, cabbage, fish, and sulfur.
- Turbid urine may contain RBCs or WBCs, bacteria, fat, or chyle and may reflect renal infection.
- Low-specific gravity (< 1.005) is characteristic of diabetes insipidus, nephrogenic diabetes insipidus, acute tubular necrosis, and pyelonephritis.
- Fixed-specific gravity, in which values remain 1.010 regardless of fluid intake, occurs in chronic glomerulonephritis with severe renal damage.
- High-specific gravity (> 1.035) occurs in nephrotic syndrome, dehydration, acute glomerulonephritis, heart failure, liver failure, and shock.
- Alkaline urine pH may result from Fanconi's syndrome, UTI caused by urea-splitting bacteria (*Proteus* and *Pseudomonas*), and metabolic or respiratory alkalosis.
- Acid urine pH is associated with renal tuberculosis, pyrexia, phenylketonuria, alkaptonuria, and acidosis.
- Glycosuria usually indicates diabetes mellitus, but may result from pheochromocytoma, Cushing's syndrome, impaired tubular reabsorption, advanced renal disease, and increased intracranial pressure.

- Ketonuria occurs in diabetes mellitus when cellular energy needs exceed available cellular glucose. In the absence of glucose, cells metabolize fat for energy. Ketone bodies — the end products of incomplete fat metabolism — accumulate in plasma and are excreted in the urine.
- Ketonuria may also occur in starvation states, low- or no-carbohydrate diets, and following diarrhea or vomiting.
- Bilirubin in urine may occur in liver disease resulting from obstructive jaundice or hepatotoxic drugs or toxins or from fibrosis of the biliary canaliculi (which may occur in cirrhosis).
- Increased urobilinogen in the urine may indicate liver damage, hemolytic disease, or severe infection.
- Decreased levels may occur with biliary obstruction, inflammatory disease, antimicrobial therapy, severe diarrhea, or renal insufficiency.
- Hematuria indicates bleeding within the genitourinary tract and may result from infection, obstruction, inflammation, trauma, tumors, glomerulonephritis, renal hypertension, lupus nephritis, renal tuberculosis, renal vein thrombosis, renal calculi, hydronephrosis, pyelonephritis, scurvy, malaria, parasitic infection of the bladder, subacute bacterial endocarditis, polyarteritis nodosa, and hemorrhagic disorders.
- Strenuous exercise or exposure to toxic chemicals may also cause hematuria.
- An excess of WBCs in urine usually implies urinary tract inflammation, especially cystitis or pyelonephritis.
- WBC and WBC casts in urine suggest renal infection or noninfective inflammatory disease.
- Numerous epithelial cells suggest renal tubular degeneration, such as heavy metal poisoning, eclampsia, and kidney transplant rejection.
- Casts form in the renal tubules and collecting ducts by agglutination of protein cells or cellular debris and are flushed loose by urine flow.

- Excessive numbers of casts indicate renal disease.
- Hyaline casts are associated with renal parenchymal disease, inflammation, trauma to the glomerular capillary membrane, and some physiologic states (such as after exercise); epithelial casts, with renal tubular damage, nephrosis, eclampsia, amyloidosis, and heavy metal poisoning; coarse and fine granular casts, with acute or chronic renal failure, pyelonephritis, and chronic lead intoxication; fatty and waxy casts, with nephrotic syndrome, chronic renal disease, and diabetes mellitus; RBC casts, with renal parenchymal disease (especially glomerulonephritis), renal infarction, subacute bacterial endocarditis, vascular disorders, sickle cell anemia, scurvy, blood dyscrasias, malignant hypertension, collagen disease, and acute inflammation; and WBC casts, with acute pyelonephritis and glomerulonephritis, nephrotic syndrome, pyogenic infection, and lupus nephritis.
- Numerous calcium oxalate crystals suggest hypercalcemia or ethylene glycol ingestion. Cystine crystals (cystinuria) reflect an inborn error of metabolism.
- Bacteria, yeast cells, and parasites in urine sediment reflect genitourinary tract infection or contamination of external genitalia.
- The most common parasite in sediment is *Trichomonas vaginalis,* which causes vaginitis, urethritis, and prostatovesiculitis.

Urinary calculi test

- Strains urine to remove any urinary calculi, so they can be chemically analyzed to reveal their cause
- Also known as *urolithiasis* or *urinary stones:* insoluble substances formed when mineral salts (such as calcium oxalate, calcium phosphate, magnesium ammonium phosphate, urate, or cystine) accumulate around the nuclei of bacteria, fibrin, blood clots, or epithelial cells (see *Types and causes of calculi*)
- Calculi usually formed in kidney, pass into ureter, and excreted in urine; variable size (microscopic to several centimeters); those that don't pass spontaneously may require surgical extraction or pulverization
- Can result from reduced urinary volume, increased excretion of mineral salts, urinary stasis, pH changes, and decreased protective substances
- Symptoms including hematuria, severe flank pain, dysuria, and urinary retention, frequency, and urgency

PURPOSE
- To detect and analyze calculi in the urine

PREPARATION
- No dietary restrictions are required.

Teaching points
- Tell the patient that this test detects urinary calculi; explain that laboratory analysis will reveal their composition.
- Tell the patient that his urine will be collected and strained.
- Advise the patient that he doesn't need to restrict food and fluids.
- Inform the patient that he will receive medication to control pain.

DIAGNOSTIC PROCEDURE

KEY STEPS
- Confirm the patient's identity using two patient identifiers according to facility policy.

- Have the patient void into the strainer.
- Inspect the strainer carefully because calculi may be minute, appearing like gravel or sand.
- Document the appearance of the calculi and the number, if possible.
- Place the calculi in a properly labeled container.

POSTPROCEDURE CARE
- Observe the patient for severe flank pain, dysuria, and urinary retention, frequency, or urgency. Hematuria should subside.
- Keep the strainer and urinal or bedpan within the patient's reach if he has received analgesics because he may be drowsy and unable to get out of bed to void.

PRECAUTIONS
- Send the container to the laboratory immediately for analysis.

COMPLICATIONS
- None

INTERPRETATION

NORMAL RESULTS
- No calculi are present.

ABNORMAL RESULTS
- More than 50% of all calculi in urine are of mixed composition, containing two or more mineral salts; calcium oxalate is the most common component.
- Determining the composition of calculi helps identify various metabolic disorders. This guides proper treatment and prevention measures.

Types and causes of calculi

A
Calcium oxalate calculi usually result from idiopathic hypercalciuria, a condition that reflects absorption of calcium from the bowel.

B
Calcium phosphate calculi usually result from primary hyperparathyroidism, which causes excessive reabsorption of calcium from bone.

C
Cystine calculi result from primary cystinuria, an inborn error of metabolism that prevents renal tubular reabsorption of cystine.

D
Urate calculi result from gout, dehydration (causing elevated uric acid levels), acidic urine, or hepatic dysfunction.

E
Magnesium ammonium phosphate calculi result from the presence of urea-splitting organisms, such as *Proteus*, which raises ammonia concentration and makes urine alkaline.

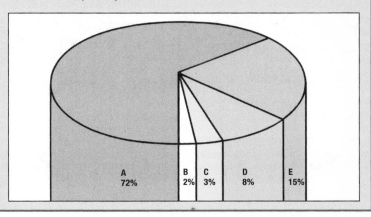

A	B	C	D	E
72%	2%	3%	8%	15%

Urine culture

DESCRIPTION

◆ Evaluates urinary tract infection (UTI), usually bladder infection
◆ Identifies pathogenic fungi such as *Coccidioides immitis*
◆ May use quick urine screen to determine if urine contains high bacteria or white blood cell (WBC) counts; only urine with bacteria or WBCs is processed for culture
◆ Preferred method of obtaining a urine specimen is clean-voided midstream collection, rather than suprapubic aspiration or catheterization
◆ To distinguish between true bacteriuria and contamination: need number of organisms in 1 milliliter of urine, estimated by a culture technique known as a colony count; additional quick centrifugation test determines origin of UTI (see *Quick centrifugation test*)
◆ Specimen collection performed on three consecutive mornings for patients with suspected urogenital tuberculosis

PURPOSE

◆ To diagnose UTI
◆ To monitor microorganism colonization after urinary catheter insertion

PREPARATION

◆ Make sure the patient has signed an appropriate consent form.
◆ Note and report all allergies.
◆ Check the patient's history for current use of antimicrobial drugs.
◆ Obtain the urine specimen before beginning antibiotic therapy.
◆ Maintain asepsis during the procedure as indicated.

Teaching points

◆ Explain that the test requires a urine specimen.
◆ Teach the patient how to collect a clean-voided midstream specimen. Stress the importance of cleaning the external genitalia thoroughly.
◆ Warn the patient of possible discomfort during specimen collection by catheterization.

KEY STEPS

◆ Confirm the patient's identity using two patient identifiers according to facility policy.
◆ Collect the first-voided urine specimen.
◆ Collect at least 3 ml of urine, but don't fill the specimen cup more than halfway.
◆ Record the suspected diagnosis, the collection time and method, current antimicrobial therapy, and fluid- or drug-induced diuresis on the laboratory request.
◆ Seal the cup with a sterile lid and send it to the laboratory at once.

POSTPROCEDURE CARE

◆ Answer the patient's questions.

PRECAUTIONS

◆ If transport is delayed for more than 30 minutes, store the specimen at 39.2° F (4° C) or place it on ice unless the urine transport tube contains a preservative.
◆ Inform the practitioner of abnormal results.

COMPLICATIONS

◆ Possible infection when specimens are obtained by catheterization

---

Quick centrifugation test

The quick centrifugation test can determine whether the source of a urinary tract infection is in the lower tract (bladder) or the upper tract (kidneys). The test involves centrifugation of urine in a test tube, followed by staining of the sediment with fluorescein. If one-quarter of the bacteria fluoresce when viewed under a fluorescent microscope, an upper tract infection is present; if bacteria don't fluoresce, a lower tract infection is present.

NORMAL RESULTS

◆ Sterile urine with no bacterial growth is noted.

ABNORMAL RESULTS

◆ Bacterial count of 100,000 or more organisms of a single microbe species per milliliter suggest UTI; less than 100,000/ml may be significant based on the patient's age, sex, history, and other individual factors.
◆ Bacterial count less than 10,000/ml usually suggest that the organisms are contaminants, except in symptomatic patients or those with urologic disorders.
◆ Isolation of *Mycobacterium tuberculosis* in a special test for acid-fast bacteria suggests tuberculosis of the urinary tract.
◆ Isolation of more than two species of organisms or of vaginal or skin organisms usually suggests contamination and requires a repeat culture.

Urine hydroxyproline level

DESCRIPTION

◆ Determines hydroxyproline levels colorimetrically on a timed urine sample or by ion-exchange or gas-liquid chromatography
◆ Measures total urine levels of hydroxyproline, an amino acid found mainly in collagen (a component of skin and bone); good index of bone matrix turnover because levels increase when collagen breaks down during bone resorption
◆ In children: bone matrix turnover and hydroxyproline levels rise during periods of rapid skeletal growth; levels also rise in disorders that increase bone resorption, such as Paget's disease, metastatic bone tumors, and certain endocrine disorders
◆ Collagen-restricted diet essential because hydroxyproline levels reflect collagen intake
◆ Free hydroxyproline — small component of total hydroxyproline and sensitive indicator of dietary collagen intake — measured to validate results

PURPOSE

◆ To monitor treatment for disorders characterized by bone resorption, including Paget's disease, metastatic bone tumors, certain endocrine disorders (hyperthyroidism), rheumatoid arthritis, and osteoporosis
◆ To help diagnose disorders characterized by bone resorption

PREPARATION

◆ Notify the laboratory and practitioner of drugs the patient is taking that may affect test results; they may be restricted.
◆ Inform the patient to follow a collagen-free diet and to avoid eating ice cream, candy, meat, fish, poultry, jelly, and any foods containing gelatin for 24 hours before the test and during the test period.
◆ Note the patient's age and sex on the laboratory request.

Teaching points

◆ Explain that the urine hydroxyproline test helps monitor treatment or detect an amino acid disorder related to bone formation.
◆ Tell the patient that the test requires urine collection over a 2-hour or 24-hour period, and teach him the correct collection technique.
◆ Inform the patient to follow a collagen-free diet and to avoid eating ice cream, candy, meat, fish, poultry, jelly, and any gelatin-containing foods for 24 hours before and during the test period.

KEY STEPS

◆ Confirm the patient's identity using two patient identifiers according to facility policy.
◆ Collect the patient's urine over a 2- or 24-hour period. In a 24-hour collection, discard the first sample and retain the last.
◆ Use a container that has a preservative to prevent hydroxyproline degradation.

POSTPROCEDURE CARE

◆ Inform the practitioner of abnormal results.
◆ Tell the patient to resume his usual diet and medications.

PRECAUTIONS

◆ Refrigerate the specimen or keep it on ice during the collection period.
◆ Send the specimen to the laboratory immediately after the collection is complete.

COMPLICATIONS

◆ None

NORMAL RESULTS

◆ Level is 1 to 9 mg/24 hours (SI, 1 to 3.4 International Units/d).

ABNORMAL RESULTS

◆ Decreased levels may occur during therapy for bone resorption disorders.
◆ Increased levels may indicate bone disease, metastatic bone tumors, or endocrine disorders that stimulate hormonal secretion.

✦ *INTERFERING FACTORS Agents used to treat Paget's disease (ascorbic acid, vitamin D, aspirin, glucocorticoids, antineoplastics, calcium gluconate, corticosteroids, estradiol, propranolol, calcitonin, and mithramycin (may decrease levels); burns (may increase levels because of collagen turnover); growth hormone, parathyroid hormone, phenobarbital, and sulfonylureas (may increase levels)*

Urine urobilinogen level test

DESCRIPTION

- Detects impaired liver function by measuring urine levels of urobilinogen — colorless, water-soluble product resulting from reduction of bilirubin by intestinal bacteria
- Quantitative analysis that involves addition of a reagent to a 2-hour urine specimen
- Resulting color reaction read promptly by spectrophotometry

PURPOSE

- To help diagnose extrahepatic obstruction such as blockage of the common bile duct
- To aid in the differential diagnosis of hepatic and hematologic disorders

PREPARATION

- Notify the laboratory and practitioner of drugs the patient is taking that may affect test results; they may be restricted.
- The test requires a 2-hour urine specimen.
- Instruct the patient not to eat bananas for 48 hours before the test.

Teaching points

- Explain that the urine urobilinogen test assesses liver and biliary tract function.
- Tell the patient that the test requires a 2-hour urine specimen, and teach him the proper collection technique.
- Inform the patient that he doesn't need to restrict food and fluids, except for bananas, which he should avoid for 48 hours before the test.

KEY STEPS

- Confirm the patient's identity using two patient identifiers according to facility policy.
- Most laboratories request a random urine specimen; others prefer a 2-hour specimen, usually during the afternoon (between 1 p.m. and 3 p.m.), when urobilinogen levels peak.

POSTPROCEDURE CARE

- Inform the practitioner of abnormal results.
- Tell the patient to resume his usual diet and medications.

PRECAUTIONS

- Send the specimen to the laboratory immediately after collection.
- This test must be performed within 30 minutes of collection because urobilinogen quickly oxidizes into an orange compound called urobilin.

COMPLICATIONS

- None

NORMAL RESULTS

- Level is 0.1 to 0.8 EU/2 hours (SI, 0.1 to 0.8 EU/2 hours) or 0.5 to 4 EU/24 hours (SI, 0.5 to 4 EU/d).

ABNORMAL RESULTS

- Absence of urine urobilinogen may result from hepatic damage or dysfunction, complete obstructive jaundice, or treatment with broad-spectrum antibiotics.
- Decreased levels may result from congenital enzymatic jaundice (for example, hyperbilirubinemia syndromes) or treatment with drugs that acidify urine, such as ammonium chloride or ascorbic acid.
- Increased levels may indicate hemolysis of red blood cells, hemolytic jaundice, hepatitis, or cirrhosis.

Urine vanillylmandelic acid level

DESCRIPTION

- Determines urine levels of vanillylmandelic acid (VMA, a phenolic acid), using spectrophotofluorometry; helps detect pheochromocytoma and evaluate adrenal medulla function
- VMA: product of hepatic conversion of epinephrine and norepinephrine; catecholamine metabolite that's prevalent in urine; levels reflect endogenous production of these catecholamines
- Performed on a 24-hour urine specimen (not a random specimen) to overcome the effects of diurnal variations in catecholamine secretion
- May measure other catecholamine metabolites — metanephrine, normetanephrine, and homovanillic acid (HVA) — at the same time
- In evaluating hypertension, specimen collected during hypertensive episode

PURPOSE

- To help detect pheochromocytoma, neuroblastoma, and ganglioneuroma
- To evaluate the function of the adrenal medulla

PREPARATION

- Notify the laboratory and practitioner of drugs the patient is taking that may affect test results; they may need to be restricted.
- The test requires urine collection over 24 hours.
- The patient should avoid foods and beverages containing phenolic acid (such as coffee, tea, bananas, citrus fruits, chocolate, vanilla, and carbonated beverages) for 3 days before the test.
- The patient should avoid stressful situations and excessive physical activity during the urine collection period.

Teaching points

- Explain that the urine VMA test evaluates hormonal secretion.
- Tell the patient that the test requires collection of urine over a 24-hour period, and teach him the proper collection technique.

- Instruct the patient to restrict foods and beverages containing phenolic acid, such as coffee, tea, bananas, citrus fruits, chocolate, vanilla, and carbonated beverages for 3 days before the test.
- Advise the patient to avoid stressful situations and excessive physical activity during the urine collection period.

DIAGNOSTIC PROCEDURE

KEY STEPS

- Confirm the patient's identity using two patient identifiers according to facility policy.
- Collect the patient's urine over a 24-hour period, discarding the first specimen and retaining the last. Use a bottle containing a preservative to keep the specimen at a pH of 3.0.

POSTPROCEDURE CARE

- Tell family members of a patient with confirmed pheochromocytoma that they, too, should receive a careful evaluation for multiple endocrine neoplasia.
- Inform the practitioner of abnormal results.
- Tell the patient to resume his usual activities, diet, and medications.

PRECAUTIONS

- Refrigerate the specimen or keep it on ice during the collection period.
- Send the specimen to the laboratory immediately after the collection is completed.

COMPLICATIONS

- None

INTERPRETATION

NORMAL RESULTS

- Level is 1.4 to 6.5 mg/24 hours (SI, 7 to 33 µmol/d).

ABNORMAL RESULTS

- Increased levels may result from a catecholamine-secreting tumor. Further testing, such as measurement of urine HVA levels to rule out pheochromocytoma, is needed for precise diagnosis. (See *Diagnosing catecholamine-secreting tumors.*)
- If pheochromocytoma is confirmed, the patient should be tested for multiple endocrine neoplasia, an inherited condition commonly associated with pheochromocytoma.

Diagnosing catecholamine-secreting tumors

Pheochromocytoma is a catecholamine-producing tumor, causing hypersecretion of epinephrine and norepinephrine by the adrenal medulla; however, not every patient with this disorder has elevated urine catecholamine levels. Moreover, hypertension, a prime clue in this condition, is sometimes absent. Thus, an analysis of one or more catecholamine metabolites is helpful in confirming the diagnosis.

INTERPRETING TEST RESULTS

When urine catecholamine levels remain normal in patients with hypertension, elevated urine vanillylmandelic acid (VMA) levels may signal a tumor. Alternatively, metanephrine may be high when VMA and catecholamines are essentially unchanged. VMA assay is also an alternative method when catecholamine

analysis has been compromised by interfering food or drugs. Increased excretion of homovanillic acid (HVA) typically indicates malignant pheochromocytoma, although the incidence of malignancy is low.

Measurement of urine VMA is also useful for diagnosing two neurogenic tumors — neuroblastoma, a common soft-tissue tumor that's a leading cause of death in infants and young children, and ganglioneuroma, a well-defined tumor of the sympathetic nervous system that occurs in older children and young adults. Both tumors primarily produce dopamine and thus show the expected high readings of dopamine's metabolite, HVA, especially in their malignant forms. However, both tumors also show abnormal increases in urine VMA levels.

Uroflowmetry

DESCRIPTION

- Detects and evaluates dysfunctional voiding patterns by a simple, noninvasive test
- Involves voiding into funnel containing an uroflowmeter; measures flow rate (volume of urine voided per second), continuous flow (time of measurable flow), and intermittent flow (total voiding time, including interruptions)
- Gravimetric system: weighs urine as it's voided and plots the weight against time; simple to use and widely available
- Other uroflowmeters: rotary disc, electromagnetic, and spectrophotometric systems

PURPOSE

- To evaluate lower urinary tract function
- To demonstrate bladder outlet obstruction

PREPARATION

- Make sure the patient has signed an appropriate consent form.
- Note and report all allergies.
- Stop drugs that may affect bladder and sphincter tone.
- Provide complete privacy during the test.

Teaching points

- Explain the purpose of the test and how it's done.
- Explain who will perform the test and where it'll be done.
- Instruct the patient not to urinate for several hours before the test and to increase fluid intake so he'll have a full bladder and a strong urge to void.
- Instruct the patient to remain still while voiding during the test to help ensure accurate results.
- Tell the patient that the test takes 10 to 15 minutes.

KEY STEPS

- Confirm the patient's identity using two patient identifiers according to facility policy.
- The test procedure is the same with all types of equipment.
- Ask a male patient to void while standing.
- Ask a female patient to void while sitting.
- Instruct the patient to avoid straining to empty the bladder.
- Check cable connections, and leave the patient.
- The patient pushes the START button on the commode chair, counts for 5 seconds, and voids.
- When finished, he counts for 5 seconds and pushes the button again.
- The volume of urine voided is then recorded and plotted as a curve over the time of voiding.
- Note the patient's position and the route of fluid intake (oral or I.V.).

POSTPROCEDURE CARE

- Teach self-catheterization if indicated.
- Provide bladder training as needed.
- Monitor the patient for urine retention and bladder distention.
- Monitor the patient's intake and output.
- Tell the patient to resume his medications.

PRECAUTIONS

- The transducer must be level and the beaker must be centered beneath the funnel.
- The beaker must be large enough to hold all urine; overflow can invalidate results and damage the transducer.

COMPLICATIONS

- None

NORMAL RESULTS

- Results vary by age, sex, and the volume of urine voided.

ABNORMAL RESULTS

- An increased flow rate suggests reduced urethral resistance, which may be associated with external sphincter dysfunction.
- A high peak on the curve plotted over the voiding time suggests decreased outflow resistance, which may be associated with stress incontinence.
- A decreased flow rate suggests outflow obstruction or hypotonia of the detrusor muscle.
- More than one distinct peak in a normal curve suggests abdominal straining, which may result from pushing against an obstruction to empty the bladder.

Venereal Disease Research Laboratory test

DESCRIPTION

◆ Flocculation test to screen for primary and secondary syphilis
◆ Has diagnostic significance during first two stages of syphilis; transient or permanent biologic false-positive reactions can make accurate interpretation difficult
◆ Serum sample usually used; may use cerebrospinal (CSF) specimen to test for tertiary syphilis

◆ Less sensitive than fluorescent treponemal antibody absorption test (see *Serodiagnostic tests for untreated syphilis*)
◆ Rapid plasma reagin test: may be used to diagnose syphilis (see *Rapid plasma reagin test*)

PURPOSE

◆ To screen for primary and secondary syphilis
◆ To confirm primary or secondary syphilis in the presence of syphilitic lesions
◆ To monitor the patient's response to treatment

PREPARATION

◆ No dietary restrictions are required, other than withholding alcohol.
◆ The test requires a blood sample.

Teaching points

◆ Explain that the test detects syphilis.
◆ Explain who will perform the test and where it'll be done.
◆ Inform the patient that the disease usually goes undetected in the general population because most infected people don't know they're infected, and thus remain untreated.
◆ Tell the patient that he doesn't need to restrict food, fluids, or medications but should abstain from alcohol for 24 hours before the test.
◆ Tell the patient that the test requires a blood sample and that he may experience slight discomfort from the tourniquet and needle puncture.
◆ Tell the patient that the test takes less than 5 minutes.

(continued)

Serodiagnostic tests for untreated syphilis

The fluorescent treponemal antibody absorption (FTA-ABS) test — which uses a strain of the *Treponema pallidum* antigen itself as a reagent — is more sensitive than the Venereal Disease Research Laboratory (VDRL) test or the rapid plasma reagin (RPR) test in detecting all stages of untreated syphilis (as shown in the graph below). However, the test's complexity and the incidence of false-positive results make it an impractical screening tool. The VDRL and RPR tests are preferred for wide-scale screening and also when primary- or secondary-stage disease is suspected. With advanced syphilis, when the VDRL test may be negative for more than one-third of infected people, the FTA-ABS test is preferred for sensitivity.

The VDRL test can also be used to monitor response to treatment. Untreated syphilis pro-

duces titers that are low in the primary stage (less than 1:32), elevated in the secondary stage (greater than 1:32), and variable in the tertiary stage. Successful therapy markedly reduces titers, with two-thirds of patients reverting to a negative VDRL, especially during the first two stages of the disease. Third-stage therapy seldom produces a nonreactive VDRL, but maintenance of low-reactive values during the 6- to 12-month posttherapy period indicates success. A subsequent rise signals reinfection. By comparison, FTA-ABS test results usually remain positive following treatment.

A significant number of patients with infectious diseases show temporary false-positive VDRL test results. Chronic false-positive VDRL and FTA-ABS test readings are associated with the immune complex diseases.

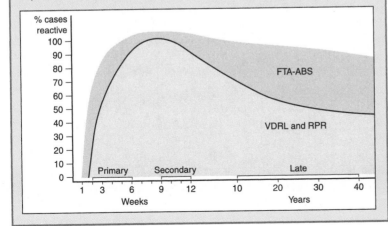

Rapid plasma reagin test

The rapid plasma reagin (RPR) test is a rapid, macroscopic serologic test that's an acceptable substitute for the Venereal Disease Research Laboratory (VDRL) test in diagnosing syphilis. The RPR test, available as a kit, uses a cardiolipin antigen to detect reagin, the antibody relatively specific for *Treponema pallidum*, the causative agent of syphilis.

In the RPR test, the patient's serum is mixed with cardiolipin on a plastic-coated card, rotated mechanically, and then examined with the unaided eye. If flocculation occurs, the test sample is diluted until no visible reaction occurs. The last dilution to show visible flocculation is the titer of the reagin antibody.

In the RPR test, as in the VDRL test, normal serum shows no flocculation.

DIAGNOSTIC PROCEDURE

KEY STEPS
- Confirm the patient's identity using two patient identifiers according to facility policy.
- Perform a venipuncture and collect the sample in a 7-ml clot-activator tube.

POSTPROCEDURE CARE
- Apply direct pressure to the venipuncture site until bleeding stops.
- If the test is reactive, report the results to state public health authorities and prepare the patient for mandatory inquiries.
- If the test is nonreactive or borderline, but syphilis hasn't been ruled out, instruct the patient to return for follow-up testing. Explain that borderline test results don't mean that he's free from the disease.
- If the test is reactive, explain the importance of proper treatment. Provide the patient with further information about sexually transmitted diseases and how they're spread and stress the need for antibiotic therapy.
- If the test is reactive, but the patient shows no clinical signs of syphilis, explain that uninfected people may show false-positive reactions. Stress the need for further specific tests to rule out syphilis.

PRECAUTIONS
- Handle the specimen gently to prevent hemolysis.

COMPLICATIONS
- Hematoma at venipuncture site

INTERPRETATION

NORMAL RESULTS
- Normal serum shows no flocculation and is reported as a nonreactive test.

ABNORMAL RESULTS
- Definite flocculation is reported as a reactive test; slight flocculation is reported as a weakly relative test.
- A reactive venereal disease research laboratory (VDRL) test occurs in about 50% of patients with primary syphilis and in almost all patients with secondary syphilis.
- If syphilitic lesions exist, a reactive VDRL test is diagnostic.
- If no lesions are evident, a reactive VDRL test necessitates repeated testing.
- A nonreactive test doesn't rule out syphilis because *Treponema pallidum* causes no detectable immunologic changes in the serum for 14 to 21 days after infection.
- Dark-field microscopy of exudate from suspicious lesions can provide early diagnosis by identifying the causative spirochetes.
- A reactive VDRL test using a CSF specimen indicates neurosyphilis, which can follow the primary and secondary states in patients who remain untreated.

Venography, leg

DESCRIPTION

◆ Radiographically examines veins in the leg to assess deep leg veins after injection of a contrast medium; used when duplex ultrasound findings are equivocal
◆ Not used for routine screening because it exposes the patient to relatively high doses of radiation and can cause phlebitis, local tissue damage, and, occasionally, deep vein thrombosis (DVT)
◆ Also known as *ascending contrast phlebography*

PURPOSE

◆ To confirm a diagnosis of DVT
◆ To distinguish clot formation from venous obstruction (such as a large tumor of the pelvis impinging on the venous system)
◆ To evaluate congenital venous abnormalities
◆ To assess deep vein valvular competence (helpful in identifying underlying causes of leg edema)
◆ To locate a suitable vein for arterial bypass grafting
◆ To evaluate chronic venous disease

PREPARATION

◆ Have the patient sign a consent form.
◆ Tell the patient that this test evaluates deep leg veins.
◆ Note and report all allergies.
◆ Report hypersensitivity to iodine, iodine-containing foods, or contrast media.
◆ Stop anticoagulant therapy.
◆ Give the patient a sedative.
◆ Withhold food and give only clear liquids for 4 hours before the test.

Teaching points

◆ Explain who will perform the study and where it'll be done.
◆ Explain the purpose of the study and how it's done.
◆ Instruct the patient to restrict food and drink only clear liquids for 4 hours before the test.

◆ Reassure the patient that contrast media complications are rare, but tell him to promptly report nausea, severe burning or itching, constriction in the throat or chest, or dyspnea.
◆ Warn the patient that he might experience a burning sensation in the leg when the contrast medium is injected and some discomfort during the procedure.
◆ Tell the patient that the test takes 30 to 45 minutes.

DIAGNOSTIC PROCEDURE

KEY STEPS

◆ Confirm the patient's identity using two patient identifiers according to facility policy.
◆ Position the patient on a tilting X-ray table so that the leg being tested doesn't bear any weight.
◆ Tie a tourniquet around the ankle to expedite venous filling.
◆ Normal saline solution is injected into a superficial vein in the dorsum of the patient's foot, and a contrast medium is injected after placement has been confirmed.
◆ Using a fluoroscope, the distribution of the contrast medium is monitored, and spot films of the thigh and femoroiliac regions are taken from the anteroposterior and oblique views.
◆ Overhead films are taken of the calf, knee, thigh, and femoral area.
◆ After filming, reposition the patient horizontally, quickly elevate the leg being tested, and infuse normal saline solution to flush the contrast medium from the veins.
◆ The fluoroscope is checked to confirm complete emptying.
◆ After the needle is removed, apply a dressing to the injection site.

POSTPROCEDURE CARE

◆ Give the patient analgesics.
◆ Encourage fluids.
◆ If DVT is documented, start therapy (heparin infusion, bed rest, and leg elevation or support).
◆ Monitor vital signs and fluid intake and output.

◆ Monitor the injection site for bleeding, infection, hematoma, and erythema.
◆ Tell the patient to resume his usual diet and medications, as ordered.

PRECAUTIONS

◆ Because of the high volume of contrast used, especially if bilateral venography is needed, monitor renal function and hydration status carefully.

⚡ **WARNING** *Because most allergic reactions to contrast media occur within 30 minutes of injection, observe the patient for signs and symptoms of anaphylaxis, such as flushing, urticaria, and laryngeal stridor.*

COMPLICATIONS

◆ Adverse reactions to contrast media or drugs
◆ Thrombophlebitis
◆ Local tissue damage
◆ Renal insufficiency or failure
◆ Small extravasations of contrast media (less than 10 ml) don't usually pose a problem, but tissue necrosis and ulceration may occur, especially with larger extravasations and in patients with arterial insufficiency

INTERPRETATION

NORMAL RESULTS

◆ Steady opacification of the superficial and deep vasculature with no filling defects is noted.

ABNORMAL RESULTS

◆ Consistent filling defects, abrupt termination of a column of contrast material, unfilled major deep veins, or diversion of flow (through collaterals, for example) suggest DVT.
◆ Improper needle placement in a superficial vein, weight bearing or muscle contraction, or use of tourniquets can produce artifacts of poor filling.
◆ Diagnosis errors often result from incomplete filling.
◆ Fluoroscopy is essential for establishing that the contrast medium has reached the vessels being filmed and that opacification is adequate.

Vertebral radiography

DESCRIPTION

◆ Radiographically shows all or part of the vertebral column to determine bone density, texture, erosion, and changes in bone relationships
◆ X-rays of bone cortex: reveal widening or narrowing and signs of irregularity
◆ Joint X-rays: reveal fluid, spur formation, narrowing or widening of the cortex, and changes in joint structure
◆ Type and extent dependent on patient's condition (for example, patients with lower back pain require a study of lumbar and sacral segments only)

PURPOSE

◆ To detect vertebral fractures, dislocations, subluxations, and deformities
◆ To detect vertebral degeneration, infection, and congenital disorders
◆ To detect disorders of the intervertebral disks
◆ To determine the vertebral effects of arthritic and metabolic disorders
◆ To follow the progression of certain disorders (such as scoliosis in children)

PREPARATION

◆ Make sure the patient has signed an appropriate consent form.
◆ Note and report all allergies.
◆ No dietary restrictions are required.

Teaching points

◆ Explain that this test evaluates bone structure in the vertebral column.
◆ Explain the purpose of the study and how it's done.
◆ Tell the patient that he doesn't need to restrict food and fluids.
◆ Inform the patient that positioning for the radiographic films may cause slight discomfort and that his cooperation will ensure accurate results.
◆ Stress the importance of remaining still and holding his breath for film exposure during the procedure.
◆ Tell the patient that the test takes 15 to 30 minutes.

KEY STEPS

◆ Confirm the patient's identity using two patient identifiers according to facility policy.
◆ The procedure varies considerably, depending on which vertebral segment is being examined.
◆ Assist the patient into a supine position on the X-ray table for an anteroposterior view.
◆ Reposition the patient for lateral or right and left oblique views; specific positioning depends on the vertebral segment or adjacent structures of interest.
◆ X-rays are obtained as required.

POSTPROCEDURE CARE

◆ Answer the patient's questions.

PRECAUTIONS

◆ Exercise extreme caution when handling trauma patients with suspected spinal injuries, especially of the cervical area. Such patients should be filmed while on the stretcher to avoid further injury during transfer to the X-ray table.

COMPLICATIONS

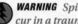 **WARNING** *Spinal injury may occur in a trauma patient.*

NORMAL RESULTS

◆ Vertebrae are without fractures, subluxations, dislocations, abnormal curvatures, or other abnormalities.
◆ Specific positions and spacing of the vertebrae vary with the patient's age. In the lateral view, adult vertebrae are aligned to form four alternately concave and convex curves.
◆ The cervical and lumbar curves are convex anteriorly; the thoracic and sacral curves are concave anteriorly.
◆ Although the structure of the coccyx varies, it usually points forward and downward.
◆ Neonatal vertebrae form only one curve, which is concave anteriorly.

ABNORMAL RESULTS

◆ Spondylolisthesis, fractures, subluxations, dislocations, wedging are noted.
◆ Deformities of the spine, such as kyphosis, scoliosis, and lordosis, are seen.
◆ There's an absence of sacral or lumbar vertebrae (congenital abnormalities).
◆ Hypertrophic spurs and osteoarthritis (degenerative processes) are noted.
◆ Thinning of the bone (osteoporosis) is observed.
◆ Intervertebral discs and adjacent surfaces of vertebral bodies are destroyed by lesions (tuberculosis).
◆ Benign or malignant intraspinal tumors are visible.

Visual acuity test

DESCRIPTION
- Evaluates a patient's ability to distinguish the form and detail of an object
- For all patients with eye complaints: letters read on a standardized visual chart (Snellen chart) from a distance of 20' (6.1 m)
- For young children and those who can't read: charts with letter "E" in various positions and sizes used (see *Visual acuity charts*)
- The smaller the symbol the patient can identify, the sharper his visual acuity
- Patient's near (reading) vision tested with standardized chart such as the Jaeger card (card with print in graded sizes)
- Near-vision test: routine test for those complaining of eyestrain or reading difficulty and for persons older than age 40
- Results serve as a baseline for treatments, follow-up examinations, and referrals

PURPOSE
- To test distance and near visual acuity
- To identify refractive errors in vision

PREPARATION
- If the patient wears glasses, tell him to bring them to the examination.

Teaching points
- Tell the patient that these tests evaluate distance and near vision.
- Explain who will perform the test and where it'll be done.
- Tell the patient that the test takes less than 10 minutes.

DIAGNOSTIC PROCEDURE

KEY STEPS
- Confirm the patient's identity using two patient identifiers according to facility policy.

Distance visual acuity
- Have the patient sit 20' (6.1 m) away from the eye chart. If he's wearing glasses, tell him to remove them so his uncorrected vision can be tested first.
- Begin with the right eye unless vision in the left eye is known to be more acute.
- Have the patient occlude the left eye; then ask him to read the smallest line of letters he can see on the chart.
- Encourage him to try to read lines he can't see clearly because intelligent guesses usually indicate that the patient can recognize some details of the symbols.
- If using the "E" chart, have the preschool child compare the letter to a table with three legs. Then ask the child to point to the direction in which the legs of the table are pointing.
- Record the number of the smallest line the patient can read; this number is expressed as a fraction. The numerator is the distance between the patient and the chart; the denominator is the distance from which a patient with normal vision can read the line. The greater the denominator, the poorer the vision.
- If the patient makes an error on a line, record the results with a minus number. For example, if the patient reads the 20/40 line but makes one error, record his vision as 20/40 –1. If the patient reads the 20/40 line and one symbol on the next line, record his vision as 20/40 +1.

Visual acuity charts

The most commonly used charts for testing vision are the Snellen alphabet chart (left) and the Snellen E chart (right), which is used for young children and adults who can't read.

SNELLEN ALPHABET CHART

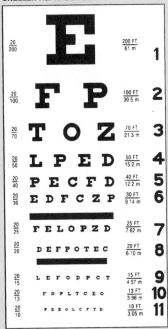

SNELLEN E CHART

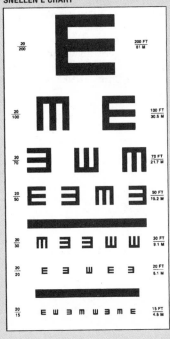

(continued)

- Have the patient occlude the right eye; then repeat the test for the left eye. To minimize recall, use a different set of symbols or have the patient read the lines backward.
- If the patient wears glasses, test his corrected vision using the same procedure. If he normally wears glasses but doesn't have them with him, note this on the test results.
- In recording the patient's responses, indicate which eye was tested and whether corrective lenses were worn.

Near visual acuity
- Have the patient remove his glasses and occlude the left eye. Ask him to read the Jaeger card at his customary reading distance.
- Test both eyes, with and without corrective lenses.
- In reporting near visual acuity, specify the size of the smallest print legible to the patient and the nearest distance at which reading is possible.

POSTPROCEDURE CARE
- If the patient can't read the largest letter on the chart, further testing is needed.

PRECAUTIONS
- None

COMPLICATIONS
- None

NORMAL RESULTS
- Distance visual acuity, 20/20 (the smallest symbol the patient can identify at 20' [6.1 m] is the same symbol a patient with normal vision can identify from the same distance).
- Near visual acuity, 14/14 (a person can read at 14" [36 cm] what a person with normal vision can read from the same distance).

ABNORMAL RESULTS
- If the denominator is more than 20 (for example, 40), his visual acuity is less than normal. In this case, it means he reads at 20' what a person with normal vision can read at 40' (12.2 m).
- A person with visual acuity of 20/200 in the better eye is considered legally blind. Similarly, if the denominator is less than 20, the patient's distance visual acuity is better than normal. For example, 20/15 vision means that the patient can read at 20' (6.1 m) what a person with normal visual acuity can see at 15' (4.6 m).
- Decreased near visual acuity is indicated by a larger denominator. For example, 14/20 near vision means that the patient can read at 14" (36 cm) what a person with normal vision can read at 20" (50.8 cm).

- Normal or better-than-normal visual acuity doesn't necessarily indicate normal vision. For example, a visual field defect may be present if the patient consistently misses the letters on one side of all the lines.
- A field defect exists if the patient states that one or more of the letters disappear or become illegible when he's looking at a nearby letter. This indicates the need for further visual field testing, such as Amsler's grid test or the tangent screen examination.
- Patients with less-than-normal visual acuity require further testing (including refraction and complete ophthalmologic examination) to determine whether visual loss is from injury, disease, or a need for corrective lenses.

Vitamin A and carotene level test

DESCRIPTION

- Measures serum levels of vitamin A (retinol) and its precursor, carotene
- Quantitative and qualitative information provided by color reactions when vitamin A and related compounds react with reagents
- Vitamin A: fat-soluble vitamin found in diet (for example, fruits, vegetables, eggs, poultry, meat, and fish); important for reproduction, vision (especially night), and epithelial tissue and bone growth
- Carotene: occurs in leafy green vegetables and in yellow fruits and vegetables

PURPOSE

- To investigate suspected vitamin A deficiency or toxicity
- To help diagnose visual disturbances, especially night blindness and xerophthalmia
- To help diagnose skin diseases, such as keratosis follicularis or ichthyosis
- To screen for malabsorption

PREPARATION

- Withhold food for 8 hours before the test.
- The test requires a blood sample.

Teaching points

- Explain that this test measures the vitamin A level in blood.
- Explain who will perform the test and where it'll be done.
- Instruct the patient to fast overnight, but tell him that he doesn't need to restrict water intake.
- Tell the patient that the test requires a blood sample and that he may experience slight discomfort from the tourniquet and needle puncture.
- Tell the patient that the test takes less than 5 minutes.

KEY STEPS

- Confirm the patient's identity using two patient identifiers according to facility policy.
- Perform a venipuncture and collect the sample in a chilled 7-ml siliconized tube.
- Protect the sample from light because vitamin A absorbs light.

POSTPROCEDURE CARE

- Apply direct pressure to the venipuncture site until bleeding stops.
- Tell the patient to resume his usual diet.

PRECAUTIONS

- Maintain standard precautions while collecting the sample.
- Keep the specimen on ice.
- Handle the sample gently and send it to the laboratory immediately.

COMPLICATIONS

- Hematoma at the venipuncture site

NORMAL RESULTS

- Vitamin A, 30 to 80 mcg/dl (SI, 1.05 to 2.8 µmol/L).
- Carotene, 10 to 85 mcg/dl (SI, 0.19 to 1.58 µmol/L).

ABNORMAL RESULTS

- Decreased vitamin A levels (hypovitaminosis A) may indicate impaired fat absorption, such as in celiac disease, infectious hepatitis, cystic fibrosis of the pancreas, or obstructive jaundice; chronic nephritis; or protein-calorie malnutrition (marasmic kwashiorkor).
- Increased vitamin A levels (hypervitaminosis A) usually indicate chronically excessive intake of vitamin A supplements or of foods high in vitamin A; other causes are hyperlipemia and hypercholesterolemia of uncontrolled diabetes mellitus.
- Decreased serum carotene levels may result from pregnancy or from impaired fat absorption or, rarely, insufficient dietary intake of carotene.
- Increased carotene levels indicate grossly excessive dietary intake.

Vitamin B$_2$ level, serum

OVERVIEW

DESCRIPTION
◆ Evaluates serum levels of vitamin B$_2$ (riboflavin); essential for growth and tissue function
◆ More reliable than urine test, which can produce artificially high values in patients after surgery or prolonged fasting

PURPOSE
◆ To detect vitamin B$_2$ deficiency

PREPARATION
◆ No dietary restrictions are required.
◆ The test requires a blood sample.

Teaching points
◆ Explain that this test evaluates vitamin B$_2$ levels.
◆ Explain who will perform the test and where it'll be done.
◆ Instruct the patient to maintain a normal diet before the test.
◆ Tell the patient that the test requires a blood sample and that he may experience slight discomfort from the tourniquet and needle puncture.
◆ Tell the patient that the test takes less than 5 minutes.

DIAGNOSTIC PROCEDURE

KEY STEPS
◆ Confirm the patient's identity using two patient identifiers according to facility policy.
◆ Perform a venipuncture and collect the sample in a 4.5-ml siliconized tube.

POSTPROCEDURE CARE
◆ Apply direct pressure to the venipuncture site until bleeding stops.
◆ Inform the patient with vitamin B$_2$ deficiency that good dietary sources of vitamin B$_2$ are milk products, organ meats (such as liver and kidneys), fish, green leafy vegetables, legumes, and fortified breads and cereals.

PRECAUTIONS
◆ Handle the sample gently to prevent hemolysis.
◆ Don't refrigerate or freeze the sample.
◆ Send the sample to the laboratory immediately.

COMPLICATIONS
◆ Hematoma at the venipuncture site

INTERPRETATION

NORMAL RESULTS
◆ Level is 3 to 15 mcg/dl.

ABNORMAL RESULTS
◆ Level less than 2 mcg/dl indicates vitamin B$_2$ deficiency, from insufficient dietary intake of vitamin B$_2$, malabsorption syndrome, or conditions that increase metabolic demands such as stress.

Vitamin B$_{12}$ level test

OVERVIEW

DESCRIPTION
- Radioisotope assay of competitive binding to quantitatively analyze serum levels of vitamin B$_{12}$ (also called *cyanocobalamin, antipernicious anemia factor,* or *extrinsic factor*); usually performed with measurement of serum folic acid levels
- Water-soluble vitamin containing cobalt; essential to hematopoiesis, deoxyribonucleic acid synthesis and growth, myelin synthesis, and central nervous system (CNS) integrity
- Occurs almost exclusively in animal products, such as meat, shellfish, milk, and eggs

PURPOSE
- To aid in the differential diagnosis of megaloblastic anemia, which may be caused by a vitamin B$_{12}$ or folic acid deficiency
- To aid in the differential diagnosis of CNS disorders that are affecting peripheral and spinal myelinated nerves

PREPARATION
- Check the patient's history for drugs that may alter test results, and note these on the laboratory request.
- Withhold food and fluid for 8 hours before the test.
- The test requires a blood sample.

Teaching points
- Explain that this test determines the amount of vitamin B$_{12}$ in blood.
- Explain who will perform the test and where it'll be done.
- Instruct the patient to fast overnight before the test.
- Tell the patient that the test requires a blood sample and that he may experience slight discomfort from the tourniquet and needle puncture.
- Tell the patient that the test takes less than 5 minutes.

DIAGNOSTIC PROCEDURE

KEY STEPS
- Confirm the patient's identity using two patient identifiers according to facility policy.
- Perform a venipuncture and collect the sample in a 4.5-ml siliconized tube.

POSTPROCEDURE CARE
- Apply direct pressure to the venipuncture site until bleeding stops.
- Tell the patient to resume his usual diet, as ordered.

PRECAUTIONS
- Handle the sample gently to prevent hemolysis.
- Send the sample to the laboratory immediately.

COMPLICATIONS
- Hematoma at the venipuncture site

INTERPRETATION

NORMAL RESULTS
- Level is 200 to 900 pg/ml (SI, 148 to 664 pmol/L).

ABNORMAL RESULTS
- Decreased serum vitamin B$_{12}$ levels may indicate inadequate dietary intake, especially in strictly vegetarian patients; malabsorption syndromes such as celiac disease; isolated malabsorption of vitamin B$_{12}$; hypermetabolic states such as hyperthyroidism; pregnancy; and CNS damage (for example, posterolateral sclerosis or funicular degeneration).
- Increased serum vitamin B$_{12}$ levels may result from excessive dietary intake; hepatic disease (such as cirrhosis or acute or chronic hepatitis) and myeloproliferative disorders such as myelocytic leukemia.

Vitamin C level test

DESCRIPTION

◆ Chemical assay that measures plasma levels of vitamin C (ascorbic acid)
◆ Water-soluble vitamin: needed for collagen synthesis and cartilage and bone maintenance; promoting iron absorption and influencing folic acid metabolism; and withstanding stresses of injury and infection
◆ Occurs in citrus fruits, berries, tomatoes, raw cabbage, green peppers, green leafy vegetables, and fortified juices
◆ Severe deficiency (scurvy): causes capillary fragility, joint abnormalities, and multisystemic symptoms

PURPOSE

◆ To help diagnose scurvy, scurvylike conditions, and metabolic disorders, such as malnutrition and malabsorption syndromes

PREPARATION

◆ Withhold food and fluid for 8 hours before the test.
◆ The test requires a blood sample.

Teaching points

◆ Explain that this test detects the amount of vitamin C in the patient's blood.
◆ Explain who will perform the test and where it'll be done.
◆ Instruct the patient to fast overnight before the test.
◆ Tell the patient that the test requires a blood sample and that he may experience slight discomfort from the tourniquet and needle puncture.
◆ Tell the patient that the test takes less than 5 minutes.

KEY STEPS

◆ Confirm the patient's identity using two patient identifiers according to facility policy.
◆ Perform a venipuncture and collect the sample in a 4.5-ml heparinized tube.

POSTPROCEDURE CARE

◆ Apply direct pressure to the venipuncture site until bleeding stops.
◆ Tell the patient to resume his usual diet.

PRECAUTIONS

◆ Avoid rough handling or excessive agitation of the sample to prevent hemolysis.
◆ Send the sample to the laboratory immediately.

COMPLICATIONS

◆ Hematoma at the venipuncture site

NORMAL RESULTS

◆ Level is 0.2 to 2 mg/dl (SI, 11 to 114 µmol/L).

ABNORMAL RESULTS

◆ Decreased levels may be caused by pregnancy, infection, fever, or anemia and may result in scurvy.
◆ Increased levels may indicate increased ingestion of vitamin C. Excess vitamin C is converted to oxalate, which is excreted in the urine. Excessive oxalate levels can produce urinary calculi.

Vitamin D₃ level, serum

DESCRIPTION
- Competitive protein-binding assay that determines serum levels of 25-hydroxycholecalciferol after chromatography separates it from other vitamin D metabolites and contaminants; usually done with measurement of serum calcium and alkaline phosphatase levels
- Vitamin D₃ (cholecalciferol): major form of vitamin D; endogenously produced in the skin from the sun's ultraviolet rays and occurs naturally in fish liver oils, egg yolks, liver, and butter

PURPOSE
- To evaluate skeletal disease, such as rickets and osteomalacia
- To help diagnose hypercalcemia
- To detect vitamin D toxicity
- To monitor therapy with vitamin D₃

PREPARATION
- Check for drugs that alter test results (such as corticosteroids or anticonvulsants); they may be restricted. If the patient must continue them, note this on the laboratory request.
- Withhold food and fluid for 8 hours before the test.
- The test requires a blood sample.

Teaching points
- Explain that this test measures vitamin D in the body.
- Explain who will perform the test and where it'll be done.
- Instruct the patient to fast for 8 to 12 hours before the test.
- Tell the patient that the test requires a blood sample and that he may experience slight discomfort from the tourniquet and needle puncture.
- Tell the patient that the test takes less than 5 minutes.

KEY STEPS
- Confirm the patient's identity using two patient identifiers according to facility policy.
- Perform a venipuncture and collect the sample in a 4.5-ml siliconized tube.

POSTPROCEDURE CARE
- Apply direct pressure to the venipuncture site until bleeding stops.
- Tell the patient to resume his usual diet and medications.

PRECAUTIONS
- Handle the sample carefully to prevent hemolysis.

COMPLICATIONS
- Hematoma at the venipuncture site

NORMAL RESULTS
- Level is 10 to 60 ng/ml (SI, 25 to 150 nmol/L).

ABNORMAL RESULTS
- Low or undetectable levels may result from poor diet, decreased exposure to the sun, or impaired absorption of vitamin D (from hepatobiliary disease, pancreatitis, celiac disease, cystic fibrosis, or gastric or small-bowel resection); or from various hepatic, parathyroid, and renal diseases. This deficiency can cause rickets or osteomalacia.
- Levels above 100 ng/ml (SI, > 250 nmol/L) may indicate toxicity caused by excessive self-medication or prolonged therapy; increased levels linked to hypercalcemia may be from hypersensitivity to vitamin D, as in sarcoidosis.

Voiding cystourethrography

OVERVIEW

DESCRIPTION

- Uses contrast medium that's instilled by gentle syringe or gravity into the bladder through a urethral catheter
- Uses fluoroscopic films or overhead X-rays to demonstrate bladder filling and excretion of the contrast as the patient voids
- Used to investigate possible causes of chronic urinary tract infection
- Other indications: suspected congenital anomaly of the lower urinary tract, abnormal bladder emptying, and incontinence
- In men or boys: assesses hypertrophy of prostatic lobes, urethral stricture, and degree of compromise of a stenotic prostatic urethra

PURPOSE

- To detect abnormalities of the bladder and urethra, such as vesicoureteral reflux, neurogenic bladder, prostatic hyperplasia, urethral strictures, or diverticula

PREPARATION

- Make sure the patient has signed an appropriate consent form.
- Note and report all allergies.
- Check the patient's history for hypersensitivity to contrast media or iodine-containing foods such as shellfish; mark the chart and notify the practitioner of sensitivities.
- Give the patient a sedative.
- No dietary restrictions are required.

Teaching points

- Explain that the test requires a catheter to be inserted into the patient's bladder.
- Explain who will perform the test and where it'll be done.
- Tell the patient that he doesn't need to restrict food and fluids.
- Warn of a possible feeling of fullness and an urge to void when the contrast agent is instilled.
- Tell the patient that the test takes 45 to 60 minutes.

- Instruct the patient to report fever, chills, or lower abdominal pain occur.

DIAGNOSTIC PROCEDURE

KEY STEPS

- Confirm the patient's identity using two patient identifiers according to facility policy.
- Assist the patient into a supine position and insert an indwelling urinary catheter into the bladder.
- Contrast medium is instilled through the catheter until the bladder is full. The catheter is clamped and radiographic films are obtained with the patient in supine, oblique, and lateral positions.
- The catheter is removed, and the patient assumes the right oblique position — right leg flexed to 90 degrees, left leg extended, and in men or boys, penis parallel to the right leg — and begins to void.
- High-speed exposures of the bladder and urethra, coned down to reduce radiation exposure, are obtained during voiding.
- If the right oblique view doesn't delineate both ureters, the patient is asked to stop urinating and to begin again in the left oblique position.
- The most reliable voiding cystourethrograms are obtained with the patient recumbent.
- Patients who can't urinate in the recumbent position may void standing (not sitting).
- Young children who can't void on command may need to undergo expression cystourethrography under general anesthesia.

POSTPROCEDURE CARE

- Encourage the patient's oral fluid intake.
- Prepare the patient for surgery if indicated.
- Monitor the patient's vital signs and intake and output.
- Watch for bleeding and infection.
- Observe and record the time, color, and volume of the patient's voiding.

If hematuria is present after the third voiding, notify the practitioner.
- Instruct the patient to report fever, chills, or lower abdominal pain.

PRECAUTIONS

- The test is contraindicated in patients with an acute or exacerbated urethral injury, or acute urethral or bladder infection.
- Difficulties encountered in bladder catheterization, especially in children, may prevent completion of the study.

COMPLICATIONS

- Bleeding
- Infection
- Adverse reaction to contrast media

INTERPRETATION

NORMAL RESULTS

- Delineation of the bladder and urethra shows normal structure and function, with no reflux of contrast medium into the ureters.

ABNORMAL RESULTS

- Structural and anatomical abnormalities suggest possible urethral stricture, vesical or urethral diverticula, ureterocele, prostatic enlargement, vesicoureteral reflux, or neurogenic bladder.

White blood cell count and differential

DESCRIPTION

- Part of a complete blood count that indicates the number of white blood cells (WBCs) in a microliter (μl, or cubic millimeter) of whole blood
- May vary by as much as 2,000 cells/μl (SI, 2×10^9/L) on any day because of strenuous exercise, stress, or digestion
- May increase or decrease significantly in certain diseases but is diagnostically useful when the patient's WBC differential and condition are considered
- Also called a *leukocyte count*

PURPOSE

- To determine infection or inflammation
- To detect and identify various types of leukemia (see *Performing a LAP stain*)
- To determine the need for further tests, such as the WBC differential or bone marrow biopsy
- To monitor response to chemotherapy or radiation therapy

PREPARATION

- Notify the laboratory and practitioner of drugs the patient is taking that may affect test results; they may be restricted.
- Give the patient a light meal before the test and limit exercise in the 24 hours before the test.
- The test requires a blood sample.

Teaching points

- Explain that the WBC test detects an infection or inflammation.
- Explain who will perform the test and where it'll be done.
- Tell the patient to avoid strenuous exercise for 24 hours before the test. Also tell him to avoid eating a heavy meal before the test.
- Tell him that the test requires a blood sample and that he may experience slight discomfort from the tourniquet and needle puncture.
- If the patient is being treated for an infection, advise him that this test will be repeated to monitor his progress.
- Tell the patient that the test takes less than 5 minutes.

DIAGNOSTIC PROCEDURE

KEY STEPS

- Confirm the patient's identity using two patient identifiers according to facility policy.
- Perform a venipuncture and collect the sample in a 3- or 4.5-ml EDTA tube.
- Completely fill the sample collection tube.
- Invert the sample gently several times to mix it with the anticoagulant.

POSTPROCEDURE CARE

- Make sure subdermal bleeding has stopped before removing pressure.
- If a large hematoma develops at the venipuncture site, monitor pulses distal to the site.
- Inform the practitioner of abnormal results.
- Tell the patient to resume his usual diet, activity, and medications.

PRECAUTIONS

- Maintain standard precautions while collecting the sample.
- Patients with severe leukopenia may have little or no resistance to infection and require protective isolation.

COMPLICATIONS

- Hematoma at the venipuncture site

Performing a LAP stain

Levels of leukocyte alkaline phosphatase (LAP), an enzyme found in neutrophils, may be altered by infection, stress, chronic inflammatory diseases, Hodgkin's disease, and hematologic disorders. Most of these conditions elevate LAP levels; only a few—notably chronic myelogenous leukemia (CML)—depress them. Thus, this test is usually used to differentiate CML from other disorders that produce an elevated white blood cell count.

PROCEDURE

To perform the LAP stain, a blood sample is obtained by venipuncture or fingerstick. The venous blood sample is collected in a 7-ml *green-top* tube, transported immediately to the laboratory, where a blood smear is prepared; the peripheral blood sample is smeared on a 3″ glass slide and fixed in cold formalin-methanol. The blood smear is then stained to show the amount of LAP present in the cytoplasm of the neutrophils. One hundred neutrophils are counted and assessed; each is assigned a score of 0 to 4, according to the degree of LAP staining. Normally, values for LAP range from 40 to 100, depending on the laboratory's standards.

IMPLICATIONS OF RESULTS

Depressed LAP values typically indicate CML; however, values may also be low in paroxysmal nocturnal hemoglobinuria, aplastic anemia, and infectious mononucleosis. Elevated levels may indicate Hodgkin's disease, polycythemia vera, or a neutrophilic leukemoid reaction—a response to such conditions as infection, chronic inflammation, or pregnancy.

After a diagnosis of CML, the LAP stain may also be used to help detect onset of the blastic phase of the disease, when LAP levels typically rise. However, LAP levels also increase toward normal in response to therapy; because of this, test results must be correlated with the patient's condition.

(continued)

INTERPRETATION

NORMAL RESULTS

◆ Value is 4,000 to 10,000/μl (SI, 4 to 10 × 10⁹/L).

◆ For normal values for the five types of WBCs classified in the differential, see *Interpreting WBC differential values*.

ABNORMAL RESULTS

◆ An increased count (leukocytosis) commonly signals infection, such as an abscess, meningitis, appendicitis, or tonsillitis; or may result from leukemia and tissue necrosis caused by burns, myocardial infarction, or gangrene.

◆ A decreased count (leukopenia) indicates bone marrow depression that may result from viral infections or from toxic reactions, such as those following treatment with antineoplastics, ingestion of mercury or other heavy metals, or exposure to benzene or arsenicals. It may also indicate influenza, typhoid fever, measles, infectious hepatitis, mononucleosis, or rubella.

◆ Abnormal differential patterns provide evidence for many disease states and other conditions. (See *Influence of disease on blood cell count.*)

⬥ ***INTERFERING FACTORS*** *Most antineoplastics; such anti-infectives as metronidazole and flucytosine; anticonvulsants such as phenytoin derivatives; thyroid hormone antagonists; and such nonsteroidal anti-inflammatory drugs as indomethacin (cause decreased counts)*

Interpreting WBC differential values

The differential count measures the types of white blood cells (WBCs) as a percentage of the total WBC count (the relative value). The absolute value is obtained by multiplying the relative value of each cell type by the total WBC count. The relative and absolute values must be considered to obtain an accurate diagnosis.

For example, consider a patient whose WBC count is 6,000/μl (SI, 6 × 10⁹/L) and whose differential shows 30% (SI, 0.3) neutrophils and 70% (SI, 0.7) lymphocytes. His relative lymphocyte count seems to be quite high (lymphocytosis), but when this figure is multiplied by his WBC count (6,000 × 70% = 4,200 lymphocytes/μl), (SI, [6 × 10⁹/L] × 0.7 = 4.2 × 10⁹/L lymphocytes), it's well within the normal range.

However, this patient's neutrophil count (30%; SI, 0.3) is low; when this figure is multiplied by the WBC count (6,000 × 30% = 1,800 neutrophils/ml) (SI, [6 × 10⁹/L] × 0.30 = 1.8 × 10⁹/L neutrophils), the result is a low absolute number, which may mean depressed bone marrow.

The normal percentages of WBC type in adults are:
Neutrophils — 54% to 75% (SI, 0.54 to 0.75)
Eosinophils — 1% to 4% (SI, 0.01 to 0.04)
Basophils — 0% to 1% (SI, 0 to 0.01)
Monocytes — 2% to 8% (SI, 0.02 to 0.08)
Lymphocytes — 25% to 40% (SI, 0.25 to 0.4).

Influence of disease on blood cell count

CELL TYPE	HOW AFFECTED

Neutrophils

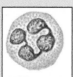

Increased by:
- Infections: osteomyelitis, otitis media, salpingitis, septicemia, gonorrhea, endocarditis, smallpox, chickenpox, herpes, Rocky Mountain spotted fever
- Ischemic necrosis due to myocardial infarction, burns, carcinoma
- Metabolic disorders: diabetic acidosis, eclampsia, uremia, thyrotoxicosis
- Stress response due to acute hemorrhage, surgery, excessive exercise, emotional distress, third trimester of pregnancy, childbirth
- Inflammatory diseases: rheumatic fever, rheumatoid arthritis, acute gout, vasculitis, myositis

Decreased by:
- Bone marrow depression due to radiation or cytotoxic drugs
- Infections: typhoid, tularemia, brucellosis, hepatitis, influenza, measles, mumps, rubella, infectious mononucleosis
- Hypersplenism: hepatic disease and storage diseases
- Collagen vascular disease such as systemic lupus erythematosus (SLE)
- Folic acid or vitamin B_{12} deficiency

Eosinophils

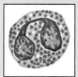

Increased by:
- Allergic disorders: asthma, hay fever, food or drug sensitivity, serum sickness, angioneurotic edema
- Parasitic infections: trichinosis, hookworm, roundworm, amebiasis
- Skin diseases: eczema, pemphigus, psoriasis, dermatitis, herpes
- Neoplastic diseases: chronic myelocytic leukemia (CML), Hodgkin's disease, metastases and necrosis of solid tumors

Decreased by:
- Stress response
- Cushing's syndrome

Basophils

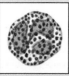

Increased by:
- CML, Hodgkin's disease, ulcerative colitis, chronic hypersensitivity states

Decreased by:
- Hyperthyroidism
- Ovulation, pregnancy
- Stress

Lymphocytes

Increased by:
- Infections: tuberculosis (TB), hepatitis, infectious mononucleosis, mumps, rubella, cytomegalovirus
- Thyrotoxicosis, hypoadrenalism, ulcerative colitis, immune diseases, lymphocytic leukemia

Decreased by:
- Severe debilitating illnesses: heart failure, renal failure, advanced TB
- Defective lymphatic circulation, high levels of adrenal corticosteroids, immunodeficiency due to immunosuppressives

Monocytes

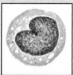

Increased by:
- Infections: subacute bacterial endocarditis, TB, hepatitis, malaria
- Collagen vascular disease: SLE, rheumatoid arthritis
- Carcinomas
- Monocytic leukemia
- Lymphomas

Decreased by:
- Overwhelming infection
- Some types of breast cancer

Wound culture and sensitivity

DESCRIPTION

- Microscopic analysis of a specimen from a lesion to confirm infection
- May be aerobic (for detection of organisms that require oxygen to grow and typically appear in a superficial wound) or anaerobic (for organisms that need little or no oxygen and exist in areas of poor tissue perfusion, such as postoperative wounds, ulcers, or compound fractures)

PURPOSE

- To identify an infectious microbe in a wound

PREPARATION

- Make sure the patient has signed an appropriate consent form.
- Note and report all allergies.

Teaching points

- Tell the patient that this test confirms the presence of an infection.
- Explain who will perform the procedure and where it'll be done.
- Tell the patient that the test takes only a few minutes.

DIAGNOSTIC PROCEDURE

KEY STEPS

- Confirm the patient's identity using two patient identifiers according to facility policy.
- Maintain aseptic technique during the procedure.
- Wear personal protective equipment during the procedure.
- Prepare a sterile field.
- Clean the area around the wound with antiseptic solution.
- For an aerobic culture: Express the wound and swab as much exudate as possible, or insert the swab deep into the wound and gently rotate. Immediately place the swab in the aerobic culture tube.

- For an anaerobic culture: Insert the swab deep into the wound, gently rotate it, and immediately place it in the anaerobic culture tub. (See *Anaerobic specimen collector.*)
- Record recent antimicrobial therapy, the source of the specimen, and the suspected organism on the laboratory request.
- Label the specimen container appropriately with the patient's name, practitioner's name, hospital number, wound site, and time of specimen collection.

POSTPROCEDURE CARE

- Clean the area around the wound thoroughly to limit contamination of the culture by normal skin flora.
- Make sure no antiseptic enters the wound.
- Re-dress the wound.
- Inform the practitioner of abnormal results.

PRECAUTIONS

- Because some anaerobes die in the presence of oxygen, place the specimen in the culture tube quickly; take care that no air enters the tube, and check that the double stoppers are secure.
- Keep the specimen container upright and send it to the laboratory within 15 minutes to prevent growth or deterioration of microbes.

COMPLICATIONS

- Spread of any existing infection

INTERPRETATION

NORMAL RESULTS

- No pathogenic organisms are found.

ABNORMAL RESULTS

- The presence of *Staphylococcus aureus*, group A beta-hemolytic streptococci, *Proteus* species, *Escherichia coli,* and other *Enterobacteriaceae,* and some *Pseudomonas* species suggests an aerobic wound infection.
- The presence of *Clostridium, Bacteroides, Peptococcus,* and *Streptococcus* species suggests an anaerobic wound infection.

Anaerobic specimen collector

Some anaerobes die when exposed to oxygen. To facilitate anaerobic collection and culturing, tubes filled with carbon dioxide (CO_2) or nitrogen are used for oxygen-free transport.

The anaerobic specimen collector shown here consists of a rubber-stopper tube filled with CO_2, a small inner tube, and a swab attached to a plastic plunger. The tube before specimen collection is shown on the left. The small inner tube containing the swab is held in place by the rubber stopper.

After specimen collection (shown on the right), the swab is quickly replaced in the inner tube, and the plunger is depressed. This separates the inner tube from the stopper, forcing it into the larger tube and exposing the specimen to the CO_2-rich environment.

The tube should be kept upright.

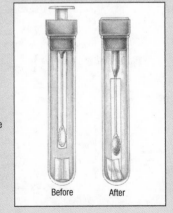

Before   After

Zinc level test

DESCRIPTION

◆ Measures serum zinc levels through analysis by atomic absorption spectroscopy; deficiency can impair body metabolism, growth, and development
◆ Zinc: important trace element; integral component of more than 80 enzymes and proteins; plays critical role in enzyme catalytic reactions
◆ Occurs naturally in water and in most foods; high levels found in meat, seafood, dairy products, whole grains, nuts, and legumes

PURPOSE

◆ To detect zinc deficiency or toxicity

PREPARATION

◆ There are no dietary restrictions required.
◆ The test requires a blood sample.

Teaching points

◆ Explain that this test determines the level of zinc in blood.
◆ Explain who will perform the test and where it'll be done.
◆ Inform the patient that he doesn't need to restrict food and fluids.
◆ Tell the patient that the test requires a blood sample and that he may experience slight discomfort from the tourniquet and needle puncture.
◆ Tell the patient that the test takes less than 5 minutes.

KEY STEPS

◆ Confirm the patient's identity using two patient identifiers according to facility policy.
◆ Perform a venipuncture and collect a 7- to 10-ml sample in a zinc-free collection tube.

POSTPROCEDURE CARE

◆ Apply direct pressure to the venipuncture site until bleeding stops.
◆ Inform the practitioner of abnormal results.

PRECAUTIONS

◆ Handle the sample gently to prevent hemolysis.
◆ Send the sample to the laboratory immediately. Reliable analysis must begin before platelet disintegration can alter test results.

COMPLICATIONS

◆ Hematoma at the venipuncture site

NORMAL RESULTS

◆ Level is 70 to 120 mcg/dl (SI, 10.7 to 18.4 µmol/L).

ABNORMAL RESULTS

◆ A decreased serum zinc level may result from an acquired deficiency (such as from insufficient dietary intake or an underlying disease), a hereditary deficiency; or from alcoholic cirrhosis of the liver, myocardial infarction, ileitis, chronic renal failure, rheumatoid arthritis, or hemolytic or sickle cell anemia.
◆ An extremely decreased zinc level may result from leukemia because of impaired zinc-dependent enzyme systems.
◆ An increased or potentially toxic zinc level may result from accidental ingestion or industrial exposure.

The abnormal laboratory test values listed here have immediate life-or-death significance to the patient. Report such values to the patient's physician immediately.

TEST	CRITICAL LOW VALUE	COMMON CAUSES AND EFFECTS	CRITICAL HIGH VALUE	COMMON CAUSES AND EFFECTS
Ammonia	<15 mcg/dl (SI,< 8.8 µmol/L)	Renal failure	>50 mcg/dl (SI, >29.3 µmol/L)	Severe hepatic disease: hepatic coma, Reye's syndrome, GI hemorrhage, heart failure
Bicarbonate	<10 mEq/L (SI,< 10 mmol/L)	Complex pattern of metabolic and respiratory factors	>40 mEq/L (SI, >40 mmol/ L)	Complex pattern of metabolic and respiratory factors
Calcium, serum	<6 mg/dl (SI, <1.75 mmol/L)	Hypoalbunemia, vitamin D or parathyroid hormone deficiency; tetany, seizures	>13 mg/dl (SI, > 3.2 mmol/L)	Hyperparathyroidism: coma, tetany
Creatine kinase isoenzymes (CK-MB)	None	None	>5%	Acute myocardial infarction (MI)
Creatinine, serum	0.4 mg/dl (SI, 35 µmol/L)	Severe liver disease	>2.8 mg/dl (SI, >247 µmol/ L)	Dehydration, rhabdomyolosis, renal failure: coma
D-dimer, serum or cerebrospinal fluid (CSF)	None	None	>250 mcg/ml (SI, >1.37 mmol/L)	Disseminated intravascular coagulation (DIC), pulmonary embolism, arterial or venous thrombosis, subarachnoid hemorrhage (cerebrospinal fluid [CSF] only), secondary fibrinolysis
Glucose, blood	<70 mg/dl (SI, <3.9 mmol/L)	Insulin overdose: brain damage	>300 mg/dl (SI, >16.6 mmol/L) (with ketonemia and electrolyte imbalance)	Diabetes, pancreatitis, steroid administration: diabetic coma
Gram stain, CSF	None	None	Gram-positive or gram-negative	Bacterial meningitis
Hemoglobin	<7 g/dl (SI, < 70 g/L)	Hemorrhage or vitamin B_{12} or iron deficiency; heart failure	>20 g/dl (SI, >200 g/L)	Dehydration, chronic obstructive pulmonary disease: thrombosis, polycythemia vera
International Normalized Ratio	None	None	>3.0	DIC, uncontrolled oral anticoagulation
Partial pressure of carbon dioxide, in arterial blood	<20 mm Hg, (SI, < 2.7 kPa)	Complex pattern of metabolic and respiratory factors	>77 mm Hg (SI, < 10.2 kPa)	Complex pattern of metabolic and respiratory factors
Partial pressure of oxygen, in arterial blood	<40 mm Hg, (SI < 5.3 kPa)	Complex pattern of metabolic and respiratory factors	None	None
Partial thromboplastin time	None	None	>40 seconds (>78 seconds for patient on heparin)	Anticoagulation factor deficiency: hemorrhage

TEST	CRITICAL LOW VALUE	COMMON CAUSES AND EFFECTS	CRITICAL HIGH VALUE	COMMON CAUSES AND EFFECTS
pH, arterial blood	<7.2 (SI, < 7.2)	Complex pattern of metabolic and respiratory factors	>7.6 (SI, > 7.6)	Complex pattern of metabolic and respiratory factors
Platelet count	<40,000/µl (SI, <40 $\times 10^3$/L)	DIC, bone marrow suppression; hemorrhage	> 1,000,000/µl (SI, > 10,000 $\times 10^8$/mm^3)	Leukemia, reaction to acute bleeding: hemorrhage
Potassium, serum	<2.8 mEq/L (SI, < 2.8 mmol/L)	Vomiting and diarrhea, diuretic therapy: cardiotoxicity, arrhythmia, cardiac arrest	>6,5 mEq/L (SI, >6.5 mmol/L)	Renal disease, burns, diuretic therapy: cardiotoxicity, arrhythmia
Prothrombin time	None	None	>14 seconds (>20 seconds for patient on warfarin)	Anticoagulant therapy, anticoagulation factor deficiency: hemorrhage
Sodium serum	<120 mEq/L (SI, < 120 mmol/L)	Burns, GI suction, diuretic therapy: cardiac failure	>160 mEq/L (SI, >160 mmol/L)	Dehydration, cardiac failure
Troponin	None	None	>1.5 ng/ml (SI > 1.5 µg/L)	Acute MI
White blood cell (WBC) count	<2,000/µl (SI, <2 $\times 10^9$/L)	Bone marrow suppression: infection	>20,000/µl (SI, >20 $\times 10^9$/L)	Leukemia: infection
WBC count, CSF	None	None	> 20 /µl (SI, >0.0012 $\times 10^9$/L)	Meningitis, encephalitis: infection

LABORATORY VALUE CHANGES IN ELDERLY PATIENTS

Standard normal laboratory values reflect the physiology of adults ages 20 to 40. However, normal values for older patients usually differ because of age-related physiologic changes.

Certain test results, however, remain unaffected by age. These include partial thromboplastin time, prothrombin time, serum acid phosphatase, serum carbon dioxide, serum chloride, aspartate aminotransferase, and total serum protein. You can use this chart to interpret other changeable test values in your elderly patients.

TEST VALUES AGES 20 TO 40	AGE-RELATED CHANGES	CONSIDERATIONS
Serum		
Albumin 3.4 to 5.4 g/dl (SI, 34 to 54 g/L)	Under age 65: Higher in males Over age 65: Equal levels that then decrease at same rate	Increased dietary protein intake needed in older patients if liver function is normal; edema: a sign of low albumin level
Alkaline phosphatase 45 to 115 International Units/ml (SI, 45 to 115 units/L)	Increases 8 to 10 International Units/L	May reflect liver function decline or vitamin D malabsorption and bone demineralization
Beta globulin 0.7 to 1.1 g/dl (SI, 7 to 11 g/L)	Increases slightly	Increases in response to decrease in albumin if liver function is normal; increased dietary protein intake needed
Blood urea nitrogen Men: 10 to 25 mg/dl (SI, 3.6 to 9.3 mmol/L) Women: 8 to 20 mg/dl (SI, 2.9 to 7.5 mmol/L)	Increases, possibly to 69 mg/dl (SI, 25.8 mmol/L)	Slight increase acceptable in absence of stressors, such as infection or surgery
Cholesterol Men: <205 mg/dl (SI, < 5.30 mmol/L) Women: <190 mg/dl (SI, < 4.90 mmol/L)	Men: Increases to age 50, then decreases Women: Lower than men until age 50, increases to age 70, then decreases	Rise in cholesterol level (and increased cardiovascular risk) in women as a result of postmenopausal estrogen decline; dietary changes, weight loss, and exercise needed
Creatine kinase 55 to 170 units/L (SI, 0.94 to 2.89 μkat/L)	Increases slightly	May reflect decreasing muscle mass and liver function
Creatinine 0.6 to 1.3 mg/dl (SI, 53 to 115 μmol/L)	Increases, possibly to 1.9 mg/dl in men (SI, 168 μmol/L)	Important factor to prevent toxicity when giving drugs excreted in urine
Creatinine clearance Men: 94 to 140 ml/min/1.73 m^2 (SI, 0.91 to 1.35 ml/s/m^2) Women: 72 to 110 ml/min/1.73 m^2 SI, 0.69 to 1.06 ml/s/m^2)	Men: Decreases; formula: ([140 – age) x kg body weight]/(72 x serum creatinine) Women: 85% of men's rate	Reflects reduced glomerular filtration rate; important factor to prevent toxicity when giving drugs excreted in urine
Hematocrit Men: 45% to 52% (SI, 0.45 to 0.52) Women: 37% to 48% (SI, 0.37 to 0.48)	May decrease slightly (unproven)	Reflects decreased bone marrow and hematopoiesis, increased risk of infection (because of fewer and weaker lymphocytes and immune system changes that diminish antigen-antibody response)

TEST VALUES AGES 20 TO 40	AGE-RELATED CHANGES	CONSIDERATIONS
Serum (continued)		
Hemoglobin Men: 14 to 18 g/dl (SI, 140 to 180 g/L) Women: 12 to 16 g/dl (SI, 120 to 160 g/L)	Men: Decreases by 1 to 2 g/dl Women: Unknown	Reflects decreased bone marrow, hematopoiesis, and (for men) androgen levels
High-density lipoprotein Men: 37 to 70 mg/dl (SI, 0.96 to 1.8 mmol/L) Women: 40 to 85 mg/dl (SI, 1.03 to 2.2 mmol/L)	Levels higher in women than in men but equalize with age	Compliance with dietary restrictions required for accurate interpretation of test results
Lactate dehydrogenase 71 to 207 units/L (SI, 1.2 to 3.52 µkat/L)	Increases slightly	May reflect declining muscle mass and liver function
Leukocyte count 4,000 to 10,000/µl (SI, 4 to 10 x 109/L)	Decreases to 3,100 to 9,000/µl (SI, 3.1 to 9 x 10^9/L)	Decrease proportionate to lymphocyte count
Lymphocyte count 25% to 40% (SI, 0.25 to 0.40)	Decreases	Decrease proportionate to leukocyte count
Platelet count 140,000 to 400,000/µl (SI, 140 to 400 x 109/L)	Change in characteristics: decreased granular constituents, increased platelet-release factors	May reflect diminished bone marrow and increased fibrinogen levels
Potassium 3.5 to 5.5 mEq/L (SI, 3.5 to 5.5 mmol/L)	Increases slightly	Requires avoidance of salt substitutes composed of potassium, vigilance in reading food labels, and knowledge of hyperkalemia's signs and symptoms
Thyroid-stimulating hormone 0 to 15 µIU/ml (SI, 15 mU/L)	Increases slightly	Suggests primary hypothyroidism or endemic goiter at much higher levels
Thyroxine 5 to 13.5 mcg/dl (SI, 60 to 165 mmol/L)	Decreases 25%	Reflects declining thyroid function
Triglycerides Men: 44 to 180 mg/dl (SI, 0.44 to 2.01 mmol/L) Women: 10 to 190 mg/dl (SI, 0.11 to 2.21 mmol/L)	Increases slightly	Suggests abnormalities at any other levels, requiring additional tests such as serum cholesterol
Triiodothyronine 80 to 220 ng/dl (SI, 1.2 to 3 nmol/L)	Decreases 25%	Reflects declining thyroid function

TEST VALUES AGES 20 TO 40	AGE-RELATED CHANGES	CONSIDERATIONS
Urine		
Glucose 0 to 15 mg/dl (SI, 0 to 8 mmol/L)	Decreases slightly	May reflect renal disease or urinary tract infection (UTI); unreliable check for older diabetics because glucosuria may not occur until plasma glucose level exceeds 300 mg/dl
Protein 50 to 80 mg/24 hours (SI, 50 to 80 mg/d)	Increases slightly	May reflect renal disease or UTI
Specific gravity 1.032 (SI, 1.032)	Decreases to 1.024 (SI, 1.024) by age 80	Reflects 30% to 50% decrease in number of nephrons available to concentrate urine

Selected references

American Diabetes Association. "Diagnosis and Classification of Diabetes Mellitus," *Diabetes Care* 27(Suppl 1):S5-S10, January 2004.

Bickley, L.S., and Szilagyi, P.G. *Bates' Guide to Physical Examination and History Taking,* 8th ed. Philadelphia: Lippincott Williams & Wilkins, 2003.

Bolotin, G., et al. "Use of Intraoperative Epiaortic Ultrasonography to Delineate Aortic Atheroma," *Chest* 127(1):60-65, January 2005.

Carr, J.J., et al. "Calcified Coronary Artery Plaque Measurement with Cardiac CT in Population-Based Studies: Standardized Protocol of Multi-Ethnic Study of Atherosclerosis (MESA) and Coronary Artery Risk Development in Young Adults (CARDIA) Study," *Radiology* 234(1):35-43, January 2005.

Chernyshev, O.Y., et al. "Yield and Accuracy of Urgent Combined Carotid/Transcranial Ultrasound Testing in Acute Cerebral Ischemia," *Stroke* 36(1):32-37, January 2005.

Chojnowksi, D. "The Latest in Cardiac Care," *Nursing Management* Suppl:16-18, 2004.

Durston, S. "The ABC's and More of Hepatitis," *Nursing Made Incredibly Easy* 2(4):22-31, July-August 2004.

Edelman, D., et al. "Utility of Hemoglobin A_{1c} in Predicting Diabetes Risk," *Journal of General Internal Medicine* 19(12):1175-180, December 2004.

Fischbach, F.T. *A Manual of Laboratory and Diagnostic Tests,* 7th ed. Philadelphia: Lippincott Williams & Wilkins, 2004.

Hoffman, R., et al. *Hematology Basic Principles and Practice,* 4th ed. New York: Churchill Livingstone, Inc., 2005.

Jacquemier, J., et al. "Protein Expression Profiling Identifies Subclasses of Breast Cancer and Predicts Prognosis," *Cancer Research* 65(3):767-79, February 2005.

Kasper, D.L., et al., eds. *Harrison's Principles of Internal Medicine,* 16th ed. New York: McGraw-Hill Book Co., Inc., 2005.

Koenig W., et al. "Prognostic Value of Apolipoprotein B and A-I in the Prediction of Myocardial Infarction in Middle-aged Men and Women: Results from the MONICA/KORA Augsburg Cohort Study," *European Heart Journal* 26(3):271-78, February 2005.

Kozier, B., et al. *Fundamentals of Nursing Concepts, Process, and Practice,* 7th ed. Upper Saddle River, N.J.: Prentice Hall Health, 2004.

Lippincott Manual of Nursing Practice Diagnostic Tests. Philadelphia: Lippincott Williams & Wilkins, 2006.

Min, R.J., et al. "Duplex Ultrasound Evaluation of Lower Extremity Venous Insufficiency," *Journal of Vascular & Interventional Radiology* 14(10):1233-241, October 2003.

Nursing Procedures, 4th ed. Philadelphia: Lippincott Williams & Wilkins, 2004.

Pagana, K.D., and Pagana, T.J. *Mosby's Diagnostic and Laboratory Test Reference,* 7th ed. St. Louis: Mosby–Year Book, Inc., 2005.

Phipps, W.J., et al. *Medical Surgical Nursing: Health and Illness Perspectives,* 7th ed. St. Louis: Mosby–Year Book, Inc., 2003.

Professional Guide to Diagnostic Tests. Philadelphia: Lippincott Williams & Wilkins, 2005.

Rakel, R., and Bope, E.T. *Conn's Current Therapy 2004.* Philadelphia: W.B. Saunders Co., 2004.

Rapid Assessment: A Flowchart Guide to Evaluating Signs & Symptoms. Philadelphia: Lippincott Williams & Wilkins, 2003.

Rempher, K.J., and Little, J. "Assessment of Red Blood Cell and Coagulation Laboratory Data," *AACN Clinical Issues* 15(4):622-37, October-December 2004.

Tiernet, L., et al. *Current Medical Diagnosis and Treatment,* 43rd ed. New York: McGraw-Hill/Appleton & Lange, 2004.

Vetrivel, K.S., and Thinakaran, G. "Amyloidogenic Processing of Beta-amyloid Precursor Protein in Intracellular Compartments," *Neurology* 66(2 Suppl 1):S69-S73, January 2006.

Waugh, J.J., et al. "Accuracy of Urinalysis Dipstick Techniques in Predicting Significant Proteinuria in Pregnancy," *Obstetrics & Gynecology* 103(4):769-77, April 2004.

Woods, S., et al. *Cardiac Nursing,* 5th ed. Philadelphia: Lippincott Williams & Wilkins, 2005.

World Health Organization. "Recommended Laboratory Tests to Identify Avian Influenza A Virus in Specimens from Humans," *WHO Geneva,* June 2005.

Yueh, B., et al. "Screening and Management of Adult Hearing Loss in Primary Care," *JAMA* 289(15):1976-985, April 2003.

WEB RESOURCES

Columbia Presbyterian Medical Center and Allen Pavilion Laboratories: *www.cpmclabinfo.cpmc.columbia.edu/*

Quest Diagnostics: *www.questdiagnostics.com*

Index

---

i refers to an illustration; t refers to a table.

i refers to an illustration; t refers to a table.

i refers to an illustration; t refers to a table.

i refers to an illustration; t refers to a table.

i refers to an illustration; t refers to a table.

i refers to an illustration; t refers to a table.

i refers to an illustration; t refers to a table.

i refers to an illustration; t refers to a table.

i refers to an illustration; t refers to a table.

Gastrointestinal bleeding
scan for, 238
sites and causes of, 215i
Gastrointestinal cancer tumor
marker, 97
Gastrointestinal tract
endoscopic biopsy of, 455
pathogens of, 464
upper, series for, 513-514
Gaze nystagmus test, 191
Gene-based test for human immunodeficiency virus, 274
German measles, antibody tests for,
436, 489
Given diagnostic imaging system, 239
Globulin levels. *See also* Immunoglobulins.
abnormal, implications of, 398i
alpha$_1$- and alpha$_2$-, 18
beta, age-related changes in, 546t
cryo-, 162
gamma, 115t, 232
protein electrophoresis for, 398
thyroxine-binding, 486
Glucagon level test, 240
Glucocorticoids, urine hydroxyproline
and, 521
Glucose
in cerebrospinal fluid, 115t
for hyperkalemia, 386
in peritoneal fluid, 369t
plasma
crisis values for, 544t
fasting, 212
lactose tolerance test and, 347
oral tolerance test for, 346
two-hour postprandial, 502
in synovial fluid, 469, 470t
urine
age-related changes in, 547t
tests for, 241, 346
Glucose enzymatic test strip, 241
Glucose loading, 246
Glucose oxidase test, 241
Glucose-6-phosphate dehydrogenase
test, 242
Glucose tolerance test, oral, 346
Glycosylated hemoglobin test, 243
Goiter, 414t

Gold salts, lupus erythematosus cell
preparation and, 311
Gonads, shielding during X-ray, 292
Gonorrhea culture, 244-245
Gout, synovial fluid in, 468-469t
Gram stain, cerebrospinal fluid,
115t, 544t
Graves' disease, 414t
Gray-scale ultrasonography of pelvic
area, 509
Griseofulvin, lupus erythematosus cell
preparation and, 311
Growth hormone. *See* Human growth
hormone.
Guthrie screening test, 374

H

Hageman factor, 126, 127t
Ham test, 247
Hantaan virus, 72t
Haptoglobin level test, 248
Hearing tests. *See under* Ear.
Heart. *See also* Echocardiography; Electrocardiography.
blood pool imaging of, 102
catheterization of, 103-104
computed tomography scan of, 137
magnetic resonance imaging of, 105
multiple-gated acquisition scan
of, 332
positron emission tomography
of, 106
technetium-99m pyrophosphate
scan of, 474
thallium imaging of, 370, 478
Heart block
bundle-branch, exercise stress test
and, 184
first-degree, 183i
Heart failure
B-type natriuretic peptide in, 91t
lactate dehydrogenase in, 293t
Heart rate, fetal
external monitoring of, 209-210
internal monitoring of, 285-286
Heavy chain disease, 281t
Heinz bodies test, 249
Helicobacter pylori, tests for, 250
Hematest, 215-216

Hematocrit
age-related changes in, 546t
test for, 251-252
Hematoma
celiac or mesenteric arteriography
and, 112
cerebral angiography and, 113
Heme, 252
Hemoccult test, 216
Hemocytoblasts, 252
Hemodilution, red blood cell count
and, 418
Hemoglobin
age-related changes in, 547t
crisis values for, 544t
electrophoresis of, 253
fetal, 219
glycosylated, 243
life cycle of, 252
mean corpuscular, 418, 419
total, 254, 492
unstable, 512
urine, 255
variations of type and distribution
of, 253t
Hemoglobin S test, 446
Hemolysis
haptoglobin level and, 248
international normalized ratio
and, 287
osmotic fragility and, 352
Hemolytic anemia, lactate dehydrogenase in, 293t
Hemorrhage. *See also* Bleeding.
small-bowel biopsy and, 456
thoracoscopy and, 480
Hemorrhagic fever, 72t
Hemorrhoidal bleeding, fecal occult
blood test and, 216
Hemosiderin level, urine, 256
Heparin
acid mucopolysaccharide value
and, 5
thrombin time and, 482
thyroxine level and, 487
triiodothyronine level and, 498i
Hepatitis
antibodies in, 43t, 44t
cancer tumor markers and, 97
immunoglobulin levels in, 281t
lactate dehydrogenase in, 293t

i refers to an illustration; t refers to a table.

i refers to an illustration; t refers to a table.

Increased intracranial pressure, cere-
brospinal fluid removal and, 308
Indirect Coombs' test, 34, 150
Indirect immunofluorescence for
Epstein-Barr virus, 198
Indomethacin, white blood cell count
and, 538
Infants. *See* Neonates or infants.
Infarct avid imaging, 474
Infection
fungal, serology for, 228, 229t
plasma glucose and, 502
postbiopsy bone, 79
Infectious agents
bioterrorism, 72-73
gastrointestinal, 464
Inheritance patterns in sickle cell
anemia, 446i
In-line trap for suctioning, 463i
Inspiratory capacity, 404t, 405, 406
Inspiratory depth, chest radiograph
quality and, 118
Instant-View fecal occult blood
test, 216
Insulin
antibody test for, 40
glucagon level and, 240
for hyperkalemia, 386
hypoglycemic reactions to, 284
serum, 283
Insulinoma, hypoglycemic reactions
and, 283
Insulin tolerance test, 284
Intact parathyroid hormone assay, 358
Internal fetal monitoring, 285-286
International normalized ratio
crisis values for, 544t
test for, 287
Intracranial computed tomography
scanning, 136
Intracranial pressure, increased, cerebrospinal fluid removal and, 308
Intraocular pressure, measurement
of, 488
Intrauterine catheter, 285, 286i
Intravenous infusion
hemodilution by, 418
for potassium imbalance, 386
Intravenous pyelography, 208

In vitro lymphocyte transformation
tests, 317
Iodides
thyroxine level and, 487
triiodothyronine level and, 498i
Iodine
hypersensitivity to, 134
radioactive, uptake test for, 410
Ionized calcium, 93
Iontophoresis, pilocarpine, 467
Iron
fecal occult blood test and, 216
role of, 252
serum, 288
Iron deficiency anemia, 419t
Ischemia-modified albumin
necrosis markers and, 289i
test for, 289
Isoniazid, lupus erythematosus cell
preparation and, 311
Ivy method for bleeding time, 75

J
Jaeger card, 529, 530
Jaundice, drug-induced, antibodies
in, 44t
Juvenile arthritis, antinuclear anti-
bodies in, 43t
Juxtaglomerular apparatus, 426i

K
Ketoacidosis, anion gap in, 31
Keto-Diastix and Ketostix tests, 291
17-ketogenic steroids, urine, 290
Ketones
serum, 70
urine, 291
Kidneys
angiography of, 422-423
biopsy of, 362
computed tomography scan of, 139
nephrotomography of, 338
radionuclide imaging of, 412
ultrasonography of, 506
venography of, 424-425
Kidney-ureter-bladder radiography,
292
Ki67 protein in breast cancer, 86
Klinefelter's syndrome, 442t

L
Lactate dehydrogenase
age-related changes in, 547t
isoenzyme variations for, 293t
test for, 293-294
Lactic acid test, 295
Lactose tolerance test, oral, 347
Laënnec's cirrhosis, immunoglobulin
levels in, 281t
Laparoscopy, 296-297
Large intestine, X-ray of, 65i
Laryngeal edema, bronchoscopy
and, 89
Laryngoscopy, direct, 298
Laryngospasm
bronchoscopy and, 89
nasopharyngeal culture and, 336
Latex agglutination for cryptococcosis,
229t
Left/right shift in neutrophils test, 339
Leg
postangiography monitoring of, 113
venography of, 307, 527
venous plethysmography of, 113
Lesions, auditory, tests for, 449-450
Leucine aminopeptidase level test, 299
Leukemia, immunoglobulin levels
in, 281t
Leukoagglutinins test, 300
Leukocyte alkaline phosphatase stain,
performing, 537
Leukocyte count, 537-539. *See also*
Lymphocyte count.
age-related changes in, 547t
for cerebrospinal fluid, 115t, 545t
crisis values for, 545t
influence of disease on, 539t
for peritoneal fluid, 369t
for synovial fluid, 468-469t, 470t
for urine, 517, 518
Leukocytes
blood smear for, 77
differential values for, 470t, 537-538
Leukocytosis and leukopenia, 538
Levodopa
plasma catecholamines and, 109
urine ketones and, 291
Levothyroxine, thyroxine level and, 487
Licorice, total carbon dioxide content
and, 490

---

i refers to an illustration; t refers to a table.

i refers to an illustration; t refers to a table.

Microscopic examination of spermatozoa, 440
Milk-alkali syndrome, 95t
Milk intake
  ionized calcium level and, 93
  phenylalanine screening and, 374
Minute volume, 404t, 406
Mithramycin, urine hydroxyproline and, 521
Mitochondria, antibody test for, 41, 44t
Mitogen assay for lymphocyte transformation, 317
Mixed lymphocyte culture assay, 317
M-mode echocardiography, 177
Modified Thayer-Martin medium, 244i
Monoamine oxidase inhibitors
  dexamethasone suppression test and, 171
  urine homovanillic acid and, 270
Monoclonal test for cytomegalovirus, rapid, 417
Monocyte count, 331
  differential, 538
  influence of disease on, 539t
  for synovial fluid, 470t
Monospot test, 198
Mono-Vacc test, 501
Morphine, dexamethasone suppression test and, 171
Mucin clot in synovial fluid, 468t, 470t
Mucopolysaccharides, acid, 5
Multiple-gated acquisition scanning, 332
Multiple myeloma
  immunoglobulin levels in, 281t
  urine calcium and phosphorus in, 95t
Multiple sclerosis, visual evoked potentials in, 206i
Multipuncture tests, tuberculin, 501
Multistix for urine hemoglobin, 255
Mumps antigen for hypersensitivity skin test, 168, 169i
Muramidase test, 318
Muscle, smooth, antibody test for, 44
Muscle mass, serum creatinine and, 158
Myasthenia gravis or myasthenic crisis, Tensilon test for, 475

Mycobacterium tuberculosis for hypersensitivity skin test, 168, 169i
Myelocytic leukemia, immunoglobulin levels in, 281t
Myelography, 333
Myocardial imaging
  cold spot, 478
  hot spot, 474
Myocardial infarction, pulmonary function tests and, 406
Myocardial injury, antibody test for, 42
Myocardial perforation, pericardiocentesis and, 366, 367
Myocardial perfusion scan, 478
Myocarditis, lactate dehydrogenase in, 293t
Myoglobin
  cardiac ischemia and, 289i
  serum, 334
  urine, 335
Myxedema, 414t

N
Nasal culture, 481
Nasopharyngeal culture, 336
Nasopharyngeal specimen
  obtaining, 336i
  for SARS virus test, 437
Natriuretic peptide
  atrial, 61
  B-type, 91
Near visual acuity, 529, 530
Necrosis markers, ischemia-modified albumin and, 289i
Needle biopsy
  of bone marrow, 81, 82
  of breast, 85
  of liver, 361i
  of lung, 309
  of pleura, 381i
  of thyroid, 483
Neisseria gonorrhoeae, culturing for, 244i
Neonates or infants
  aspartate aminotransferase level in, 60
  bilirubin level for, 71
  direct Coombs' test for, 39, 149
  phenylalanine screening for, 374
  siderocyte level in, 288

Neonates or infants *(continued)*
  thyroid-stimulating hormone test for, 337
Neoplasms. *See* Tumors.
Nephritis and nephrosis, urine calcium and phosphorus in, 95t
Nephrotic syndrome, immunoglobulin levels in, 281t
Nephrotomography, 338
Nephrotoxic drugs
  serum potassium and, 386
  urine hemoglobin and, 255
Nerve conduction studies, 187
Nerve injury, thoracoscopy and, 480
Neuroblastoma, 523
Neurography, 324
Neurologic system, magnetic resonance imaging of, 323-324
Neutrophil count
  differential, 538
  influence of disease on, 539t
  in synovial fluid, 468t, 470t
Neutrophils
  function tests for, 317
  leukocyte alkaline phosphatase stain for, 537
  test for, 339
Nitroblue tetrazolium test, 317
Non-Hodgkin's lymphoma, staging, 315
Nonsteroidal anti-inflammatory drugs
  bleeding time and, 75
  white blood cell count and, 538
Nonstress test, fetal monitoring for, 209, 210
Norepinephrine
  plasma, 109
  urine, 110
N-telopeptide level, 84
N-terminal fragment parathyroid hormone assay, 358
Nuclear antibodies, tests for, 43, 46
Nuclear antigen, extractable, antibody test for, 211
Nuclear matrix protein 22, 74
Nuclear medicine scanning, 340. *See also* Radionuclide imaging; *specific test.*
Nucleic acid test for human immunodeficiency virus and hepatitis C, 274

i refers to an illustration; t refers to a table.

---

i refers to an illustration; t refers to a table.

i refers to an illustration; t refers to a table.

i refers to an illustration; t refers to a table.

i refers to an illustration; t refers to a table.

i refers to an illustration; t refers to a table.

i refers to an illustration; t refers to a table.

i refers to an illustration; t refers to a table.

i refers to an illustration; t refers to a table.

X

X and Y chromosomes
anomalies of, 442-443t
test for, 442-443
X-rays. *See* Radiography.

Y

Yellow fever, 72t
Yersinia enterocolitica, 464
Yersinia pestis, 72t

Z

Zinc level test, 541

i refers to an illustration; t refers to a table.